Master Techniques in Orthopaedic Surgery

Reconstructive Knee Surgery

Third Edition

Master Techniques in Orthopaedic Surgery

Editor-in-Chief
Bernard F. Morrey, MD

Founding Editor
Roby C. Thompson, Jr., MD

Volume Editors

Surgical Exposures
Bernard F. Morrey, MD

The Hand
James Strickland, MD
Thomas Graham, MD

The Wrist
Richard H. Gelberman, MD

The Elbow
Bernard F. Morrey, MD

The Shoulder
Edward V. Craig, MD

The Spine
David S. Bradford, MD
Thomas L. Zdeblick, MD

The Hip
Robert L. Barrack, MD

Reconstructive Knee Surgery
Douglas W. Jackson, MD

Knee Arthroplasty
Paul A. Lotke, MD
Jess H. Lonner, MD

The Foot & Anke
Harold B. Kitaoka, MD

Fractures
Donald A. Wiss, MD

Pediatrics
Vernon T. Tolo, MD
David L. Skaggs, MD

Soft Tissue Surgery
William Cooney, MD
Steven L. Moran, MD

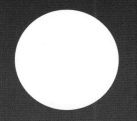

Master Techniques in Orthopaedic Surgery

Reconstructive Knee Surgery

Third Edition

Editor

Douglas W. Jackson

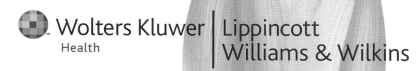

Health

Philadelphia, Pennsylvania

Acquisitions Editor: Robert Hurley
Developmental Editor: Keith Donnellan, Dovetail Content Solutions
Managing Editor: David Murphy, Jr.
Marketing Manager: Sharon Zinner
Project Manager: Fran Gunning
Design Coordinator: Doug Smock
Production Service: Maryland Composition

© 2008 by LIPPINCOTT WILLIAMS & WILKINS, a WOLTERS KLUWER business
530 Walnut Street
Philadelphia, PA 19106 USA
LWW.com

Printed in China

Library of Congress Cataloging-in-Publication Data
978-0-7817-6563-3
0-7817-6563-3

Reconstructive knee surgery / editor, Douglas W. Jackson. — 3rd ed.
   p. ; cm. — (Master techniques in orthopaedic surgery)
 Includes bibliographical references and index.
 ISBN 978-0-7817-6563-3
 1. Knee—Surgery. I. Jackson, Douglas W. II. Series: Master techniques in orthopaedic surgery
(3rd ed.)
  [DNLM: 1. Knee Injuries—surgery. 2. Arthroscopy—methods. 3. Knee Joint—surgery
WE 870 R3115 2007]
 RD561.R39 2007
 617.5'82059--dc22
                2007031772

To purchase additional copies of this book, call our customer service department at (800) 638-3030 or fax orders to (301) 223-2320. International customers should call (301) 223-2300.

Visit Lippincott Williams & Wilkins on the Internet: at LWW.com. Lippincott Williams & Wilkins customer service representatives are available from 8:30 am to 6 pm, EST.

10 9 8 7 6 5 4 3 2 1

To
My wife, Sandi,
and the spouses of the other contributors,
who have fostered an environment
that makes special projects possible.

Contents

Contributors

Frederick M. Azar, MD
Professor
Director, Residency Program
Director, Sports Medicine
Fellowship, University of Tennessee—Campbell Clinic
Department of Orthopaedic Surgery
Memphis, Tennessee

Sue D. Barber-Westin, BS
Director, Clinical and Applied Research
Cincinnati SportsMedicine Research and Education
Foundation
Cincinnati, Ohio

John A. Bergfeld, MD
Director, Operating Room Management Team
Cleveland Clinic
Cleveland, Ohio

Kevin F. Bonner, MD
Associate Professor
Eastern Virginia Medical School
Norfolk, Virginia

Petros J. Boscainos, MD
Clinical Fellow, University of Toronto
Division of Orthopaedic Surgery
Toronto East General Hospital
Research Fellow, Division of Orthopaedic Surgery
Mount Sinai Hospital
Toronto, Ontario

William D. Bugbee, MD
Associate Professor
Department of Orthopaedics
University of California
Attending Physician
Scripps Clinic
La Jolla, California

Anthony M. Buoncristiani, MD
Sawtooth Orthopaedics and Sports Medicine
St. Luke's Hospital
Ketchum, Idaho

E. Lyle Cain, Jr., MD
Fellowship Director
Orthopaedic Surgeon
American Sports Medicine Institute Center
Birmingham, Alabama

S. Terry Canale, MD
Professor
Chairman
University of Tennessee—Campbell Clinic
Department of Orthopaedic Surgery
Memphis Tennessee

Brett M. Cascio, MD
LSU Health Sciences Center
School of Medicine at New Orleans
Department of Orthopaedics
New Orleans, Louisiana

Guglielmo Cerullo, MD
Orthopaedic Surgeon
Clinica Valle Giulia
Roma, Italy

Edward Y. Cheng, MD
Mairs Family Professor
University of Minnesota
Chief, Department of Orthopaedic Surgery
University of Minnesota Medical Center
Minneapolis, Minnesota

Massimo Cipolla, MD
Università di Roma La Sapienza
Roma, Italy

William G. Clancy, Jr., MD, PhD
Orthopedic Associates of Aspen
Aspen Valley Hospital
Aspen, Colorado

Struan H. Coleman
Assistant Attending Orthopaedic Surgeon
Hospital for Special Surgery
Instructor in Orthopaedics
Weill Medical College of Cornell University
New York, New York

Andrew J. Cosgarea, MD
Director, Sports Medicine and Shoulder Surgery
Associate Professor
Department of Orthopaedic Surgery
Johns Hopkins University
Baltimore, Maryland

Brad A. Cucchetti, DO
Director, Sports Medicine
Florida Orthopaedic Institute
Tampa, Florida

Zsófia Duska
Physiotherapist, Human Kinesiologist
Orthopaedic and Trauma Department
Uzsoki Hospital
Budapest, Hungary

Craig J Edson, MS, PT, ATC
Geisinger/Healthsouth Rehabilitation Hospital
Danville, Pennsylvania

Gianni Enrico, MD
Clinica Valle Giulia
Roma, Italy

Gregory C Fanelli, M.D.
Chief, Arthroscopic Surgery and Sports Medicine
Fanelli Sports Injury Clinic
Department of Orthopaedic Surgery
Geisinger Clinic Medical Center
Danville, Pennsylvania

Mario Ferretti, M.D.
Ferguson Laboratory for Orthopaedic Rearch
Department of Orthopaedic Surgery
University of Pittsburgh
Pittsburgh, Pennsylvania

Vittorio Franco, MD
Policlinico Umberto I
Roma, Italy

Freddie Fu, MD, DSc, DPS
David Silver Professor and Chairman
Department of Orthopaedic Surgery
University of Pittsburgh Medical Center
Pittsburgh, Pennsylvania

John P. Fulkerson, M.D.
Orthopedic Associates of Hartford, P.C.
Clinical Professor and Sports Medicine Fellowship Director
University of Connecticut School of Medicine
Farmington, Connecticut

Seth Gasser, MD
Director, Sports Medicine
Florida Orthopaedic Institute
Tampa, Florida

Allen E. Gross, MD, FRCSC, O.Ont.
Orthopaedic Surgeon
Division of Orthopaedic Surgery
Mount Sinai Hospital
Professor of Surgery
Faculty of Medicine
University of Toronto
Toronto, Ontario

László Hangody, MD, PhD, DSc
Clinical Professor
Orthopaedic and Trauma Department
Uzsoki Hospital
Budapest, Hungary

Christopher D. Harner, MD
University of Pittsburgh
Medical Director
UPMC Center for Sports Medicine
Pittsburgh, Pennsylvania

Stephen Hendricks
Alaska Orthopedic Labs
Anchorage, Alaska

Stephen M. Howell, MD
Associate Professor
Department of Mechanical and Aeronautical Engineering
University of California—Davis
Davis, California

Douglas W. Jackson, MD
President
Memorial Orthopaedic Surgical Group, Inc.
Southern California Center for Sports Medicine
Medical Director
Orthopaedic Research Institute
Long Beach, California

Zoltán Kárpáti, MD
Orthopaedic and Trauma Department
Uzsoki Hospital
Budapest, Hungary

Catherine F. Kellett
Clinical Fellow
University of Toronto
Division of Orthopaedic Surgery
Mount Sinai Hospital
Toronto, Ontario

Bryan T. Kelly
Department of Orthopaedic Surgery
The Hospital for Special Surgery
New York, New York

Jason L. Koh, MD
Fellow
Sports Medicine
Cleveland Clinic
Cleveland, Ohio

Peter R. Kurzweil, MD
Fellowship Director
Southern California Center for Sports Medicine
Long Beach, California

Roger V. Larson, MD
Associate Professor
Orthopaedic and Sports Medicine
University of Washington
Seattle, Washington

Keith W. Lawhorn, MD
Advanced Orthopaedics and Sports Medicine Institute
Inova Fair Oaks Hospital
Fairfax, Virginia

David A. McGuire, MD
Affiliate Professor
University of Alaska, Anchorage
Healthsouth Alaska Surgery Center
Anchorage, Alaska

Frank R. Noyes, MD
President and Medical Director
Cincinatti SportsMedicine and Orthopaedic Center
Clinical Professor
Department of Orthopaedic Surgery
University of Cincinnati College of Medicine
Cincinnati, Ohio

Richard D. Parker, MD
Professor of Surgery
Education Director
Cleveland Clinic Foundation
Cleveland, Ohio

Lars Peterson, MD, PhD
Professor of Orthopaedics
University of Göteborg
Clinical Director
Gothenburg Medical Center
Gothenburg, Sweden

Christopher S. Proctor, MD
Alta Orthopaedics
Santa Barbara, California

Giancarlo Puddu, MD
Clinica Valle Giulia
Roma, Italy

Michael A. Rauh, MD
State University of New York at Buffalo
Clinical Assistant Professor of Orthopaedic Surgery
Department of Orthopaedic Surgery
University Sports Medicine
Buffalo, New York

Brant Richardson, PAC
Alta Orthopaedics
Santa Barbara, California

William G. Rodkey, DVM
Diplomat
American College of Veterinary Surgeons
Director
Basic Science Research and Senior Scientist
Steadman Hawkins Research Foundation
Vail Vally Medical Center
Vail, Colorado

Vineet Sharma
Fellow
Adult Reconstruction
Ranawat Orthopaedic Center
New York, New York

Wei Shen, MD, PhD
Post-Doctoral Research Associate
Department of Orthopedic Surgery
University of Pittsburgh Medical Center
Pittsburgh, Pennsylvania

Manno Steckel, MD
University of Goettingen
Department of Orthopaedic Surgery
Goettingen, Germany

Fotios Paul Tjoumakaris, MD
Fellow
Center for Sports Medicine
University of Pittsburgh Medical Center
Pittsburgh, Pennsylvania

Albert Mu-Hong Tsai, MD
Memorial Orthopaedic Surgical Goup
Long Beach, California

William H. Warden, III, MD
Southern California Center for Sports Medicine
Long Beach, California

Blaine Warkentine, MD
Southern California Center for Sports Medicine
Long Beach, California

Russell F. Warren, MD
Professor of Orthopaedics
Weill Cornell Medical College
Attending Surgeon-in-Chief Emeritus
Hospital for Special Surgery
New York, New York

William M. Wind, Jr., MD
Clinical Assistant Professor
State University of New York at Buffalo
Department of Orthopaedic Surgery
Buffalo, New York

Series Preface

Since its inception in 1994, the *Master Techniques in Orthopaedic Surgery* Series has become the gold standard for both physicians in training and experienced surgeons. Its exceptional success may be traced to the leadership of the original series editor, Roby Thompson, whose clarity of thought and focused vision sought "to provide direct, detailed access to techniques preferred by orthopaedic surgeons who are recognized by their colleagues as 'masters' in their specialty," as he stated in his series preface. It is personally very rewarding to hear testimonials from both residents and practicing orthopaedic surgeons on the value of these volumes to their training and practice.

A key element of the success of the series is its format. The effectiveness of the format is reflected by the fact that it is now being replicated by others. An essential feature is the standardized presentation of information replete with tips and pearls shared by experts with years of experience. Abundant color photographs and drawings guide the reader through the procedures step by step.

The second key to the success of the *Master Techniques* series rests in the reputation and experience of our volume editors. The editors are truly dedicated "masters" with a commitment to share their rich experience through these texts. We feel a great debt of gratitude to them and a real responsibility to maintain and enhance the reputation of the *Master Techniques* Series that has developed over the years. We are proud of the progress made in formulating the third edition volumes and are particularly pleased with the expanded content of this series. Six new volumes will soon be available covering topics that are exciting and relevant to a broad cross-section of our profession. While we are in the process of carefully expanding *Master Techniques* topics and editors, we are committed to the now-classic format.

The first of the new volumes will be *Relevant Surgical Exposures,* which I will edit. The second new volume is *Essential Procedures in Pediatrics.* Subsequent new topics to be introduced are *Soft Tissue Reconstruction, Management of Peripheral Nerve Dysfunction, Advanced Reconstructive Techniques in the Joint*, and finally *Essential Procedures in Sports Medicine.* The full library thus will consist of 16 useful and relevant titles.

I am pleased to have accepted the position of series editor, feeling so strongly about the value of this series to educate the orthopaedic surgeon in the full array of expert surgical procedures. The true worth of this endeavor will continue to be measured by the ever-increasing success and critical acceptance of the series. I remain indebted to Dr. Thompson for his inaugural vision and leadership, as well as to the *Master Techniques* volume editors and numerous contributors who have been true to the series style and vision. As I indicated in the preface to the second edition of *The Hip* volume, the words of William Mayo are especially relevant to characterize the ultimate goal of this endeavor: "The best interest of the patient is the only interest to be considered." We are confident that the information in the expanded *Master Techniques* offers the surgeon an opportunity to realize the patient-centric view of our surgical practice.

Bernard F. Morrey, MD

PREFACE

Symptoms and injuries related to the knee joint are responsible for more people visiting an orthopaedic surgeon's office than any other joint. These patients have high expectations for overcoming their knee complaints and returning to their desired activity level. They have read about knee injuries in the sports page every day and athletes returning to their sports following their injuries. As a result of lay articles in the print and electronic media and marketing efforts to the public, patients have come to expect less-invasive surgical approaches that preserve their uninvolved anatomy and result in faster rehabilitation. The reconstructive knee surgery procedures and techniques presented in this text focus on the latest arthroscopic and less-invasive surgical applications. The procedures described in this edition comprise a significant percentage of the total operative cases performed by orthopaedic surgeons. These new and updated chapters focus on the current state of surgical procedures and techniques for extensor mechanism and patellofemoral disorders, for torn and damaged menisci, for articular cartilage lesions, and for reconstructive ligament surgery of the knee. In addition, the evolving role of allografts in knee surgery as well as computer-assisted applications account for six of the new chapters in this edition.

Since the publication of the first edition of this book in 1995, there have been many advances in the surgical treatment of the knee. This edition updates the important, time-tested operations from the first and second editions and introduces many new procedures that have emerged. There are 15 new chapters in this edition in addition to the 20 other updated chapters. Experts share their approach to meniscal repair and fixation; meniscal transplantation; cruciate ligament tunnel placement and fixation; graft harvesting; the role of allografts; the latest techniques for ACL, PCL, MCL and poterolateral corner reconstruction; opening-wedge osteotomy; computer-assisted surgery; arthroscopic chondroplasty; microfracture; osteochondral plugs; chondrocyte transplantation; and pigmented villonodular synovitis resection.

The surgeons contributing to this volume were carefully chosen for their expertise and experience in the clinical application of the latest techniques and technology of specific procedures. They present surgical innovations, clinical judgment, experience, operating room methodology, and decision making. They share their indications and contraindications, as well as the pitfalls that may occur during surgery. Each chapter includes systematic details with pictorial amplifications of essential points designed to give the reader an operating room experience.

Because each chapter represents a selected individual author's approach to a specific knee problem, the references at the end of each chapter are limited. It is neither a review of the subject, nor a discussion of why the authors do not do it differently. The chapters depict how carefully selected experts perform the surgeries they find most beneficial in their experience.

My involvement in both selecting the authors and reviewing and editing these chapters has improved the surgical care that I am able to offer my patients. I am convinced that this book will be a benefit and will help the reader master these surgical techniques.

Douglas W. Jackson, MD

EXTENSOR MECHANISM— PATELLOFEMORAL PROBLEMS

1 Arthroscopic Lateral Release of the Patella with Radiofrequency Ablation

Seth I. Gasser and Brad A. Cucchetti

INDICATIONS/CONTRAINDICATIONS

Arthroscopic lateral release of the patella with electrocautery was first reported in the literature in 1982 (10). Its prime advantage over standard lateral release procedures is the potential to minimize postoperative bleeding and subsequent hemarthrosis. The reported rate of significant postoperative hemarthrosis decreased from more than 15% to less than 5% with the use of electrocautery (6). Other advantages of this technique include improved arthroscopic visualization during transection of the lateral retinaculum and a decrease in postoperative pain by minimizing the potential for significant postoperative hemarthrosis. This allows the patient to participate in an earlier, aggressive rehabilitation program that may improve the ultimate results of surgery.

The indications for arthroscopic lateral release of the patella have changed over the past decade and are much narrower today than in the past. The procedure has significant potential complications and should be performed only in selected cases. Our current indications for arthroscopic lateral release of the patella include patients with recalcitrant anterior knee pain unresponsive to conservative treatment with:

- Tightness of the lateral retinaculum associated with lateral patellar tilt (excessive lateral pressure syndrome)
- Patellofemoral arthritis with lateral patellar and/or trochlear chondral damage and associated lateral patellar tilt
- Recurrent patellar subluxations/dislocations (typically performed in conjunction with either reconstruction of the medial patellofemoral ligament or a distal bony realignment)
- Painful bipartite patella with associated lateral pressure syndrome

The exact mechanism whereby lateral release is effective in relieving pain is unknown. Current theories include:

- Decreased tension in the lateral retinaculum
- Partial denervation of the patella
- Correction of patellar tilt with decreased loading of the lateral patella/trochlea

Arthroscopic lateral release of the patella is not indicated for the treatment of chronic anterior knee pain in adolescents with normal patellar tracking.

Conservative therapy is successful in treating most cases of anterior knee pain syndrome. This therapy ideally consists of 6 to 12 months of activity modification, selective use of anti-inflammatory agents, and a carefully structured exercise and stretching program. Patients are instructed to limit those activities that exacerbate their symptoms. They are encouraged to substitute other pain-free activities to maintain muscle strength, flexibility, and aerobic fitness. The therapeutic exercise program begins with the stretching of tight muscle–tendon units (e.g., hamstrings, triceps surae, iliotibial band, hip flexors) as well as the strengthening of weak muscles [e.g., quadriceps, vastus medalis oblique (VMO), hip external rotators]. Initially, isometric exercises are performed at or near full extension. Later, short-arc isotonic exercises and closed-chain quadriceps exercises are added. Emphasis should be on pain-free functional exercises for the entire lower extremity kinetic chain.

Various mechanical devices may also be used, including a Polumbo-style brace, a neoprene patellar sleeve, or orthotics to prevent excessive foot pronation. McConnell taping may be helpful during therapy sessions and when exercising to improve patellar tracking and relieve lateral facet compression (5). Braces that attempt to simulate the effects of McConnell taping are available. Additional braces have been introduced for patients with recalcitrant anterior knee pain who demonstrate tightness of the iliotibial band (Ober test) and hip flexors (Thomas test), with anterior pelvic tilt on physical examination. These braces have provided mixed results in treating patients with patellofemoral pain in our practice. Likewise, ultrasonography, phonophoresis, and iontophoresis have not been very helpful in our therapeutic programs for anterior knee pain. We have used them to treat localized soft-tissue areas that are symptomatic.

The great majority of patients with anterior knee pain will respond to a nonsurgical protocol (4). Once the symptoms have improved, we encourage a maintenance exercise program done a minimum of three times per week, and a gradual return to full activity. Surgery is offered only after attempts at nonsurgical treatment have failed and the patient is unwilling to live with the persisting symptoms (8). It is important that patients have realistic expectations of the success and failure rate of a lateral release in relieving their anterior knee pain.

PREOPERATIVE PLANNING

Patient evaluation begins with a careful detailed history. It is important to note whether the onset of the presenting pain was insidious or related to a specific or repetitive trauma. Acute anterior knee pain associated with a large hemarthrosis can be associated with a recent patellar subluxation or dislocation. These patients should also be evaluated for injury to the anterior cruciate ligament, since both can occur secondary to hyperextension of the knee. Rupture of the quadriceps or patellar tendon is an infrequent finding but needs to be ruled out, particularly in older patients. Localization of the type and character of pain is quite helpful, including location, duration, frequency, exacerbating activities, alleviating maneuvers, and previous treatments. Subtle malalignment may be associated with anterior knee pain that is typically worse with squatting, stair climbing, and prolonged knee flexion. Teenage females commonly experience self-limited anterior knee pain that resolves over a period of time. A history of recurrent effusions may suggest articular cartilage degeneration of the undersurface of the patella and/or trochlea.

The history usually provides a good indication of the diagnosis, which is then confirmed by a thorough physical examination. Key points of the physical examination include assessment of the sitting Q angle, patellar inhibition test, patellar apprehension test, active and passive patellar tracking, and specific muscle tightness. The Q angle has traditionally been measured with the knee in full extension. A sitting Q angle (tubercle sulcus angle) is a better measure of the relationship of the two vectors of the quadriceps and the patellar tendon. At 90 degrees of knee flexion, the tibial tubercle should be directly under the center of the femoral sulcus, or at an angle of 0 degrees. If it is lateral, or at a valgus angle, this indicates lateralization of the tibial tubercle (3). In addition, the presence of VMO atrophy or hypoplasia should be assessed. Comparison of the VMO musculature to the vastus lateralis should be noted, as well as whether the contraction is concentric. The patella should track smoothly through an active range of motion, without abrupt or sudden movements. Crepitus with flexion and extension may be present but does not always correlate with pain or the degree of chondromalacia. Facet tenderness and retinacular pain should also be documented.

The evaluation for patellar tilt and glide is an important part of the physical examination. Patellar tilt is performed with the patient in the supine position and the knee in full extension. Normally, the lateral side of the patella can be elevated above the horizontal. Inability to do this indicates tightness of lateral restraints, and correlates with a higher success rate with surgery in symptomatic patients who undergo lateral release. Testing of the patellar glide is performed with the knee in 30 degrees of flexion. A lateral glide of greater than 75% of the patellar width suggests incompetent medial restraints, whereas a medial glide of less than 25% indicates tightness of the lateral restraints (5).

Hamstring tightness may be associated with increased loads on the patellofemoral joint. This can be assessed by measuring the popliteal angle with the patient supine and the hip flexed to 90 degrees. With the patient supine, flex the hip and knee to 90 degrees. Then slowly extend the knee until muscle resistance is felt, keeping the low back flat. The knee should be fully extended. If the hamstrings are tight, the knee will remain flexed, and this angle short of full extension can be recorded. An Ober test should be performed to rule out iliotibial band contracture. This is performed with the patient on his side with the involved leg uppermost. The leg is abducted with the knee flexed to 90 degrees while keeping the hip joint in neutral to slight extension. With release of the abducted leg, the thigh should drop to an adducted position if the iliotibial tract is normal. However, the thigh will remain abducted if there is a contracture of the iliotibial band. Hip flexor tightness should be evaluated by performing a Thomas test. The patient should be supine with his pelvis level. Both hips are maximally flexed to the chest. Have the patient hold the uninvolved leg on the chest while letting the involved leg down until it is as straight as possible. The extent of a hip flexion contracture can be estimated by observing the angle between the leg and the table. Recently, anterior pelvic tilt with hip muscular strength abnormalities has been shown to be associated with patellofemoral pain. Reducing postural habits that cause anterior pelvic tilt while strengthening hip flexors and abductors may be effective in this group of patients. Weakness of the hip musculature can be evaluated via a single leg squat test.

In general, both extremities should be examined for side-to-side differences, and routine evaluation for meniscal and ligamentous pathology should be performed. Foot pronation is associated with obligatory internal tibial rotation and may contribute to anterior knee pain in patients with flatfoot deformity. These patients may benefit from orthotics. Referred pain from the low back or hip should be excluded by performing a straight-leg raise test and examining hip range of motion. In addition, the patient should be checked for generalized ligamentous laxity, which may be associated with patella alta and lateral subluxation or dislocation of the patella.

Radiographic evaluation consists of a standing PA view in 30 degrees of flexion, a lateral view in 30 degrees of flexion, and a Merchant tangential view. These radiographs should be evaluated for bipartite patella, occult fractures, tibiofemoral arthritis, patella alta, and patellar malalignment. Abnormalities in patellar height can be associated with symptomatic anterior knee pain. Insall and Salvati's ratio, normally 0.8 to 1.2, can be calculated from the lateral view in 30 degrees of flexion. It is determined by the diagonal length of the patella divided by the length of the patellar tendon (Fig. 1-1). A ratio of 0.8 or less demonstrates patella alta, whereas a ratio of greater than 1.2 indicates patella baja. The lateral radiograph can also be used to measure trochlear depth and dysplasia. Galland and coworkers defined three types of trochlear dysplasia based on where the line of the intercondylar groove crossed the shadow of the medial and lateral condyles (11).

The Merchant view is obtained with the patient supine and the knee flexed 45 degrees in a Merchant frame (9). The x-ray beam is directed from cephalad to caudad, 30 degrees from the horizontal. Both patellofemoral joints are imaged on a single cassette, allowing calculation of the sulcus

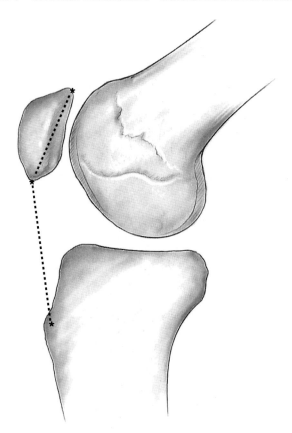

FIGURE 1-1

Insall and Salvati's ratio (P/PT). Normal values with the knee in 30 degrees flexion range from 0.8 to 1.2.

angle (normal: 130 degrees; range: 126 to 150 degrees; standard deviation: 6 degrees) and the congruence angle (normal: −6 degrees; standard deviation: 11 degrees). The congruence angle is determined by bisecting the sulcus angle to establish a reference line. A second line is then drawn from the apex of the sulcus to the lowest point on the articular ridge of the patella. A negative value is designated if the apex lies medial to the reference line (Fig. 1-2). Any angle greater than +16 degrees is associated with patellofemoral malalignment (9). All radiographic measurements have significant shortcomings, and we do not routinely measure angles and draw lines on every radiograph taken. Furthermore, abnormalities on radiographs do not necessarily correlate with clinical symptoms and must be viewed in the context of the entire history and physical examination.

Computerized tomography (CT) has gained increasing popularity in evaluating patellar alignment and tracking. CT cuts at 0, 15, 30, and 45 degrees allow the relationship of the patella to the tibial tubercle to be established, as well as calculation of the patellar tilt angle. Furthermore, CT scans of the hip, patella, and tibial tubercle can be used to calculate the Q angle.

Magnetic resonance imaging (MRI) scans may show abnormalities of articular cartilage and are helpful in evaluating other suspected intra-articular pathology. Sophisticated imaging studies, including stress radiographs, bone scans, and kinematic MRI, are available for more difficult diagnostic cases but are rarely needed.

SURGERY

Patient Positioning

The patient is placed on the operating table in the supine position. Under IV sedation, the knee is sterilely prepped and injected with 50 mL of a 1:1 mixture of 1% lidocaine with epinephrine and 0.25% Marcaine. An additional 10 mL is instilled into the region of the anteromedial and anterolateral portals, as well as the soft tissue over the lateral retinaculum. The surgeon then scrubs while the entire extremity is prepped and draped, allowing the local anesthesia time to take full effect. Routine diagnostic arthroscopy is performed using two standard portals. A commercially available pump with appropriate cannulas allows inflow through the same portal as the arthroscope. The anesthesiologist can titrate the amount of IV sedation needed during the procedure so the patient does

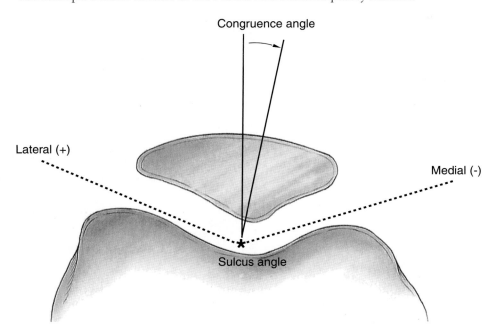

FIGURE 1-2

Calculation of the congruence angle.

not experience pain. The use of epidural or general anesthesia depends on patient and surgeon preference.

Since a leg holder may bind the quadriceps and alter patellofemoral mechanics, we prefer a lateral post to assist in the arthroscopic assessment of the entire knee joint. We do not use a tourniquet for several reasons. First, with meticulous hemostasis, we have not found one to be necessary. Second, we believe our patients experience more pain postoperatively when a tourniquet is used. Third, a tourniquet that is applied tightly but not inflated may act to decrease venous blood flow, which can increase bleeding and diminish visualization.

Technique

During the diagnostic arthroscopy, particular attention is paid to patellar tracking (tilt and subluxation) and to articular cartilage wear. The patella should centralize in the femoral groove at 30 to 45 degrees of knee flexion. Failure of the midpatellar ridge to seat centrally in the femoral groove at 45 degrees of knee flexion suggests lateral tracking (8) (Fig. 1-3). A separate superolateral viewing portal can also be used to assess tracking, and may assist in the decision to proceed with arthroscopic

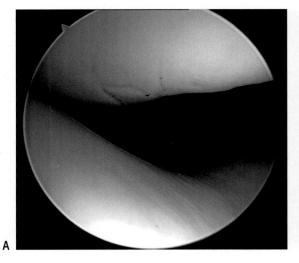
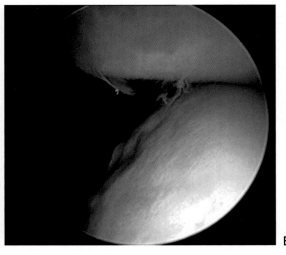

FIGURE 1-3

A: Failure of the midpatellar ridge to seat centrally with the knee flexed 45 degrees. Note the cartilage fissures on the central ridge of the patella. **B:** Lateral overhang of the lateral patellar facet on the femoral condyle.

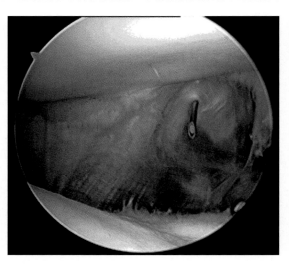

FIGURE 1-4

An 18-gauge needle placed through the lateral patellar retinaculum, just proximal to the level of the superior pole of the patella, denotes the upper level of retinacular release.

lateral release. However, we have not found this portal necessary and no longer use it. Any of the currently available radiofrequency ablation devices are satisfactory for the procedure.

An 18-gauge needle may be placed through the lateral patellar retinaculum just proximal to the level of the superior pole of the patella for orientation. This denotes the upper level of the retinacular release (Fig. 1-4). The arthroscopic and working portals are then switched; the radiofrequency wand is inserted through the anterolateral portal and the arthroscope anteromedially (Fig. 1-5). Using the ablation mode on the lowest effective setting, the lateral retinaculum is released from a proximal to distal direction, beginning at the level of the needle, 1 cm proximal and lateral to the superior edge of the patella, with the knee in full extension.

The tissue is released in layers in a controlled and well-visualized manner. The vessels can often be seen before their transection and are immediately coagulated. The lateral superior geniculate artery must be cauterized if it is transected at the superolateral border of the patella. The radiofrequency devices allow ablation and coagulation with the same wand by simply stepping on the appropriate control pedal. The proximal release is not extended into the muscle fibers of the vastus lateralis or quadriceps tendon. The release is continued distally to just below the inferior pole of the patella, effectively to the level of the tib/fib joint (Fig. 1-6). The capsular or retinacular bands run-

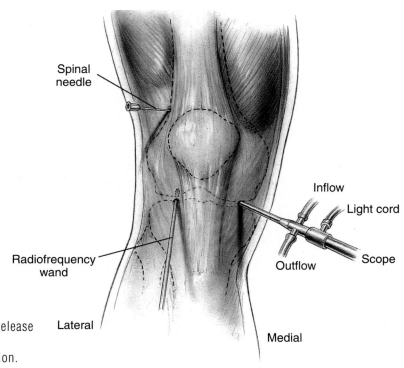

Spinal needle

Inflow

Light cord

Radiofrequency wand

Outflow

Scope

Lateral

Medial

FIGURE 1-5

Portals used for arthroscopic lateral release of the patella with radiofrequency ablation.

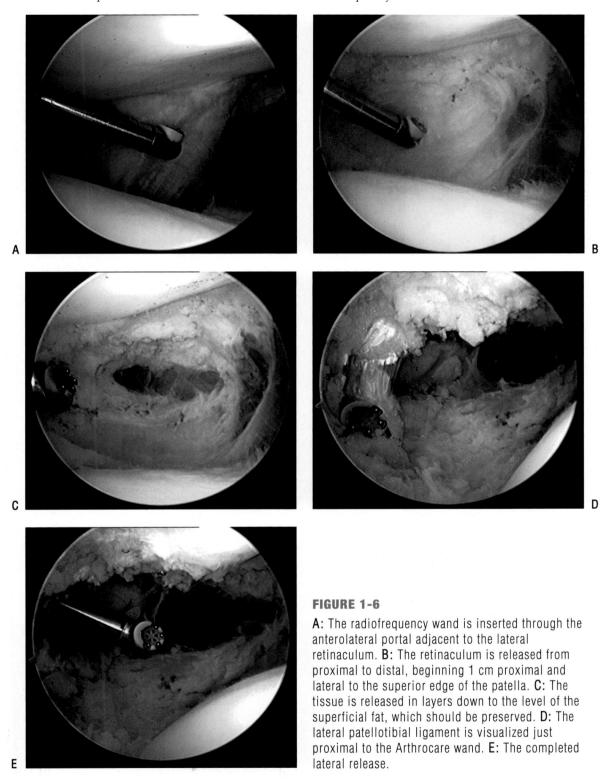

FIGURE 1-6

A: The radiofrequency wand is inserted through the anterolateral portal adjacent to the lateral retinaculum. **B:** The retinaculum is released from proximal to distal, beginning 1 cm proximal and lateral to the superior edge of the patella. **C:** The tissue is released in layers down to the level of the superficial fat, which should be preserved. **D:** The lateral patellotibial ligament is visualized just proximal to the Arthrocare wand. **E:** The completed lateral release.

ning from the inferolateral pole to the lateral tibial plateau should be released (Fig. 1-7). Removing a portion of the fat pad in this area with a full-radius resector enhances visualization and helps ensure that the distal aspect of the release is complete. The resection should proceed stepwise through the tissue layers until the superficial fat is seen. This layer should be preserved. Upon completion of the release, the positive inflow pressure is reduced and supplemented with gentle suction to allow identification and coagulation of any additional source of bleeding. Patellar tracking should be reassessed (Fig. 1-8). After a full release has been completed, there should be strong outflow of irrig-

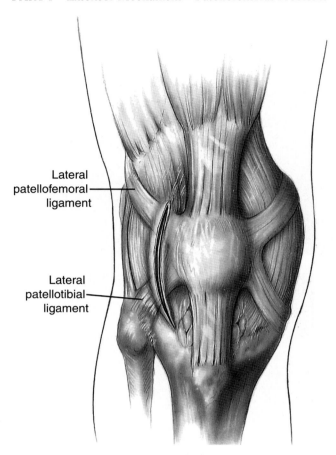

FIGURE 1-7

The lateral patellofemoral and patellotibial ligaments should be released.

ant from the inferior lateral portal once the wand has been removed. Complete correction of patellar maltracking may not be obtained in all patients. Those with more significant subluxation should be considered for a medial plication/reconstruction and/or distal realignment. Adequate release is confirmed by the ability to manually evert the patella in the femoral groove with the knee in full extension (Fig. 1-9).

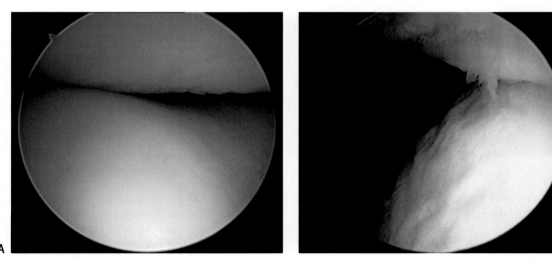

FIGURE 1-8

Patellar tracking after lateral release. **A:** Central tracking. **B:** Correction of lateral overhang.

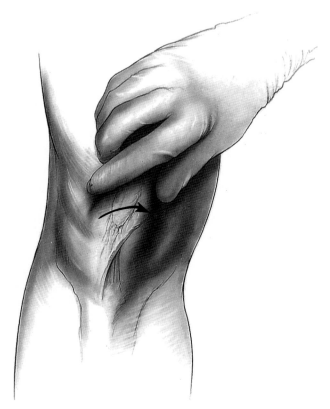

FIGURE 1-9

The patella should be manually everted 90 degrees to confirm adequate lateral release.

Pearls and Pitfalls

- Lateral release should be performed only with the appropriate surgical indications.
- A slight bend made near the tip of the radiofrequency probe facilitates ease of lateral release.
- Avoid injury to the muscle fibers of the vastus lateralis proximally.
- Mechanical debridement of the fat pad around the anterolateral portal improves visualization and ensures an adequate distal release.
- Decrease the pump pressure at the end of the procedure to help identify all bleeding vessels. Meticulous hemostasis avoids the common complication of a postoperative hemarthrosis and the associated pain that accompanies it.

POSTOPERATIVE MANAGEMENT

The immediate postoperative management and treatment is aimed at decreasing pain and swelling with rest, ice, compression, and elevation. We feel the early initiation of a specific rehabilitation program is an important part in achieving the best results following an arthroscopic lateral release of the patella. Patients are encouraged to start isometric exercises in the immediate postoperative course. They are allowed range of motion and weight bearing as tolerated. We suggest using ice and crutches for comfort and ambulation until muscle control of the extremity is re-established. Formal physical therapy usually begins at the first postoperative visit 5 to 7 days after surgery. The patient may shower within 2 days, but we recommend not immersing the knee in water for 2 weeks post-operatively. Patients can generally return to school or a sedentary job within 3 to 4 days after surgery. Crutches are recommended for several weeks for walking any distance, but shorter distances may be negotiated without crutches after only a few days. Limiting prolonged standing and walking for the first few weeks after surgery helps prevent the development of a large effusion, which may slow the recovery process. It takes 3 to 4 months for most patients to reach maximum recovery.

Electrical stimulation of the VMO and biofeedback may be selectively employed if progress is slow. Patient participation in passive patellar tilting and mobilization is instituted at the first post-operative visit. A long-term exercise program that re-establishes and maintains quadriceps strength ensures the best long-term results. The regimen begins with isometric exercises at or near full extension and progresses to short-arc isotonic quad sets, closed chain limited squats, and bicycle riding. Both closed- and open-chain exercises may be employed. Progression is individualized for each patient.

COMPLICATIONS

Complications of arthroscopic lateral release using radiofrequency ablation include:

- Hemarthrosis
- Thermal injury to the skin
- Infection
- Medial subluxation following excessive lateral release
- Patellar hypermobility
- Quadriceps weakness
- Transection or rupture of the vastus lateralis insertion and/or quadriceps tendon
- Reflex sympathetic dystrophy
- Persistent knee pain

The incidence of hemarthrosis can be reduced by careful attention to surgical detail, obtaining adequate visualization, and meticulous cauterization of all bleeding vessels. The lowest setting that allows adequate cutting and coagulation should be used to decrease the incidence of thermal injury to the overlying skin. Insertion of an 18-gauge needle at the superolateral border of the patella to delineate the starting point of the lateral release should help prevent transection of the quadriceps tendon and extension of the release too proximally into the vastus lateralis muscle fibers. Postoperative medial subluxation and patellar hypermobility occur primarily in those cases in which the lateral retinacular release is carried too proximally, or was misdiagnosed and not appreciated preoperatively. This represents a formidable treatment problem; if it exists but is not recognized preoperatively, it is often made worse by a lateral retinacular release. Surgical reattachment of the vastus lateralis with or without medial release provides unpredictable results in trying to salvage this complication.

Superficial infections require special attention because of the potential for subcutaneous accumulation of blood that communicates with an underlying hemarthrosis. Intra-articular postoperative infections are rare. If there is any question of deep infection, the patient should be returned to the operating room for formal irrigation and debridement followed by appropriate antibiotics if indicated. We also recommend restricting knee range of motion if there is any suggestion of drainage from an intra-articular effusion.

Pre-existing complex regional pain syndrome should be recognized at the stage of preoperative planning because it can be aggravated by surgery. An early rehabilitation program is important to its postoperative prevention. Patients with unusual postoperative pain and/or slow progress regaining knee motion deserve special attention. We feel any signs of complex regional pain syndrome developing in the postoperative period are best dealt with by a multidisciplinary approach. Unrecognized complex regional pain syndrome or delayed treatment for this condition can result in a postoperative disability that exceeds the patient's preoperative symptoms.

RESULTS

As the indications for arthroscopic lateral release have become more specific, outcomes have improved, but are still evolving. The literature currently reports success rates in the range of 65% to 92% (1,2,6). These statistics bring to light the fact that it is imperative to reserve lateral release for those cases with definitive clinical, radiographic, and arthroscopic findings consistent with the surgical indications previously outlined.

We believe that approximately 75% of our patients have achieved significant improvement following surgery. The degree and timing of improvement vary a great deal. Patients should have realistic expectations and understand that they may continue to have some symptoms after surgery.

RECOMMENDED READING

Fanni AS, Tartarone M, Patricola A, et al. Long-term results of lateral retinacular release. *Arthroscopy.* 2005;21(5): 526–531.

REFERENCES

1. Aderinto J, Cobb AG. Lateral release for patellofemoral arthritis. *Arthroscopy.* 2002;18(4):399-403.
2. Carson WG, James SL, Larson RL, et al. Patellofemoral disorders: physical and radiographic evaluation. *Clin Orthop.* 1984;185:165–186.
3. Friederichs MG, Burks RT. Patellofemoral disorders. In: Garrick JG, ed. *Orthopaedic knowledge update: sports medicine 3.* Rosemont, IL: American Academy of Orthopaedic Surgeons; 2004:213–221.
4. Fulkerson JP. Patellofemoral pain disorders: evaluation and management. *J Am Acad Orthop Surg.* 1994;2:124–132.
5. Fulkerson JP, Kalenak A, Rosenberg TD, et al. Patellofemoral pain. In: Eilert RE, ed. *AAOS instructional course lectures,* vol. 41. Rosemont, IL: American Academy of Orthopaedic Surgeons; 1992:57–71.
6. Gallick GS, Brna JA, Fox JM. Electrosurgery in operative arthroscopy. *Clin Sports Med.* 1987;6(3):607–618.
7. Kelly MA. Algorithm for anterior knee pain. In: Cannon WD, ed. *AAOS instructional course lectures,* vol. 47. Rosemont, IL: American Academy of Orthopaedic Surgeons; 1998:339–343.
8. Lombardo SJ, Bradley JP. Arthroscopic diagnosis and treatment of patellofemoral disorders. In: Scott WN, ed. *Arthroscopy of the knee: diagnosis and treatment.* Philadelphia: WB Saunders; 1990:155–173.
9. Merchant AC. Classification of patellofemoral disorders. *Arthroscopy.* 1988;4:235–240.
10. Miller GK, Dickason JM, Fox J, et al. The use of electrosurgery for arthroscopic subcutaneous lateral release. *Orthopaedics.* 1982;5:309–314.
11. Walsh WM. Patellofemoral joint. In: DeLee JC, Drez D, eds. *Orthopaedic sports medicine: principles and practice,* vol. 2. Philadelphia: WB Saunders; 1994;1163–1248.

2 Medial Patellofemoral Ligament Reconstruction and Repair

Andrew J. Cosgarea and Brett M. Cascio

INDICATIONS

Over the years, a large number of procedures have been described to treat patellar instability. Recently there has been a great deal of interest in procedures that address the medial patellofemoral ligament (MPFL), the primary soft tissue passive restraint to pathologic lateral patellar displacement (2,4). The MPFL is torn when the patella dislocates (10,15), and a variety of techniques have been described to repair (3,10,15) or reconstruct (5,12,16) the ligament in an attempt to restore its function as a check-rein.

History

The indication for MPFL surgery is patellar instability; therefore, the most important clinical determination to make is whether anterior knee pain is associated with instability. The much more common clinical entity of patellofemoral pain syndrome is nearly universally treated nonoperatively. Among the spectrum of disorders causing anterior knee pain, patellar instability represents a distinct clinical entity that is usually amenable to surgical treatment. Instability represents a continuum ranging from minor incidental subluxation episodes to traumatic dislocation events. Dislocations can occur from an indirect twisting mechanism as the upper body rotates while the foot remains planted on the ground. Less commonly, a direct blow along the medial aspect of the patella during sports activity drives the patella laterally. Medial dislocations are rare in patients who have not undergone previous lateral retinacular release surgery. Sometimes the patella reduces spontaneously, although on occasion a formal reduction maneuver may be necessary. With a first dislocation episode, the patient usually experiences significant pain, and swelling is caused by soft tissue and intra-articular damage. The resulting swelling and muscle weakness may take several weeks to resolve. Patients who sustain multiple episodes tend to experience less dramatic symptoms. Subluxation episodes also tend to be less dramatic. Patients may describe a feeling of instability with or without pain. Instability usually occurs with trunk rotation during physical activity, as the foot remains planted on the ground. The discomfort is usually anterior, and may be bilateral, especially in patients with malalignment or hyperlaxity.

Physical Examination

Careful physical examination can confirm patellar instability. Alignment is evaluated with the patient standing or walking. The knee is then observed for extra-articular swelling or an effusion. The soft tissues are palpated, and the examiner should try to identify an area of tenderness along the course of the MPFL, as this usually identifies the location of the tear. A thorough cruciate and collateral ligament examination is necessary to rule out concomitant pathology. Medial collateral ligament tears often occur at the same time as a patellar dislocation. The quadriceps angle (Q angle) can be measured as a gross assessment of the lateral force vector. Patellar tracking is observed as the knee is extended from a flexed position. The patella has a tendency to slip laterally as the knee approaches the last 20 degrees of extension and the patella is no longer constrained by the lateral trochlear ridge (J sign). Patellar translation is assessed by pushing on the medial side of the patella with the knee in full extension. The amount of translation is quantified in quadrants and compared to the normal contralateral knee. An indistinct endpoint suggests MPFL incompetence. A feeling of apprehension (apprehension sign) supports the diagnosis of instability. Lateral retinacular tightness is assessed by manually elevating the lateral edge of the patella (tilt test).

The standard radiograph series includes anteroposterior, lateral (30 degrees flexion), tunnel, and sunrise (30 to 45 degrees flexion) views. The tunnel view may demonstratel osteochondritis dissecans lesions or loose bodies in the notch. The sunrise view shows the degree of subluxation and tilt. Computed tomography (CT) scan axial images (20 degrees flexion) are occasionally helpful to identify subluxation and tilt. Magnetic resonance imaging (MRI) demonstrates the characteristic bone bruise pattern involving the medial facet of the patella and the proximal lateral femoral condyle in patients who have recently sustained a dislocation.

MPFL reconstruction is indicated in skeletally mature patients with symptomatic recurrent lateral subluxation or dislocation. Patients have usually failed attempts at nonoperative treatment including activity modification, physical therapy, and knee bracing. Some authors recommend MPFL repair for patients following their first patellar dislocation (15). We usually recommend treating an initial dislocation episode nonoperatively, but will repair an acute MPFL tear when surgery is necessary for concomitant intra-articular pathology (large loose body, meniscus tear). MPFL repair techniques may also be used to treat recurrent instability. The MPFL becomes attenuated and functionally incompetent with repeated instability episodes, so it is tightened by cutting, shortening, and reattaching it at the patellar or femoral insertion, or by midsubstance imbrication.

CONTRAINDICATIONS

MPFL repair and reconstruction are contraindicated in patients with medial instability or isolated anterior knee pain. Great care should be taken not to overtighten the MPFL or malposition the graft as this will result in excessive medial patellofemoral joint pressures and is likely to exacerbate patellofemoral pain, particularly in patients with medial patellofemoral chondral damage. The distal femoral growth plate is at risk for injury in skeletally immature patients. The traditional MPFL reconstruction technique can be modified so that the graft is passed around the proximal superficial medial collateral ligament (MCL), or sutured directly to adjacent soft tissue.

Tibial tuberosity osteotomy procedures, such as the Elmslie-Trillat, have a theoretical advantage in patients with greater degrees of malalignment. The Fulkerson anteromedialization osteotomy is preferred in patients with malalignment and degenerative changes involving the inferior pole of the patella or lateral facet (9). MPFL reconstruction or repair can be combined with distal osteotomy if either alone is insufficient to provide adequate stability.

SURGERY

Patient Positioning

The patient is placed supine on a standard operating room table. A vertical post is used to facilitate arthroscopic evaluation and can be removed before starting the open portion of the surgery. A tourniquet is used to facilitate hemostatis and visualization. Surgery is performed on an outpatient basis using general or regional anesthesia. Prophylactic intravenous antibiotics are administered before incision.

Exam under Anesthesia

After induction of satisfactory anesthesia, a comprehensive examination is performed. Patellar stability, translation, and tilt are usually easier to characterize when the patient is anesthetized. With the knee extended, the position of the patella is determined at rest, and with a lateral translation force applied. The amount of translation on the symptomatic side is compared to the normal lateral patellar translation in the contralateral knee (Fig. 2-1). The patella is pushed laterally, and the amount of translation and the consistency of the endpoint are assessed. The examiner everts the lateral edge of the patella to determine whether the lateral retinaculum is tight. If the patient's symptoms and exam are consistent with excessive lateral retinacular tightness, then consideration should be given to performing a concomitant arthroscopic lateral retinacular release.

Diagnostic Arthroscopy

Arthroscopy is performed first using the standard superolateral, inferomedial, and inferolateral portals. The suprapatellar pouch, the medial and lateral parapatellar gutters, and the posteromedial and posterolateral compartments are carefully assessed for loose bodies. The articular surfaces of the patella and trochlear are thoroughly scrutinized for chondral lesions. The medial facet of the patella and the proximal portion of the lateral femoral condyle are the areas most commonly injured during a traumatic patellar dislocation. Hemorrhage may be noted in the soft tissue adjacent to the medial edge of the patella in patients who have sustained a recent avulsion of the MPFL insertion. Patellar tracking in the trochlear groove is visualized as the knee is ranged. Any large chondral lesions are addressed surgically with debridement, microfracture, or repair techniques as indicated. In some circumstances, large defects should be unloaded using tibial tuberosity anteromedialization. Arthroscopic lateral retinacular release may be performed at this point, although we have not found that to be routinely necessary.

Surface Landmarks

After removing the arthroscopy equipment, a marking pen is used to identify the important bony landmarks (Fig. 2-2). Marks are made over the patella, tibial tuberosity, adductor tubercle, and medial femoral epicondyle. The pes anserine tendon insertion site is palpated, and a 3- to 4-cm oblique mark is made over the sartorial fascia insertion on the proximal medial tibia for the harvest site incision. A second 3- to 4-cm line is drawn directly over the MPFL, halfway between the medial border of the patella and the medial femoral epicondyle. The position is modified if the location of the MPFL tear has been ascertained from the preoperative examination or MRI, and an MPFL repair is planned.

The tourniquet is raised while the knee is in an extended position. A longitudinal incision is made midway between the medial edge of the patella and the medial epicondyle. Sharp and blunt dissection is used to expose the thick medial retinacular layer contiguous with the inferior border of the vastus medialis obliquus muscle. With gentle dissection, the superior and inferior borders of the MPFL are isolated (Fig. 2-3). In patients who have sustained a recent dislocation, it may be possi-

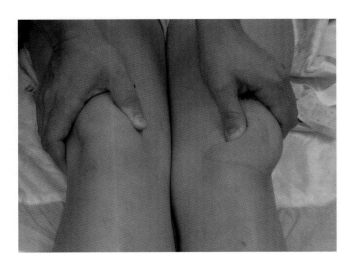

FIGURE 2-1

Comparison of patellar translation between symptomatic left and asymptomatic right knees with equal lateral forces applied under general anesthesia. Note lateral translation of the left patella is greater than two quadrants.

FIGURE 2-2

The circle is drawn over the patella. The proximal "X" is over the adductor tubercle; the distal "X" overlies the medial epicondyle. The proximal line is over the midportion of the MPFL and is where the incision is made to expose the medial border of the patella and medial femoral epicondyle. The distal line overlies the pes anserine insertion and is where the incision is made to harvest the gracilis tendon.

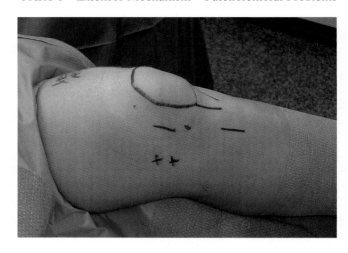

ble to identify the site of the MPFL tear at the medial border of the patella, the medial femoral epicondyle, or in midsubstance.

Medial Patellofemoral Ligament Repair

The medial edge of the patella is brought into the operative field by applying a medially directed force to the lateral border of the patella. If the MPFL is torn at this location, a direct repair can be performed using bone tunnels or suture anchors. The adductor tubercle and medial femoral epicondyle can be exposed through the same incision with posterior retraction. The torn MPFL can be repaired in this location to a stump of remaining tissue using #2 nonabsorbable sutures, or reattached directly to a freshened bony surface using 2 or 3 suture anchors. With midsubstance ruptures it is not always possible to identify the location of tissue failure. In chronic cases, it can be especially difficult to determine how much to shorten the attenuated ligament. Overtightening the ligament will cause repair failure or overconstrain the patella. We usually perform MPFL repairs in patients who have experienced recent instability episodes when acute surgical intervention is indicated for concomitant intra-articular pathology.

Graft Harvest for Medial Patellofemoral Ligament Reconstruction

A variety of different graft sources are available for reconstructing the MPFL. We prefer to use the gracilis tendon because it is adjacent to the reconstruction site and is relatively easy to harvest. An incision is made over the pes anserine insertion, and the sartorial fascia is exposed. The superior edge of the sartorial fascia is identified just anterior to the superficial medial collateral ligament. It is incised and then everted to expose the underlying gracilis and semitendinosus tendons (Fig. 2-4). The gracilis tendon is dissected free from the undersurface of the sartorial fascia. The free end of the

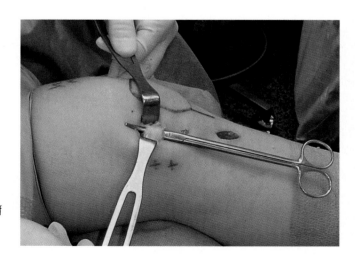

FIGURE 2-3

The superior and inferior borders of the MPFL are identified and exposed.

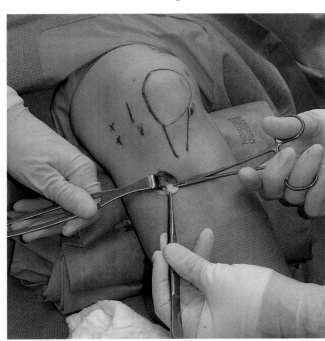

FIGURE 2-4

The sartorial fascia is incised and inverted, exposing the gracilis tendon.

tendon is then tagged and harvested using a tendon stripper (Fig. 2-5). Although the gracilis is smaller and shorter than the semitendinosus tendon, it is still significantly stronger then the native MPFL (1,2,11) and long enough to construct an adequate graft. The sartorial fascia is sutured back to its insertion on the proximal medial tibia.

Muscle is removed from the surface of the gracilis tendon (Fig. 2-6). The length and diameter are measured. A folded graft length of 9 to 10 cm is sufficient, as the length will be increased by the addition of the Continuous Loop EndoButton (Acufex, Smith & Nephew, Andover, MA) once the graft construct has been completed.

Patella Tunnel

The MPFL insertion on the medial edge of the patella is identified and a rongeur is used to clear the soft tissue and expose cancellous bone (Fig. 2-7). The proximal and distal poles of the patella are

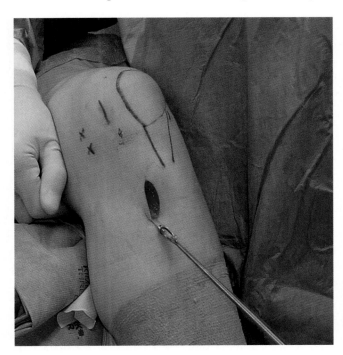

FIGURE 2-5

The gracilis tendon is tagged with a #2 Ticron suture, then harvested with a tendon striper.

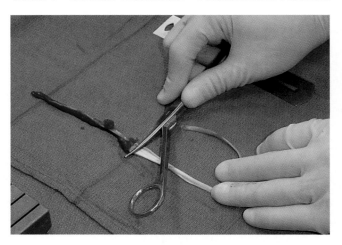

FIGURE 2-6

Muscle is removed from the gracilis tendon.

palpated, confirming that the patellar tunnel starting point is in the superior half of the patella. A 2.5-mm drill bit is advanced laterally in the midportion of the MPFL insertion, which is usually just above the equator of the patella. The surgeon must be careful while drilling not to violate either the anterior bony cortex or posterior articular surface. Lateral fluoroscopy can be used to confirm appropriate positioning (Fig. 2-8). The 2.5-mm drill bit is then replaced with a 2.0-mm eyelet K-wire, which is then overdrilled with a 4.5-mm cannulated drill bit (Fig. 2-9). The length of the tunnel is then measured with a depth gauge. The appropriate length Continuous Loop EndoButton is chosen to complete the graft construct based on the length of the tendon and the amount of graft that the surgeon wants in the patellar tunnel. The gracilis tendon is passed through the loop of the EndoButton and sutured to itself using a #2 nonabsorbable woven suture (Fig. 2-10). Sutures are woven through the femoral end of the graft, which will be used later to pull the graft into the femoral tunnel. If the graft diameter is greater than 4.5 mm, then the patellar tunnel is enlarged with the appropriate-sized cannulated drill bit (Fig. 2-11).

The sutures from the EndoButton are loaded through the eyelet of the 2.0-mm K-wire, which is then pulled out through the superolateral portal site (Fig. 2-12). With the EndoButton positioned lengthwise, the graft is pulled through the patellar tunnel. Once it clears the tunnel, tension is placed on the femoral end of the graft so that EndoButton is brought flush to the lateral edge of the patella. The position of the EndoButton can be manually manipulated so that it lies flush and lengthwise along the lateral edge of the patella, which can be confirmed with fluoroscopy if desired (Fig. 2-13).

Femoral Tunnel

A common error that occurs during MPFL reconstruction surgery is to place the femoral tunnel too far proximal. Several studies have shown that the femoral attachment site of the MPFL is at the medial epicondyle, which is approximately 1 cm distal to the adductor tubercle (13,14,17). Therefore, it is crucial to distinguish between these 2 bony prominences (Fig. 2-14). A recent biomechanical

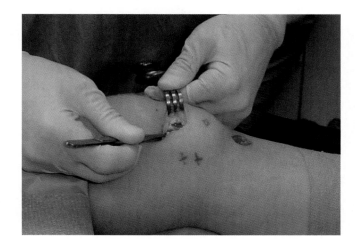

FIGURE 2-7

The attachment site of the MPFL at the medial edge of the patella is exposed in preparation for drilling the patellar tunnel.

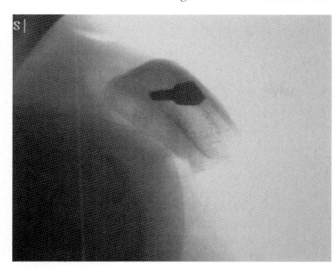

FIGURE 2-8

A 2.5-mm drill bit passed transversely from medial to lateral. Fluoroscopy can be used to confirm the appropriate position of the drill bit in the patella proximal to the equator.

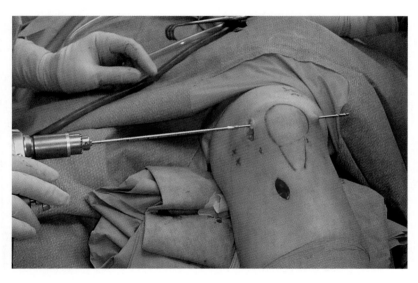

FIGURE 2-9

The 2.5-mm drill bit is replaced with a 2.0-mm eyelet K-wire, which is over-drilled with a cannulated 4.5-mm drill bit.

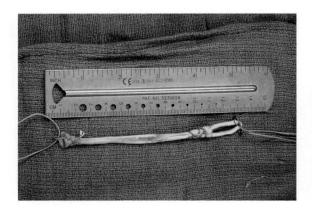

FIGURE 2-10

The gracilis tendon is passed through the loop of the EndoButton and sewn back to itself with #2 Ticron suture. A loop is sewn into the free end so that the pull-through suture can be removed at the end of the case.

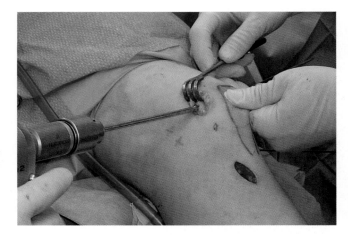

FIGURE 2-11

The patellar tunnel size is increased to the appropriate depth based on the length of the EndoButton loop and diameter of the completed graft.

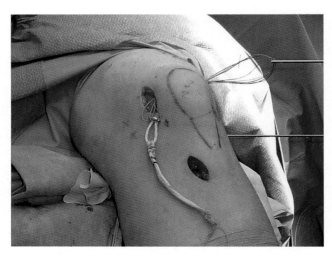

FIGURE 2-12

The graft is brought through the patellar tunnel.

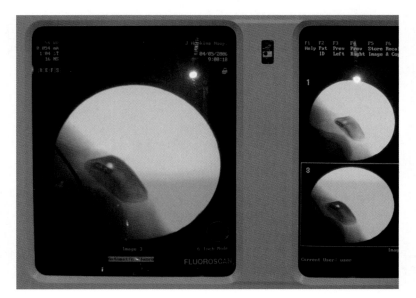

FIGURE 2-13

The position of the tunnel and EndoButton may be confirmed with fluoroscopy.

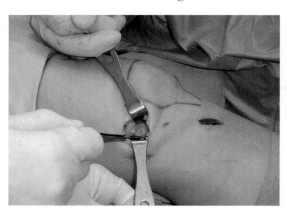

FIGURE 2-14
The anatomic insertion site of the MPFL just anterior to the medial femoral epicondyle is exposed.

study suggests that malpositioning the femoral tunnel even 5 mm too far proximal results in increased graft force and pressure applied to the cartilage of the medial patellofemoral cartilage (6).

A 2.5-mm drill bit is placed just anterior to the medial femoral epicondyle. The graft is then passed underneath the medial retinaculum and the remnant of the MPFL and then wrapped around the drill bit, allowing for assessment of graft isometry as the knee is ranged (Fig. 2-15). The position of the drill bit can be adjusted to allow for fine-tuning of tunnel positioning. Once the femoral tunnel has been determined, the drill bit is replaced with a 2.0-mm eyelet K-wire. The K-wire is then over drilled with a 6.0-mm cannulated drill bit to the correct depth based on the remaining length of the graft. The suture ends are then passed through the eyelet of the K-wire and pulled into the femoral tunnel as the K-wire exits the lateral side of the knee.

Graft Tensioning and Fixation

With tension placed on the free suture ends, the surgeon moves the knee several times through a full range of motion. As the knee is ranged, graft isometry can be ascertained by feeling tension on the free suture ends. In addition, the graft is directly palpated and visualized through the medial incision. It is crucial not to overconstrain the graft. Next, the knee is placed in full extension, and the patella is pushed laterally. An attempt is made to identify the graft length, which allows the same amount of lateral translation noted on the normal contralateral side. Once the appropriate graft length is identified, fixation is obtained using a 7.0-mm bioabsorbable cannulated femoral interference screw (Fig. 2-16) and can be augmented by suturing the graft to the adjacent soft tissue. The surgeon should then confirm that the knee has full range of motion, the patella is no longer dislocatable, and the graft provides a firm checkrein to pathologic lateral translation.

The wound is closed in layers. A subcuticular skin closure allows for excellent cosmesis (Fig. 2-17). A cryotherapy unit is used to help control pain and swelling. A compressive dressing is then applied, followed by a thigh-high compression stocking and a postop brace locked in full extension.

The procedure's surgical steps are summarized in Table 2-1.

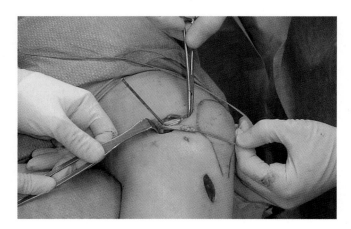

FIGURE 2-15
The femoral end of the EndoButton is wrapped around the K-wire and graft tension is assessed as the knee is ranged. The femoral tunnel position may be modified if necessary.

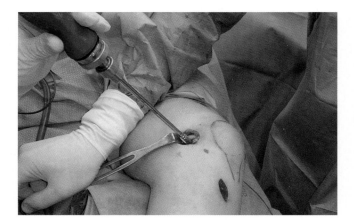

FIGURE 2-16

Once the correct femoral tunnel position is determined, it is drilled with a 6.0-mm cannulated drill bit to the appropriate depth, based on the remaining length of the graft. Fixation is achieved using 7.0-mm bioabsorbable interference screw.

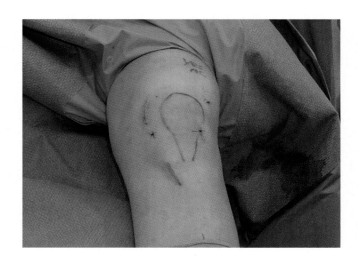

FIGURE 2-17

Subcuticular wound closure allows for excellent cosmesis.

TABLE 2-1. Surgical Steps for MPFL Reconstruction	
• Exam under anesthesia	• Soft tissue tunnel passage
• Arthroscopic evaluation	• Femoral tunnel preparation
• Hamstring graft harvest	• Femoral tunnel graft passage
• MPFL exposure	• Graft tensioning
• Patellar tunnel preparation	• Femoral interference screw fixation
• Hamstring graft preparation	• Wound closure
• Graft passage and EndoButton fixation	

Pearls and Pitfalls

- An incision over the midportion of the MPFL allows exposure of both the medial border of the patella and the medial femoral epicondyle.
- The correct location of the patellar tunnel is on the medial border of the patella proximal to the equator.
- The patellar tunnel should be initially drilled with a 2.5-mm drill bit and the position confirmed with fluoroscopy before overdrilling with a 4.5-mm drill bit to minimize the risk of patellar fracture.
- When the free ends of the hamstring graft are sewn together, a suture loop is created so that the passing suture that is used to pull the graft into the femoral tunnel can be completely removed where it exits percutaneously on the lateral side of the knee.
- The femoral tunnel should be distal to the adductor tubercle and anterior to the medial epicondyle.
- Final femoral fixation should occur at the knee flexion angle that causes the greatest amount of tension in the graft with the goal of reproducing the same amount of lateral patellar translation as was appreciated on the contralateral normal side with the knee extended during the examination under anesthesia.
- It is better to leave the reconstructed MPFL graft slightly loose than to overconstrain the patellofemoral joint by making the graft too tight.

POSTOPERATIVE MANAGEMENT

Patients are instructed in quadriceps sets and straight leg raises in the recovery room and are allowed to ambulate with crutches and touchdown weight-bearing status. The brace remains locked in full extension for 1 week, and then patients are encouraged to begin knee range of motion and to progress as tolerated. Patients are instructed to attend formal physical therapy 3 times per week, where knee range of motion and quadriceps strengthening are emphasized. Weight bearing progresses as tolerated, and the brace is unlocked for ambulation as soon as quadriceps strength is sufficient. Patients are encouraged to reach 120 degrees of knee flexion by 4 weeks postop, and the brace is generally discontinued by 6 weeks. Full knee range of motion should be achieved by 8 weeks. Patients are allowed to progress to jogging and sports-specific drills by 12 weeks, and most patients are able to return to sports by 4 to 5 months. A rehabilitation plan is outlined in Table 2-2.

COMPLICATIONS

As with most patellofemoral reconstruction procedures, the most common postoperative complication is loss of motion. Motion deficits may be secondary to inadequate postoperative rehabilitation. Loss of flexion may also be secondary to intraoperative technical errors such as malpositioning or overtensioning the graft. These errors could also overload the medial patellofemoral joint articular surfaces and result in arthrosis, especially if there is a pre-existing medial patellar chondral lesion. The saphenous nerve is at risk for injury during exposure of the femoral tunnel. Other potential complications include recurrent instability secondary to graft failure, painful hardware, and patella fracture.

TABLE 2-2. **Postoperative Rehabilitation**
• Postop: Touchdown weight bearing in brace locked in extension, quadriceps sets, and straight leg raises
• Week 1: Physical therapy referral, progress with knee range of motion, weight bearing, and strengthening
• Week 6: Discontinue brace
• Week 8: Should have full range of motion
• Week 12: Jogging program
• Week 16: Sports-specific drills
• Week 20: Return to sports when strength and agility allow

RESULTS

Outcome following MPFL repair or reconstruction has been generally favorable (5,7,8,10,15). Although these studies generally have been limited by small numbers of patients, retrospective design, and the lack of control groups, most report satisfactory outcome (good and excellent) in the range of 86% to 96% (5,7,8,10).

REFERENCES

1. Amis AA, Firer P, Mountney J, et al. Anatomy and biomechanics of the medial patellofemoral ligament. *Knee*. 2003;10:215–220.
2. Conlan T, Garth WP Jr, Lemons JE. Evaluation of the medial soft-tissue restraints of the extensor mechanism of the knee. *J Bone Joint Surg Am*. 1993;75:682–693.
3. Davis DK, Fithian DC. Techniques of medial retinacular repair and reconstruction. *Clin Orthop Relat Res*. 2002;402: 38–52.
4. Desio SM, Burks RT, Bachus KN. Soft tissue restraints to lateral patellar translation in the human knee. *Am J Sports Med*. 1998;26:59–65.
5. Drez D Jr, Edwards TB, Williams CS. Results of medial patellofemoral ligament reconstruction in the treatment of patellar dislocation. *Arthroscopy*. 2001;17:298–306.
6. Elias JJ, Cosgarea AJ. Technical errors during medial patellofemoral ligament reconstruction could overload medial patellofemoral cartilage. *Am J Sports Med*. 2006;34:1478–1485.
7. Ellera Gomes JL. Medial patellofemoral ligament reconstruction for recurrent dislocation of the patella: a preliminary report. *Arthroscopy*. 1992;8:335–340.
8. Ellera Gomes JL, Stigler Marczyk LR, Cesar de Cesar P, et al. Medial patellofemoral ligament reconstruction with semitendinosus autograft for chronic patellar instability: a follow-up study. *Arthroscopy*. 2004;20:147–151.
9. Fulkerson JP, Becker GJ, Meaney JA, et al. Anteromedial tibial tubercle transfer without bone graft. *Am J Sports Med*. 1990;18:490–496; disc 496–497.
10. Garth WP Jr, DiChristina DG, Holt G. Delayed proximal repair and distal realignment after patellar dislocation. *Clin Orthop Relat Res*. 2000;377:132–144.
11. Hamner DL, Brown CH Jr, Steiner ME, Hecker AT, Hayes WC. Hamstring tendon grafts for reconstruction of the anterior cruciate ligament: biomechanical evaluation of the use of multiple strands and tensioning techniques. *J Bone Joint Surg*. 1999;81A:549–557.
12. Muneta T, Sekiya I, Tsuchiya M, et al. A technique for reconstruction of the medial patellofemoral ligament. *Clin Orthop Relat Res*. 1999;359:151–155.
13. Nomura E, Horiuchi Y, Kihara M. Medial patellofemoral ligament restraint in lateral patellar translation and reconstruction. *Knee*. 2000;7:121–127.
14. Nomura E, Inoue M. Surgical technique and rationale for medial patellofemoral ligament reconstruction for recurrent patellar dislocation. *Arthroscopy*. 2003;19:E47.
15. Sallay PI, Poggi J, Speer KP, et al. Acute dislocation of the patella. A correlative pathoanatomic study. *Am J Sports Med*. 1996;24:52–60.
16. Schock E, Burks R. Medial patellofemoral ligament reconstruction using a hamstring graft. *Op Tech Sports Med*. 2001; 9:169–175.
17. Smirk C, Morris H. The anatomy and reconstruction of the medial patellofemoral ligament. *Knee*. 2003;10: 221–227.

3 Anteromedial Tibial Tubercle Transfer

John P. Fulkerson

INDICATIONS/CONTRAINDICATIONS

The best candidate for anteromedial tibial tubercle transfer (2,5–6) (Fig. 3-1) is a patient with lateral patellar tilt (and/or subluxation) associated with grade III or IV articular degeneration localized on the lateral and/or distal medial patellar facets following the failure of nonsurgical therapy. If there is no articular degeneration or pain, there is no need to anteriorize the tibial tubercle, and a straight medial transfer of the tibial tubercle as described by Trillat (11) and reviewed by Carney, Mologne, Muldoon, and Cox (1) is more appropriate for correcting subluxation. However, some patients have distal and/or lateral patella articular softening (grade I) or cartilage breakdown (grade II–IV).

In such patients, the surgeon may wish to anteriorize the extensor mechanism to some extent at the time of realignment. An oblique osteotomy will transfer load off an area of articular degeneration, particularly when damage is noted on the distal aspect of the patella (anteriorization "tips" up the distal patella, thereby unloading it). Anteromedial tibial tubercle transfer is appropriate whenever the surgeon wishes to shift contact stress on the patella from the lateral and distal aspects of the patella to the more proximal and medial patellar articular cartilage. Most important is to recognize that tibial tubercle anteriorization at the time of medialization gives the added benefit of removing articulation with the distal patella, which is often a fragmented or softened source of pain.

Before considering anteromedial tibial tubercle transfer, alternative nonsurgical treatment methods must fail. In particular, a well-structured program of rehabilitation should be tried involving mobilization of a lateralized and tight extensor mechanism supplemented by patellar bracing (9). I use the Tru-Pull braces (DJOrtho, Vista, CA). A tight extensor mechanism and hamstrings should be mobilized through stretching and strengthening. Prone quadriceps stretching has been very helpful and is easy for patients to do at home. Lower extremity core stability including hip stabilization exercises is important in these patients. Nonsteroidal anti-inflammatory medication is often helpful for symptomatic treatment during the period of nonsurgical therapy.

Failed lateral release is another potential indication for anteromedial tibial tubercle transfer. If a patient is left with residual articular pain or symptomatic lateral malalignment of the patella following lateral release, anteromedial tibial tubercle transfer may be helpful.

Contraindications to anteromedial tibial tubercle transfer include:

- Diffuse patella articular breakdown. Particularly if the cartilage loss involves the proximal medial patella (dashboard or crush injury), patients are less likely to benefit from anteromedial tibial tubercle transfer.
- Tilt alone and no significant subluxation or lateral facet collapse. Such patients may benefit from simple lateral retinacular release; therefore anteromedial tibial tubercle transfer is not recommended as a first procedure.
- Reflex sympathetic dystrophy and chronic pain syndrome.
- Patients with a bleeding tendency or history of deep venous thrombosis are less desirable candidates for this type of surgery.
- Poor healing capacity, diabetes, gross obesity, and smoking are relative contraindications for tibial tubercle transfer.

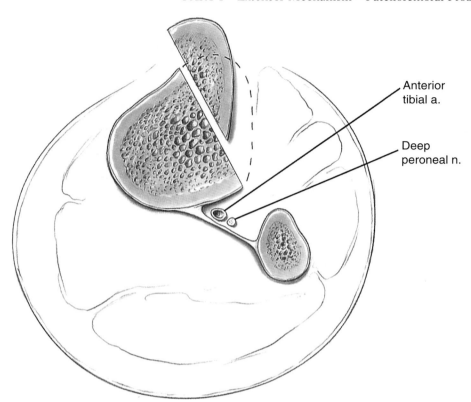

Anterior
tibial a.

Deep
peroneal n.

FIGURE 3-1

Anteromedial tibial
tubercle transfer.

PREOPERATIVE PLANNING

Clinical examination is important in preoperative planning for anteromedial tibial tubercle transfer.
The examination should include compression of the patella while flexing and extending the knee to
see if articular pain can be elicited (Fig. 3-2). The examining surgeon should also rule out other
nonarticular causes of pain such as neuroma, isolated retinacular pain, patellar tendonitis, referred
pain, plica, meniscus derangement, synovitis, and osteochondritis dissecans. The physical examination should be done with the patient in both standing and supine positions. The examiner should look
for evidence of lateralization of the extensor mechanism and tilt. Passive patellar tilt and tightness
of the lateral retinaculum should be noted (2). Pain on compression of the patella with flexion and
extension of the knee is likely to have an articular source. If this is associated with lateralization and
lateral tilt of the patella, the patient may be a candidate for anteromedial tibial tubercle transfer, particularly if the compression pain is prominent in early knee flexion, indicating a distal patella articular lesion that will be completely unloaded on anteriorization of the tibial tubercle. It is important
to be certain that pain is not due to a retinacular neuroma, painful scar, or intra-articular cause that
might be corrected by a smaller surgical procedure or injection.

Standard anteroposterior and lateral radiographs should be taken on all surgical candidates and
supplemented with an axial (tangential) view. A standard axial (10) view (knee flexed 45 degrees
and x-ray beam 30 degrees from the horizontal plane) provides a good idea of patella orientation in
the trochlea and is our view of choice. If a specific malalignment pattern is identifiable on the axial
radiograph, no further radiographic evaluation is necessary. On the other hand, some patients with
significant malalignment of the extensor mechanism will demonstrate a normal axial radiograph yet
have significant lateral subluxation and/or tilt on computed tomography (CT) of the patellofemoral
joint.

A true lateral radiograph of the knee (posterior condyles superimposed) at 0 and 30 degrees knee
flexion will help greatly in understanding trochlea morphology from top to bottom.

CT of the patellofemoral joint should be done with normal standing alignment of the patient re-
produced in the scanner gantry. Midpatellar transverse tomographic images should be made with the

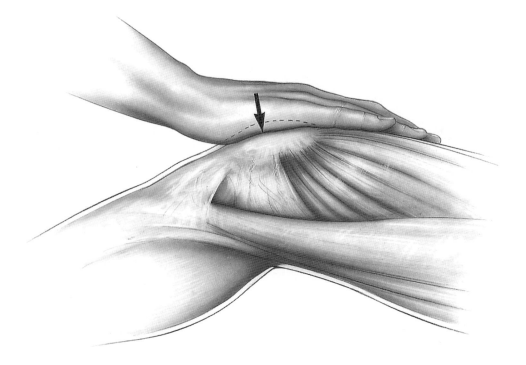

FIGURE 3-2

Compression of the patella while passing the knee through a range of motion will give an impression of the extent of articular damage and pain emanating from the articular surfaces of the patellofemoral joint.

CT cut directed to include the posterior condyles of the femur (Fig. 3-3). These tomographic slices should be taken with the knees flexed 15, 30, and 45 degrees (5). The patella is significantly tilted if the patellar tilt angle (the angle created by lines drawn along the lateral facet of the patella and the posterior femoral condyles) is less than 12 degrees on the tomographic image with the knee flexed 15 degrees. The patella should be centered in the trochlea on the tomographic image in which the knee is flexed at 15 degrees. (In other words, the congruence angle [10] should be 0 or slightly negative). Furthermore, CT provides an ideal opportunity to understand the relationship of the tibial tubercle to the central trochlea (TT-TG index as described by Goutallier [7]). As the TT-TG index rises, TT transfer becomes increasingly desirable, particularly when it exceeds 20 mm.

Following full clinical evaluation and radiographic study, the surgeon will know whether the patella is malaligned and will have some idea of the degree of articular degeneration, particularly as demonstrated by pain and crepitation on flexion/extension of the knee while compressing the patella. If appropriate nonsurgical treatment has failed, the patient may be a candidate for anteromedial tibial tubercle transfer, given significant malalignment (tilt and/or subluxation) and evidence of pain coming from the patellar articular surface (particularly if articular degeneration is distal and/or lateral).

SURGERY

The patient is positioned supine on the operating room table, and the anesthesiologist may apply a percutaneous nerve stimulator over the femoral nerve at the groin level. A tourniquet is applied on the proximal thigh and the patient is prepped from the tourniquet level down to and including the toes. Impermeable drapes are used.

Technique

An arthroscopy is routine at the outset of anteromedial tibial tubercle transfer. A superomedial portal, two finger-breadths above the medial proximal pole of the patella, allows an excellent view of the patellar articular surfaces (Fig. 3-4), but standard arthroscopic evaluation using medial and lateral infrapatellar portals is often sufficient. By distending the knee to 60 mm Hg pressure, the sur-

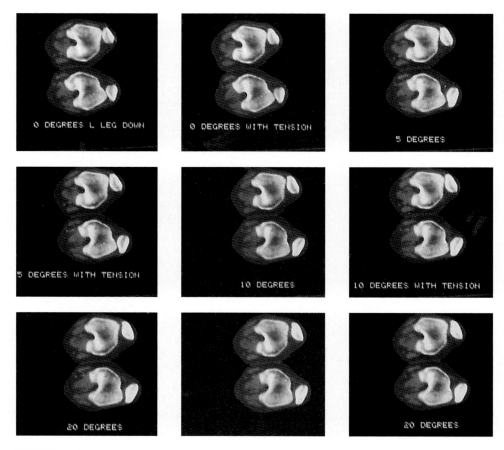

FIGURE 3-3

Computed tomographic imaging of the patellofemoral joint should include precise midpatellar transverse cuts directed through the posterior femoral condyles.

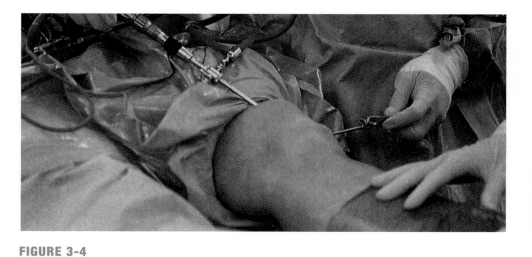

FIGURE 3-4

Arthroscopy of the patellofemoral joint using the superomedial approach gives an excellent view of the entire patellar articular surface as well as the medial and lateral recesses.

geon can determine the extent of articular damage as well as the extent and location of articular breakdown. Reducing the fluid inflow pressure gives an idea of the extent of patellar subluxation and/or tilt with flexion and extension of the knee. The femoral nerve may be stimulated (to brief tetany) with the knee in progressive flexion to help determine the dynamic alignment/malalignment. The arthroscopy is completed through an infrapatellarportal to evaluate the rest of the knee and to confirm the patellar findings noted if a proximal approach was used.

The surgeon must first characterize and document (by print or video) the nature and location of any articular lesion. A precise description of all articular lesions and their location should be dictated later in the operation report.

Loose flaps of articular cartilage or fibrillated cartilage can be removed most easily at the time of arthroscopy. Abrasion or resection of exposed sclerotic bone can also be done at the time of arthroscopy or with the knee open at the time of anteromedial tibial tubercle transfer. Drilling of the patella is best accomplished after lateral release. Debridement of inflamed synovium, preferably using cautery, and removal of loose bodies are best accomplished arthroscopically.

Most important at the time of arthroscopy is a critical assessment of whether anteromedial tibial tubercle transfer will remove the loading from soft or fragmented articular surfaces and transfer it to better cartilage. Experience has shown that patients in whom the proximal medial facet is preserved are those most likely to benefit from anteromedial tibial tubercle transfer. The operation effectively transfers load from the more lateral and distal aspects of the patella onto proximal medial articular cartilage. Since most patients with chronic patellar malalignment have breakdown of the lateral facet or distal patella, anteromedial tibial tubercle transfer is helpful to many if not most patients with patellar articular degeneration related to chronic malalignment. Patients with dashboard injuries, which occur with the knee flexed, often have destruction of proximal patellar cartilage and may be less amenable to anteromedial tibial tubercle transfer, since this operation transfers load onto proximal and medial patellar cartilage. Failure of straight medial tibial tubercle transfer may result from a failure to unload a distal patella articular pain source.

In performing an anteromedial tibial tubercle transfer, a longitudinal incision is made immediately along the patellar tendon and extended to a point 6 cm distal to the tibial tubercle at the anterior midline (Fig. 3-5). The patellar tendon is identified by sharp dissection (Fig. 3-6) and a lateral retinacular release is accomplished, taking care to dissect away the subcutaneous tissues (Fig. 3-7) bluntly and to release all components of the lateral retinaculum (6) and distal vastus lateralis obliquus (9), but *not the main vastus lateralis tendon.* In fact, it is best to do a limited lateral release, only to the level of the top of the patella, in most patients, to minimize the risk of creating a medial subluxation problem. At this time also release any indurated fat pad that might tether the distal patella and limit

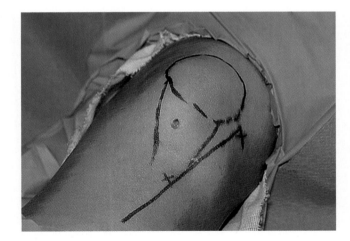

FIGURE 3-5

The incision for anteromedial tibial tubercle transfer should extend from the lateral patella to a point 6 cm distal to the tibial tubercle at the midline.

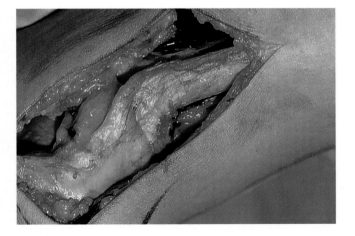

FIGURE 3-6

The patellar tendon is identified by sharp dissection.

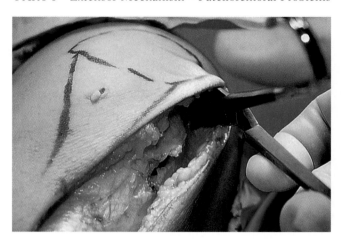

FIGURE 3-7

The lateral retinacular release should extend through the entire retinaculum, with care taken to release any tight fibrous bands in the retropatellar fat-pad area. The lateral release should extend only to the superior pole of the patella, avoiding the main tendon of the vastus lateralis. Do not overrelease. Leaving some of the proximal muscle/vastus lateralis obliquus attached to the main vastus lateralis tendon is a good idea in most cases.

free movement of the patella anteriorly after the osteotomy is completed. Inspect the patellar surface and debride carefully to remove loose cartilage flaps while abrading or drilling eburnated bone (Fig. 3-8). Also at this time, determine the need for any autologous, allogeneic, or synthetic osteochondral allograft resurfacing. Place Kelly clamp behind the patellar tendon (Fig. 3-9), and incise longitudinally into the periosteum parallel to the anterior crest of the tibia, just medial to the crest and lateral at the muscle origin of the anterior compartment, reflecting the periosteum and muscle belly to expose the entire lateral tibia for 8 to 10 cm. Periosteum is elevated carefully, and a drill guide is used to define the osteotomy plane, allowing a cut close to the anterior tibial crest medially (Fig. 3-10). A special drill guide with a cutting slot, such as the Tracker guide (Mitek), can make this process easier. The drill bits are pointed posterolaterally, with the most proximal drill bit penetrating the lateral tibial cortex under direct visualization and with careful retraction of the tibialis anterior (Fig. 3-11). Multiple parallel drill holes are made (Figs. 3-12 and 3-13). The angle can be modified according to the desired degree of anteriorization and medialization of the tibial tuberosity. The drill bits should be aligned to limit the depth of the distal tibial pedicle tip to 2 mm, so that fracture of the distal pedicle will be possible. Great care must be taken to avoid drill penetration too far posteriorly into the posterior neurovascular structures. Although the pedicle of bone deep to the tibial tubercle is fairly thick, it tapers anteriorly to the tip of the pedicle distally.

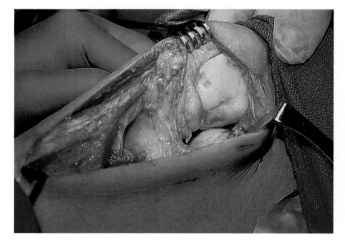

FIGURE 3-8

The patella can be inspected thoroughly following lateral release.

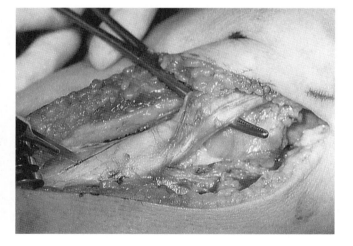

FIGURE 3-9

The patellar tendon insertion is carefully identified and elevated with a Kelly clamp.

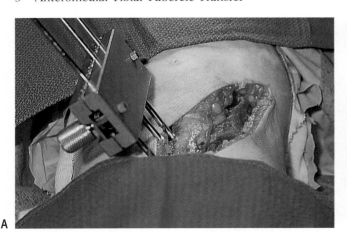
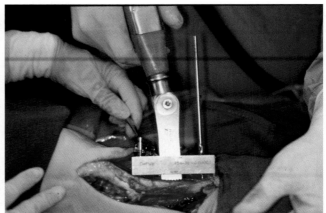

A   B

FIGURE 3-10

A: A drill guide allowing parallel drill placement along the osteotomy plane allows for precise definition of the osteotomy plane. It is most important to taper the osteotomy distally toward the anterior cortex, leaving only 1 to 2 mm of cortical bone at the distal anterior aspect of the bone pedicle. **B:** The Mitek Tracker guide is ideal for this purpose.

An oscillating saw or osteotomes are used to carefully fashion a cut connecting the drill holes (Figs. 3-14 and 3-15), adding an oblique cut from the most proximal drill hole to a spot just proximal to the insertion of the lateral patellar tendon (Fig. 3-16). This avoids cutting into the broad metaphyseal region of the tibia. The osteotomy must be made in the defined plane only, and care should be taken to work at all times in the osteotomy plane. The cut is completed at about 5 to 8 cm from the tibial tuberosity. The length of this bone pedicle should provide good surface contact and avoid tilting the fragment medially. With great care, the bone fragment is carefully mobilized (Fig. 3-16) and displaced anteromedially along the osteotomy plane (Fig. 3-17). If advancement of the tuberosity is desired, a segment of the distal pedicle may be removed and the remaining fragment advanced slightly to compensate for patella alta. This may also be desirable if significant laxity of the patellar tendon is noted following anteromedialization or if there is patella alta. Once the best position for

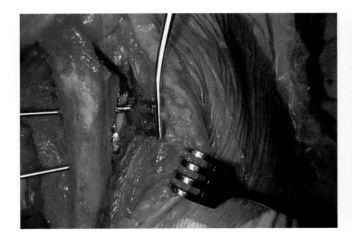

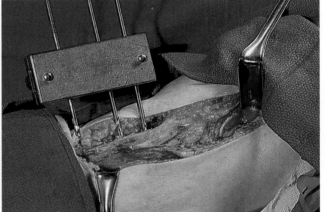

FIGURE 3-11

Exiting of the drill bits at the lateral tibial cortex must be directly visualized by carefully retracting the tibialis anterior muscle from the lateral tibia. The deep peroneal nerve and anterior tibial artery are just behind the posterolateral corner of the tibia.

FIGURE 3-12

The obliquity of the osteotomy plane is demonstrated.

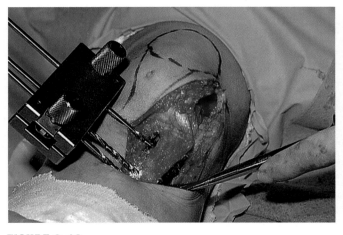

FIGURE 3-13

Great care must be taken to place the drill bits parallel to each other so that an accurate osteotomy will be defined before cutting the anterior tibial bone pedicle. The Mitek Tracker guide works very well for this purpose and has a cutting slot for an oscillating saw.

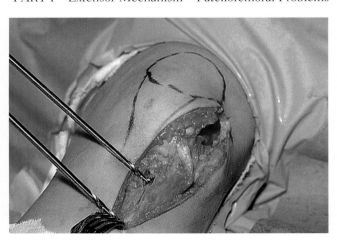

FIGURE 3-14

The proximal and distal drill bits are left in place to help define the plane while cutting the bone pedicle.

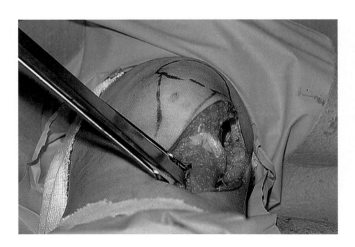

FIGURE 3-15

A sharp, broad osteotome works well for fashioning the osteotomy. The surgeon may wish to use an oscillating saw.

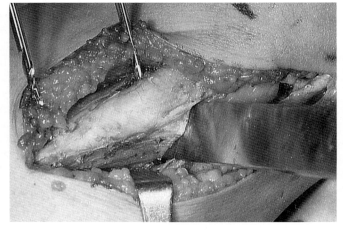

FIGURE 3-16

An osteotome or oscillating saw is used to connect the proximal drill bit tip with the tibial bone posterior and proximal to the patellar tendon insertion. Full visualization of the cutting tool as it exits the lateral tibia is mandatory. Note taper of the osteotomy toward the anterior cortex.

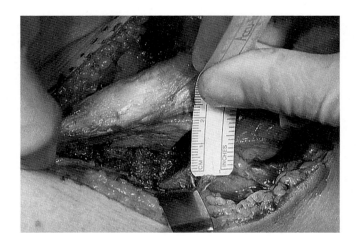

FIGURE 3-17

The bone pedicle will be displaced in an anteromedial direction, usually giving 12 to 17 mm of anteriorization as well as some medialization, depending on the obliquity of the osteotomy.

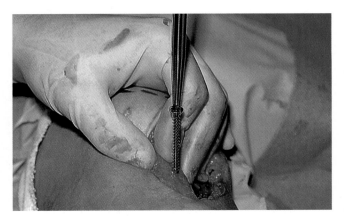

FIGURE 3-18

Cortical lag screws are used to lock the pedicle in the corrected position, placing the screws into the posterior tibial cortex for secure fixation. Keep the proximal screw at least 1 to 2 cm distal to the patella tendon insertion.

the tibial tuberosity is determined, a drill hole is made through the pedicle and into the posterior cortex of the tibia distal to the tuberosity, and a cortical lag screw is passed into the posterior cortex of the tibia, applying only slight compression (Fig. 3-18). The anterior tibial cortex must be overdrilled slightly to create a slight lag effect, and a second screw is added for additional stability, also using lag technique (Fig. 3-19). Anteriorization of the tibial tuberosity by about 15 mm is most desirable when there is a primary patellofemoral arthritis problem. In some patients, if subluxation persists, careful advancement of the medial patellofemoral ligament and vastus medialis obliquus may be desirable to selectively, but not so much that the patella is pulled posteriorly or a medial articular lesion is loaded.

When careful surgical technique is used, technical problems are uncommon. The surgeon must be careful to taper the distal osteotomy anteriorly so as not to remove too much of the tibial diaphyseal bone at the distal extent of the osteotomy. The osteotomy should be very flat, thereby maintaining excellent bone-to-bone contact on transfer of the bone pedicle. All drill holes must be made very carefully, taking care to avoid the deep peroneal nerve and anterior tibial artery just behind the prox-

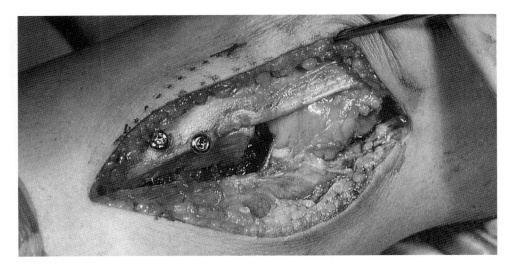

FIGURE 3-19

In most cases, two cortical lag screws are used to give firm fixation of the transferred bone pedicle.

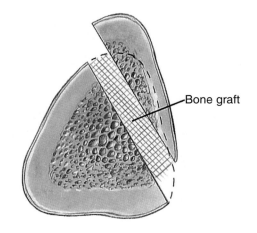

FIGURE 3-20

A local bone graft taken from the tibial metaphysis may be placed in the osteotomy plane, thereby displacing the osteotomy in an anterolateral direction, producing net anterior displacement of the tibial tubercle. Direct anteriorization with less bone graft can be achieved using this technique. A sagittal cut in the tibia as described in the text will also permit straight anteriorization.

imal posterolateral tibia. Once the bone pedicle has been shifted in an anteromedial direction, it must be held securely in the corrected position both while making the initial drill hole and subsequently. Shifting of the transferred pedicle may make engagement of the posterior cortex difficult and necessitate extra drill holes, thereby weakening the posterior tibia. Once the first screw is secured to the posterior cortex, the pedicle is quite secure and the second screw is easy to place.

The surgeon may choose to use an "offset bone graft" (Fig. 3-20) if straight anterior displacement of the tibial tubercle is needed. By placing a 4- to 5-mm–thick section of corticocancellous auto- or allograft bone in the oblique osteotomy plane, any medial displacement of the tibial tubercle will be "offset" and slight additional anteriorization of the tubercle achieved. If the patella appears to be located too medially following anteromedial tibial tubercle transfer, an offset bone graft may be added. Also, because this gives additional anteriorization, the offset bone graft may be used selectively if there is need to further unload the distal, medial portion of the patella. Care must be used when an offset bone graft is added in the osteotomy site. Because this adds to anteriorization, the surgeon must be careful not to anteriorize excessively. In our experience, 2 cm of anteriorization is maximal to avoid undue "tenting" of the skin and risk of skin slough. In a consecutive series of over 600 anteromedial tibial tubercle transfers, I have not had a skin slough.

Another option for achieving straight anteriorization is to make a sagittal plane cut into the tibia, followed by a back cut from the lateral side, both tapered to an anterior point distally, thereby permitting a straight anterior transfer of the tibial tubercle along the osteotomy plane. This transferred bone pedicle can then be fixated with medial-lateral cortical screws.

The skin should close without tension, provided that no bone graft is added. We use a full subcutaneous closure with 2-0 absorbable suture, followed by skin clips or subcuticular closure and the application of full-length 0.5-inch Steri-strips, followed by infiltration with 0.5% Marcaine. A suction drain may be used but is not usually necessary. If one anteriorizes more than 2 cm, one may wish to consult preoperatively with a plastic surgeon.

Using careful surgical technique, a precise flat osteotomy, secure fixation of the transferred pedicle with two screws, appropriate anteriorization, meticulous hemostasis, appropriate patient selection, early range of motion, and good postoperative rehabilitation, anteromedial tibial tubercle transfer will give uniformly good results.

POSTOPERATIVE MANAGEMENT

Assuming secure two-screw fixation of the transferred bone pedicle (as described), patients are started on immediate, once-daily active and passive range-of-motion exercises of the knee but are maintained in a knee immobilizer for 4 weeks on crutches. Continuous passive motion has not been necessary except in unusual circumstances, such as concomitant release of arthrofibrosis. Cryotherapy is helpful in the immediate postoperative period. A cryocuff is applied immediately after surgery (Fig. 3-21) and maintained for 3 to 4 days. This has helped diminish pain and facilitate early mobilization by minimizing swelling and pain.

Elevation is encouraged for the first 72 hours, and patients are allowed to ambulate with toe-touch weight bearing, using crutches. The drain, if used, is removed at 18 to 24 hours after surgery if bleeding has subsided. Most patients are given antibiotic coverage preoperatively, and this may be con-

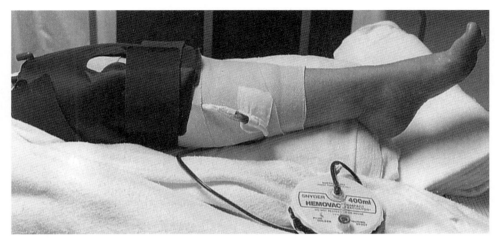

FIGURE 3-21

Cryotherapy will help reduce swelling and pain postoperatively. A Hemovac may be left in the wound for 2 to 24 hours, as needed.

tinued for 5 days selectively. We recommend postoperative aspirin daily for 6 to 8 weeks. Most patients can be discharged the day of surgery as long as they are mobile, swelling and pain are controlled, and there is no evidence of fever, calf tenderness, or any complication. Most patients need only a light dressing and knee immobilizer (4 weeks) over the wound as long as they are competent and appropriately cautious on crutches. The immobilizer should be taken off once each day to permit knee flexion. After 4 weeks, the patient may switch to a Tru-pull brace. Eighty-nine to ninety percent of patients have an objectively good or excellent result (4). Those patients with more advanced articular breakdown, however, can expect a 75% chance of a good result. Excellent results appear to be uncommon in patients with extensive articular breakdown. With 5 years minimum follow-up, results are maintained in most patients. Follow-up for 8 to 10 years has shown sustained improvement.

Some patients complain of prolonged discomfort along the anterior aspect of the tibia. Generally, this resolves by 6 to 12 months from the time of surgery. Most patients have some discomfort from the screws, and removal of the screws at 6 to 12 months after surgery is common. Most patients benefit from physical therapy, but some can recover on a home program, progressing to exercise bicycling, swimming, and progressive physical activity as tolerated after healing of the transferred bone pedicle. Active and passive motion are important in the first few weeks after surgery, and full range of motion of the knee should be achieved by 4 to 8 weeks from the time of surgery. Physical therapy may be very helpful to those patients with less motivation or who are progressing slowly. Full active work on quadriceps strengthening will generally start at 8 to 12 weeks from the time of surgery, but light quadriceps exercise, leg lifts, and range-of-motion exercises may be started immediately after surgery.

COMPLICATIONS, PEARLS, AND PITFALLS

Serious complications after properly performed anteromedial tibial tubercle transfer have been very uncommon. The surgeon should watch carefully for evidence of infection or thrombophlebitis. Although aspirin prophylaxis is routine, the threshold for initiating coumadin should be low if there is any concern about thrombophlebitis. Anterior compartment syndrome is a concern because of the subperiosteal elevation of the tibialis anterior muscle from the lateral side of the tibia and open cancellous bone from the osteotomy that can bleed into the anterior compartment. Although full anterior or posterior fasciotomy has not been necessary in our experience, a low threshold for performing fasciotomy must be maintained if a compartment syndrome is suspected.

Technical complications include fracture through a screw hole, nonunion, tibial fracture, neurovascular injury, deep venous thrombosis, overcorrection, skin slough, undercorrection, and incisional neuroma. Another potential complication is failure to achieve pain relief because of extensive articular degeneration.

Fracture of the tibia is avoidable by using careful technique but will require cast immobilization if it does occur. The period of immobilization, however, should be kept as short as possible.

In the event of undercorrection, the tubercle transfer procedure can be repeated at 6 to 12 months after the initial operation, with additional anteriorization and/or medialization. After removing the screws, the operative technique is the same as that used initially. This has been very uncommon.

In the event of overcorrection, careful lateral transfer of the healed tibial tubercle may be necessary. This should not be undertaken until 6 to 12 months from the time of the initial surgery, and it is best to watch the patellar tracking carefully, with femoral nerve stimulation used at the time of surgery to balance the patella in the trochlea.

Medial subluxation, as a dynamic complication of patella realignment surgery, is always possible. Such patients may not have an obvious medial alignment of the patella. Instead, they express a devastating and very painful feeling of the patella jumping out of place (from too far medial back into the trochlea) upon early knee flexion in gait. The astute examiner will detect this by holding the patella medially with the knee extended, then abruptly flexing the knee while releasing the patella simultaneously. This reproduces the event that the afflicted patient experiences. This complication can be controlled by using a Trupull brace (DJOtho, Vista, CA), holding the patella from medial to lateral. If necessary, a repair of released lateral tissues, with or without a tenodesis on the lateral side, can control this problem.

Nonunion of the transferred pedicle may be treated by removal of the fixation screws, debridement of fibrous tissue in the osteotomy site, exposure of bleeding bone, flattening of the osteotomy plane to allow improved apposition of the pedicle to underlying bone, cancellous bone grafting, and refixation with two cortical lag screws.

Although stiffness is uncommon with the use of immediate postoperative range-of-motion exercises and ambulation, it may be treated if necessary by postoperative manipulation at 8 to 12 weeks after surgery, followed by physical therapy.

Avoiding Fracture

The key to avoiding fracture and non union after anteromedial tibial tubercle transfer osteotomy is to taper a precise osteotomy cut, at its distal extent, towards the **anterior** tibial cortex. Also, the surgeon should avoid the proximal posterior osteotomy extending into the posterior tibia. In other words, do not let the osteotomy extend into or past the posterior, lateral corner of the tibia. Excellent visualization and a precise, flat, single plane osteotomy are of paramount importance in achieving the optimal osteotomy. Furthermore, excellent bone-bone contact and secure cortical screw fixation (2 screws), well seated into good bone, using excellent technique (lag effect, countersink screw heads, precise drill holes with secure grasp of posterior cortex) will improve the likelihood of the desired stable fixation. Proper technique permits early motion, earlier full weight bearing, primary bone-bone healing quickly, an excellent result, and a happy patient.

RECOMMENDED READING

Fulkerson J. Diagnosis and treatment of patients with patellofemoral pain. *Am J Sports Med.* 2002;30(3):447–456.
Saleh K, Arendt E, Eldridge J, et al. Operative treatment of patellofemoral arthritis. *J Bone Joint Surg* 2005;87A;659–671.

REFERENCES

1. Carney J, Mologne T, Muldoon M, et al. Long-term evaluation of the Roux-Elmslie-Trillat procedure for patellar instability. *Am J Sports Med.* 2005;33(8):1220–1223.
2. Fulkerson J. Awareness of the retinaculum in evaluating patellofemoral pain. *Am J Sports Med.* 1982;10:147.
3. Fulkerson J. Diagnosis and treatment of patients with patellofemoral pain. *Am J Sports Med.* 2002;30(3):447–456.
4. Fulkerson J. *Disorders of the patellofemoral joint.* Philadelphia: Lippincott Williams & Wilkins; 2004.
5. Fulkerson J, Becker G, Meany J, et al. Anteromedial tibial tubercle transfer without bone graft. *Am J Sports Med.* 1990;18:490–497.
6. Fulkerson J, Gossling H. Anatomy of the knee joint lateral retinaculum. *Clin Orthop.* 1980;153:183–188.
7. Goutallier D, Bernageau J, Lecudonnec B. The measurement of the tibial tuberosity patella groove distance: technique and results. *Rev Chir Orthop Reparatrice Appar Mot.* 1978;64:423–428.
8. Hallisey M, Doherty N, Bennett W, et al. Anatomy of the junction of the vastus lateralis tendon and the patella. *J Bone Joint Surg.* 1987;69A:545–549.
9. Powers CM, Ward SR, Chen YJ, et al. The effect of bracing on patellofemoral joint stress during free and fast walking. *Am J Sports Med.* 2004;32(1):224–231.
10. Merchant A, Mercer R, Jacobsen R, et al. Roentgenographic analysis of patellofemoral congruence. *J Bone Joint Surg.* 1974;56A:1391–1396.
11. Trillat A, Dejour H, Coutette A. Diagnostique et traitement des subluxations recidivantes de la routle. *Rev Chir Orthop.* 1964;50:813–824.

4 Patellectomy

Christopher S. Proctor and Douglas W. Jackson

INDICATIONS/CONTRAINDICATIONS

The role of patellectomy in the treatment of patellofemoral disorders is a subject of controversy. The popularity of this procedure was great initially when there was little understanding of its biomechanics. Today, indications for patellectomy have narrowed with the knowledge that the patella is vital to the normal function of the knee joint; now more emphasis is placed on its preservation.

Major functions of the patella include lengthening the quadriceps lever arm, thereby facilitating knee extension (8,10,11,14,15); decreasing the compressive stresses on the patellofemoral joint; and providing a smooth, nearly frictionless surface that is resistant to wear (16). Patellectomy has been shown to alter knee-joint mechanics. Clinically, the most apparent effect of patellectomy is a decrease in the quadriceps muscle lever arm, necessitating a 30% increase in force to maintain the same torque during knee extension (10,11). We believe that every effort should be made to preserve the patella and have found that alternatives to patellectomy exist (12,13).

Patellectomy has been described as the treatment for a variety of patellofemoral disorders (7,9,13,15). Primary patellectomy is often the treatment of choice for cases of trauma with severe comminution *not* amenable to osteosynthesis, and for rare tumors of the patella. However, when evaluating patellar fractures consideration should *first* be given to obtaining an adequate reduction with internal fixation. Partial patellectomy is the surgical procedure chosen for comminuted fractures of the patella that are not amenable to osteosynthesis but in which one pole of the patella *can* be saved. In the debate over which pole of the patella to save, we recommend saving the pole with the greatest amount of articular cartilage, irrespective of which pole this is. Better results and postoperative function are obtained if more of the patella can be saved (5,6,17).

Despite the limited indications as a primary procedure, patellectomy can be a useful secondary or "salvage" procedure. Satisfactory results have been described for the following disorders:

- Chondromalacia patella
- Recurrent patellar dislocations
- Patellofemoral osteoarthritis
- Patellar osteomyelitis
- Failed prosthetic replacement of the patella

The indication for patellectomy in these conditions is limited to those cases with persistent pain and disability not relieved by other avenues of treatment, including vigorous rehabilitation, medical treatment, arthroscopic surgery, and surgery to realign the extensor mechanism. If pain and disability continue despite these measures, a patellectomy may be considered.

PREOPERATIVE PLANNING

A complete history and physical examination are required as part of the preoperative evaluation. Radiographs obtained should include anteroposterior, lateral, and Merchant views of the knee. The diagnosis of patellar pain is made after other causes of knee pain are ruled out. Other treatment options should be exhausted, including rehabilitation, medical treatment, and limited surgical management. If pain and disability persist, a patellectomy may be considered.

SURGERY

Complete Patellectomy

Patient Positioning   The patient is in a supine position on the operating room table. A well-padded tourniquet is applied on the proximal thigh, and the patient is prepped from the tourniquet level down the entire lower extremity with a Betadine (povidone/iodine) scrub. Drape the lower extremity free from the level of the mid thigh.

Surgical Procedure   Make a midline anterior incision through the skin and subcutaneous tissue starting 5 cm above the superior pole of the patella and proceeding distally to below the level of the tibial tubercle (Fig. 4-1). We favor a midline longitudinal incision, since it is not limiting to future surgical procedures. Elevate medial and lateral full-thickness skin flaps using blunt dissection to expose the quadriceps, patella, and patellar tendon. Split the midportion of the quadriceps and patellar tendons and the expansion of the extensor mechanism over the patella in line with their fibers (Fig. 4-2). Place retractors proximal and distal into the joint to protect the trochlear articular surface, and then split the patella longitudinally into equal halves with an osteotome or saw (Fig. 4-3). Grasp each half of the patella in turn with a towel clip and enucleate it from the quadriceps mechanism (Fig. 4-4). When enucleating the patella, use sharp dissection starting from the under surface

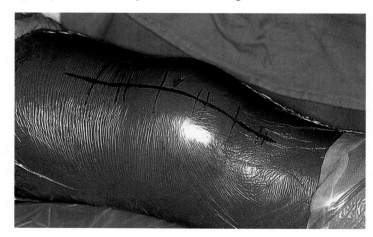

FIGURE 4-1

Make a midline incision anteriorly starting 5 cm above the superior pole of the patella and proceeding distally to below the level of the tibial tubercle.

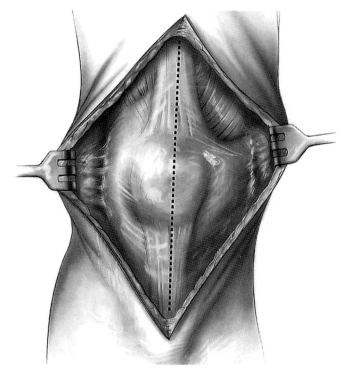

FIGURE 4-2

Mark the midline of the quadriceps tendon, patellar tendon, and extensor expansion over the patella and split longitudinally in line with the fibers.

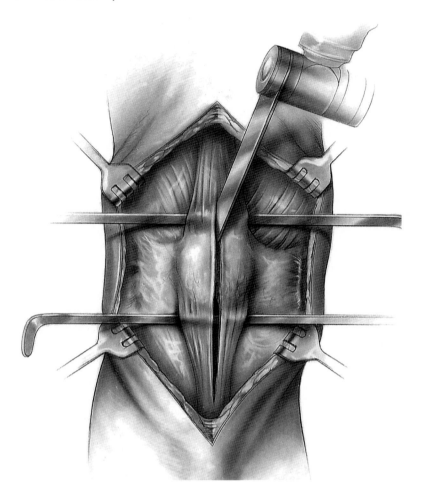

FIGURE 4-3

Place retractors underneath the patellar and quadriceps tendons to protect the underlying articular surfaces. Then split the patella longitudinally with an osteotome or saw into two equal halves.

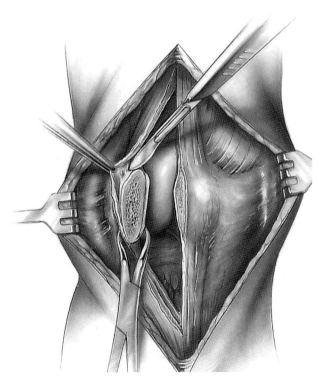

FIGURE 4-4

Grasp the patella with a towel clip and sharply enucleate it, taking care to preserve intact the surrounding soft tissues.

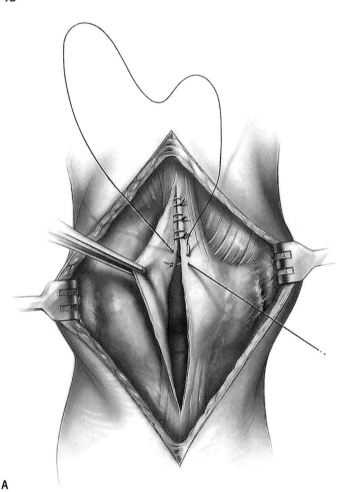

A

FIGURE 4-5

A: Retract the lateral one half of the extensor mechanism and suture the medial one half to its undersurface. **B:** Fold the lateral one half over the top of the medial portion and suture in place in a pants-over-vest fashion.

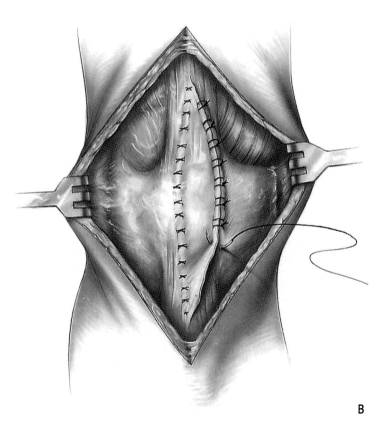

B

of the patellar and quadriceps tendons. This will preserve the expansion of the quadriceps tendon over the patella and preserve the continuity of the quadriceps and petellar tendons. Once the patella is removed, inspect the anterior compartment of the knee joint; remove any loose bodies and address any other intra-articular pathology at this time. If indicated, the patellar tendon may be split to the tibial tubercle and the quadriceps tendon split 10 cm proximal to the patella. Release the tourniquet and obtain hemostasis before closing the rent in the tendon. Use nonabsorbable, interrupted figure-eight sutures to close one side of the tendon over the other in a pants-over-vest fashion so that a double row of sutures is obtained (Fig. 4-5). Once the tendon is repaired, flex the knee to 90 degrees to ensure that there is no undue stress on the suture line and that the tendon tracks in the midline of the trochlear groove. If lateral displacement of the patellar tendon is noted, advance the vastus medialis obliquus laterally and distally over the sutured defect. If the tendon is still not centralized, consider performing a limited lateral release. Close the subcutaneous tissue with interrupted absorbable sutures and the skin with absorbable suture material using a running subcuticular technique. Cover the wound with a sterile dressing and apply a long leg-support hose. Place the lower extremity in a knee immobilizer or a brace locked in extension.

Partial Patellectomy

The surgical technique for the treatment of comminuted fractures of the patella by partial patellectomy differs from the technique described earlier for total patellectomy. Make an identical approach to expose the patella, but divide the extensor apparatus over the patella transversely (Fig. 4-6). Retain the largest fragment of the patella and subchondral surface, and remove all remaining fragments by sharp dissection, taking care to cause as little injury to the soft tissues as possible (Fig. 4-7). Debride and make smooth the edges of the remaining patellar fragment. Next, drill parallel holes transversely across the patella such that they exit at the junction of the anterior and middle thirds of the patella (Fig. 4-8). Suture the patellar or quadriceps tendon to the anterior one third of the retained fragment using No. 1 nonabsorbable suture and a horizontal mattress technique (Fig. 4-9). Although some authors recommend suturing the tendon to the posterior one third of the patella at the articular margin (6,13), we obtain superior results by attaching the tendon to the anterior one third of the patella. Recent experimental data confirm that an anterior reattachment minimizes the decrease in patellofemoral contact area and the increased contact pressure associated with patellectomy (16). Next, carefully repair the expansion of the extensor apparatus over the patella using 3-0 absorbable sutures. The remainder of the surgical technique is as described earlier; postoperatively, place the extremity in a knee immobilizer or locked knee brace for 6 weeks.

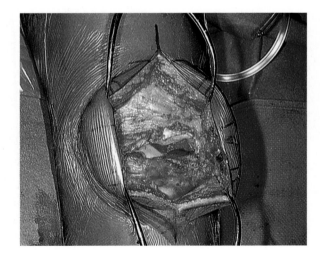

FIGURE 4-6
For a partial patellectomy use a midline incision, as for total patellectomy. Divide the extensor apparatus transversely to expose the patellar fragments.

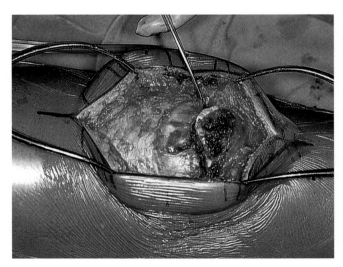

FIGURE 4-7

Retain the larger fragment and remove the smaller fragments via sharp dissection, causing as little soft-tissue damage as possible.

Pearls and Pitfalls

- The trochlear cartilage can easily be damaged when splitting the patella longitudinally into halves. It is, therefore, important to protect the underlying cartilage with retractors.
- Preserving the expansion of the quadriceps tendon over the patella is important for successful reconstruction.
- With partial patellectomy, the best results are obtained by anatomically reconstructing the patellar or quadriceps tendon to the anterior edge of the patella.

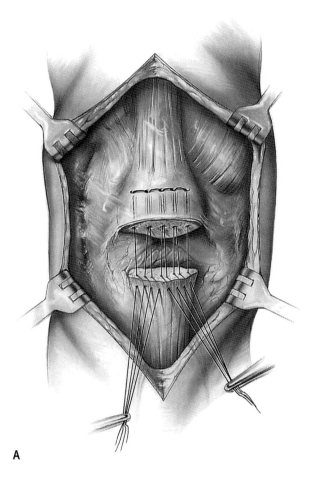

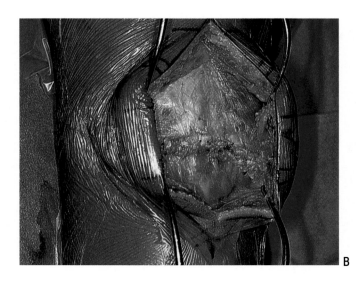

B

A

FIGURE 4-8

Drill holes transversely across the patella (A) such that they exit the patella at the junction of its anterior and middle thirds (B); then suture the tendon to the center of the patella using a horizontal mattress technique.

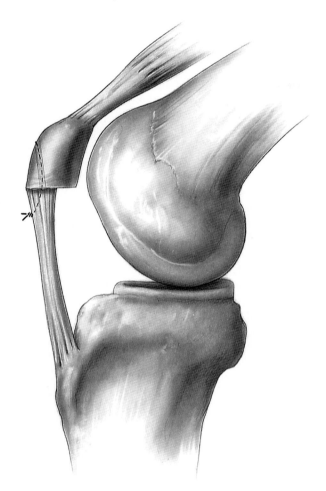

FIGURE 4-9

The tendon is sutured to the anterior one third of the retained fragment. This minimizes the decrease in patellofemoral contact area and the increase in contact pressure associated with partial patellectomy.

POSTOPERATIVE MANAGEMENT

Complete Patellectomy

Maintain the knee in a knee immobilizer or brace locked in extension. On postoperative day 1, start quadriceps-strengthening exercises. Our preference is to remove the immobilizer on postoperative day 5 and begin passive flexion and active extension. Protective weight bearing is allowed in the immediate postoperative period. Encourage progression to full, unprotected weight bearing when adequate quadriceps strength is demonstrated. We expect that most patients will obtain at least 90 degrees of passive flexion by the second to third postoperative week, and full active flexion by 8 to 10 weeks. Full extension with good muscle power is slower to obtain and often requires as long as 5 to 6 months of an active, supervised exercise program.

Partial Patellectomy

Maintain the knee in a knee immobilizer or locked knee brace for 3 weeks, allowing weight bearing as tolerated. Begin straight leg-raising exercises during the first postoperative week. Passive flexion exercises are started at 3 weeks. We expect a full range of knee flexion in 8 to 10 weeks with full extension established by 3 to 4 months. Loss of 10 to 20 degrees of symmetric flexion may still be associated with a functional recovery.

COMPLICATIONS

Although patellectomy may be unavoidable in certain cases, the change in anatomy has significant consequences.

- Extensor lag/weak extensor power (20,21) is the most common complication. The lever mechanism of the quad muscle becomes less efficient without the patella, and it may result in failure to achieve full extension.
- Decreased range of motion is often seen following long periods of immobilization and with transverse repair of the quadriceps and patellar tendons (2). If motion is not restored with aggressive rehabilitation, an arthroscopic lysis of adhesions and re-establishment of the suprapatellar notch should be coupled with a gentle manipulation under anesthesia. This should be done as soon as it becomes apparent that no progress restoring motion is being made over a 2- to 4-week period postoperatively.
- Continued anterior knee pain is not uncommon in patients who have undergone patellectomy. Treatment choices for patients are to have the patient live with the pain or to try anteriorization of the tibial tubercle in selected cases.
- One of the more serious complications following patellectomy is disruption of tendon repair. This most commonly occurs with transverse repairs of the tendon; it may also be seen in longitudinal repairs in association with infection.
- Subluxation of the extensor mechanism can arise with failure to recognize and correct malalignment (3). The loss of the spacer effect of the patella leaves the quadriceps tendon prone to dislocation. The increase in laxity leaves the femoral joint surface vulnerable without the bony protection of the patella. The femoral cartilage is easily damaged by knocks and falls.
- Damage to the infrapatellar branch of the saphenous nerve may occur during patellectomy. If the nerve is cut, the identified end should be buried in fat in a nonprominent area to minimize the formation of a symptomatic neuroma.
- Calcification at the patellectomy site has been described, but we have found it to be of little consequence (3,6).

RESULTS

As stated previously, patellectomy has a deleterious effect on normal knee function and may be unpredictable in providing pain relief in terms of the patient's underlying disease. Recent studies have demonstrated good or excellent results in only about 53% to 72% of patients (1,13,15,16). When evaluating the results of patellectomy, it is important to remember that they may be different for different conditions (7). Furthermore, it is important to note that better results are obtained with patellectomy if the patellofemoral joint is the sole joint involved.

In our hands, the results of patellectomy for these indications have been variable. Patients are not symptom-free, are seldom able to do running or jumping activities, and often have difficulty with normal gait progression on stairs. In patients with otherwise normal extensor mechanisms, patellectomy for severely comminuted patellar fractures and for failed prosthetic replacements of the patella provides more satisfactory short- and long-term results. Justifiably a terminal procedure, a well-performed patellectomy is, for selected patients, a consideration in the management of severe patellofemoral pain.

RECOMMENDED READING

Jensen DB, Hansen LB. Patellectomy for chondromalacia. *Acta Orthop Scand.* 1989;60:17–19.
Marder RA, Swanson TV, Sharkey NA, et al. Effects of partial patellectomy and reattachment of the patellar tendon on patellofemoral contact areas and pressures. *J Bone Joint Surg.* 1993;75:35–45.

REFERENCES

1. Ackroyd CE, Polyzoides AJ. Patellectomy for osteoarthritis. *J Bone Joint Surg.* 1978;60:353–357.
2. Baker CL, Hughston JC. Miyakawa patellectomy. *J Bone Joint Surg.* 1988;70:1489–1494.
3. Boucher HH. Results of excision of the patella. *J Bone Joint Surg.* 1952;34:516.
4. Boyd HB, Hawkins BL. Patellectomy—a simplified technique. *Surg Gynecol Obstet.* 1948;86:357–358.
5. Bröstrom A. Fractures of the patella. *Acta Orthop Scand.* 1972;143(suppl):1.
6. Duthie HL, Hutchinson JR. The results of partial and total excision of the patella. *J Bone Joint Surg.* 1975;40:75.

7. Fulkerson JP, Hungerford DS. *Disorders of the patellofemoral joint.* 2nd ed. Baltimore: Williams & Wilkins; 1990.

8. Haxton H. The function of the patella and the effects of its excision. *Surg Gynecol Obstet.* 1945;80:389.

9. Ivey FM, Bazina ME, Fox JM, et al. Reoperation following patellectomy for chondromalacia. *Orthopaedics.* 1979;2:136–137.

10. Kaufer H. Mechanical function of the patella. *J Bone Joint Surg.* 1971;53:1551–1560.

11. Kaufer H. Patellar biomechanics. *Clin Orthop.* 1979;144:51–54.

12. Kelly MA, Insall JN. Patellectomy. *Orthop Clin North Am.* 1986;17:289–295.

13. Kelly MA, Proctor CS. Patellectomy. *Semin Orthop.* 1990;4:149–154.

14. Lewis MN, Fitzgerald PF, Jacobs B, et al. Patellectomy. An analysis of one hundred cases. *J Bone Joint Surg.* 1976;58A:736.

15. Maquet PCJ. *Biomechanics of the knee with application to the pathogenesis and surgical treatment of osteoarthritis.* Berlin; Springer-Verlag; 1976.

16. Mow VC, Proctor CS, Kelly MA. Biomechanics of articular cartilage. In: Nordin M, Frankel, V, eds. *Basic biomechanics of the musculoskeletal system.* 2nd ed. Philadelphia: Lea and Febiger, 1989:31–58.

17. Saltzman CL, Goulet JA, McClellan T, et al. Results of treatment of displaced patellar fractures by partial patellectomy. *J Bone Joint Surg.* 1990;72A:1279–1285.

18. Sutton FS, Thompson CH, Lipke J, et al. The effect of patellectomy on knee function. *J Bone Joint Surg.* 1976;58:537–540.

19. Watkins MP, Harris BS, Wender S, et al. Effect of patellectomy on the function of the quadriceps and hamstrings. *J Bone Joint Surg.* 1983;65A:390–395.

5 Patella and/or Extensor Mechanism Allograft Reconstruction

William H. Warden III and Douglas W. Jackson

INDICATIONS

A chronic dysfunctional extensor mechanism with an associated symptomatic extensor lag that persists after multiple repair or reconstruction attempts may be amenable to allograft reconstruction. Potential allograft techniques for reconstructing a portion or all of the extensor mechanism involve using an allograft that includes the quadriceps tendon with or without a patella, patellar tendon, and tibial tubercle. The allograft is used to fill defects and provide continuity by replacing or supplementing deficient tissue. If the patient's patella is usable, we prefer using an Achilles tendon allograft with attached bone block to replace the nonfunctional quadriceps and/or patellar tendon.

Extensor mechanism disruption can occur as result of a traumatic event, tendon degeneration, or as a complication of knee surgery. Primary and secondary techniques for repair or reconstruction of specific portions of a deficient extensor mechanism have been described and are often successful. If multiple attempts at direct repair and reconstruction fail and the patient still has an extensor lag, allograft replacement of the extensor mechanism becomes a consideration.

The main indication is a symptomatic extension lag related to a deficiency in the extensor mechanism that has failed at least one primary repair and/or reconstruction using autogenous tissue, for example, failed quadriceps and patellar tendon repairs with large palpable tendon defects. Other causes of irreparable extensor deficits include disruption of the extensor mechanism during or following procedures such as:

- patellectomy
- total knee arthroplasty
- patellar realignment procedures
- lysis of adhesions for arthrofibrosis
- correction of patella infera or infrapatellar adhesions

CONTRAINDICATIONS

- Current infection in the knee or underlying bone
- An extensor mechanism that can be reconstructed using primary repair and/or reconstruction with local autogenous tissue
- A patient who does not wish to accept restricted knee flexion
- A patient who is unwilling to accept to accept a minimum of 6 to 8 weeks or longer of bracing and an involved postoperative rehabilitation
- A patient who is averse to possibly a manipulation, arthroscopic lysis of adhesions, and/or further open repair of portions of the graft
- A patient who is not willing to accept the possibility of effusion and low-grade inflammatory response that may persist for a long period after a large allograft (entire extensor mechanism)
- A patient who is unwilling to accept that an allograft may fail or need to be removed

PREOPERATIVE PLANNING

A history and physical examination of the knee and extremity includes a review of the duration and severity of the patient's symptoms and extensor mechanism dysfunction in relation to the patient's surgical history. Particular attention is given to prior extensor mechanism procedures and includes the number performed and the success or failure of each of those surgeries. Prior operative reports are reviewed; previous history of infection is explored as well as associated potential risk factors (e.g., diabetes, renal failure, collagen diseases, immune deficiencies, chronic medications, and smoking history). These and any factors that may delay wound healing are discussed with the patient. The current symptoms related to the extensor lag, episodes and frequency of giving-way, disability with stairs, and arising from the seated position are documented.

The complete physical examination of the lower extremities includes documentation of active and passive range of motion, evaluation of the use of assisted walking devices, and gait pattern. Special attention is paid to the prior surgical incisions over and around the knee. In addition, the degree of extensor lag and any restriction in passive extension (fixed flexion contractures) are documented. The tracking of the extensor mechanism during active and passive range-of-motion testing is assessed. The ideal candidate for this reconstruction will have 120 degrees or more of active flexion.

Radiographs include four views of the knee with standing (anteroposterior and 30 degrees flexed), lateral, and Merchant views. These are evaluated for degenerative arthritis in all three compartments, as well as for patella infera, patella alta, and the presence or absence of a patella. They are also evaluated for hardware and hetereotopic bone. If an associated knee replacement has been performed, it is assessed for alignment, loosening, and the status of the patella, if present, and its alignment. Further studies may be necessary to evaluate rotational alignment if malrotation is a contributing factor to the extensor mechanism dysfunction.

Laboratory studies may include an erythrocyte sedimentation rate, serum C-reactive protein level, and white blood cell count if there is a possibility of chronic infection. If an effusion is present, a knee aspiration is performed and sent for cell count, crystal analysis, and synovial fluid cultures. Radiographs are sent to the tissue bank for sizing of the entire allograft if a patella allograft is to be part of the reconstructed extensor mechanism.

SURGERY

Technique

Ancef 1 g (or alternative antibiotic) is given intravenously 1 hour before surgery if there is no history of allergy or other contraindication. The knee to be reconstructed is marked and observed by professional staff. This is done even when the patient has multiple scars and a palpable defect at the surgical site. The patient is placed in the supine position on the operating table with a pneumatic tourniquet high around the thigh of the involved lower extremity that has been marked and again checked in the operating room by the staff and physician. The extremity is then prepped and draped separately in the usual orthopaedic manner.

The previous surgical incisions as well as a line for the incision are marked with methylene blue before the application of the Steri-Drape. Once ready for the incision, the tourniquet is inflated after extremity elevation and with the knee flexed 90 degrees. We prefer a midline skin incision if possible; however, we may use a previous incision and extend it as needed proximally and/or distally to obtain adequate exposure. If there are multiple incisions present, it is our preference to use the most lateral incision and not cross a previous surgical incision in a manner that may compromise the blood supply to a section of skin. The dissection is carried down in the midline elevating skin and subcutaneous flaps, with consideration for blood supply preservation determining the extent of exposure. The medial and lateral patellar retinaculum, quadriceps, and patellar tendon are exposed. The medial and lateral gutters and suprapatellar pouch spaces are re-established. The defect(s) in the extensor mechanism is defined. The midline incision is carried proximally into the host quadriceps maintaining a medial and lateral margin of tendon to suture to in the repair. This can be difficult if there is minimal host quadriceps tendon remaining proximally. The incision is carried in the midline distally to expose the host tibial tubercle. It is important to maintain as much of the host soft tissue medial and lateral to the incision as possible.

The allograft specimen to be used is prepared on a side table (see Chapter 17, Allograft Preparation for ACL Reconstruction) during the surgical exposure and preparation for the eventual graft. The trough in the patient's tibial tubercle is not prepared until the allograft tibial block has been shaped and sized. The allograft tibial block shape is matched to a rectangular trough drawn out with methylene blue. It is cut out using a micro-saw and will be approximately 6 cm long, 2 cm wide, and 2 cm deep. The allograft block is further trimmed and downsized once the graft site is prepared to facilitate a press-fit (Fig. 5-1). Two No. 2 Ethibond sutures as described by Krackow et al are placed along the medial and lateral aspects of the allograft proximal quadriceps tendon (5). These sutures are used to apply traction and test how well the allograft bone is secured to the tibial bed. Once prepared, the graft is wrapped with a sterile saline-soaked sponge and stored in a protected area until ready for implantation.

The host proximal tibial trough is positioned to provide the desired height of the patella in relation to the femoral sulcus and in comparison to the contralateral patella height. Ideally, the tibial tubercle anatomy is duplicated by the new patella tendon block at the original insertion and level. Care is taken to leave the prox-

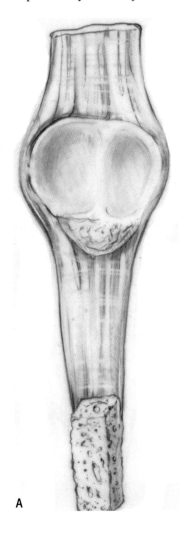

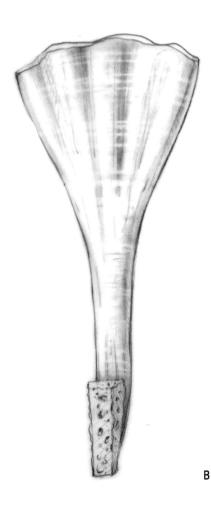

A

B

FIGURE 5-1

An artist's depiction of a tibial-patellar tendon-patella-quadriceps graft **(A)** and an Achilles graft **(B)**. The bone plugs are approximately 6×2×2 cm in size.

imal portion of the host tibia trough intact as it serves as the buttress against proximal migration. The rectangular tibial trough is marked out in methylene blue and cut to a length of 5 cm, a width of just less than 2 cm, and a depth of 2 cm. The final prepared host site is slightly smaller than the allograft bone block, to allow a press-fit placed with use of a bone punch. Once the allograft tibial bone is press fit, it is drilled and tapped for a cortical screw that further fixes and compresses it into the host tibia (Fig. 5-2). Usually one well-placed screw gives good fixation. We do not use a washer and slightly countersink the head so that it is flush. The traction placed on the graft is perpendicular to the graft. The press-fit, well-shaped proximal tibial buttress and screw fixation can tolerate greater forces than the graft will experience for several weeks. The tibial bone graft is biologically fixed within 6 to 8 weeks and has not been a problem in late displacement or migration. We confirm the screw length and tibial position of the graft using a mini-C arm image intensifier at this point before proceeding with the soft tissue fixation and tensioning (Fig. 5-3). Patients with at total knee and tibial stems may require other fixation techniques. However, we have found slightly angled screw fixation satisfactory in the limited cases we have done following total knee replacement. In those patients who have had their extensor mechanisms reconstructed before their total knee replacement, we have simply removed the screw at the time of surgery. Alternate fixation of the tibial block should be considered if the extensor mechanism surgery is done simultaneously with the total knee replacement revision.

It is important to prepare and maintain medial and lateral soft-tissue sleeves along the entire area the graft will touch. Our preference is to deflate the tourniquet before soft tissue suturing. The sleeves (adjacent residual tendon, retinaculum, and soft tissue) are sutured to and used to cover the allograft where possible (Fig. 5-4). The side-to-side sutures provide additional fixation until the allografts are incorporated. When they are approximated to the allograft, the quadriceps sutures are pulled snuggly with the knee in full extension. It is important to place the sutures securely into the remaining host quadriceps tendon and secure the proximal aspect of the allograft. The medial and lateral side-to-side closure is then completed. When possible the repair of the host retinaculum is brought over the top of the allograft. It is often difficult to get complete coverage if an allograft patella is used in the reconstruction. If sutures and bulky tissue are left on the surface of the patella, they can be a source of constant irritation.

Prior to closure, we prefer to flex the knee at least 45 degrees (Fig. 5-5), directly visualizing the repair, patella tracking, and bone block. This should occur without sutures pulling out and without displacement of the distal bone block. Even in the knee brace locked in extension, there will be up to 20 degrees of knee motion possible during the healing phase. We want to make certain the graft repair will hold until biologic fixation takes over (estimated 4 to 6 weeks). The subcutaneous tissues

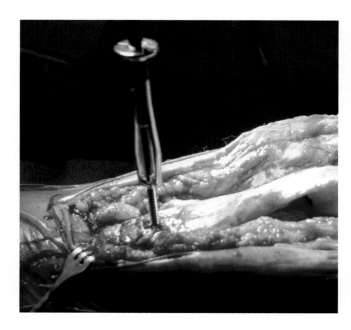

FIGURE 5-2
Once the allograft tibial bone is press fit, it is drilled, tapped, and slightly countersunk for a cortical screw that further fixes and compresses it into the host tibia.

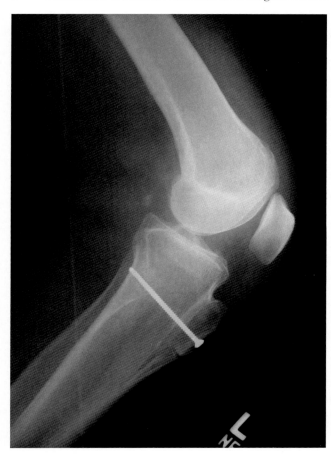

FIGURE 5-3
We confirm the screw length and tibial position of the graft using a mini-C arm image intensifier at this point before proceeding with the soft tissue fixation and tensioning. This is a postoperative radiograph of an allograft patellar reconstruction in a patient with a previous Maquet procedure.

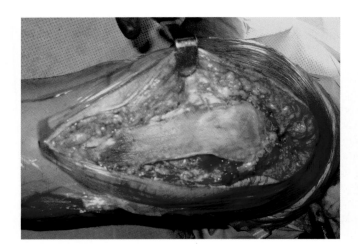

FIGURE 5-4
Adjacent residual tendon, retinaculum, and soft tissue are sutured to and used to cover the allograft. The side-to-side sutures provide additional fixation until the allograft is incorporated.

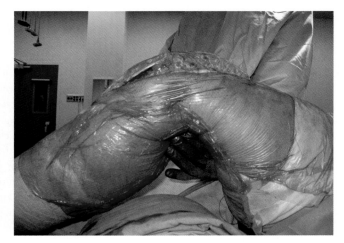

FIGURE 5-5
Prior to closure, the knee is flexed at least 45 degrees, assessing fixation.

are closed in routine fashion. The skin is closed with staples unless the skin is fragile and then 3-0 nylon vertical mattress sutures are used.

Pearls and Pitfalls

- We prefer a fresh-frozen, nonirradiated allograft specimen from a well-established tissue bank consisting of a quadriceps tendon, patella, patellar tendon, and tibial bone. It is preferable to have the patella sized in comparison to the contralateral patella and the recipient femoral groove.
- Be sure to specify right or left in your allograft request and check that you have an allograft for the appropriate side. Contralateral images or magnetic resonance images used for sizing can lead to confusion! Furthermore, it can be difficult to distinguish a right patella from a left.
- Have at least 5 cm of quadriceps tendon allograft for suture repair into the host quadriceps mechanism. This requires talking with the tissue bank or their representative. We like to see a drawing and the graft dimensions.
- If the patient's patella is acceptable and can be used, we prefer using an Achilles tendon with attached bone block for the reconstruction.
- If the native patella is present, we prefer to leave it and use soft tissue around and over it. An effort should be made to maintain what blood supply there is to the existing patella.
- The most difficult reconstructions have been those that have had more than one quadriceps repair attempted with very little or no functional host quadriceps tendon to repair to. Preoperative magnetic resonance imaging of the quadriceps tendon is helpful in determining whether this is a potential problem.
- It is important that the knee be able to be passively brought to full extension preoperatively or at minimum at the time of surgery.
- We prefer to press fit the allograft tibial bone into the recipient bone trough and transfix it with at least one cortical screw (see Fig. 5-2). Care should be taken to have an adequate bone block that will not split with the drilling, tapping, and screw placement. We have not had difficulty with migration if attention is given to placement and fixation.
- The allograft is sutured in place tensioned with the knee in extension.
- As much of the patient's adjacent soft tissue (retinaculum and tendon) as possible is sutured to the graft to obtain additional fixation.
- During the repair and at the completion of placing the allograft, we prefer to flex the knee under direct visualization of the repair. We want at least 45 degrees of flexion with the fixation and sutures holding well.
- The knee is immobilized in a brace in extension and weight bearing is progressed as tolerated in extension.

POSTOPERATIVE MANAGEMENT

The knee is placed in a hinged brace locked in full extension. We place it over a long leg support stocking that holds the dressings in place. We maintain the knee in full extension within the brace, realizing there is some passive motion in the brace. The patient is started the following day on toe-touch weight bearing and allowed to progress to full weight bearing as tolerated in the brace with the knee in extension. Staples are removed 2 weeks after surgery assuming the wounds are closed and healing as desired. We encourage isometric static quadriceps contractions. It is usually 2 to 3 weeks or longer before the patient is comfortable bearing full weight in the brace around the house. We encourage crutches when outside for 4 to 6 weeks. After 6 weeks 30 degrees of active flexion is permitted, under the supervision of a physical therapist, with the patient wearing a hinged knee brace with a lockout against further flexion. During weight bearing, we lock the brace in full extension. The brace is worn for 8 weeks when ambulating and sleeping. It can be off during the day for periods of time. At 12 weeks, we allow further active flexion up to a maximum of 90 degrees, and gentle quadriceps strengthening exercises are initiated. Passive flexion is limited to minimize the chance of graft failure or early attenuation. If there is concern over the tissue quality or fixation at the quadriceps, we are more conservative with our rehabilitation.

COMPLICATIONS

Extensor mechanism allografts are a large transplant of bone (patella and tibia) and soft tissue to the front of the knee. Although fresh-frozen allografts do not have living cells within the transplanted tissue, they do contain cellular remains including residual nuclear material. These donor cellular residuals have to be degraded further and removed by the host. This occurs as the tissue is repopulated by recipient cells. Certain individuals may have significantly more inflammatory reactions, with chronic effusions and malaise for several weeks. It is possible that the inflammatory and/or low-grade immune reaction would be so significant the graft would need to be removed.

If the host does not have sufficient residual proximal quadriceps tendon to hold sutures, the allograft quadriceps tendon can pull away from the quadriceps muscle resulting in an extension lag. There is often loss of some knee flexion as a result of prolonged immobilization associated with the secondary reconstruction of the quadriceps tendon portion of the allograft. Knee flexion may not be completely re-established even after rigorous physical therapy, surgical lysis of adhesions, and/or manipulation under anesthesia.

RESULTS

The patients that may benefit from an allograft reconstruction of their extensor mechanism represent a varied population. There are those with a deficient quadriceps tendon and patella tendon that have failed recurrent attempts at primary repair and reconstruction using autogenous tissue. The repairs may require replacement of tissue that both covers and allows fixation to the existing patella. The patella tendon may benefit from fixation into the tibial bone at its attachment site. Allograft extensor mechanism reconstructions are usually reasonable in re-establishing full extension but may limit the patient's flexion range. Patients are usually willing to accept this if they have extension power back. These patients often have had multiple previous surgeries and have underlying degenerative articular cartilage disease. They do not end up with a normal knee but a more functional knee.

Reconstruction with the patella, quadriceps, and patellar tendon is a much more extensive procedure than a soft tissue reconstruction. The patella takes a long time to revascularize, if ever (Fig. 5-6). The underlying articular cartilage will degenerate with time. The graft requires matching to the underlying femoral sulcus for tracking and sizing. This is a salvage procedure. Once again the goals are eliminating the extension lag enabling the patient to be more functional. It also prepares the patient for a future knee replacement or helps salvage the current or revised one.

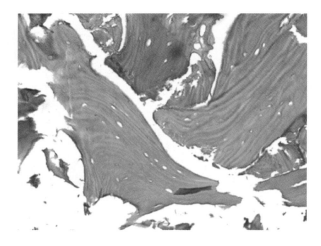

FIGURE 5-6

A biopsy specimen of a patellar allograft with no viable cells in the bone.

RECOMMENDED READING

Burnett RS, Fornasier VL, Haydon CM, et al. Retrieval of a well-functioning extensor mechanism allograft from a total knee arthroplasty. Clinical and histological findings. *J Bone Joint Surg Br.* 2004;86:986–990.

Burnett RS, Berger RA, Paprosky WG, et al. Extensor mechanism allograft reconstruction after total knee arthroplasty. A comparison of two techniques. *J Bone Joint Surg Am.* 2004;86:2694–2699.

Emerson RH Jr, Head WC, Malinin TI. Extensor mechanism reconstruction with an allograft after total knee arthroplasty. *Clin Orthop Relat Res.* 1994;303:79–85.

Jackson DW, Simon TM. Donor cell survival and repopulation after intraarticular transplantation of tendon and ligament allografts. *Microscopy Research and Techniques.* 2002;58(1):25–33.

Krackow KA, Thomas SC, Jones LC. Ligament-tendon fixation analysis of a new stitch and comparison with standard techniques. *Orthopedics.* 1988;11:909–917.

6 Acute Quadriceps Tendon Repair

Christopher S. Proctor and Brant L. Richardson

INDICATIONS/CONTRAINDICATIONS

Quadriceps tendon rupture is uncommon, occurring much more frequently in males than in females (3,4,6) and more often in patients over 40 years of age. Rupture of the quadriceps tendon is a serious injury that we believe should be surgically repaired within 2 weeks of injury. Beyond 2 weeks, quadriceps contracture and scarring can begin to make the repair more difficult, and postoperative strength and patient satisfaction are adversely affected (4). Some studies have found a loss of range of motion (ROM) with delayed repair as well (5,6). Complete ruptures that go unrepaired produce a lower extremity with a poorly performing extensor mechanism; however, even chronic tears stand to make significant gains through repair (4). We feel that repair is indicated in all acute cases of complete rupture other than the medically unstable patient and those patients who were not ambulatory prior to the injury.

The first step in treating a quadriceps rupture is a prompt and accurate diagnosis. Unfortunately, quadriceps tendon rupture often goes unrecognized in the family practice and emergency setting, leading to delayed diagnoses and repair. Patients with a quadriceps rupture will generally present with suprapatellar gap, suprapatellar pain, and an inability to extend the knee. Diagnosis is complicated by hematoma filling the suprapatellar gap and an unwillingness by some evaluators to thoroughly palpate the tender area. Medical providers often rely on radiography, which can show patella baja if bilateral radiographs are obtained, but more often the case is a normal appearing unilateral series. In some patients, systemic medical issues lead to tendon degeneration and relatively little pain on rupture with a low-energy mechanism of injury. Bilateral ruptures are more likely to have a medical predisposition for tears, such as autoimmune diseases, gout, diabetes mellitus, rheumatoid arthritis, hyperparathyroidism, long-term steroid use, and end-stage renal disease (1–3). Further complicating diagnosis is the case of tendon rupture with an intact retinaculum, which allows weak knee extension to be maintained. If the retinaculum is torn at all the patient will lose some ROM (6). Prompt diagnosis and surgical repair will afford the best opportunity for a successful recovery after quadriceps rupture.

PREOPERATIVE PLANNING

A full history and physical examination are required as part of the preoperative evaluation. Anteroposterior and lateral radiographs of the knee should also be obtained. Magnetic resonance imaging (MRI) is helpful to determine the extent of the tear and to prepare the surgeon for other injuries that may need to be addressed; however, surgery should not be delayed to obtain an MRI.

SURGERY

Patient Positioning

We position the patient supine on the operating table with a well-padded tourniquet fitted snugly high on the thigh. The entire lower extremity is then prepared with Hibiclens solution, and the lower extremity is draped free from the level of the mid thigh.

Technique

A midline longitudinal incision is made starting 15 cm above the proximal patella and is extended to the tibial tubercle. Medial and lateral full-thickness skin flaps are elevated using blunt dissection to expose the extensor mechanism. If the retinaculum is intact, it is split longitudinally. Irrigation is used to dislodge any hematoma, allowing the tear to be assessed. The osteotendinous junction at the patella is the most common site of the rupture. The tendon is then debrided of all necrotic and frayed tissues. The quadriceps tendon is carefully mobilized from any surrounding adhesions. Once tendon length has been maximized, we place sutures in the tendon as follows: starting at the tear, No. 5 nonabsorbable sutures are placed in a running Bunnel configuration along the edges of the tendon to 3 cm proximal of the tear, then run back down closer to the midline (Fig. 6-1). The anterior proximal pole of the patella is then debrided of soft tissue and lightly roughened with a bur to provide a bed for the tendon. A 2-mm hole is drilled longitudinally down the midline of the patella and out the distal pole. Two parallel holes are drilled medially and laterally, in a similar fashion, approximately 1 cm from the midline. A suture passer is then used to pass the two central sutures down the central drill hole and the medial and lateral sutures through the medial and lateral drill holes, respectively (Fig. 6-2). We then tie the sutures over the bone bridge, securing the tendon to the patella. As much of the retinaculum as possible is then repaired with No. 2-0 absorbable sutures.

More recently we have also been using suture anchors to secure the tendon to the patella rather than drill holes. Using this technique, the tear is exposed and the proximal pole of the patella is prepared as previously discussed. Two suture anchors double loaded with No. 2 FiberWire sutures (Arthrex, Inc., Naples, FL) are then inserted into the patella dividing it into approximately equal thirds (Fig.

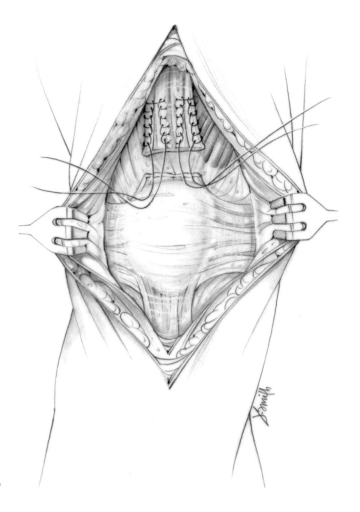

FIGURE 6-1

Running sutures placed in a running Bunnel configuration, producing four free strands.

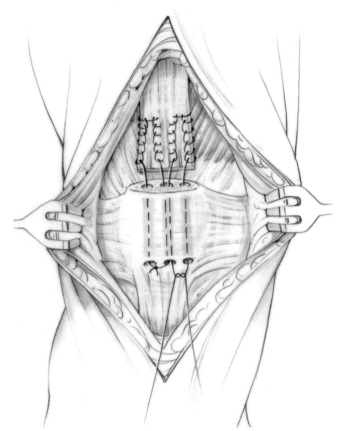

FIGURE 6-2

Sutures placed through three longitudinal drill holes in the patella are tightened, pulling the quadriceps to the patella.

6-3). Each of the four sutures is then secured to the tendon using a modified Mason-Allen technique. The remainder of the repair then proceeds as previously described. To aid our postoperative planning, we then range the knee to determine how much the knee can be flexed without overly stressing the repair. At this time, patellar alignment is also assessed and lateral release performed if necessary.

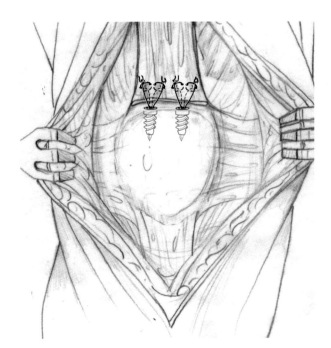

FIGURE 6-3

Suture anchors buried in the patella are made visible in this figure for clarity. Each anchor is loaded with 2 pairs of FiberWire sutures; the sutures are tied to the tendon using a modified Mason-Allen technique.

Pearls and Pitfalls

Tension across the suture line is minimized during repair by extending the knee completely, deflating the tourniquet, and pulling the tendon distally. Careful attention must be paid to anatomic alignment of the quadriceps tendon and patella to help prevent future patellofemoral complications. Repair of the lateral retinaculum can be forgone and a more extensive lateral release performed if patellar alignment demands it.

POSTOPERATIVE MANAGEMENT

We believe it is important for patients to take an early and active role in their recovery to give them a sense of control while they are disabled and to promote the mind-set that their full recovery relies on their own hard work in physical therapy. Postoperatively, we keep the leg locked in extension with a dial lock brace and keep the patient non–weight bearing until they are examined at 1 week. After the first week, the patient is allowed to partially weight bear with crutches. Patients are encouraged to do quad sets and straight leg raises at home and are started in physical therapy for gentle, passive ROM at 2 weeks. At 3 weeks, patients are made full weight bearing but continue to be locked in extension. At rest, they are encouraged to unlock their brace and work on passive ROM. At 6 weeks, active ROM is begun. Patients are allowed to ambulate with the brace unlocked up to their active ROM. Progressive increases of 10 to 15 degrees per week should yield full ROM by 12 to 16 weeks. Patients begin full resistance exercise, move on to light jogging, and by 20 weeks can start full running.

COMPLICATIONS

Although most patients regain a functional ROM, loss of motion is the most common problem after quadriceps repair. Patients must work diligently in physical therapy for a prolonged period to regain full function, and many find it easier to live with a less-than-perfect lower extremity. Atrophy of the extensor mechanism is also not uncommon but is usually not associated with overt weakness compared to the uninjured leg (7). Delayed surgery increases the likelihood of extensor lag, need for ambulatory aids, and poor stair-climbing ability (7).

RESULTS

Quadriceps tendon rupture is an infrequent but serious injury most often occurring in men over 40 years of age. Most patients recover full ROM, near full strength, and are able to return to their former occupation. If the quadriceps rupture is diagnosed and repaired promptly, most patients can expect a satisfactory return of extensor mechanism function. Rigorous, extended physical therapy is necessary for complete recovery and a return to sports, although 50% of patients perform sports at a decreased level. It is not surprising that any delay in surgical repair can lead to increased weakness and disability postoperatively.

RECOMMENDED READING

Gelberman R, Woo SL, Buckwalter JA. Injury and repair of the musculoskeletal soft tissues. *Amer Acad Ortho Surg.* 1988;21–23.
Ramseier LE, Werner CML, Heinzelmann M. Quadriceps and patellar tendon rupture. *Int J Care Injured.* 2006;37:516–519.
Richards DP, Barber AF. Repair of quadriceps tendon ruptures using suture anchors. *J Arthro Rel Surg.* 2002;18:556–559.
Woo SL, Vogrin TM, Abramowitch SD. Healing and repair of ligament injuries in the knee. *J Am Acad Orthop Surg.* 2000;8:364–372.

REFERENCES

1. Ilan DI, Tejwani N, Keschner M, et al. Quadriceps tendon rupture. *J Am Acad Orthop Surg.* 2003;11(3):192–200.
2. Konrath AG, Chen D, Lock T, et al. Outcomes following repair of quadriceps tendon rupture. *J Orthop Trauma.* 1998;12:273–279.
3. Puranik GS, Faraj A. Outcomes of quadriceps tendon repair. *Acta Orthop Belg.* 2006;72:176–178.
4. Rougraff BT, Reek CC, Essenmacher J. Complete quadriceps tendon ruptures. *Orthopedics.* 1996;19:509–514.
5. Scuderi G. Ruptures of the quadriceps tendon: study of 20 tendon ruptures. *Am J Surg.* 1958;91;626–635.
6. Siwek CW, Rao JP. Ruptures of the extensor mechanism of the knee joint. *J Bone Joint Surg.* 1981;63:932–937.

7 Patellar Tendon Repair

Albert M. Tsai

INDICATIONS/CONTRAINDICATIONS

Isolated rupture of the patellar tendon is a rare injury occurring primarily in patients less than 40 years old. Most ruptures occur as the result of a rapid forceful contraction of the quadriceps muscle with a flexed knee, and a history of stumbling or giving way of the knee can often be elicited along with a sudden pop and acute onset of pain. It has been demonstrated that normal tendons usually do not rupture without significant trauma (2). A certain degree of tendon degeneration is often present, the result of cumulative microtrauma or the degenerative changes associated with aging. The injury can also be associated with systemic diseases, such as chronic renal failure, rheumatoid arthritis, systemic lupus erythematosus, or diabetes mellitus, and occurs with little or no trauma in these patients. Rarely, iatrogenic patellar tendon rupture has been reported after harvesting the middle third of the tendon for anterior cruciate ligament reconstruction (1,3).

Surgical repair of an acutely ruptured patellar tendon is the standard of care and is necessary to reestablish continuity of the extensor mechanism of the knee. Neglected injuries can lead to proximal retraction of the quadriceps and patella with resultant adhesions and extensor mechanism insufficiency. Contraindications to acute surgical repair include acute infection, medical comorbidities that make the surgical risk prohibitive, or soft tissue loss that makes primary repair impossible.

PREOPERATIVE PLANNING

The first step in assessing the injured knee is a thorough history and physical examination. There is generally swelling and ecchymosis about the knee as well as tenderness along the patellar tendon or at the inferior aspect of the patella. There may also be a palpable defect in the tendon. Occasionally the patient will be able to perform a straight leg raise maneuver through an intact extensor retinaculum. However, the diagnosis should still be apparent as there will usually be an extensor lag and weakness when compared to the uninjured extremity.

Imaging of the knee should include routine radiographs to rule out fractures. On a lateral view of the knee, patella alta can be seen (Fig. 7-1). Magnetic resonance imaging (MRI) is not usually necessary in acute injuries but may be helpful in chronic neglected ruptures, in those few acute cases where the diagnosis is unclear, or to diagnose suspected concomitant intra-articular pathology (Fig. 7-2).

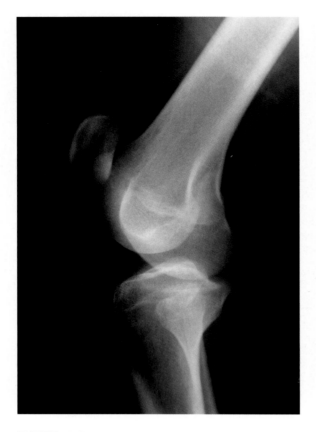

FIGURE 7-1

Lateral radiograph of patellar tendon rupture demonstrating patella alta.

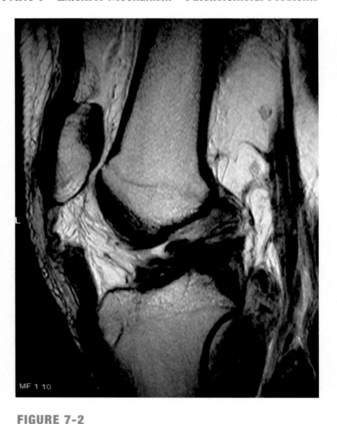

FIGURE 7-2

Magnetic resonance imaging clearly shows disruption of the patellar tendon. MRI was performed in this patient because of associated injuries to the anterior cruciate ligament, posterior cruciate ligament, and posterolateral corner.

SURGERY

Patient Positioning

The patient is placed in the supine position, and a small bump is placed under the ipsilateral hip to keep the patella pointing toward the ceiling. A tourniquet is placed on the proximal thigh but is usually not inflated during the procedure. The entire extremity is then sterilely prepped and draped free.

Technique

A midline skin incision is made centered over the defect in the patellar tendon. If the disruption is an avulsion off the inferior pole of the patella, the incision may extend more proximally. In the case of a midsubstance tear or tibial tubercle avulsion, the incision may extend more distally. Routine dissection is carried sharply down through skin and subcutaneous tissue. At this point, the knee joint is frequently visualized through the ruptured tendon. The joint is thoroughly irrigated to remove old hematoma and soft tissue debris, and the articular surfaces can be examined for any injury. If possible, the paratenon should be identified and incised to further dissect out the patellar tendon in preparation for repair.

Most commonly, the patellar tendon is avulsed from the inferior aspect of the patella, along with tears of the medial and lateral retinaculum (Fig. 7-3). The frayed, tattered stump of patellar tendon is sharply debrided with dissecting scissors or a sharp scalpel to freshen up the tendon and remove any nonviable tissue. Next, a Rongeur is used to debride the inferior pole of the patella, removing soft tissue remnants and providing a healthy bleeding bone surface for the repaired tendon. A total of two No. 2 FiberWire (Arthrex, Inc., Naples, FL) sutures are woven into the end of the tendon using a Krackow-type locking stitch. One suture is woven into the medial half of the tendon, working

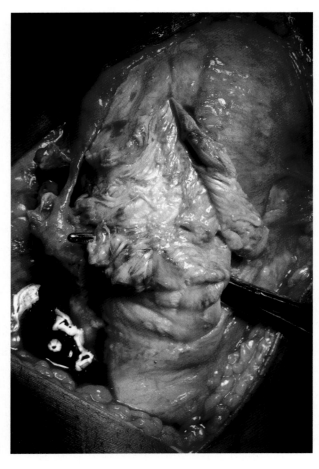

FIGURE 7-3

In this patient there is a near complete avulsion of the patellar tendon from the inferior aspect of the patella. The clamp lies behind the proximal patellar tendon.

from proximal to distal and then back up in the medial central portion of the tendon. The second suture is similarly woven down the lateral half of the tendon and back up the lateral central portion of the tendon, leaving four suture strands exiting the tendon (Fig. 7-4). These sutures are marked with hemostats so that they can later be passed through drill holes in the patella. For ease of identification, the central sutures can be cut shorter than the peripheral ones and clamped together (Fig. 7-5).

Next, a total of three parallel drill holes are made in the patella from distal to proximal, using a 2-mm drill bit. When drilling, the flat end of an Army-Navy retractor can be used to locate the drill bit as it exits the superior border of the patella and the quadriceps tendon (Fig. 7-6). After withdrawing the drill bit, often it is difficult to locate the hole in the superior aspect of the patella to place a suture passer from proximal to distal. Instead, a suture passer is used from distal to proximal to pass a loop of 0 PDS suture. This loop of PDS can then be used to pass the FiberWire sutures through their appropriate drill holes (Fig. 7-7). The lateral suture is passed through the lateral drill hole, the medial suture through the medial drill hole, and the two shorter central sutures through the central drill hole. After passing these sutures, they can be tied with the knee in extension, the medial suture to the medial central suture and the lateral suture to the lateral central suture (Fig. 7-8). The tendon should contact the previously prepared inferior pole of the patella, but care should be taken not to overtighten the repair and cause patella baja. If there is any question, an intraoperative lateral radiograph can be taken and compared to the contralateral knee.

The medial and lateral retinacular defects are then closed with No. 1 absorbable suture. A No. 2-0 absorbable suture is used for the paratenon, if possible, as well as the subcutaneous layer, and surgical staples or a running subcuticular stitch are used to approximate the skin. A routine sterile dressing is placed and the patient is placed into a range of motion brace, which is locked in extension.

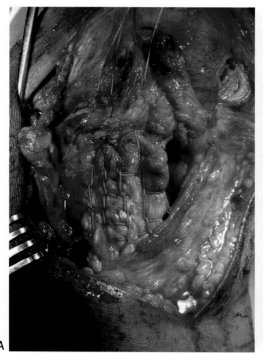
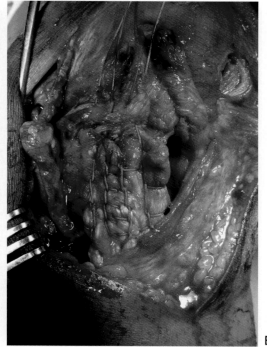

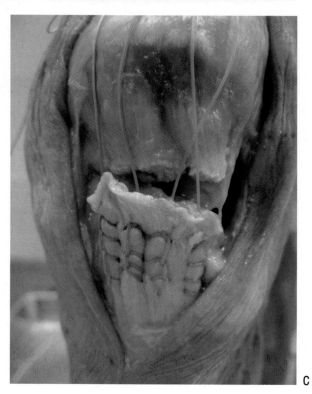

FIGURE 7-4

A,B: No. 2 FiberWire suture is woven into the stump of patellar tendon using medial and lateral Krackow locking stitches. **C:** Cadaver specimen demonstrating medial and lateral Krackow locking stitches for patellar tendon rupture.

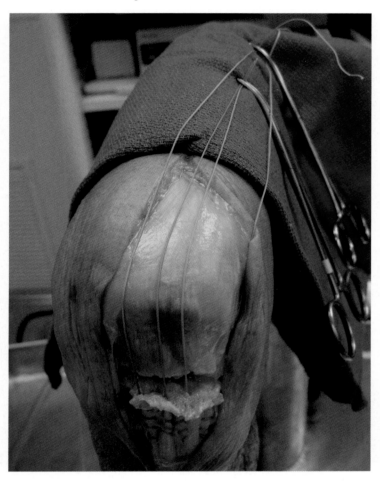

FIGURE 7-5
The central strands of the medial and lateral Krackow stitches can be cut short and clamped together for ease of identification.

A similar surgical technique is used for patellar tendon disruption from the tibial tubercle, except the sutures are passed through transosseous tunnels in the tubercle and tied over medial and lateral bony bridges. For a midsubstance tendon rupture, direct tendon-to-tendon repair is performed with a total of four No. 2 FiberWire sutures—medial and lateral Krackow-type locking stitches in both the proximal and distal tendon stumps (Fig. 7-9). The patellar tendon suture line is oversewn with interrupted No. 2-0 absorbable suture. Retinacular repair and closure are the same as for proximal avulsion injuries.

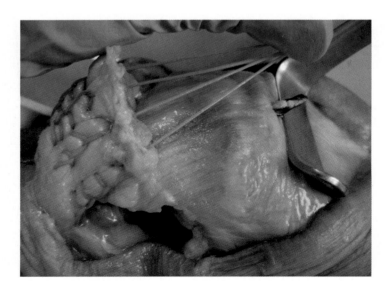

FIGURE 7-6
An Army-Navy retractor helps locate the exiting drill bit.

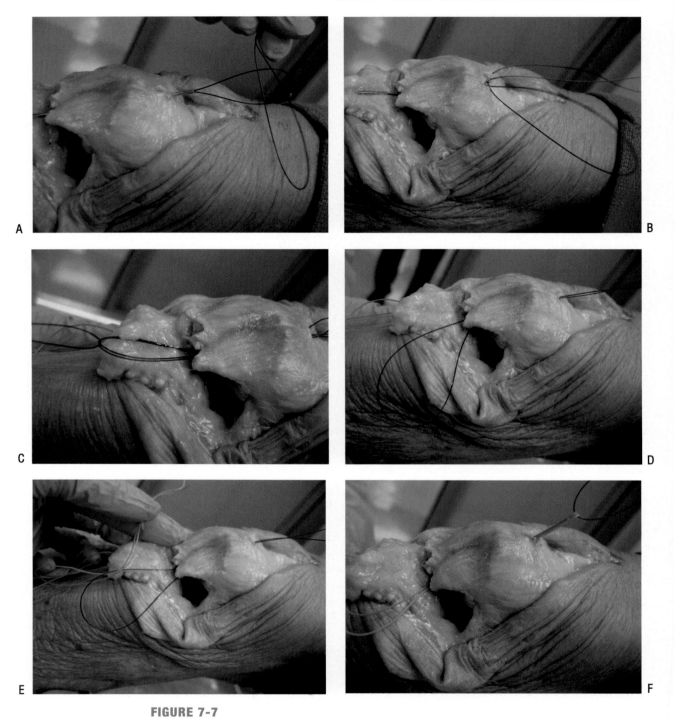

FIGURE 7-7

A: Hewson suture passer used from distal to proximal. **B,C,D:** Loop of 0 PDS suture passed from proximal to distal. **E,F:** FiberWire suture passed through drill hole using PDS loop.

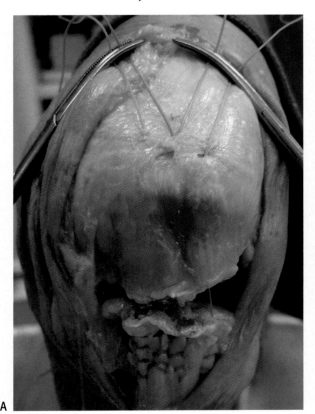

A

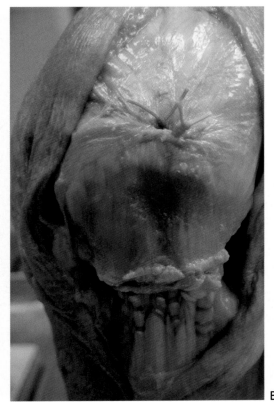

B

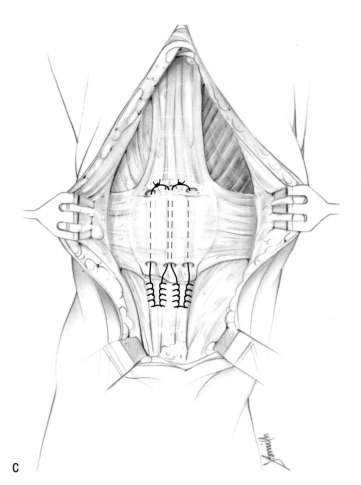

C

FIGURE 7-8

A,B: Cadaver specimen demonstrating patellar tendon repair with sutures passed through patellar drill holes. **C:** Schematic illustrating patellar tendon repair.

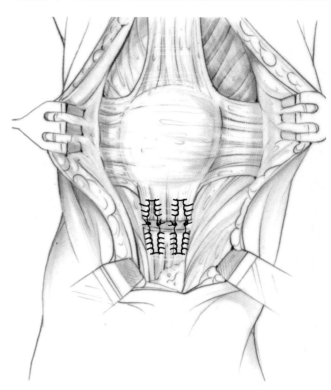

FIGURE 7-9
Midsubstance patellar tendon repair
with sutures.

Pearls and Pitfalls

- When drilling the three parallel drill holes, take care to start the holes closer to the articular sur-face rather than the dorsal surface of the patella. This will prevent inward tilting of the distal pole of the patella when the repair is tightened, which could lead to increased contact pressure in the patellofemoral joint.
- After drilling holes through the patella, it is difficult to pass a suture passer from proximal to distal. Use a suture passer from distal to proximal to pass a loop of 0 PDS. The loop can then be used to pass the FiberWire from distal to proximal.
- Overtightening the repair can lead to patella baja and a poor result. If in doubt, obtain an in-traoperative lateral radiograph and compare it to the contralateral knee.
- A good repair of the medial and lateral retinacular tissue is a key portion of the procedure. This relieves much of the stress on the central repair and allows for aggressive postoperative range of motion and strengthening.

POSTOPERATIVE MANAGEMENT

Immediate full weight bearing is initiated after surgery with crutches and the range of motion brace locked in extension. Isometric quadriceps and hamstring exercises are also initiated on the first day after surgery. Surgical staples are removed in the office at 10 to 14 days after surgery, at which time supervised physical therapy is begun with active flexion and passive extension of the knee. The range of motion is started at 0 to 30 degrees and advanced 30 degrees every 2 weeks with the goal of 90 degrees at 6 weeks. The range of motion brace is gradually unlocked to coincide with the in-creases in flexion allowed and is discontinued when 90 degrees of flexion is achieved at 6 weeks. A supervised strengthening program is then started, with full return to sports activity prohibited until 6 months after surgery or until the patient demonstrates full range of motion of the knee and at least 80% of the strength of the contralateral knee with isokinetic testing.

COMPLICATIONS

Decreased Motion

Decreased range of motion is most likely a result of the initial injury itself, rather than any technical problems related to the surgical procedure. To overcome this, a secure repair allows an aggressive postoperative therapy program emphasizing early range of motion and strengthening. Significant lack of motion at 2 to 3 months is uncommon with acute primary repair but can be treated with manipulation under anesthesia to improve flexion or arthroscopic lysis of adhesions for loss of passive extension.

Wound Problems

Wound dehiscence or infection is uncommon, but may occur distally, where skin coverage is the thinnest. Local wound care and appropriate antibiotics if necessary are usually sufficient to resolve these problems.

Hemarthrosis

Postoperative bleeding may cause an uncomfortable hemarthrosis, which usually resolves spontaneously but can limit mobility and progress with postoperative physical therapy. Meticulous hemostasis during surgery can help prevent this problem. If a tourniquet is used, this should be deflated and hemostasis achieved prior to wound closure.

Missed Diagnosis

Delayed treatment of a neglected patellar tendon rupture will often necessitate reconstruction of the extensor mechanism. Lack of adequate soft tissue and native tendon often precludes primary repair, and quadriceps muscle contracture and adhesions often prevent the patella from being brought distally to an acceptable position. During the preoperative evaluation, a lateral radiograph should be obtained of the contralateral knee to be used in estimating patellar height during the reconstruction.

Patient positioning is the same as for acute repair cases. A generous midline incision is used to fully delineate the anatomy and address the quadriceps contracture. If significant patella alta is present, the quadriceps mechanism may need fractional lengthening with a pie-crusting technique or formal V-Y advancement. Either Achilles or patellar tendon allograft can be used to reconstruct the extensor mechanism in the absence of acceptable native tissue.

When using Achilles tendon allograft, a rectangular plug of calcaneus with attached Achilles tendon is press fit into a matching rectangular trough made in the tibial tubercle. This bone plug is fixed with 4.5-mm bicortical screws. The soft tissue of the Achilles tendon is then split into two grafts and brought through two transosseous patellar tunnels and sewn into the quadriceps mechanism (Fig. 7-10).

Alternatively, patellar tendon allograft allows bony fixation on both the tibial and patellar sides. A large rectangular plug from the allograft tibia is inserted into a matching trough in the patient's tibial tubercle and fixed with 4.5-mm bicortical screws. On the patellar side, the inferior pole of the patient's patella is removed to match a large portion of the inferior pole of the allograft patella that has been left with the graft. Naturally, the appropriate size and length patellar tendon allograft must be selected during the preoperative planning, which can be facilitated with a lateral radiograph of the contralateral knee. Patellar fixation is achieved with Kirschner wires or cannulated 4.0-mm screws and a figure-of-eight tension band wire or No. 5 nonabsorbable suture (Fig. 7-11).

With reconstruction of chronic tears, a No. 5 nonabsorbable suture, or 5-mm Mersilene tape placed through a transosseous drill hole in the tibial tubercle and then up and over the patella through the quadriceps mechanism will help relieve stress on the repair. A cerclage wire accomplishes the same task but frequently breaks when range of motion is initiated, occasionally necessitating removal.

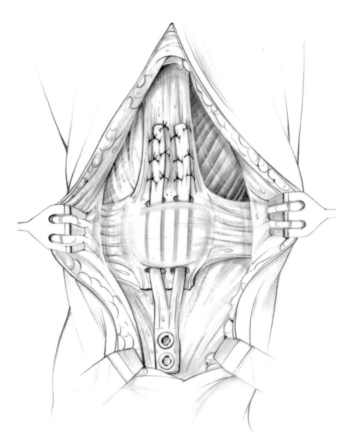

FIGURE 7-10

Achilles tendon allograft for patellar tendon reconstruction. The calcaneal bone plug is fixed with 4.5-mm screws. The soft tissue is passed through 7-mm transosseous tunnels and sutured to the quadriceps mechanism.

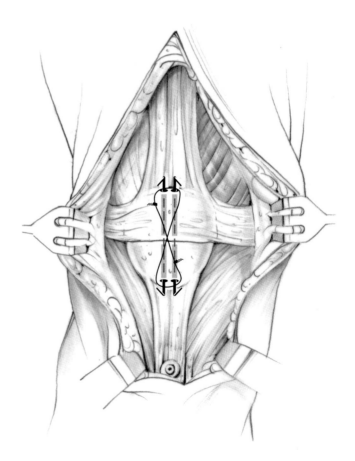

FIGURE 7-11

Patellar tendon reconstruction using patellar tendon allograft.

RESULTS

Results after patellar tendon repair are most closely correlated with the amount of time that has passed between injury and surgical treatment. The overwhelming majority of patients that undergo timely primary repair of an acute patellar tendon rupture will have excellent results, with full range of motion and normal quadriceps strength. Mild quadriceps atrophy may persist but should not affect the return of strength. The results for patients that undergo delayed reconstruction are less satisfactory, with loss of full knee flexion and a decrease in quadriceps strength more likely. However, a functional extensor mechanism can still be re-established.

RECOMMENDED READINGS

Greis PE, Holmstrom MC, Lahav A. Surgical treatment options for patella tendon rupture, Part I: acute. *Orthopedics.* 2005;28(7):672–679.

Greis PE, Lahav A, Holmstrom MC. Surgical treatment options for patella tendon rupture, Part II: chronic. *Orthopedics.* 2005;28(8):765–769.

Kuechle DK, Stuart MJ. Isolated rupture of the patellar tendon in athletes. *Am J Sports Med.* 1994;22(5):692–695.

Matava MJ. Patellar tendon ruptures. *J Am Acad Orthop Surg.* 1996;4(6):287–296.

REFERENCES

1. Busfield BT, Safran MR, Cannon WD. Extensor mechanism disruption after contralateral middle-third patellar tendon harvest for anterior cruciate ligament revision reconstruction. *Arthroscopy.* 2005;21(10):1268.e1–1268.e6.
2. Kannus P, Josza L. Histopathological changes preceding spontaneous rupture of a tendon. A controlled study of 891 patients. *J Bone Joint Surg Am.* 1991;73:1507–1525.
3. Marumoto JM, Mitsunaga MM, Richardson AB, et al. Late patellar tendon ruptures after removal of the central third for anterior cruciate ligament reconstruction. A report of two cases. *Am J Sports Med.* 1996:24(5):698–701.

PART TWO

MENISCUS SURGERY

8 Meniscus Repair: Inside-Out Suture Technique

Kevin F. Bonner

INDICATIONS/CONTRAINDICATIONS

In an effort to preserve meniscal function, meniscus repair should be performed when there is a reasonably good chance the meniscus will heal and maintain its function. Patient age, activity level, knee stability, type, location, and chronicity of the tear are important factors when considering meniscal repair versus resection. In general, active patients under the age of 45 years with a longitudinal tear within 3 to 5 mm of the meniscocapsular junction are good candidates for repair. Radial tears going to the meniscocapsular junction are also typically repaired in a young patient (more common lateral). The younger the patient, the more likely I am to attempt repairing a tear considered to have marginal healing capacity. Degenerative type tears or tears with minimal healing capacity are treated with partial meniscectomy. Anterior cruciate ligament (ACL) reconstruction is strongly recommended in the setting of a repairable meniscus tear and instability.

Although all-inside meniscus repair devices are becoming much more popular as the result of their ease of use, the inside-out technique is the most versatile and still considered the "gold standard." Although I have also used suture-based all-inside meniscus repair devices for several years, I still often use the inside-out repair technique.

PREOPERATIVE PLANNING

The diagnosis of a meniscus tear can be made with reasonable certainty with a thorough history, physical examination, and radiographs. Magnetic resonance imaging (MRI) is not required but is often helpful in differentiating between meniscal versus articular cartilage pathology and in the assessment of associated injuries in the acute setting. We can also get a fairly good idea whether a tear may be repairable based on signal patterns; but certainly the final decision between meniscectomy and repair is not made until the time of surgery (Fig. 8-1).

If a patient has a potentially repairable meniscus it is important to have all of the equipment and personnel available. A skilled assistant is required to perform an inside-out repair. Even for surgeons who prefer an all-inside repair technique, it is important to be proficient and ready with the alternative technique of inside-out repair, since some tears are not as amenable to all-inside repair. It is important to discuss with the patient the risks and benefits, as well as the difference in the rehabilitation protocol, for a meniscus repair versus a meniscectomy.

SURGERY

Preoperatively in the holding area, the correct side is confirmed and the patient's knee is signed. Within 1 hour prior to surgery, the anesthesiologist intravenously administers 1 g (2 g if patient >80 kg) of a first-generation cephalosporin (Cefazolin) if the patient is not allergic. Alternatively, the patient is given Clindamycin 600 to 900 mg intravenously. Regional versus general anesthesia is decided by the patient and the anesthesiologist.

Patient Positioning

The patient is placed in a supine position with the leg resting straight on the operating room table. A tourniquet is placed on the proximal thigh, and lateral thigh post is used to allow a valgus stress to improve visualization of the medial compartment. A pillow is placed under the contralateral knee. The knee is positioned distal to the break in the table, allowing posteromedial access if the foot of the table is flexed during the procedure. After adequate anesthesia, an examination under anesthesia is performed comparing both knees.

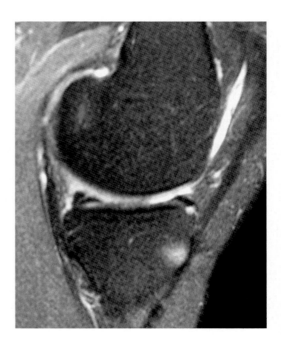

FIGURE 8-1
MRI of a potentially repairable medial meniscus tear in a 22-year-old woman.

The portal sites and any additional incision sites are infiltrated with 0.25% Marcaine with 1:200,000 epinephrine. The meniscus repair (with or without ACL reconstruction) may be performed with or without a tourniquet. If a tourniquet is used, the leg is exsanguinated with an esmark wrap, and the tourniquet is inflated to 300 mm Hg. If an ACL reconstruction is to be performed in the same setting, I will harvest the graft prior to performing knee arthroscopy. A diagnostic arthroscopy is performed first if there is any uncertainty regarding the status of the ACL. Allografts are also used fairly frequently in my practice. All of these grafts will be prepared at the back table by the assistant. The assistant will work on the graft until he or she is needed for the meniscus repair.

Diagnostic Arthroscopy

The diagnostic arthroscopy is started with placement of the anterolateral portal adjacent to the patellar tendon 1 cm below the inferior pole of the patella. The arthroscope is gently inserted into the joint through the anterolateral portal with the knee in 70 to 90 degrees of flexion. With the arthroscope focused in the medial compartment, the anteromedial portal is created with the aid of an 18-gauge spinal needle. The anteromedial portal should be just to the medial side of the patellar tendon. Depending on the side of the meniscus tear, the medial portal can be adjusted appropriately. For a medial sided tear, the spinal needle is placed adjacent to the patellar tendon just superior to the anterior horn of the medial meniscus confirming optimal access to the posterior horn. If preoperatively it is determined that the lateral meniscus is most likely going to require repair, I may delay making the anteromedial portal until the knee is in the figure-of-4 position. In this setting, use the spinal needle as a probe to help determine if a medial tear is present. Optimal placement of the anteromedial portal for a lateral meniscus repair is typically more superior than for a medial meniscus repair, since the suture cannula will need to avoid the tibial eminence.

I will initially assess the tear and determine the feasibility of a successful repair. The younger the patient the more prudent to attempt repair. A probe is used to characterize the size of the tear, degree of instability, quality of the tissue, and zone of the tear (i.e., red-red, red-white, white-white). The width and integrity of the meniscal rim is evaluated in a far peripheral tear to determine if an all-inside device may be an option. Far posterior tears may need to be assessed with a 70-degree scope placed posterior through the notch. Once the diagnostic arthroscopy is complete, the meniscus repair will proceed in a step-wise fashion.

Tear Preparation

A meniscal rasp (Acufex, Andover, MA) is used to debride granulation tissue on both sides of the tear (Fig. 8-2). Alternatively, a 3.5-mm shaver may be used to debride the edges of the tear site. It is important to take quite a bit of time in preparing the edges to healthy tissue since this step is crucial in optimizing the healing potential. Rasp the perimeniscal synovium both superior and inferior to the tear site. In the case of a displaced repairable bucket handle tear, it is often useful to debride the edges of the tear prior to reduction (Fig. 8-3). This will give you direct visualization and access to both sides of the tear. Once the tear edges are abraded back to healthy tissue, the meniscus is reduced into an anatomic position. After the meniscus site is prepared, the posteromedial or posterolateral incision is created.

Preparation of a peripheral, far posterior tear may require access through a posteromedial or posterolateral portal. These portals are made approximately 1 cm above the joint line with the knee at 90 degrees of flexion. The 70 scope is placed posterior through the notch, and a spinal needle is used to direct posterior portal placement. Alternatively, I prefer to make a small portal through the capsule once the posteromedial or posterolateral approach has been made. A rasp or shaver is used through the posterior portal to access the tear site.

Technique for Medial Meniscus Repair

Optimal positioning of the skin incision can be enhanced with translumination of the posteromedial joint line by placing the arthroscope in the medial compartment with the room lights dimmed (Fig. 8-4). The knee should be flexed between 60 and 90 degrees for the exposure. A 3- to 4-cm vertical incision is created along the posteromedial joint line posterior to the medial collateral ligament (Fig. 8-5). Approximately two thirds of the incision should be distal to the joint line because the needles

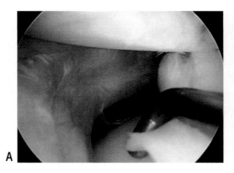
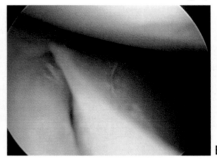
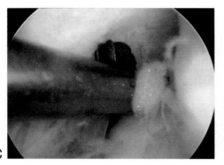
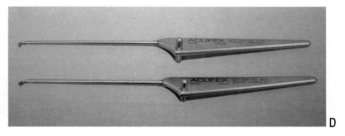

FIGURE 8-2

A–C: Evaluation and preparation of a lateral meniscus tear using a meniscal rasp (Acufex, Andover, MA) **(D)**.

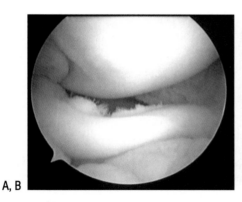
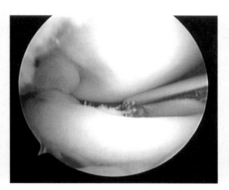
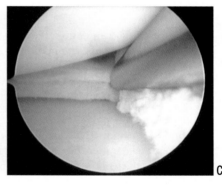

FIGURE 8-3

A: Displaced bucket handle medial meniscus tear in a 15-year-old. **B:** Tear edge of the displaced fragment is prepared with a shaver prior to reduction. **C:** Posterior rim is prepared with the fragment displaced anterior allowing optimal visualization.

FIGURE 8-4

Translumination of the medial or lateral compartment may assist in planning posterior incision site.

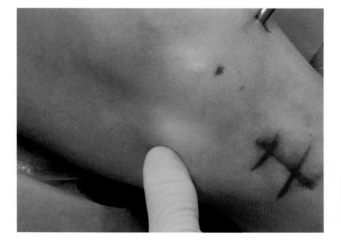

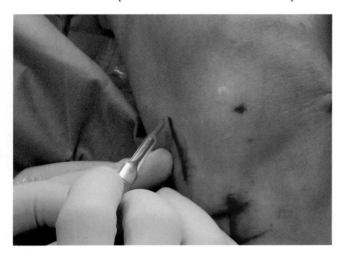

FIGURE 8-5

A 3- to 4-cm incision is made posterior to the MCL. Two thirds of the incision is below the joint line.

tend to angle downward as they exit the meniscus and capsule. The saphenous vein should be posterior to the incision and can often be seen by translumination through the joint.

On dissection through the subcutaneous tissue, the oblique pes fascia is identified. An incision is made anterior within the fascia, which should be split proximal and distal using Metzenbaum scissors (Fig. 8-6). Care is taken to retract the sartorius, gracilis, and semitendinosis tendons along with the saphenous nerve posteromedial (Fig. 8-7). The saphenous nerve will lie within the posterior border of the sartorius and with retraction of the tendons should be protected. Knee flexion will relax the pes tendons and aid in retraction. If a hamstring autograft will be used for an ACL reconstruction, it is very helpful to harvest the grafts first, allowing for much easier dissection and retraction.

The deep dissection is continued in the interval between the medial head of the gastrocnemius and the joint capsule. Keep the knee in flexion to relax the hamstrings and the medial head of the gastrocnemius. Separating the muscle off the capsule is facilitated by starting distal. Start with a pair of Metzenbaum scissors, followed by placing an index finger to help expand this interval. By dorsiflexing and plantar flexing the ankle, the surgeon should be able to palpate the gastrocnemius on the posterior side by his or her finger (Fig. 8-8). This will assist in verifying the proper plane. Once developed, a posterior retractor is positioned anterior to the medial gastrocnemius muscle (Fig. 8-9). By retracting the medial head of the gastrocnemius lateral and posterior, the neurovascular structures will be protected (Fig. 8-10). Various retractors may be used; I prefer a Henning retractor or half of a pediatric speculum, although a bent spoon can be used as a retractor as well (Fig. 8-11). The retractor needs to be angled so the needles piercing through the posterior capsule are deflected medial toward the assistant.

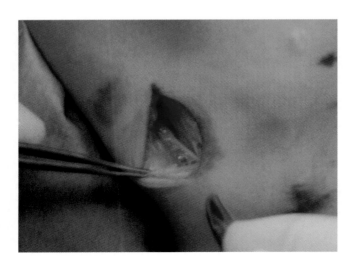

FIGURE 8-6

The pes fascia is identified, incised, and split proximal and distal.

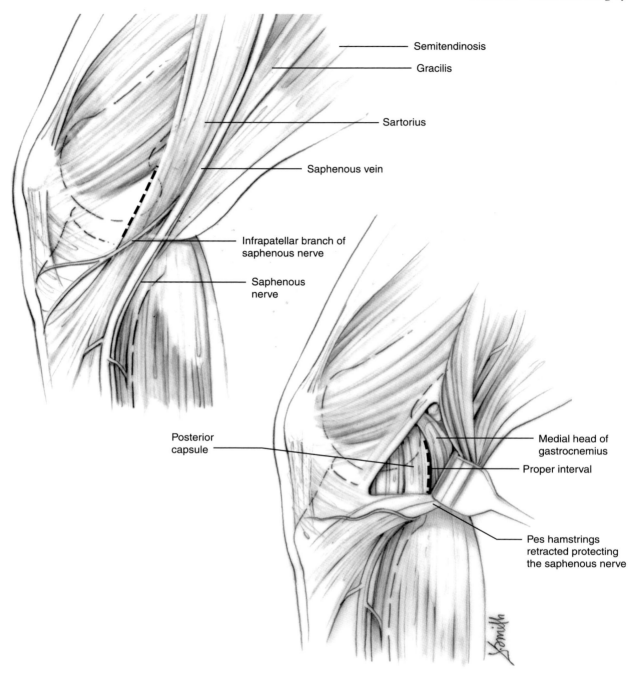

FIGURE 8-7

The saphenous nerve should be protected with posterior retraction of the pes hamstring tendons.

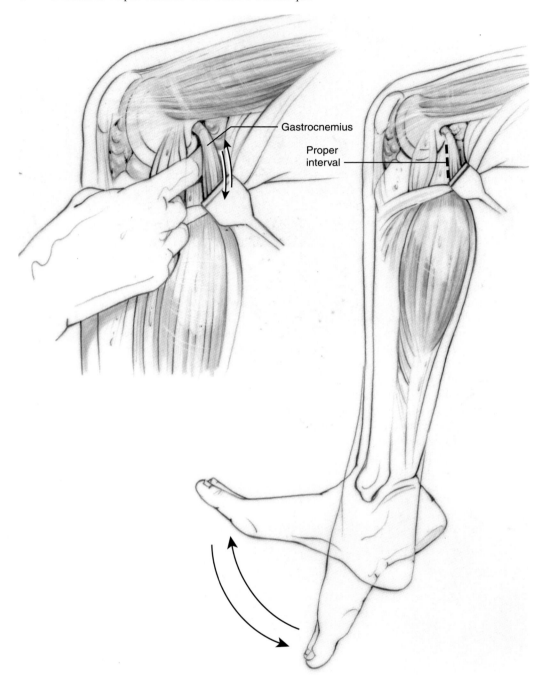

Gastrocnemius

Proper interval

FIGURE 8-8

Confirmation of the proper interval anterior to the gastrocnemius can be made by dorsiflexion and plantarflexion of the ankle. Palpate the motion of the gastrocnemius on the posterior side of your finger.

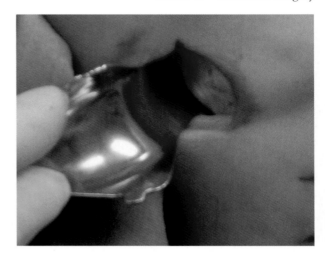

FIGURE 8-9

The posterior retractor is positioned revealing the posteromedial joint capsule. The hamstrings and medial head of the gastrocnemius are posterior to the retractor.

Once the retractor is placed, the knee is kept between 20 and 60 degrees of flexion. Knee extension will enhance arthroscopic visualization of the posterior horn of the meniscus, but consequently makes posterior retraction and visualization more difficult. Increasing knee flexion relaxes the hamstrings and gastrocnemius, thus improving posterior retraction and visualization of exiting needles.

I always prefer to place sutures into the medial meniscus through a cannula entering the anterolateral portal. This angulation tends to improve the direction of exiting needles toward the medial exposure. However, far posterior tears near the meniscal root may require use of a curved cannula entering through the anteromedial portal with the curve directed medial (away from midline). Sutures are typically placed from posterior to anterior. Even if you begin with the suture cannula in the medial portal, as the repair proceeds anterior it is easier to switch portals and place the majority of sutures with the cannula entering from the anterolateral portal.

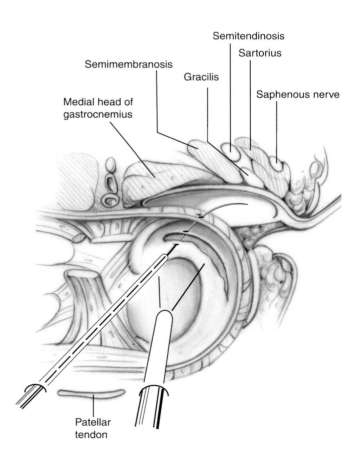

FIGURE 8-10

Retracting the medial head of the gastrocnemius lateral and posterior will protect the neurovascular structures.

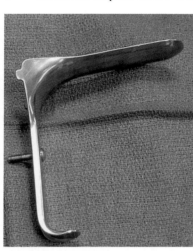

FIGURE 8-11

Half of a pediatric speculum may be used as a posterior retractor.

Single- or double-lumen zone-specific suture cannulas are commercially available (Fig. 8-12). These come straight and with varying curvatures to address different zones of the meniscus. I prefer single-lumen cannulas since they allow greater mobility and independence when placing sutures. However, this does increase the risk of damage to the suture as the second needle is being placed adjacent to the suture. Ten-inch flexible needles with attached 2.0 Ethibond suture are used for the repair (Ethicon, Inc., Somerville, NJ) (Fig. 8-13). I prefer nonabsorbable sutures, since there are data to suggest these sutures may improve clinical healing rates.

Flexing the foot of the table will allow your assistant improved access to the posteromedial exposure (Fig. 8-14). The assistant should "toe in" on the retractor and be prepared to retrieve with a needle driver. With the surgeon applying a valgus force to the knee and directing the cannula under arthroscopic visualization, the inside-out sutures can be placed (Fig. 8-15).

Under direct visualization, place the suture cannula against the meniscus in the desired location. I use a second assistant to help pass the needles through the cannula. Pass the needle to the end of the cannula which is against the meniscus. Visualize the tip of the needle by slightly retracting (3 to 5 mm) the cannula within the joint. Pierce the unstable meniscus fragment with the needle tip. The needle can then be used to aid in the tear reduction. Confirming the tear is anatomically reduced; proceed with delivering the needle into the peripheral rim fragment and through the capsule. Place the needles through the meniscus with the knee flexed approximately 10 to 20 degrees. Once the needle is through the meniscus, it is helpful to flex the knee to 45 to 60 degrees, which will facilitate posterior retrieval.

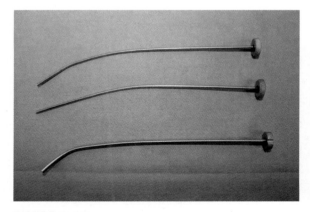

FIGURE 8-12

Commercially available single- and double-lumen suture cannulas (Acufex, Andover, MA).

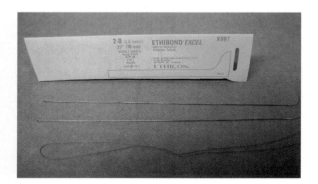

FIGURE 8-13

Ten-inch flexible needles with attached 2.0 Ethibond suture are used for the repair (Ethicon, Inc., Somerville, NJ).

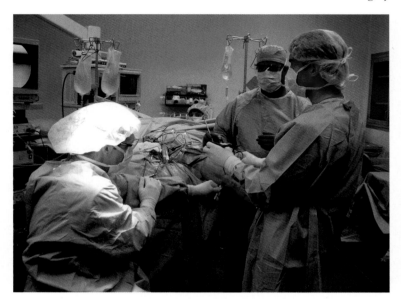

FIGURE 8-14

The foot of the table is flexed to allow the assistant improved access to receive needles through the medial approach.

Slowly advance the needles, paying strict attention to how far they are inserted. If the needle is inserted approximately 1 to 1.5 cm and the needle tip cannot be visualized, the needle is retracted and retractor placement is reassessed (look further inferior and lateral). Sutures are typically placed from posterior to anterior. Alternatively, an anterior suture may be placed giving the retrieving assistant a reference point for placement of additional posterior sutures. Once the first needle tip is visualized, it is grasped with the needle driver by the assistant and pulled out of the posterior capsule (often bending the needles) (Fig. 8-16).

Once the first needle is delivered out of the incision, the single-barrel cannula is redirected. To help avoid laceration to the suture, slight tension is applied to the suture and the second needle is delivered down the cannula adjacent to the suture (Fig. 8-17). In a similar fashion, the second needle is placed, thus creating either a vertical, oblique, or horizontal stitch. Care is taken to ensure the sutures will anatomically reduce the tear. Multiple sutures are passed in a similar fashion (Fig. 8-18).

The assistant sequentially cuts off the needles and tags the sutures with a hemostat. You can either tie as you go or clamp several sutures before tying. If greater than 3 or 4 sutures are placed, it is helpful to tie this group and then proceed, so as to avoid tangling (Fig. 8-19). When tying medial sutures, the knee should be held in full extension with the meniscus reduced under direct visualization. This will avoid imbrication of the posteromedial capsule which may cause a postoperative flexion contracture. Be careful not to overtighten the sutures.

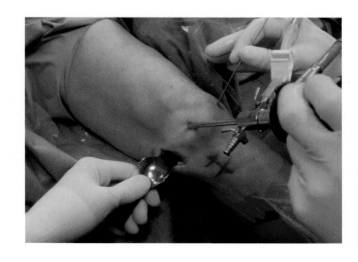

FIGURE 8-15

A valgus stress is applied to the knee by the surgeon while holding the scope in the medial portal and directing the suture cannula from the lateral portal.

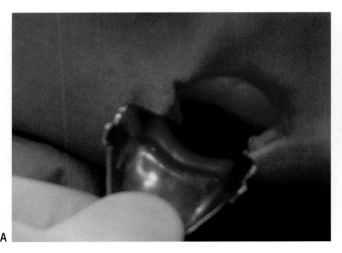 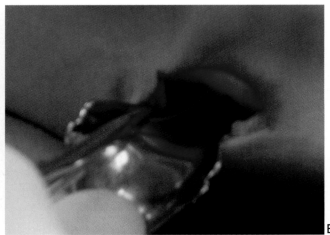

FIGURE 8-16

A: The first needle pierces through the posterior capsule. **B:** The 10-inch needle is pulled through with a needle driver.

A vertical suture pattern is the preferred technique due to increased capture of the strong circumferential fibers of the meniscus. However, it is very useful to often use an oblique or horizontal pattern and to place these sutures both on the femoral and tibial side of the meniscus (Fig. 8-20). Sutures should be placed approximately 3 to 5 mm apart. The number of sutures will depend on the character and stability of the repair.

Biologic Augmentation

There are different methods to potentially improve the biologic healing capacity of a meniscus repair (Table 8-1). In the setting of marginal vascularity, I will create vascular access channels using an 18-gauge spinal needle. The needle (bend to help maneuver) is used from inside-out through the meniscus after the repair has been performed. Perforate into the meniscocapsular junction to pro-

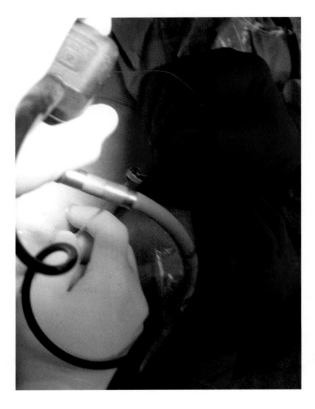

FIGURE 8-17

The second needle is delivered down the single-lumen cannula adjacent to the suture, which is placed on slight tension.

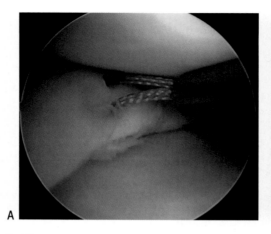
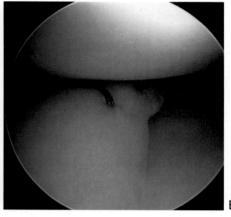

FIGURE 8-18

A: The single-lumen suture cannula is used to place a vertical stitch. **B:** The loop of Ethibond suture is pulled through the cannula.

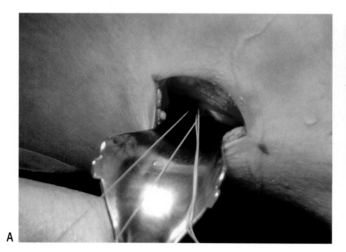
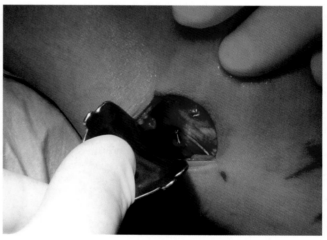

FIGURE 8-19

A: Sutures are delivered and tagged through the posteromedial incision. **B:** With the knee in full extension, sutures are tied over the posteromedial joint capsule.

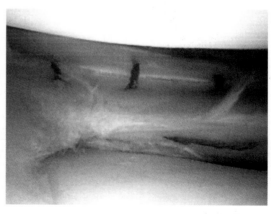

FIGURE 8-20

Sutures are placed on both the femoral and tibial sides of the meniscus.

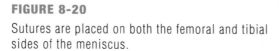

TABLE 8-1.   **Biologic Augmentation Techniques for Meniscus Repair**
• Vascular access channels • Fibrin clot* • Limited notchplasty (creation of hemarthrosis)* • Platelet-rich plasma*
*Option if not combined with ACL reconstruction.

mote bleeding and vascular inflow. Be careful not to damage sutures and do not go through the capsule behind the posterior horn of the lateral meniscus (popliteal vessels). If the repair is not combined with an ACL reconstruction, I will create a postoperative hemarthrosis by performing a limited notchplasty of the lateral femoral condyle. A 5.5-mm full radius shaver is used to create a bleeding cancellous bone bed being careful not to injure the ACL (Fig. 8-21). I have evolved to using this technique instead of placing a fibrin clot.

The subcutaneous tissue and skin are closed in separate layers. Drains are not used in the joint or posterior incisions. The joint and incisions are injected with 20 to 30 ml of 0.5% plain Ropivacaine combined with 5 mg of Duramorph. Alternatively, 0.5% plain Marcaine may be substituted for Ropivacaine. After the dressing is applied, a cold therapy device and postoperative brace locked in full extension are placed in the operating room.

Technique for Lateral Meniscus Repair

The general principles for a lateral meniscal repair are the same as for a medial repair. The anteromedial portal often needs to be slightly superior to avoid obstruction from the tibial eminence when placing suture cannulas to the posterior horn of the lateral meniscus. Use a spinal needle to plan this portal with the leg in the figure-of-4 position. If necessary, you can always make a second anteromedial portal more superior. Once the meniscal edges are prepared, the posterolateral approach is made. The knee is placed into a figure-of-4 position, which places the knee in approximately 70 to 90 degrees of flexion. This will take tension off the peroneal nerve, biceps tendon, and lateral head of the gastrocnemius and place a varus stress on the joint. Alternatively, it is often helpful to place the leg over the side of the table, flexing the knee to 90 degrees. In this position, the surgeon can perform the posterolateral dissection in a less awkward position. Once the dissection is carried out and the retractor is placed, the leg can be repositioned into the figure-of-4 with the foot on the table.

A vertical incision is placed just posterior to the lateral collateral ligament (LCL). Translumination through the joint may aid in identifying the proper plane and level. With the knee in a figure-of-4 position, the LCL can typically be palpated from the fibular styloid to the lateral epicondyle. The incision is 3 to 4 cm with two thirds of the incision below the joint line. The interval between the iliotibial band and biceps tendon is incised. The biceps tendon is a valuable landmark since the peroneal nerve, which is at risk during this procedure, is located posteromedial to the biceps tendon. By staying anterior to the biceps tendon and lateral head of the gastrocnemius, the nerve should be protected. Carrying the dissection deeper, identify the interval between the lateral head of the gastrocnemius and the posterolateral joint capsule. Once the interval is started with Metzenbaum scissors, the muscle can be bluntly dissected off the capsule using either a blunt key elevator or your finger.

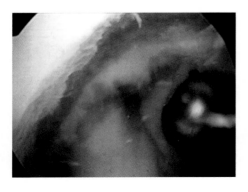

FIGURE 8-21

Postoperative hemarthrosis is created by performing a limited notchplasty.

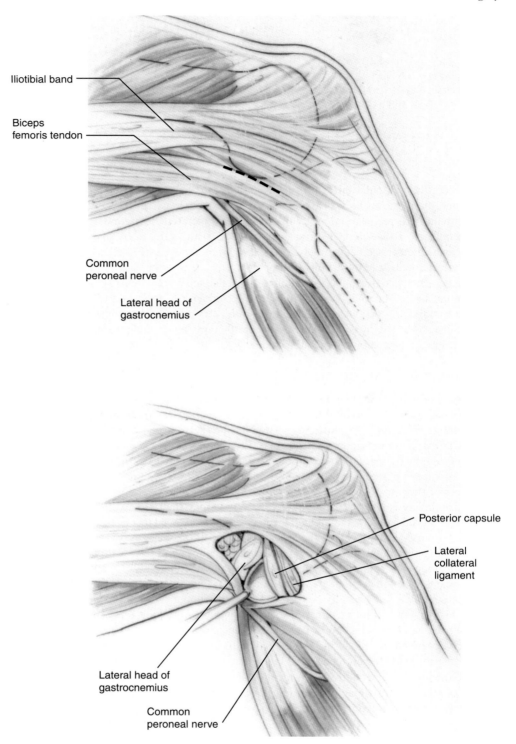

Iliotibial band

Biceps
femoris tendon

Common
peroneal nerve

Lateral head of
gastrocnemius

Posterior capsule

Lateral
collateral
ligament

Lateral head of
gastrocnemius

Common
peroneal nerve

A

FIGURE 8-22

A: The proper interval dissection for the posterolateral approach. Note the location of the peroneal nerve, which is at risk during this approach. **B:** Retractor placement in relation to the neurovascular structures.

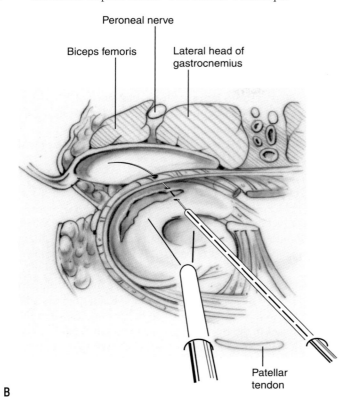

Peroneal nerve

Biceps femoris   Lateral head of
                        gastrocnemius

Patellar
tendon

B

FIGURE 8-22
(Continued)

The interval development is facilitated by starting distal to the joint line. Similar to the medial side, you may use your index finger to confirm you are anterior to the lateral head of the gastrocnemius by plantar flexing and dorsiflexing the foot. Once in the proper interval directly against the postero-lateral joint capsule, the popliteal retractor should be placed to protect the neurovascular structures (Fig. 8-22). The suture cannulas are placed through the anteromedial portal. Debridement of the fat pad will facilitate passage of the cannula. Suture cannulas are not used from the anterolateral portal due to the potential risk to the popliteal vessels, which are just posterior to the posterior horn of the lateral meniscus. The assistant receiving needles sits on a stool. It is often helpful to elevate the table and remove the lateral post to improve the assistant's comfort and visualization. Sutures are placed in a similar fashion to the medial side. Do not to advance the needle beyond 1 to 1.5 cm before vi-sualizing the needle coming through the posteromedial capsule or reflecting into the surgical field off the posterior retractor. Once retrieved, sutures can either be clamped or tied individually. Cap-ture of the posterolateral capsule is typically not an issue as on the medial side and therefore the su-tures are tied with the knee in 70 to 90 degrees of flexion. Although some authors have advocated tying the sutures after the ACL reconstruction is performed, I have found it helpful to tie them at the time of the meniscus surgery. This tends to save time by avoiding the need to re-expose and replace retractors later in the case. One difference between the lateral side and the medial side is dealing with the popliteus tendon. I place sutures adjacent to the popliteus tendon, but not through the tendon. However, other authors have not reported problems with placing sutures through the tendon.

Closure is similar to the medial side except that the interval between the iliotibial band and biceps is closed using vicryl sutures.

Pearls and Pitfalls

- Debride the edges of a bucket handle tear with the tear displaced anterior (allows direct visu-alization).

- Perform the posterolateral approach with the knee flexed over the side of the table. Once the retractor is placed, place the leg into the figure-of-4 position.
- Dissecting gastrocnemius off the posterior joint capsule is facilitated by starting distal.
- Always place suture cannulas through the anteromedial portal for a lateral repair.
- Pass the needles through the medial meniscus in greater extension (10 to 20 degrees) and once through the meniscus, flex the knee to 60 degrees to retrieve the needles posterior.
- If you have difficulty visualizing needles coming through the posterior capsule, place a more anterior suture (easier to locate) and use this suture as a guide for posterior sutures.
- A limited notchplasty is an easy way to create a postoperative hemarthrosis (similar to ACL reconstruction)

POSTOPERATIVE MANAGEMENT

A postoperative long leg hinged knee brace locked in full extension is worn at night and when ambulating for the first 6 weeks. The brace should be removed by the patient, as well as the therapist, for range of motion exercises up to 90 degrees for the first 6 weeks. The brace is discontinued at 6 weeks.

The patient is allowed immediate weight bearing as tolerated with the knee locked in full extension. Weight bearing with flexion is not allowed during the first 6 weeks. Radial repairs are kept non–weight bearing for the first 6 weeks followed by progressive weight bearing. Range of motion exercises between 0 and 90 degrees are allowed in the first 6 weeks. For tenuous repairs, motion is limited from 0 to 60 degrees for the first 4 weeks (isolated repair only). Between 6 and 12 weeks, range of motion is progressively increased. Closed kinetic chain quadriceps exercises and hamstring exercises are started at 4 to 6 weeks, but no resistance exercises beyond 80 degrees of flexion are allowed for 6 months. Squatting is not allowed for 6 months postoperatively. Straight line running is allowed at 4 to 4-1/2 months. Return to full sports for an isolated repair is 6 months as long as strength is adequate. Repairs performed in conjunction with an ACL reconstruction follow the ACL protocol with the addition of no squatting for 6 months.

COMPLICATIONS

Injury to the saphenous nerve can be avoided by careful dissection and retraction of the nerve with the sartorius muscle.

Injury to the peroneal nerve can occur when inadvertently placing needles without adequate retraction. This should be avoided by taking tension off the nerve with knee flexion and by adequately protecting the nerve behind the biceps and lateral head of the gastrocnemius with the popliteal retractor.

To avoid popliteal vessel injury, needles should always be directed away from the midline toward the posterior exposure. Be extremely careful when placing needles into the posterior horn of the lateral meniscus. Always bring suture cannulas from the anteromedial portal across for a lateral repair.

To prevent limitation of motion, tie the posteromedial sutures with the knee in extension, avoiding imbrication of the posterior capsule, which may subsequently cause a flexion contracture. Immediate range of motion should be instituted when combined with an ACL reconstruction, since this group is at higher risk for this complication.

Infection rates are relatively low (0% to 2%). The hospital staff should wash down the suture cannulas to properly sterilize.

RESULTS

Studies have reported successful meniscus repair in more than 90% of patients who have inside-out repairs performed in conjunction with ACL reconstruction. In contrast, a 40% to 50% failure rate is expected when performed in the setting of persistent functional ACL instability. Isolated repairs (intact ACL) have an approximately 70% to 85% clinical success rate. In general, lateral meniscal repairs have improved healing rates when compared with medial repairs. Nonabsorbable sutures have been reported to have lower clinical failure rates compared with absorbable sutures. Recent reports show that even in patients over the age 40, over 85% of repairs were asymptomatic at the latest follow-up (most combined with ACL reconstruction).

RECOMMENDED READING

Baratz ME, Fu FH, Mengato R. Meniscal tears: the effect of meniscectomy and of repair on intra-articular contact areas and stress in the human knee. *Am J Sports Med.* 1986;14:270–275.

Cannon WD, Vittori JM. The incidence of healing in arthroscopic meniscal repairs in anterior cruciate ligament reconstructed knees versus stable knees. *Am J Sports Med.* 1992;20:176–181.

Lindenfeld T. Inside-out meniscus repair. *Instr Course Lect.* 2005;54:331–336.

Morgan CD, Wojtys EM, Casscells CD, et al. Arthroscopic meniscal repair evaluated by second-look arthroscopy. *Am J Sports Med.* 1991;17:632–638.

O'Shea JJ, Shelbourne KD. Repair of locked bucket handle meniscus tears in knees with chronic anterior cruciate ligament deficiency. *Am J Sports Med.* 2003;31:216–220.

Rosenberg TD, Scott SM, Coward DP, et al. Arthroscopic meniscal repair evaluated with repeat arthroscopy. *Arthroscopy.* 1984;2:14–20.

Rubman MH, Noyes FR, Barber-Westin SD. Arthroscopic repair of meniscal tears that extend into the avascular zone. A review of 198 single and complex tears. *Am J Sports Med.* 1998;26:1987–1995.

Tenuta JJ, Arciero RA. Arthroscopic evaluation of meniscal repairs. Factors that affect healing. *Am J Sports Med.* 1994;22:797–802.

Watson FJ, Arciero RA. Inside-out meniscus repair. *Oper Tech Sports Med.* 2003;11(2):104–126.

Wolf BR, Rodeo SA. Arthroscopic meniscus repair with suture: inside-out with fibrin clot. *Sports Med Arthrosc.* 2004;12:15–24.

9 Meniscal Repair with Meniscal Fixators

Peter R. Kurzweil

The fixation of meniscal tears has undergone a revolution since the introduction of fixators into arthroscopic surgery a decade ago. The simplicity and ease of insertion of these devices led to their popularity for the repair of torn menisci. The only alternative was the traditional suture technique, which required additional incisions, prolonged operative time, and the risk of neurovascular injury.

The first fixators on the market were somewhat rigid devices made of a variety of bioabsorbable materials, with varying resorption times. They are supplied in varying lengths, with the appropriate size chosen depending on the location of the tear. They were designed with barbs, heads, or screw threads to engage meniscal tissue, and therefore are not well suited for the most peripheral tears or capsular detachments. Compression at the tear site is often difficult to achieve and nearly impossible to adjust after insertion. Among the most popular first-generation fixators are the Arrow, the Hornet, the Clearfix Screw, and the Dart.

With increasing reports of unsatisfactory long-term results and the inability to repair peripheral tears to the capsule, a second generation of meniscal fixators was developed to more closely mimic suture repairs. The two suture-based implants currently available are the Fast-Fix (Smith & Nephew, Endoscopy Division, Andover, MA) and the RAPIDLOC (Mitek Surgical Products, Westwood, MA) (Fig. 9-1A,B). Both of these implants consist of two small polymer T-bar anchors connected by a pre-tied, locking, sliding knot, which has eliminated the need for arthroscopic knot tying. Both Fast-Fix anchors and one of the RAPIDLOC anchors are designed to be deployed across the capsule, then rotate to engage the capsule when the connecting suture is pulled, analogous to EndoButton (Smith & Nephew, Andover, MA) fixation. Since the suture length between the two anchors adjusts during implantation to allow compression of the tear, these fixators come in only one size. The only variability is the angle of the needle delivery system. But, like other fixators, the anchors deployed across the capsule cannot be removed arthroscopically once inserted.

The Fast-Fix Delivery Needle is supplied with three angles: 0, +22, and −22 degrees (Fig. 9-1D). The −22-degree needle allows suture placement on the undersurface of the meniscus. The device requires that each anchor be deployed across the capsule, and at least one also pass through the tear. This allows for a vertical or horizontal suture orientation. The Rapid-Loc comes with needle tips of 0, 12, and 27 degrees (Fig. 9-1C). It is designed to be placed on the superior surface of the meniscus. Its insertion requires only one pass of the "backstop" anchor across the tear and through the capsule. Both fixators come with anchors and sutures that are permanent or bioabsorbable. The choice depends on surgeon preference. I prefer permanent material, as is my choice when doing the traditional inside-out or outside-in suture repair techniques.

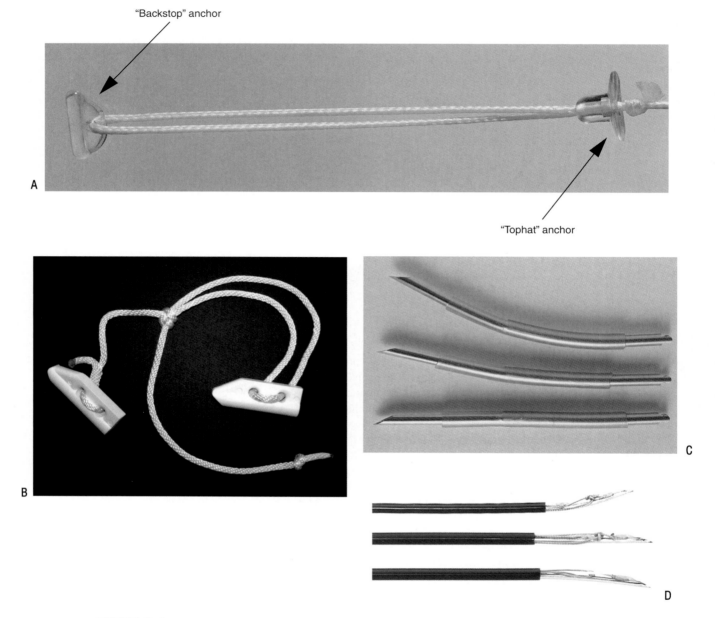

FIGURE 9-1

A: The Rapid-Loc is made of two anchors called the "top-hat" and "backstop," which are connected by a pre-tied, sliding suture of No. 2 nonabsorbable Ethibond (Ethicon, Somerville, NJ). Note that it is also available with absorbable components using a PDS "top-hat" and Panacryl suture. **B:** The Fast-Fix is made of two 5-mm anchors also connected by a pre-tied, sliding No. 0 suture of nonabsorbable, braided polyester. **C:** The angles for the insertion needles for the Rapid-Loc are 0, 12, and 27 degrees. **D:** The Fast-Fix is supplied with three insertion angles of 0, +22, and −22 degrees.

INDICATIONS/CONTRAINDICATIONS

The indication for meniscal repair should remain the same regardless of technique. Fixators are not ideal to use for every tear location and orientation. My preference is to use outside-in suture repairs for anterior third tears, and once started, I will often stretch this to the anterior two thirds of the meniscus. Fixators are most ideal for the posterior third, where the traditional inside-out technique would have required a posterior incision to protect neurovascular structures. For tears entirely in the posterior half of the meniscus, I will generally use suture-based fixators only. However, there is no reason to commit to just one method of fixation. I frequently use hybrid fixation, with outside-in sutures anteriorly and fixators posteriorly. Cost is an issue, and these second-generation fixators are far more expensive than using sutures.

In my experience, unstable bucket-handle tears, which are found displaced in the notch, have sometimes failed when fixators alone were used. Although these failures were seen with first-generation fixators, this led me to favor the traditional suture repair techniques for this scenario. Recently, I have been more confident with hybrid repairs using suture-based fixators and outside-in sutures for these displaced bucket-handle tears.

Tear orientation is also important. Ideally, fixators (and sutures) should be inserted into the meniscus so that they are perpendicular to the tear, making vertically oriented tears ideal. Horizontal cleavage tears and radial tears are less suited for fixators, and sutures are preferred if a repair is indicated. Some surgeons are attempting to use the Fast-Fix in these situations.

SURGERY

Patient Positioning

We prefer to have the patient supine on the operating room table, allowing the knees to rest in extension. A tourniquet is applied to the proximal thigh but is not routinely inflated. A lateral thigh post clamped to the table allows application of a valgus stress to the knee, opening the medial compartment for visualization. For viewing the lateral compartment, the leg is placed in the figure-4 position. We have also found that general anesthesia affords a little extra room in the compartments, since valgus or varus stressing to open the knee is sometimes too painful with only local anesthesia.

Meniscal Preparation

Although fixators are simple to use, they should not be inserted immediately on visualization of the tear. The tear site needs to be prepared just as it would be for any repair technique. The edges on both sides of the tear are debrided of fibrous tissue with a shaver or rasp. The capsular attachment at the meniscal–synovial border is abraded with a rasp or motorized shaver to stimulate a healing response (bleeding). The meniscus rim may also be trephinated to produce vascular access channels. This can be quickly done using an 18- or 20-gauge needle from outside in or a meniscal repair needle through a cannula introduced through a portal.

The best results are obtained when the meniscus tear is optimally reduced. Surgeons strive for an anatomic reduction with fractures, and should do the same with torn menisci. With very unstable tears, we have found it convenient to hold the reduction with temporary fixation, much like using a K-wire to for provisional fracture fixation. Use a probe under arthroscopic visualization to help reduce the tear and give counter-pressure as a small needle is inserted from outside-in across the tear (Fig. 9-2). At this point the fixators can be inserted.

Fixator Insertion

The needle angle and portal of entry are selected to provide the most perpendicular approach to the tear. This is usually best accomplished through the contralateral portal. Once again fixation of a fracture is a well-suited anaology, as screws are inserted perpendicular to the orientation of the break. Sometimes with posterior tears near the root, the best approach is through the ipsilateral portal. In these situations, particular attention needs to be given to the neurovascular bundles.

The fixator insertion needle first engages the central portion of the tear, which is manipulated to achieve the best anatomic reduction before passing the needle across the tear, through the peripheral portion of the menicus and the capsule. If the reduction of the tear is difficult to achieve with the fixator insertion device, the outside-in needle "trick" described previously can be used.

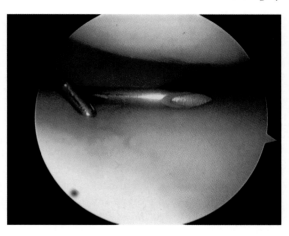

FIGURE 9-2

With unstable large meniscus tears, it is sometimes convenient to hold the reduction with temporary fixation, much like using a K-wire for provisional fracture fixation. A probe is used to manipulate the tear and give counterpressure as a small needle is inserted from outside-in across the tear.

The number of fixators used depends on the length and stability of the tear. They are generally spaced 5 to 8 mm apart. Once the repair has been completed, the knee is ranged (with the arthroscope removed) and then the tear is probed to assess stability and gapping. If the repair site gaps, supplemental fixation should be considered. In cases requiring concomitant anterior cruciate ligament (ACL) reconstruction, the meniscal pathology is addressed first.

Pearls and Pitfalls

Although the Rapid-Loc is supplied with three different angles, we almost always use the 12-degree angle. It allows the best angle of approach to the tears, whether directing the insertion needle vertically or horizontally. Also, for stocking purposes, it simplifies having to have more than one. Before inserting the fixator into the knee, the top-hat anchor is slid halfway down the loop, closer to the tip. The metal skid supplied by Mitek is introduced into the portal and carefully directed toward the tear with caution to avoid scuffing the articular cartilage. The fixator is inserted through the portal such that the curve of the needle and the top-hat anchor are angled toward the metal skid to avoid dragging the fat pad into the knee. The trailing suture is held under some tension, keeping the top-hat anchor flat against the "meniscal applier" deployment device during this manuever. The meniscus should be penetrated at least 3 mm central to the tear (Fig. 9-3A,B). After inserting the needle across the tear, with the depth of penetration limited by a built-in stop, the trigger is pressed to deploy the backstop anchor (Fig. 9-3C). The trigger is held depressed as the insertion needle is withdrawn for the knee joint, leaving the suture trailing out of the portal. This suture is loaded through the eyelet of the tensioning-cutting instrument, which is used to bring the top-hat anchor down onto the superior surface of the meniscus, just under the pre-tied, sliding knot. Compression is adjusted with a push-pull manuever. Slight dimpling of the meniscus is preferred before cutting the suture (Fig. 9-3D).

The Fast-Fix anchor, like the Rapid-Loc, is generally inserted in the portal contralateral to the tear. Occasionally, posterior horn tears are best approached through the ispilateral portal. A curved meniscal depth probe is inserted to simulate the angle of repair before selecting fixator needle angle and insertion portal. The selected portal is spread with a snap to avoid fat-pad entrapment. This device comes with a blue plastic cannula to help ensure a smooth entry into the joint, although the metal skid from the Rapid-Loc works well here, too. Once again, the straight (0-degree) device is rarely used and is generally not carried in our surgery center to facilitate stocking. Most of the time the 122-degree fixator is used. The −22-degree fixator works well to keep the meniscus from flouncing or puckering in the superior direction by placing an occasional horizontal mattress suture on the undersurface of the meniscus. When creating vertical sutures, the first pass is superior, often over

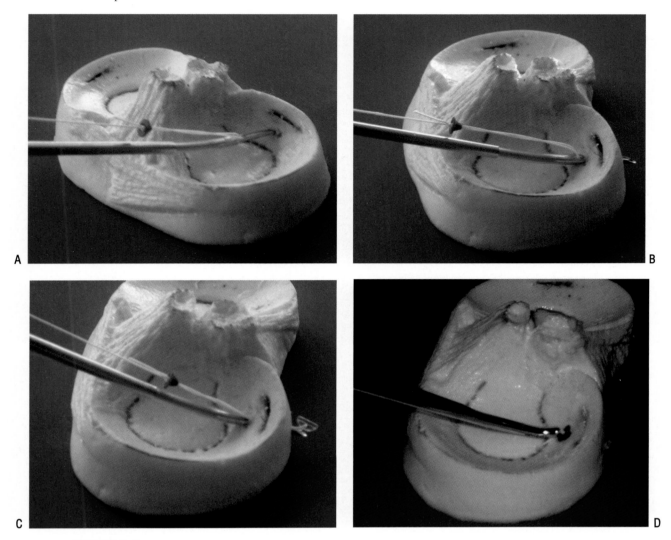

FIGURE 9-3

Rapid-Loc insertion. **A:** The delivery needle is placed 3 mm central to the tear. **B:** The insertion needle penetrates across the tear and through the capsule. **C:** The trigger is depressed to deploy the backstop anchor behind the capsule. **D:** The top-hat anchor is brought down onto the meniscus and tensioned with the pusher-cutter instrument.

the meniscus directly into the capsule. Placing the second anchor through the tear, more inferiorly, facilitates cutting and tensioning the knot, which tends to slide toward the second anchor. With horizontal suture placment, the first anchor is usually placed more anteriorly.

After the first pass, the needle is slowly retracted, leaving the first anchor behind the capsule (Fig. 9-4A,B). The pre-tied knot is usually a good reference for depth of insertion. While still in the joint and under arthroscopic visualization, the second anchor is "clicked" into position by sliding the gold trigger forward on the handle of insertion device (Fig. 9-4C). After its deployment the insertion device is removed, leaving only a single suture trailing out the portal (Fig. 9-5A). This suture is loaded on the "suture cutter and knot pusher," and the suture is pulled, advancing the sliding knot and reducing the tear (Fig. 9-5B). The knot is cinched down directly onto the meniscus and tension of the construct adjusted with a push-pull action (Fig. 9-5C). The suture/knot is appropriately tensioned before it is cut (Fig. 9-5D). The white "depth penetration limiter" is helpful in the learning phase of using this device to avoid plunging in the back of the knee. With experience, the surgeon gains confidence with the feel of the needle penetrating the capsule. I no longer use this protection sheath except when working near the root of the meniscus, or using the device through the portal ispilateral to the tear.

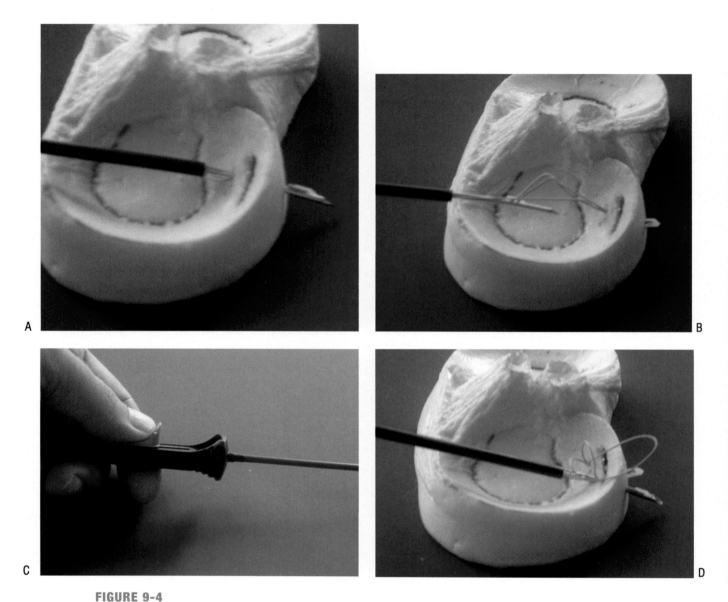

FIGURE 9-4

Fast-Fix insertion. **A:** The needle penetrates the meniscus 3 mm central and passes through the capsule. **B:** The insertion device is slowly withdrawn, leaving the first anchor behind the capsule. **C:** The gold trigger is pushed forward to advance the second anchor into the ready position. **D:** The second anchor is inserted approximately 5 mm away and deployed across the capsule.

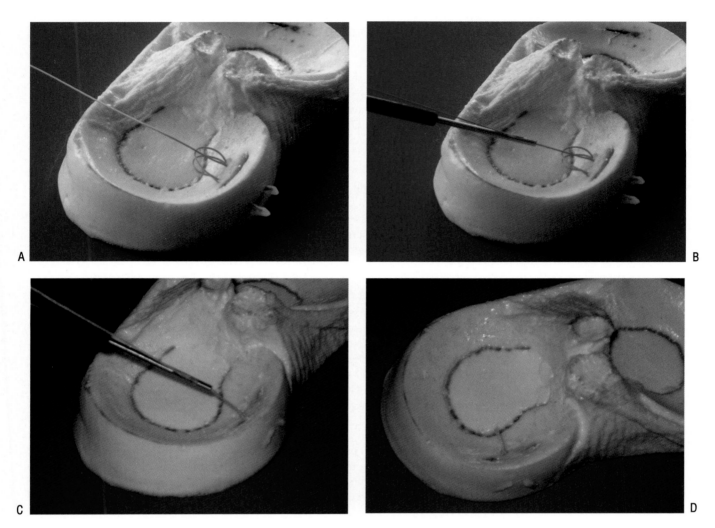

FIGURE 9-5

A: The insertion device is withdrawn from the joint, leaving a suture trailing out of the portal. **B:** The suture is loaded on the "suture cutter and knot pusher" device, although the knot is initially advanced and the meniscus reduced by just pulling on the suture. **C:** The instrument helps set the tension on the knot with a push-pull action. **D:** The suture is cut.

POSTOPERATIVE MANAGEMENT

We do not follow an "aggressive" postoperative protocol. For the first 2 weeks postsurgery, patients are instructed to use a knee immobilizer and crutches for toe-touch weight bearing. Progressive weight bearing in the knee immobilizer is allowed during weeks 3 and 4. Patients are encouraged to range the knee only when seated or supine beginning the week 3. Unrestricted walking occurs at 1 month, and use of the stationary bike is recommended. Squatting is avoided for 4 months, and return to cutting and pivoting sports is delayed 6 months. When concomitant ACL reconstruction is performed, the postoperative regimen of the meniscus repair takes precedence.

COMPLICATIONS

There are numerous reports of complications with the first-generation fixators, particularly the Arrow, as noted previously. (The Arrow has since been redesigned to have a lower profile.) Complications with the suture-based fixators are much less frequent, and often appear to be related to deployment or insertion problems. There is only one report of the top-hat anchor of the Rapid-Loc scoring the femoral articular cartilage.

RESULTS

Although short-term studies with first-generation fixators were initially favorable, the results decreased over time and were associated with various complications. Reports described scoring the overlying articular cartilage of the femoral condyle, implant breakage, and protrusion of the tip of the device at the joint line. My experience with the Arrow became quite unsatisfactory with longer follow-up. In 60 repairs followed an average of 4.5 years, we experienced failure in 28% of our cases. The failure rate rose to 42% with isolated repairs, not accompanied by an ACL reconstruction. Similar results have have been reported by others, which has led us to abandone the use of first-generation fixators.

The results of suture-based fixators appear to be more promising. One recent report showed a success rate of 91% in 54 repairs after 35 months with the Rapid-Loc. Several published studies on the Fast-Fix have also shown promising results. The success rate in these reports ranged from 86% to 91% with follow-up periods varying from 18 to 32 months.

RECOMMENDED READING

Barber FA, Herbert MA, Richards DP. Load to failure testing of new meniscal repair devices. *Arthroscopy*. 2004; 20(1):45–50.

Barber FA, Johnson DH, Halbrecht JL. Arthroscopic meniscal repair using the BioStinger. *Arthroscopy*. 2005; 21(6):744–750.

Buchalter DP, Karzel R, Friedman M, et al. Evaluation of all-inside arthroscopic meniscal repair using the FasT-Fix System (SS-35). *Arthroscopy*. 2006;22;6(suppl):e18–e19.

Haas AL, Schepsis AA, Hornstein J, et al. Meniscal repair using the FasT-Fix all-inside meniscal repair device. *Arthroscopy*. 2005;21(2):167–175.

Kotsovolos ES, Hantes ME, Mastrokalos DS, et al. Results of all-inside meniscal repair with the FasT-Fix Meniscal Repair System. *Arthroscopy*. 2006;22(1):3–9.

Kurzweil PR, Lemos MJ. Meniscal repair with first generation fixators. *Sports Med Arthrosc Rev*. 2004;12:37–43.

Kurzweil PR, Tifford CD, Ignacio EM. Unsatisfactory clinical results of meniscal repair using the meniscus arrow. *Arthroscopy*. 2005;21(8):905.e1–905.e7.

Quinby JS, Golish SR, Hart J, et al. All-inside meniscal repair using a new flexible, tensionable device (SS-37). *Arthroscopy*. 2006;22;6(suppl):e19–e20.

Sgaglione NA. Meniscus repair update: current concepts and new techniques. *Orthopedics*. 2005;28(3):280–286.

Sgaglione NA. New generation meniscus fixator devices. *Sports Med Arthrosc Rev*. 2004;12:44–59.

Sgaglione NA, Steadman JR, Shaffer B, et al. Current concepts in meniscus surgery: resection to replacement. *Arthroscopy*. 2003;19;Dec(suppl):161–188.

10 Meniscal Transplantation without Bone Plugs

Fotios P. Tjoumakaris, Anthony M. Buoncristiani, and Christopher D. Harner

The meniscus plays a vital role in the successful performance and well-being of the knee. Loss of the meniscus, in part or in total, significantly alters joint functions and predisposes the articular cartilage to degenerative change. Meniscal transplantation has been developed in an attempt to alter the natural history of the postmeniscectomy knee. The procedure is performed in hopes of forestalling progressive joint deterioration by theoretically restoring part of the meniscal function.

Surgical techniques for meniscal transplantation have evolved over the last decade from mainly open arthrotomies to arthroscopically assisted techniques, with or without the use of bone plugs (or blocks) at the meniscal horn attachments. Proper patient selection as well as realistic patient goals and expectations are vital to avoid unnecessary failures. Results from long-term outcome studies should help to further refine meniscal allograft techniques as well as its indications and improve our understanding of where this procedure belongs in the treatment algorithm of the postmeniscectomy knee.

INDICATIONS/CONTRAINDICATIONS

The ideal candidate for a meniscal allograft transplant has joint line pain secondary to meniscal deficiency and fits the following criteria: (a) documented evidence of a previous subtotal or total meniscectomy or its biomechanical equivalent; (b) ligamentously stable or concurrently performed ligament reconstruction; (c) early grade I or II articular cartilage changes as determined by the use of a 45 degrees posteroanterior (PA) flexion weight-bearing radiograph; (d) no evidence of malalignment as determined on standing long cassette views; and (e) no evidence of articular incongruity on diagnostic arthroscopy. All patients are informed during preoperative counseling that the ultimate decision to proceed with the transplant is made in the operating room. Contraindications to transplantation include grade III or IV changes in the involved compartment, ligamentous instability, malalignment that would place significant stress on the allograft, and a patient with unrealistic expectations regarding outcome.

PREOPERATIVE PLANNING

Physical Examination

Candidates being considered for meniscal transplant surgery require a comprehensive examination of both lower extremities. Height and weight should be recorded as an indication of body habitus as well as the standing alignment of the lower extremities. The patient's ability to squat and any limitations in movement and associated discomfort are noted. It is important to observe the gait of the patient for any abnormalities. Both knees are examined for the presence of an effusion.

The patella must be examined and a thorough ligamentous examination performed with special attention placed on the anterior cruciate ligament (ACL) status. This is done through the Lachman test, pivot shift, and anterior drawer in neutral, internal, and external rotation. The posterior cruciate ligament (PCL) is evaluated with the posterior drawer and posterior sag with the hip and knee flexed to 90 degrees. Posterolateral rotatory instability is ruled out through the dial test, reverse pivot shift, and the posterolateral drawer. The collaterals are tested with varus and valgus stress at 0 and 30 degrees of knee flexion. It is important to elicit the presence or absence of joint line tenderness over the involved and the uninvolved compartments as well as the presence of hyperflexion signs.

Imaging

We routinely obtain four views of the knee in meniscal transplant candidates. This includes a PA 45-degree flexion weight-bearing view, Merchant, lateral, and long cassette from the hips to the ankles to evaluate the mechanical axis. From these studies the alignment and joint space of the involved knee is calculated and compared with the opposite asymptomatic knee. Patients who have a mechanical axis deviation toward the involved compartment require a staged or combined osteotomy in addition to transplantation. We routinely obtain a magnetic resonance image (MRI) of the knee to assess the quality and amount of remaining meniscal tissue. In patients whose pain is nonspecific, a three-phase ^{99}Tc bone scan is obtained. Increased uptake in the compartment indicates early degenerative changes.

Before the definitive procedure, the amount of remaining meniscus, the quality of the articular surface, and any associated ligamentous injuries must be verified so they may be addressed at the time of surgery. If necessary, this can involve an examination under anesthesia and a diagnostic arthroscopy staged before transplantation. The plain radiographs are also used to determine the appropriate size for the allograft tissue as required for the tissue bank.

SURGERY

Positioning, Draping, and Operating Room Organization

The patient is positioned supine on a regular operating room table with a sandbag taped to the table at the foot of the bed to hold the leg at 90 degrees of knee flexion. A standard side post is used at the level of the greater trochanter to provide a fulcrum for valgus stress and to provide lateral support with the knee at 90 degrees of flexion. A tourniquet is not routinely used for the procedure. The extremity is prepped from the tourniquet distally with alcohol and betadine and draped with a nonimpervious stockinette, extremity drape, and a half sheet to cover the post. A bolster is placed between the lateral thigh and the post (Fig. 10-1).

The operating room should be organized to provide a controlled environment where traffic and the potential for contamination are kept to a minimum. It is necessary to have a separate table for graft preparation that has an oscillating saw, drill, and instruments.

Specific Approaches

All incision sites as well as the joint are marked before prepping and draping, prepped out with a betadine stick, and injected with 1% lidocaine with epinephrine. A standard arthroscopy is performed using an anterolateral-viewing portal just adjacent to the patellar tendon and above the joint line and an anteromedial working portal 1 cm medial to the medial edge of the patellar tendon. Two main approaches are used in both the medial and lateral transplants: the anteromedial or lateral and the posteromedial or lateral approaches. The anterior approach involves an extension of the arthroscopy skin incision superiorly along the patellar tendon. A medial or lateral parapatellar arthrotomy is

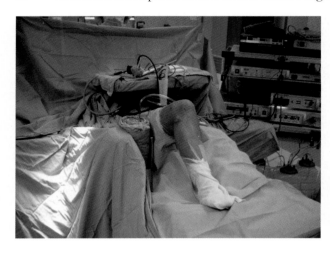

FIGURE 10-1

The extremity is prepped, draped, and positioned so that it can rest at 90 degrees of flexion.

made. Often it is necessary to remove a small amount of the fat pad to visualize the joint. The anterior horn of the remaining meniscus should be well visualized. Three No. 2 braided nonabsorbable sutures are passed around the remaining anterior horn, leaving the needles attached for later fixation to the allograft.

The posteromedial approach involves a skin incision 3 cm long just anterior to the posterior margin of the medial femoral condyle. One third of the incision should be above the joint line. Careful dissection is used to divide the subcutaneous fat, and care is taken to look for and protect the infrapatellar branch of the saphenous nerve, which typically crosses just above the joint line. The sartorial fascia (layer 1) is then divided in line with the skin incision and a posterior capsulotomy is made between the posterior border of the medial collateral ligament and the posterior oblique ligament (layer 2). Three No. 2 nonabsorbable sutures are passed around the posterior oblique ligament for later closure. The posterolateral approach involves a 3-cm skin incision just posterior to the lateral collateral ligament, two thirds below and one third above the joint line. The interval between the iliotibial band and the biceps femoris is developed using a combination of blunt and sharp dissection. The plane between the lateral head of the gastrocnemius and the posterolateral capsule is developed and a popliteal retractor is placed.

Details of Procedure

A standard arthroscopy is initially performed to evaluate the condition of the articular surface as well as the amount of remaining meniscal tissue. The graft can be thawed after this information is obtained and it is determined that the patient is a suitable candidate. The remaining edge of the meniscus is trimmed using a square-tipped biter to provide an edge to which the transplant is sutured. This is easiest to perform arthroscopically in a lateral meniscal transplant and open in the medial transplant. Care is taken to preserve a portion of the remaining meniscus for fixation to the allograft. The graft is then prepared on a separate table. We prefer to begin preparing the graft before performing the arthrotomies and trough preparation because there have been cases in which the incorrect graft has been sent. The graft preparation, trough formation, and arthrotomies can then be performed simultaneously.

Lateral Meniscal Transplant

For lateral meniscal transplants, we use a bone block technique where a block of bone is left joining the anterior and posterior insertions of the meniscus in anatomic position. A soft tissue technique without allograft bone can be used as well; however, we prefer to keep the meniscal attachments to the allgoraft for the lateral meniscus due to their proximity, and it does not significantly add to the complexity of the procedure. The bone block is trimmed of excess bone and contoured to fit into the appropriate slot of the sizing block (Fig. 10-2). Two drill holes are placed in the center of the bone block and a No. 2 braided nonabsorbable suture is passed. A second No. 2 suture is placed at the posterolateral corner of the graft to help guide the posterior horn past the lateral femoral condyle (Fig. 10-3).

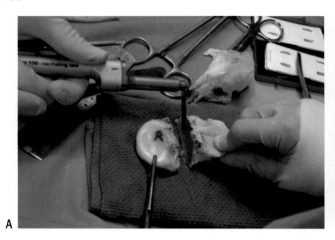
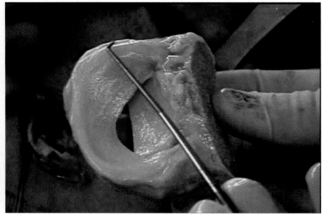

FIGURE 10-2

A: Preparation of the lateral meniscus with a small bone block that retains the meniscal root attachments. **B:** Finalized lateral meniscus allograft ready for suture placement and ultimate passage.

The arthroscopy and meniscal debridement are performed as described earlier. With the arthroscope in the lateral portal, a trough is prepared through the medial portal. A 0.25-inch curved osteotome is used to begin cutting the trough. The trough is started by using the osteotome with the curve toward the notch and immediately adjacent to the ACL (Fig. 10-4). The medial wall, lateral wall, and floor of the trough are developed to the width of the osteotome, which is approximately 7 mm. Care is taken to avoid penetration of the posterior cortex because of risk of injury to the neurovascular structures and to provide a backstop for the allograft. The trough is then progressively deepened with the quarter round and large cutting gouges to correspond to the contour, depth, and thickness of the bone plug (Fig. 10-5). The round rasp included in the set can then be used to smooth the edges of the trough. Metal templates are manufactured for each width and are placed into the trough to verify the size. The anterolateral and posterolateral open approaches are then performed as described earlier.

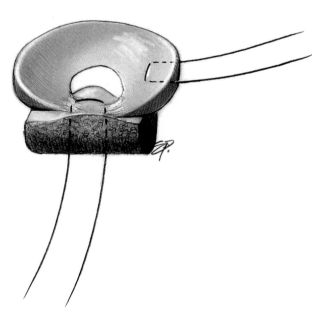

FIGURE 10-3

A prepared lateral meniscus transplant with suture placed in the posterolateral horn and through drill holes in the bone block.

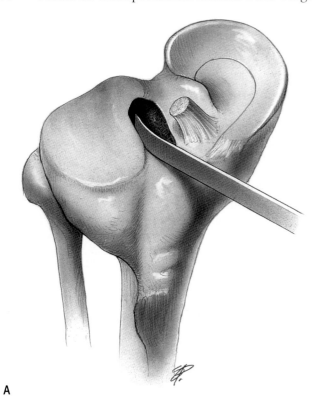

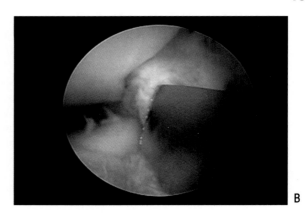

B

A

FIGURE 10-4

A: A quarter-inch curved osteotome is used through the medial portal to begin the walls and floor of the trough.
B: Arthroscopic view from the lateral portal.

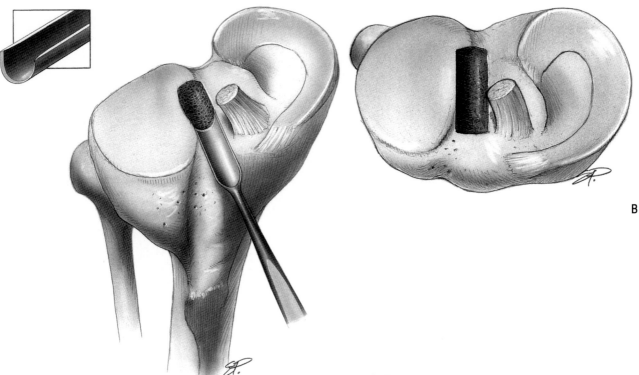

A

B

FIGURE 10-5

A,B: A large gouge deepening the trough to match the bone block size.

Transosseous holes in the tibia that are used to secure the bone block are drilled using an ACL guide. An ACL tip aimed guide is used to target the center of the trough 1 cm apart and to exit on the anteromedial tibia (Fig. 10-6). An incision is made in Langer's lines corresponding to the location of exit of the holes, and 3/32-inch K-wires are drilled. Care is taken to leave at least a 1-cm bone bridge between the exiting sutures so there is an adequate distance between them when they are tied. The K-wires are exchanged for Hewson suture passers, which are pulled into the joint and out of the medial portal.

A tonsil clamp is passed through the medial portal, punched through the posterolateral capsule, and pulled out through the posterolateral incision. This is exchanged for a suture passer, and the posterolateral suture in the graft is pulled through. The sutures in the bone block are pulled through the tibia (Fig. 10-7). Care must be taken to avoid entangling the sutures. The graft is passed into the joint through the anterolateral incision by first gently guiding the bone block into place, then pulling the meniscus into the compartment by the posterolateral suture (Fig. 10-8).

The sutures that were previously passed through the anterior horn of the native lateral meniscus are then passed in a simple fashion around the anterior horn of the transplanted meniscus and tied. Zone-specific cannulas are then used to pass suture in an inside-out technique to repair the posterior horn and body of the transplanted meniscus to the native meniscus and capsule (Fig. 10-9).

Medial Meniscus

For the medial meniscus, we use a soft-tissue technique without bone plugs. The graft is removed from the allograft tibial plateau and secured at each attachment with No. 2 bradied nonabsorbable suture in a whip stitch configuration (Fig. 10-10). Three No. 2 sutures, spaced 1 cm apart, are passed in a simple fashion through the posterior horn of the graft. The top of the graft is marked *TOP* so that there is no confusion when the graft is placed into the joint.

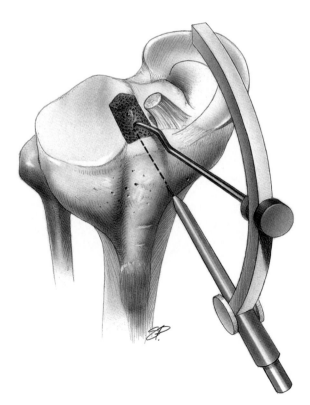

FIGURE 10-6

An ACL tip guide is used to drill two 3/32 K-wires from the anteromedial tibia to the center of the trough 1 cm apart.

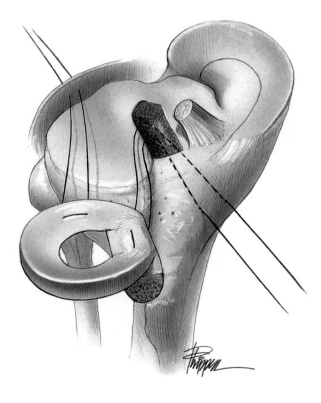

FIGURE 10-7

The K-wires are exchanged for suture passers, which are used to pull the bone block sutures through the tibia. A tonsil clamp is used to pass a suture passer, which is used to pull the posterolateral suture into the joint and out the posterolateral capsule.

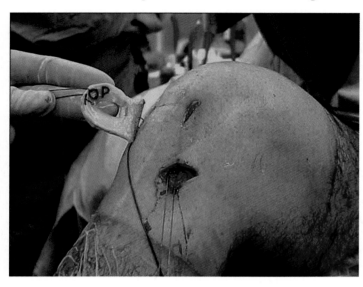

FIGURE 10-8

The passage of the lateral meniscus allograft through the anterior incision.

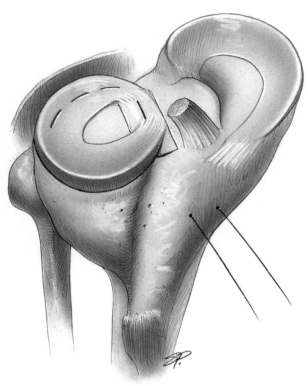

FIGURE 10-9

The reduced bone block and meniscus after inside-out repair of the posterior horn to the capsule.

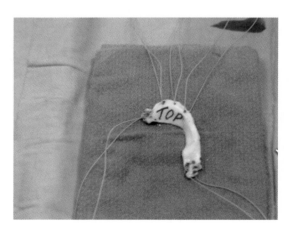

FIGURE 10-10

Preparation of the medial meniscus graft is performed without the use of bone plugs. The top portion of the graft is marked prior to removal from the plateau, and care is taken to preserve the meniscal roots in their entirety.

The arthroscopy, meniscal debridement, and open approaches are performed as described earlier. Three nonabsorbable sutures are passed around the anterior capsule and meniscus and clamped for later passage around the allograft. The ACL tip guide set at 47.5 degrees is used to pass two 3/32 K-wires from the anterolateral tibia to the anterior and posterior meniscal insertions (Fig. 10-11). The posterior insertion should be just anterior to the PCL and is easier to visualize through the postero-medial incision while the guide is placed through the anterolateral portal. An oblique incision in Langer's lines is made in the area in which the K-wires will exit. There should be a 7- to 10-mm cortical bridge between the exit of the anterior and posterior sutures. Both K-wires are replaced with suture passers that are pulled through the anterolateral incision and clamped (Fig. 10-12).

The graft is passed from the anterior incision into the joint with the assistance of a tonsil that helps to shuttle the rim sutures through the posteromedial incision. The posterior horn suture is passed through the posterior suture passer and is pulled through the tibia. The anterior suture is then shuttled in similar fashion for the anterior attachment. Tension is placed on the sutures while the fit of the meniscus is checked with the arthroscope. The sutures are then tied over the anterolateral tibial cortex. A free needle is used to pass the previously placed suture in the posterior horn of the graft around the native meniscal remnant and capsule (Fig. 10-13). The anterior horn is sutured with the previously placed sutures in the capsule/remnant. Using zone-specific cannulas, an inside-out repair is carried out for the body of the transplant. All incisions are closed in layers.

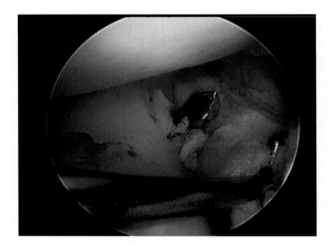

FIGURE 10-11

With the assistance of an ACL guide, a K-wire is drilled through the posterior medial meniscal root attachment for later passage of the allograft suture.

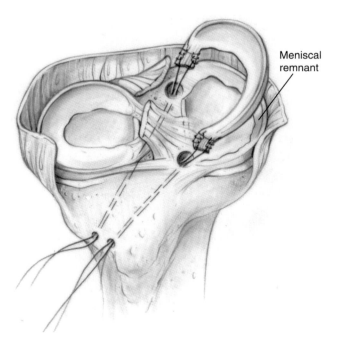

Meniscal remnant

FIGURE 10-12

The meniscus (prepared without bone plugs) and suture placement for fixation to the joint capsule.

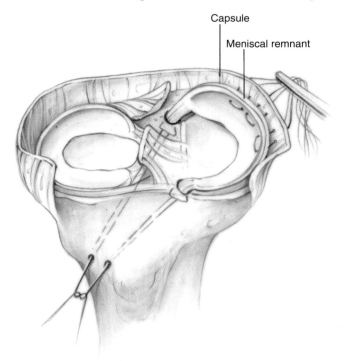

Capsule

Meniscal remnant

FIGURE 10-13

The reduced meniscus after the anterior bone plug has been pulled into place and the posterior horn is sutured to the capsule open.

Pearls and Pitfalls

- Reconfirmation of the indication for meniscal transplantation is performed with arthroscopy before thawing the graft. Subsequently, confirmation of the correct meniscus (right vs. left, medial vs. lateral) is performed before making the arthrotomies in case the incorrect meniscus has been sent and the procedure needs to be terminated.
- Portal placement is extremely important. The anteromedial portal should be just adjacent to the medial border of the patellar tendon to allow the bone trough to be created in the correct position next to the ACL. A portal that is created too medial will cause the surgeon to fight the soft tissues to prevent the osteotome from migrating into the lateral plateau.
- Adequate arthroscopic debridement of the remaining meniscus to stable, well-vascularized tissue ensures that the transplant will have the greatest potential for cell ingrowth. In the medial transplant it is simpler to perform after the arthrotomies are created using an arthroscopic punch. For the most part, the bed for the lateral transplant can be prepared arthroscopically.
- During introduction of the lateral meniscus into the joint, it is important to reduce the bone block into the trough before pulling the meniscus to the capsule and reducing it into the joint. Slack must be left on the posterior suture until the bone block is in place.
- Because the medial compartment is much tighter than the lateral compartment, the graft may be difficult to get into the compartment. Some authors have removed the medial tibial spine, partially released the medial collateral ligament, or placed an external fixator to distract the compartment to facilitate graft passage.

POSTOPERATIVE MANAGEMENT

In the immediate postoperative period up until 4 weeks, a hinged postoperative brace is kept locked in extension at all times except during range of motion (ROM) exercises. Twenty percent weight bearing is permitted with crutches. A continuous passive motion (CPM) machine is used from 0 to 45 degrees and progressed 10 to 15 degrees per week until full flexion is reached. Quadriceps rehabilitation is started using quadriceps sets and straight leg raises. Active assisted ROM using heel slides and calf pumps is also begun.

At 4 to 8 weeks postsurgery, the brace is unlocked for walking and sleeping. Weight bearing as tolerated is permitted with crutches. The CPM machine is discontinued. Isometric quadriceps rehabilitation and active assisted ROM are continued. The knee brace is removed at 6 weeks. Patients may return to sedentary work at 4 weeks.

At 8 to 12 weeks postsurgery, stationary bike and short-arc quadriceps strengthening are added. Walking with one crutch or a cane and driving are permitted.

At 3 to 6 months postsurgery, patients progress to walking without a crutch or cane. Rehabilitation progresses to include stepper exercises, treadmill walking, swimming (no breast stroke), and jogging in a pool. Closed chain and eccentric strengthening are added.

Patients who are 6 to 9 months postsurgery may begin open-chain, proprioception, and activity-specific conditioning. When patients are 9 months postsurgery, they may return to light sports and heavy labor. In general, return to high-demand, impact sports is not recommended.

COMPLICATIONS

Meniscal allograft transplantation sensitizes both the humeral and cell-mediated immune responses to create local and systemic responses to the graft. Lyophilizing and deep-freezing the grafts decreases the antigenicity, whereas cryopreservation maintains HLA antigens and host sensitization. However, based on the current studies comparing clinical success and immunogenicity, there does not appear to be any correlation between sensitization and outcome.

Complications include continued or increased compartment pain, full or partial loss of graft function, failure of peripheral healing of the meniscus, progression of degenerative arthrosis, and infection. In general, continued or increased pain, complete failure to heal, and infection require complete graft removal. Partial meniscectomy is the treatment of choice for partial tears of the graft. Significant advancement of osteoarthrosis is treated with total knee arthroplasty in suitable candidates.

RESULTS

Surgeon expectations from meniscal allograft transplantation are for greater than 90% subjective improvement in pain, instability, and function. However, objectively 20% to 40% of patients are rated as clinical failures by having repeat surgery for either partial or total graft removal. As for the goal of preventing the progression of degenerative changes of the articular surface, studies to date support this only in compartments with grade I or II changes.

RECOMMENDED READING

Cameron JC, Saha S. Meniscal allograft transplantation for unicompartmental arthritis of the knee. *Clin Orthop Rel Res.* 1997;337:164–171.

Cole BJ, Dennis MG, Lee SJ, et al. Prospective evaluation of allograft meniscus transplantation: a minimum 2-year follow-up. *Am J Sports Med.* 2006;34:919–27.

Garrett JC. Meniscal allograft transplantation. *Sports Med Arthrosc Rev.* 1993;2:164–167.

Johnson DL, Swenson TM, Harner CD. Meniscal reconstruction using allograft tissue: an arthroscopic technique. *Oper Tech Sports Med.* 1994;2:223–231.

Johnson DL, Swenson TM, Livesay GA, et al. Insertion-site anatomy of the human menisci: gross, arthroscopic, and topographical anatomy as a basis for meniscal transplantation. *Arthroscopy.* 1995;11:386–394.

Kuhn JE, Wojtys EM. Allograft meniscus transplantation. *Clin Sports Med.* 1996;15:537–556.

Milachowski KA, Weismeier K, Worth CJ, et al. Homologous meniscus transplantation: experimental and clinical results. *Int Orthop.* 1989;13:1–11.

Sekiya JK, Ellingson CI. Meniscal allograft transplantation. *J Am Acad Orthop Surg.* 2006;14:164–174.

Verdonk PC, Verstraete KL, Almqvist KF, et al. Meniscal allograft transplantation: long-term clinical results with radiological and magnetic resonance imaging correlations. *Knee Surg Sports Traumatol Arthrosc.* 2006;7:1–13.

Wirth CJ, Peters G, Milachowski KA, et al. Long-term results of meniscal allograft transplantation. *Am J Sports Med.* 2002;30:174–181.

Yoldas EA, Sekiya JK, Irrgang JJ, et al. Arthroscopically assisted meniscal allograft transplantation with and without combined anterior cruciate ligament reconstruction. *Knee Surg Sports Traumatol Arthrosc.* 2003;11:173–182.

11 Medial and Lateral Meniscus Transplantation: Arthroscopic-Assisted Techniques and Clinical Outcomes

Frank R. Noyes and Sue D. Barber-Westin

The meniscus provides important functions in the human knee, including load bearing, shock absorption, stability, and joint nutrition, that are vital for the integrity of the articular cartilage. While many meniscus tears can be successfully repaired, including complex tears that extend into the central avascular region (23), not all are salvageable, especially if considerable tissue damage has occurred. Transplantation of human menisci is hypothesized to restore partial load-bearing meniscus function, decrease patient symptoms, and provide chondroprotective effects (7,15,27). However, the procedure remains in an evolving state, as investigations of tissue-processing, secondary sterilization, and long-term function continue to evaluate its effectiveness. The optimal candidate is a young patient who has had a total meniscectomy and has pain and mild articular cartilage deterioration in the involved tibiofemoral compartment. There are few treatment options for these individuals and the goal of meniscal transplantation in the short term is to decrease pain, increase knee function, allow pain-free activities of daily living, and delay the onset of tibiofemoral arthrosis.

INDICATIONS/CONTRAINDICATIONS

The indications for a meniscus allograft are:

- Prior meniscectomy
- Age of 50 years or less
- Pain in the meniscectomized tibiofemoral compartment
- No radiographic evidence of advanced joint deterioration ($\geq$2 mm of tibiofemoral joint space demonstrated on 45-degree weight-bearing posteroanterior radiographs [22] and no or only minimal bone exposed on tibiofemoral surfaces)

Normal axial alignment and a stable joint are required, as untreated abnormal limb alignment and anterior cruciate ligament (ACL) deficiency have correlated with a high rate of meniscus allograft failure in several studies. Axial correction is recommended in knees in which the weight-bearing line is less than 45% (varus) or greater than 55% (valgus), representing a 2- to 3-degree change from normal alignment. An osteochondral autograft transfer or autologous chondrocyte implantation may be required in knees with full-thickness articular cartilage defects in the meniscectomized tibiofemoral compartment, which may be done either during or before the meniscus transplant procedure. These cartilage procedures expand the indications for meniscus transplantation in knees with femoral articular cartilage defects.

Contraindications for a meniscus allograft are:

- Advanced knee joint arthrosis with flattening of the femoral condyle, concavity of the tibial plateau, and osteophytes that prevent anatomic seating of the meniscus allograft (14)
- Varus or valgus axial malalignment
- Knee joint instability
- Knee arthrofibrosis
- Muscular atrophy
- Prior joint infection
- Symptomatic patellofemoral articular cartilage deterioration
- Obesity (>30 body mass index)

We do not recommend a prophylactic meniscus transplantation after total meniscectomy in asymptomatic patients who do not have articular cartilage deterioration, as long-term predictable success rates are not available. In addition, the operative procedure does carry a slight risk for complications that could make the patient's condition worse. There are sophisticated magnetic resonance imaging (MRI) techniques that are useful in determining the integrity of the articular cartilage and detect early deterioration prior to the onset of symptoms (20). A relative indication of meniscus transplantation is early (mild) arthritic deterioration in the involved tibiofemoral compartment in an asymptomatic patient.

PREOPERATIVE PLANNING

A thorough history is taken that includes assessment of prior operative records and current symptoms and functional limitations. The validated Cincinnati Knee Rating System (3) is used to rate pain, swelling, and giving-way of the knee as well as limitations with daily, athletic, and occupational activities. A comprehensive evaluation of the knee is conducted, which documents range of knee motion, joint effusion, tibiofemoral joint pain on palpation and during joint motion, and tibiofemoral joint crepitus. We also evaluate the patellofemoral joint, all knee ligaments, and gait abnormalities (17).

Diagnostic imaging includes bilateral anteroposterior radiographs in full extension, a 45-degree weight-bearing posteroanterior radiograph (22), and an axial view of the patellofemoral joint. The anteroposterior and lateral radiographs are taken with a magnification marker to obtain width and length measurements for the meniscus transplant (18). Axial lower limb alignment is measured using full standing hip-knee-ankle weight-bearing radiographs in knees that demonstrate varus or valgus alignment. MRI using fast-spin-echo techniques (19,20) are used in select cases to evaluate the condition of the articular cartilage and subchondral bone.

Selection of Meniscus Implant

A variety of sterilization techniques have been described for meniscus allografts, including none (fresh-frozen), irradiated, and cryopreserved, and no scientific data exist to select one type of graft processing method over another. Some authors advocate secondary sterilization using low-dose irradiation (1–2 Mrads) for purposes of bacterial sterilization (6). We recommend that allografts be obtained from tissue banks that have been accredited by the American Association of Tissue Banking and inspected by the Food and Drug Administration, where serological testing meets or exceeds the standards of these organizations (26). Importantly, donor selection criteria may vary between tissue banks, and the surgeon should understand the specific criteria used by the bank chosen to supply the transplant. Surgeons should also be aware that even though allograft tissues are generally processed aseptically, this may not prevent contamination and does not guarantee a sterile graft. We use prophylactic antibiotics intravenously before surgery and carefully monitor patients postoperatively for any signs of infection. The implications of different processing techniques on graft sterility is beyond the scope of this chapter, but have been discussed in detail by others (4,7,26).

We advise the surgeon to request that the tissue bank provide a photograph of the transplant that has been selected for the patient before surgery. A metric ruler should be placed adjacent to the transplant in the photograph to ensure that the allograft is of adequate size and width. Medial menisci may have a hypoplastic anterior horn that is narrow, inserting distal to the medial tibial surface (type III)(5); these menisci are not acceptable for implantation. The middle one third of a medial or lateral meniscus may be 8 to 10 mm in width and only suitable for small patients. The lateral meniscus may have reduced anteroposterior length, less than that calculated on the sagittal radiograph, and therefore not suitable for implantation.

SURGICAL TECHNIQUE

Transplant Preparation

The meniscus is thawed, inspected, and prepared before administration of patient anesthesia because it is difficult to detect implant defects through the plastic packaging, and the meniscus must be thoroughly evaluated. For a lateral meniscus allograft, implant preparation is accomplished first to determine the depth and width required for the tibial slot for the central bone bridge technique. The central bone portion of the lateral meniscus transplant incorporates the anterior and posterior meniscal attachments and usually measures 8 mm wide in smaller patients and 9 mm in larger patients. The length of the bone attachment is usually 35 mm, but this can be altered as required. The posterior 8 to 10 mm of tibia bone that protrudes beyond the posterior horn attachment is removed to later produce a buttress against the bone slot in the host knee. Commercially available (Stryker Endoscopy Co., Kalamazoo, MI, and Cryolife Inc., Kennesaw, GA) sizing blocks and channel cutters are helpful for appropriate sizing. There is also a dove-tail technique that the surgeon may elect, which has the advantage of providing added stability to the fixation at the tibial bone portion of the transplant (Fig. 11-1). This procedure entails cutting a trapezoidal bone block which includes a narrow, 7-mm bone bridge that preserves the ACL tibial attachment site.

Medial meniscus transplants are not prepared until it is determined if the central bone bridge technique (which is preferred) or the two-tunnel technique (separate anterior and posterior bone attachments and tunnels) will be performed, as we will describe in a following section.

It should be noted that the normal ACL tibia attachment site, or a planned ACL tibial graft tunnel, may compromise lateral or medial meniscus transplant tibial fixation in smaller patients who do not have sufficient width of the central tibial region to accommodate both the transplant and ACL tibial attachment or tunnel. Since it is not possible in these knees to use the central slot technique when an ACL reconstruction is to be performed concurrently, the two-tunnel procedure is selected for a medial meniscus transplant. More commonly, the two operations are staged by performing the ACL reconstruction first and the meniscus transplant procedure several months later.

Lateral Meniscus Transplantation

The patient is placed in a supine position on the operating room table with a tourniquet applied with a leg holder, and the table adjusted to allow 90 degrees of knee flexion. The opposite lower extrem-

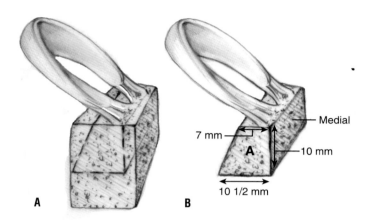

FIGURE 11-1

Dovetail meniscus allograft technique. **A:** An outline of the dovetail bone block is drawn on the end of the bone plug. An implant jig system is used to hold the meniscus implant and produce the desired bone cuts. **B:** Final appearance showing typical dimensions for the trapezoidal bone block prior to transplant insertion. (Reprinted with permission, Arthrex Meniscal Allograft Transplantation Featuring Dovetail Meniscal Allograft Technique. Carter TR. Arthrex, Naples, Florida, 2004.)

ity is placed in a thigh-high elastic stocking and is padded to maintain mild hip flexion to decrease tension on the femoral nerve. After examination under anesthesia, diagnostic arthroscopy is done to confirm the preoperative diagnosis and assess articular cartilage changes. A meniscus bed of 3 mm is retained when possible, except at the popliteal tendon region. In knees that require a cruciate ligament reconstruction, an arthroscopically assisted approach is used (11). The femoral and tibial tunnels are drilled, and the ligament graft is passed through the tunnels with femoral fixation done first, followed by the meniscal transplantation, and then tibial cruciate graft fixation. Performing ligament graft fixation at the tibia as the final step allows for maximum separation of the tibiofemoral joint during meniscal transplantation. This also prevents potential ligament fixation problems during the operation.

The tourniquet is inflated only for the two operative approaches. A limited 3-cm lateral arthrotomy is made just adjacent to the patellar tendon. Although arthroscopic techniques are available to prepare the tibial slot, we believe the limited arthrotomy provides superior visualization and avoids incising into the patellar tendon, which must be displaced medially to properly place the tibial slot. A common mistake involves placing the central tibial slot lateral to the normal attachment of the anterior horn of the lateral meniscus. A second 3-cm posterolateral incision is made just behind the lateral collateral ligament (Fig. 11-2) (10,24). The interval between the short head of the biceps muscle and the iliotibial band is identified and incised. The lateral head of the gastrocnemius is gently dissected with Metzenbaum scissors off the posterior capsule at the joint line just above the fibular head. Care is taken at this point, as dissection that extends too far proximal to the joint line at the posterolateral aspect would enter the joint capsule. If this occurs, a capsular repair is required to maintain joint integrity during the inside-out meniscal repair procedure. The inferior lateral geniculate artery, also in close proximity, is identified and preserved. The space between the posterolateral capsule and the lateral head of the gastrocnemius is further developed bluntly. An appropriately sized popliteal retractor (Stryker Co., Kalamazoo, MI) is placed directly behind the lateral meniscus bed and anterior to the lateral gastrocnemius muscle.

The width of the transplant is determined, and a template made out of aluminum foil of the same width and length is cut and inserted into the lateral compartment to determine the proper placement of the bone slot. This sizing step is important to ensure there is no lateral overhang of the meniscal body produced by not placing the bone far enough medially. A rectangular bone slot is prepared at the anterior and posterior meniscus tibial attachment sites to match the dimensions of the prepared transplant. The sequence of steps to prepare the lateral tibial slot is shown in Figure 11-3. The tibial

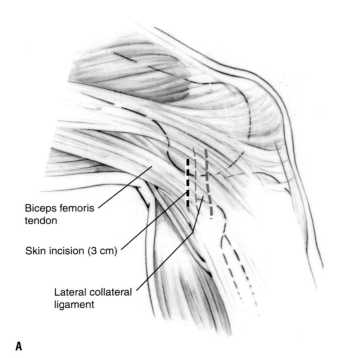

Biceps femoris tendon

Skin incision (3 cm)

Lateral collateral ligament

A

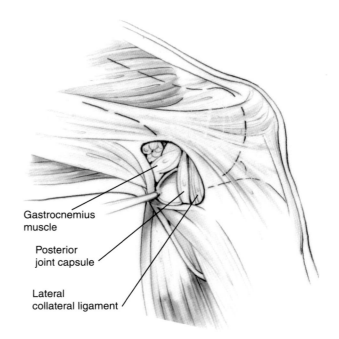

Gastrocnemius muscle

Posterior joint capsule

Lateral collateral ligament

C

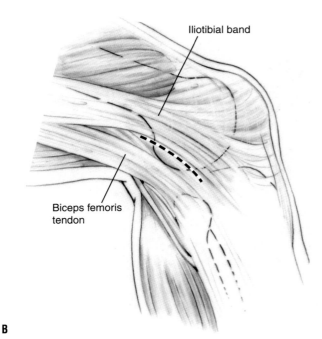

Iliotibial band

Biceps femoris tendon

B

FIGURE 11-2

A: Site of the posterolateral incision for a lateral meniscus transplant. **B:** Incision site in the interval between the posterior edge of the iliotibial band and the anterior edge of the biceps tendon. **C:** The interval between the lateral gastrocnemius and posterolateral capsule is opened bluntly, just proximal to the fibular head avoiding entering the joint capsule proximally. (Redrawn after Noyes FR, Barber-Westin SD, Rankin M. Meniscal transplantation in symptomatic patients less than fifty years old. Surgical technique. *J Bone Joint Surg Am* 2005;87(suppl 1):149-165, with permission.)

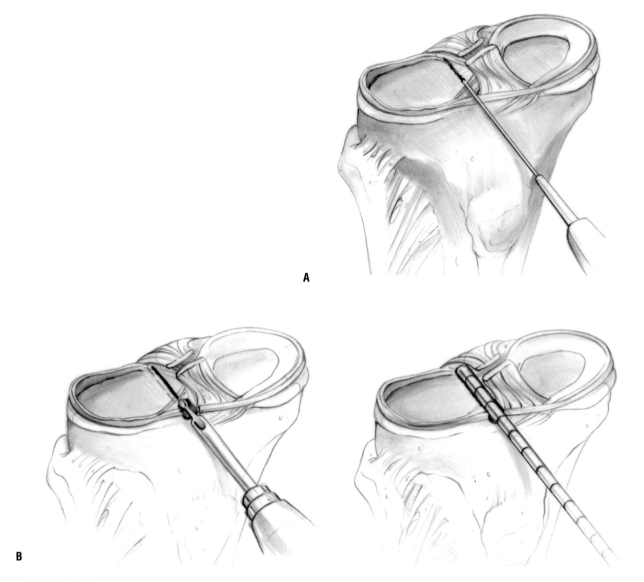

A

B

FIGURE 11-3

Tibial slot technique for lateral meniscus transplantation. The technique is shown for the lateral meniscus. An arthroscopic-assisted technique or mini-lateral arthrotomy may be used in this procedure. The authors prefer the mini-arthrotomy as it offers superior visualization and avoids incising the patellar tendon. **A:** Establish a line connecting the center of the anterior and posterior horn attachments using an electrocautery device. In the mini-open arthrotomy, a template of the meniscus coronal width is used to verify the medial-to-lateral width of the transplant to move the slot appropriately to prevent tibial overhang of the implant. **B:** A burr removes the tibial spine and creates a 4-mm straight anterior-to-posterior reference slot along the plane of the tibial slope. This calibrated guide pin sits flush with the articular cartilage. **C:** The drill guide uses a guide pin that has been marked with a laser to set the depth of a second guide pin, allowing a drill to ream 5 mm less to retain the posterior portion of the tibial slot. **D:** The 8-mm drill bit with a collar at the defined depth is used, followed by use of a box cutter to create a rectangular slot of the desired depth and width. ("Slot Instruments for Meniscal Transplantation: Surgical Technique." Farr J and Cole B. Stryker Endoscopy, San Jose, CA.) (Adapted from Noyes FR, Barber-Westin SD, Rankin M. Meniscal transplantation in symptomatic patients less than fifty years old. Surgical technique. *J Bone Joint Surg Am.* 2005;87(suppl 1):149–165, with permission.)

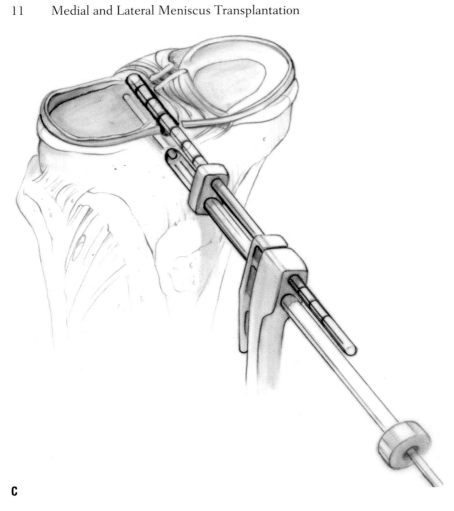

C

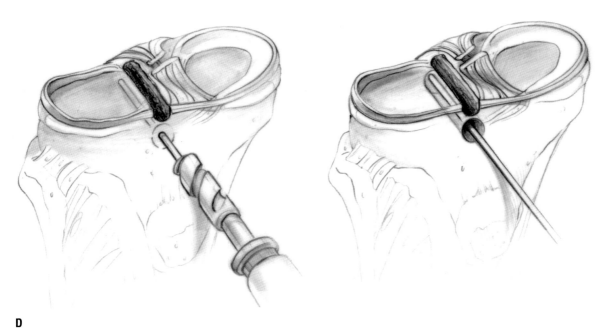

D

FIGURE 11-3
(*Continued*)

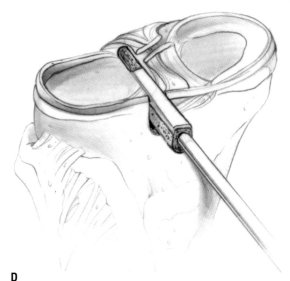

FIGURE 11-3

D

(*Continued*) **D:** The 8-mm drill bit with a collar at the defined depth is used, followed by use of a box cutter to create a rectangular slot of the desired depth and width. **E:** The lateral meniscus implant with the central bone bridge technique is ready to be placed into the tibial slot. A detailed description of the surgical steps and operative instruments is available. ("Slot Instruments for Meniscal Transplantation: Surgical Technique." Farr J and Cole B. Stryker Endoscopy, San Jose, CA.) (Adapted from Noyes FR, Barber-Westin SD, Rankin M. Meniscal transplantation in symptomatic patients less than fifty years old. Surgical technique. *J Bone Joint Surg Am.* 2005;87(suppl 1):149–165, with permission.)

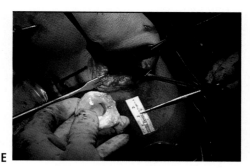

E

bone slot is 1 to 2 mm wider than the transplant to facilitate implantation. The anterior and posterior horns of the implant are placed into their normal attachment locations, adjacent to the ACL.

An alternative technique uses a starter chisel and finishing chisels to fashion the tibial slot to its final depth and width (Fig. 11-4A). A tibial slot sizing guide is used to check the length and depth (Fig. 11-4B). The allograft sizing block (Fig. 11-4C) confirms that the allograft bone bridge is of the correct width and depth.

The implant is inserted into the slot (Fig. 11-3E), and the bone portion of the graft is seated against the posterior bone buttress to achieve correct anterior-to-posterior placement of the attachment sites. A vertical suture in the posterior meniscus body is passed posteriorly to provide tension and facilitate implant placement and is later tied. The knee is flexed, extended, and rotated to confirm correct placement of the transplant has been obtained. Sutures are placed into the anterior one third of the meniscus, attaching it to the prepared meniscus rim under direct visualization.

Two fixation methods are available for the central bone attachment. Two 2-0 nonabsorbable sutures (Ticron, Davis and Beck Co., Wayne, NJ, or Ethibond, Ethicon Inc., Somerville, NJ) may be placed over the central bone bridge, brought through a drill hole, and tied to a tibial post. We prefer to place an interference screw (7 × 25 mm, comprised of an absorbable composite material) adjacent medially to the bone bridge (8). A tap is inserted over the guidewire to create a path for the interference screw with the bone bridge held in place manually. The arthrotomy is closed, and the inside-out meniscal repair is completed with multiple vertical divergent sutures, which are placed first superiorly to reduce the meniscus (Fig. 11-5), and then inferiorly in the outer one third of the implant. Sutures are not placed in the middle and inner thirds of the meniscus to avoid weakening the implant due to its limited healing capability in these regions (Fig. 11-6).

Medial Meniscus Transplantation

The patient is placed in a supine position on the operating room table with a tourniquet applied with a leg holder, and the table adjusted to allow 90 degrees of knee flexion. The opposite lower extrem-

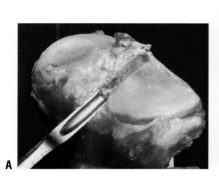
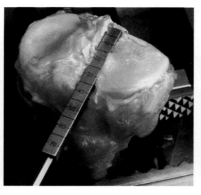
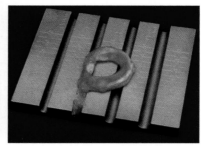

A   B, C

FIGURE 11-4

An alternative technique uses a starter chisel and finishing chisels to fashion the tibial slot to its final depth and width **(A)**. A tibial slot sizing guide is used to check the length and depth **(B)**. The allograft sizing block **(C)** confirms that the allograft bone bridge is of the desired width and depth. A detailed description of the surgical steps and operative instruments is available. ("Meniscus Reconstruction Trough Surgical Technique." Halbrecht JL. Cryolife, Inc., Kennesaw, GA) (Reprinted with permission from Noyes FR, Barber-Westin SD, Rankin M. Meniscal transplantation in symptomatic patients less than fifty years old. Surgical technique. *J Bone Joint Surg Am.* 2005; Suppl 1; 149–165.

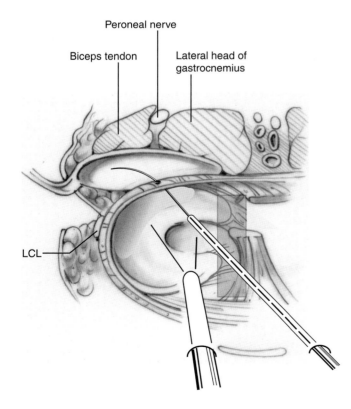

FIGURE 11-5

Cross-section showing spoon (a popliteal retractor may also be used) between the lateral gastrocnemius and the posterior capsule. A single cannula is introduced from the adjacent portal to facilitate placement of the vertical sutures into the periphery of the meniscus implant. (Adapted from Noyes FR, Barber-Westin SD, Rankin M. Meniscal transplantation in symptomatic patients less than fifty years old. Surgical technique. *J Bone Joint Surg Am.* 2005;87(suppl 1):149–165, with permission.)

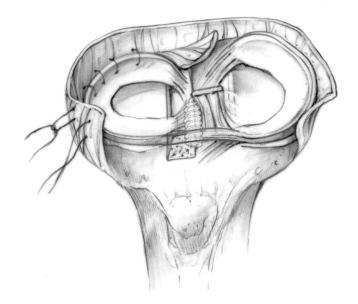

FIGURE 11-6

Lateral meniscus graft in place and sutured. (Adapted from Noyes FR, Barber-Westin SD, Rankin M. Meniscal transplantation in symptomatic patients less than fifty years old. Surgical technique. *J Bone Joint Surg Am.* 2005;87(suppl 1):149–165, with permission.)

ity is placed in a thigh-high elastic stocking and is padded to maintain mild hip flexion (to decrease tension on the femoral nerve). After examination with the patient under anesthesia, diagnostic arthroscopy is done to confirm the preoperative diagnosis and assess articular cartilage changes.

The tourniquet is inflated only for the anteromedial and posteromedial surgical approaches. A 4-cm skin anteromedial incision is made adjacent to the tibial tubercle and patellar tendon. A second 3-cm vertical posteromedial incision is made, similar to that described for inside-out meniscus repairs (10) (Fig. 11-7). The fascia is incised anterior to the sartorius muscle, and the pes anserine muscle groups are retracted posteriorly. The interval between the semimembranosus tendon and the capsule is sharply dissected. The tendon sheath of the semimembranosus is incised to facilitate exposure. The layer between the medial gastrocnemius tendon and the posterior capsule is separated with blunt dissection. Great care is taken to identify and avoid injury to the infrapatellar branches of the saphenous nerve. The two approaches are performed with the tourniquet inflated to 275 mm and usually require 15 minutes; otherwise, the tourniquet is not used.

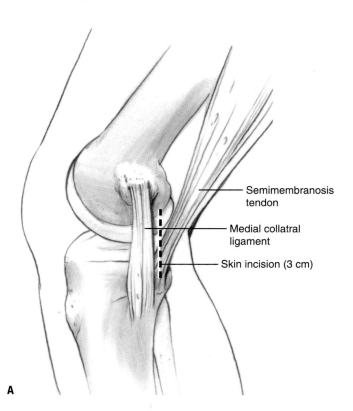

Semimembranosis tendon

Medial collatral ligament

Skin incision (3 cm)

FIGURE 11-7

The accessory posteromedial approach is shown for a medial meniscus allograft. **A:** Site of the posteromedial skin incision.

A

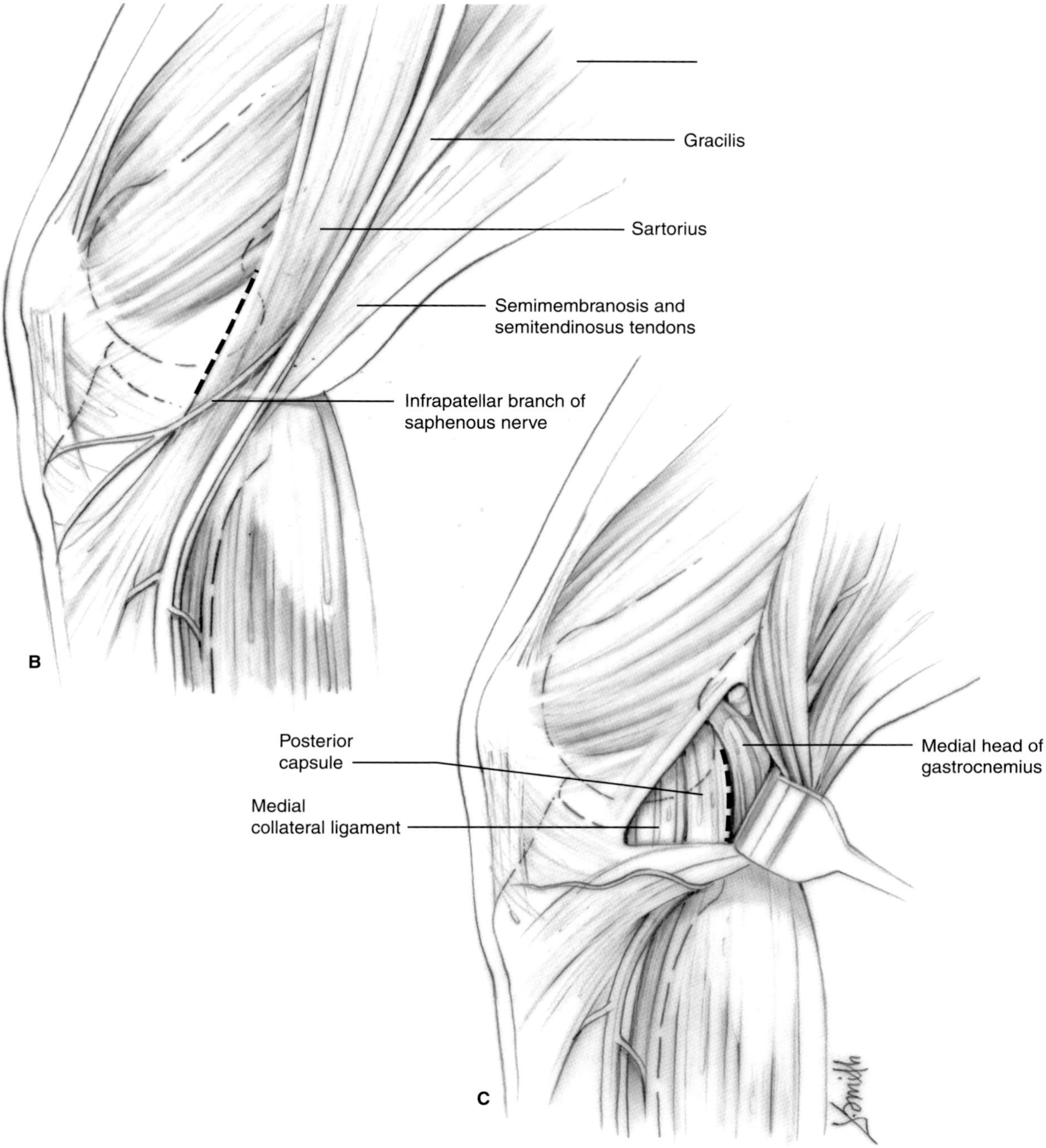

FIGURE 11-7

(Continued) **B:** The incision is shown through the anterior portion of the sartorius fascia. **C:** The interval is opened between the posteromedial capsule and the gastrocnemius tendon, just proximal to the semimembranosus tendon. The fascia over the tendon is excised to its tibial attachment to facilitate retrieval of the meniscus sutures. (Adapted from Noyes FR, Barber-Westin SD, Rankin M. Meniscal transplantation in symptomatic patients less than fifty years old. Surgical technique. *J Bone Joint Surg Am.* 2005;87(suppl 1):149–165, with permission.)

The goal of the operative procedure is to transplant the medial meniscus and bone attachments into the normal anterior and posterior attachments and to suture the transplant to maintain the desired position in the knee joint. An aluminum foil template of the medial meniscus transplant is measured according to its anterior-posterior and medial-lateral dimensions and is inserted through the anterior arthrotomy to measure the medial tibial plateau. This allows the position of the central bone slot to be marked and to determine if the meniscus implant will be properly positioned adjacent to the ACL tibial attachment without medial tibial overhang. The anterior and posterior meniscus attachment locations are verified to be at the anatomically correct sites. The central bone bridge technique removes 4 to 6 mm of the medial tibial eminence. If the implant is suitable and no medial tibial overhang is present, then the central bone bridge technique may be used. If the implant needs to be adjusted to fit to the medial tibial plateau by attaching the anterior horn placement further laterally, then the two-tunnel technique is selected. This sizing step is critical to obtain proper placement of the medial meniscus implant into the host tibia. In many knees, the central slot technique will not be possible due to a sizing problem that results in excessive medial displacement of the meniscus body or that would compromise the ACL tibial attachment. Once the appropriate technique has been determined, the meniscus allograft is prepared.

Medial Meniscus Central Bone Bridge Technique

The technique is similar as that already described for lateral meniscus transplantation. A reference slot is first made on the tibial plateau in the anteroposterior direction. A guide pin is positioned in the slot, inferiorly on the tibia, and a cannulated drill bit is placed over the pin to drill a tunnel. The final tibial slot is 8 to 9 mm wide and 10 mm deep. A rasp is used to smooth the slot to allow insertion of the allograft central bone bridge.

Alternatively, the dove-tail technique may be used, as previously discussed for a lateral meniscus transplant. The central bone bridge of the allograft is sized to a width of 7 mm (1 mm less than the dimension at the tibial site) and a depth of 10 mm (8). This allows adjustment of the central bone bridge position in the anterior-posterior direction while the meniscus is positioned to fit in the anatomically correct position relative to the femoral condyle.

A vertical suture is placed through the posterior meniscus horn and advanced through the capsule to exit through the posteromedial incision. The meniscus is passed through the arthrotomy into the knee with tension placed on the posterior suture to facilitate proper positioning in the knee joint. Care is taken to align the bone bridge with the recipient tibial slot. The knee is taken through flexion and extension and tibial rotation to align the implant. Once the appropriate anterior-posterior central bone bridge position is achieved, a guidewire is inserted between the bone bridge and the lateral side of the slot. A tap is inserted over the guidewire to create a path for an interference screw with the bone bridge held in place manually. An absorbable bone interference screw is inserted adjacent to the bone bridge. Occasionally, there will be an osteophyte on the anterior portion of the medial tibial plateau that must be resected to avoid meniscal implant compression. The anterior horn of the meniscus is sutured with vertical divergent sutures (2-0 Ethibond) under direct visualization (Fig. 11-8). The anterior arthrotomy is closed and the inside-out vertical divergent sutures are placed, as described, to suture the meniscus to the meniscus bed, removing any implant undulations and restoring circumferential meniscal tension. The central bone bridge of the implant provides for fixation of the anterior and posterior portions of the implant and subsequent healing to the host tibia (Fig. 11-9).

Medial Meniscus Two-Tunnel Technique

If it is determined that the central bone bridge technique is not acceptable, the surgeon must prepare separate anterior and posterior bone attachments for the meniscus transplant that will be secured to the normal anatomic attachment sites (Fig. 11-10). The transplant is prepared with a posterior bone plug 8 mm in diameter and 12 mm in length. Although techniques have been described that use only a soft-tissue fixation of the posterior horn by removing the bone portion of the meniscus graft to allow easier graft passage, we believe that this provides less secure fixation and leads to a higher failure rate. The anterior bone attachment is 12 mm in width, length, and depth. Two 2-0 nonabsorbable Ethibond sutures (Ethicon, Somerville, NJ) are passed retrograde through each bone attachment, with two additional locking sutures placed in the meniscus adjacent to the bone attachment for subsequent secure fixation.

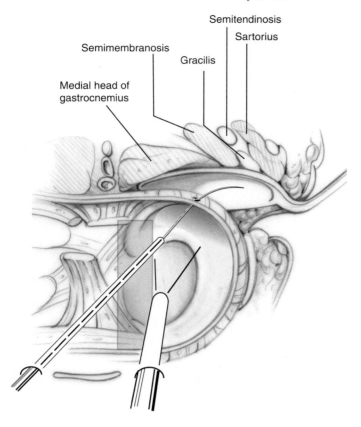

FIGURE 11-8

Cross-section showing the arthroscope, needle cannula, and spoon in place. A popliteal retractor may also be used, which the authors prefer. The meniscus is passed through the arthrotomy into the knee with tension placed on the sutures to facilitate proper positioning in the knee joint. Using a single-barrel cannula, the suture is advanced through the capsule at the corresponding attachment site of the meniscus and exits through an accessory incision. (Adapted from Noyes FR, Barber-Westin SD, Rankin M. Meniscal transplantation in symptomatic patients less than fifty years old. Surgical technique. *J Bone Joint Surg Am.* 2005;87(suppl 1):149–165, with permission.)

A guide pin is placed adjacent to the tibia tubercle and is directed to the anatomic posterior meniscus attachment. A tibial tunnel is drilled over the guidewire to a diameter of 8 mm. The bone tunnel edges are champhered and slightly enlarged with a curette to allow easier passage of the graft into the tibial tunnel. A limited medial femoral condyle notchplasty is usually required. At least 8 mm of opening adjacent to the posterior cruciate ligament (PCL) and medial femoral condyle is required to pass the posterior bone attachment of the graft. On occasion, a subperiosteal release of the long fibers of the tibial attachment of the medial collateral ligament (with later suture anchor repair) is required to open the medial tibiofemoral joint sufficiently. The meniscus bed is prepared by removing any remaining meniscus tissue, while preserving a 3-mm rim when possible. The meniscus bed is rasped for revascularization of the graft.

The graft is passed through the anteromedial arthrotomy. The surgeon is seated with a headlight in place, and the knee is flexed to 90 degrees. A guidewire is passed retrograde through the tibial tunnel, and the sutures attached to the posterior bone are retrieved. A second suture is placed into the posterior horn and is passed inside-out through the posteromedial approach to guide the meniscus.

The knee is flexed to 20 degrees under a maximum valgus load to pass the posterior bone portions of the graft, with the secondary meniscus body suture being held by an assistant. A nerve hook is

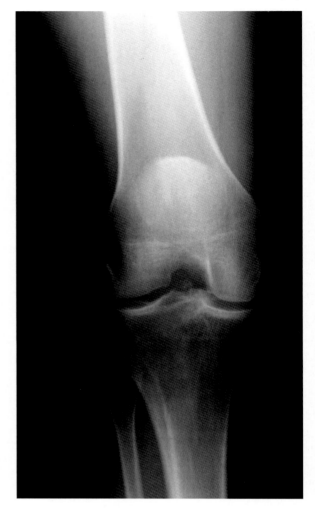

FIGURE 11-9

Weight-bearing posteroanterior radiograph of a 36-year-old woman 6 years after medial meniscus central bone bridge implantation shows incorporation of the bone bridge into the host, with preservation of the medial joint space. (Adapted from Noyes FR, Barber-Westin SD, Rankin M. Meniscal transplantation in symptomatic patients less than fifty years old. Surgical technique. *J Bone Joint Surg Am.* 2005;87(suppl 1):149–165, with permission.)

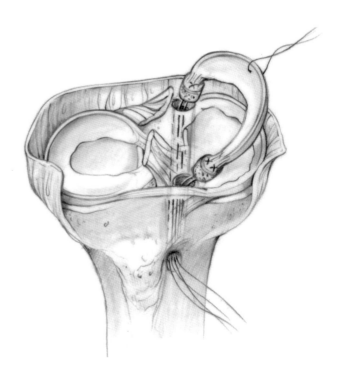

FIGURE 11-10

Two-tunnel technique for medial meniscus allografts. The illustration shows insertion of transplant, including posteromedial suture placed to facilitate meniscus reduction. The anterior and posterior bone attachments of the medial meniscus transplant are fixed into separate tibial tunnels. (Adapted from Noyes FR, Barber-Westin SD, Rankin M. Meniscal transplantation in symptomatic patients less than fifty years old. Surgical technique. *J Bone Joint Surg Am.* 87 2005; Suppl 1: 149–165, with permission.)

used to gently assist the passage of the graft. With direct visualization, it is possible to confirm appropriate meniscus graft passage and positioning into the medial tibiofemoral compartment. Care is taken not to advance the posterior meniscus body too far into the tibial tunnel, but only to seat the bone portion of the graft in order to not shorten the overall circumferential length of the meniscus graft. The posterior meniscus bone attachment sutures are tied over the tibial post to provide tension to the posterior bone attachment. One or two sutures are passed to secure the posterior horn. The knee is flexed and extended to assess meniscus fit and displacement. The optimal location for the anterior meniscal bone attachment is identified with appropriate lateral placement to restore proper meniscus position and prevent medial transplant overhang. The knee is placed in full extension, and the position of the transplant is verified to be correct. A 12-mm rectangular bone attachment is fashioned in the tibia to correspond to the anterior bone attachment of the meniscus graft. A 4-mm bone tunnel is placed at the base of this bone slot and exits at the anterior tibia just proximal to the posterior bone tunnel. The sutures are passed through the bone tunnel, and the anterior horn is seated. Full knee flexion and extension are again performed to determine proper graft placement and fit. Tension is applied to the anterior bone sutures, which are not tied at this point but are used to maintain tension in the graft during the inside-out suture repair. This meticulous seating of the meniscus transplant under circumferential tension with bone attachment of both the anterior and posterior horns is believed to be crucial for meniscus weight-bearing position and function.

The anterior arthrotomy is closed, and the arthroscope is inserted into the anterolateral portal for the posterior meniscal repair and into the anteromedial portal for the middle and anterior one-third repairs, with the single needle cannula inserted in the other anterior portal. The meniscal repair is performed in an inside-out fashion, starting with the posterior horn, with use of multiple vertical divergent sutures of 2-0 nonabsorbable Ethibond both superiorly and inferiorly, constantly tensioning the meniscus from posterior to anterior to establish circumferential tension. The assistant is seated with a headlight and retrieves the suture needles through the posteromedial approach. Each suture is placed and tied bringing the meniscus directly to the meniscus bed with observation that correct meniscus placement, fixation, and tension exist. We do not consider an alternative technique of using meniscus fixators, as this lessens the ability to precisely secure and restore tension to the meniscus transplant. The anterior arthrotomy is opened and final tensioning and fixation of the anterior horn bone attachment is performed. Occasionally, additional sutures are required to secure the most anterior one third of the meniscus to the capsular attachments. This step is performed under direct vision (Fig. 11-11). An alternative method of fixation is to use a 3.5-mm cancellous screw with a washer for fixation of the anterior horn meniscus-bone attachment.

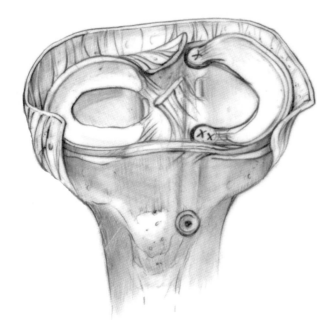

FIGURE 11-11

Final anterior and posterior tunnel fixation appearance of medial meniscus transplant and vertical divergent sutures. (Adapted from Noyes FR, Barber-Westin SD, Rankin M. Meniscal transplantation in symptomatic patients less than fifty years old. Surgical technique. *J Bone Joint Surg Am.* 2005;87(suppl 1):149–165, with permission.)

After final inspection of the graft with knee flexion and extension and tibial rotation, the operative wounds are closed in a routine fashion.

Pearls and Pitfalls

- We advise patients that the transplant will be inspected in the operating room just before the administration of anesthesia. At this time, the decision will be made to proceed if the graft is deemed suitable. There is also the remote possibility that during the operation, either the final preparation or the implantation of the transplant may not be possible due to problems with graft size or the ability to obtain correct positioning in the joint. Although these problems are rare, the patient should be advised.
- The preparation of the meniscus template is critical to obtain successful placement of the final tibial slot and ensure correct positioning of the transplant. The template is made of aluminum foil to represent the size of the implant and is inserted through the limited anterior arthrotomy incision.
- The slot placement for the transplant must be exact. Otherwise, the meniscus may be displaced at its midportion outside the joint, or positioned too far inside the joint and subsequently incur excessive compression and tearing. It is possible to realign the bony slot a few millimeters medially or laterally in the coronal plane and use an absorbable interference screw for fixation in the final coronal adjustment of the implant.
- The use of multiple vertical divergent sutures is required to position the transplant in the anatomically correct manner. There are wavy areas in the implant with loss of circumferential tension that can be successfully removed by correct placement of these sutures.
- We prefer the inside-out meniscus repair technique, which is viewed as the most precise suturing method.
- We avoid meniscal fixators, as it is not possible to provide the same secure fit and exact placement of the implant as that obtained with sutures.
- The sutures should not be placed in the middle and inner thirds of the meniscus, as this may weaken the transplant.
- A total of 12 to 15 sutures are placed both superiorly and inferiorly, in a vertical direction. Horizontal sutures have poor holding ability and are therefore not used during meniscal transplantation.
- Care is taken to avoid damaging the articular cartilage. This technique requires two surgical assistants, one dedicated to holding the lower limb to open the medial or lateral tibiofemoral compartment for visualization of the implant, and another seated to retrieve and tie the sutures at the posterior aspect of the joint.
- The suturing of the lateral posterior horn adjacent to the posterior attachment requires angulation of the suture needle away from the neurovascular structures.
- In order for the meniscus transplant to function, it must be placed at the normal anatomic insertion sites. The posterior horn attachment of the lateral meniscus, if placed too far posteriorly, will not promote load sharing (1). Alternatively, too anterior of a position of a medial meniscus transplant will produce excessive compressive forces and damage the meniscus.
- During medial meniscus transplantation, the template may indicate that the transplant is excessively wide in the medial-to-lateral direction. If this occurs, the middle one third of the transplant would rest outside of the medial tibial plateau to avoid compromising the ACL attachment. In this case, the two-tunnel technique is selected to obtain correct anatomic positioning and the desired subsequent circumferential hoop stress.
- We disagree with published techniques on medial meniscus transplantation in which the posterior bone portion of a medial meniscus implant is not retained and the fibrocartilaginous posterior horn is placed in a posterior tibial attachment tunnel. Although far easier to prepare and implant surgically, there are inadequate scientific data to support that the soft tissue ends of the meniscus implant (without the bone attachment) will heal and provide the circumferential tension in the meniscus that is required for function.
- We disagree with published reports in which meniscus transplants are used in knees with advanced tibiofemoral compartment arthrosis (25). In our experience, the transplant extrudes from the joint in these knees, and its ability to decrease symptoms or have a chondroprotective effect is lost (14).

- For medial meniscus transplants, the central bone slot is limited in its lateral-most placement by the ACL tibial attachment. The anterior horn of the medial meniscus must not be of a type III configuration (5), inserting too far distally on the anterior tibial margin. If there is a medial-to-lateral size mismatch for a medial meniscus transplant, then separate anterior and posterior bone attachments and tunnels are required. The posterior bone-meniscus transplant is placed at the normal attachment, and the anterior horn is placed in a medial-to-lateral direction to restore correct tensioning and position in the joint.
- For tight knees in which there are only a few millimeters of medial joint opening, the central bone bridge technique avoids performing a partial detachment of the distal medial collateral ligament which would otherwise be required to gain access to the joint for suturing and avoid damage to the articular cartilage.

POSTOPERATIVE MANAGEMENT

The initial goal of the postoperative rehabilitation program is to prevent excessive weight-bearing and joint compressive forces that could disrupt the healing meniscus allograft (Table 11-1). Patients are placed in a long-leg postoperative brace immediately after surgery, and the brace is worn for approximately 6 weeks. Knee range-of-motion exercises from 0 to 90 degrees are begun the first day. Knee flexion is increased 10 degrees each week to allow 135 degrees after 4 weeks. Patients are allowed only toe-touch (5 lb) weight bearing during the first 2 weeks, and then are slowly progressed to bear 50% of body weight at 4 weeks and full weight bearing at 6 weeks.

Flexibility and quadriceps strengthening exercises are begun immediately postoperatively. Balance, proprioception, and closed-kinetic chain exercises are implemented when patients achieve full weight bearing. Stationary bicycling with low resistance is begun at 8 weeks, and swimming and walking programs are initiated between 9 and 12 weeks. Return to light recreational sports is delayed for at least 12 months. Patients are advised not to return to high-impact, strenuous athletics due to the joint damage present and questionable ability of the meniscus transplant to restore normal load-bearing function.

COMPLICATIONS

We have not encountered knee arthrofibrosis or joint infection problems following meniscus transplantation, although this is always a possibility after any major knee operation. Any patient whose knee fails to achieve the extension and flexion goals is placed into an intervention program previously described in detail (16). In our series of 40 consecutive meniscus transplants, four knees required a gentle manipulation under anesthesia performed 4 to 6 weeks postoperative for a limitation of knee flexion. These patients had a concomitant ligament reconstruction or osteochondral autograft transfer procedure.

The patient is observed for any loss of meniscus repair and stabilization in the initial postoperative period. Rarely, a resuture and repeat fixation are required. Postoperative radiographs are taken to assess bony incorporation of the transplant.

RESULTS

We have previously described the clinical outcome of 40 consecutive cryopreserved and 96 fresh-frozen irradiated medial and lateral meniscus transplants in detail (12,14,15,21).

Forty cryopreserved meniscus allografts were implanted into 38 patients from November 1995 to March 2000. Four of the meniscus transplants failed and were removed before the minimum 2-year follow-up study period; these cases were included in the overall failure rate. We followed 35 patients (36 meniscus transplants; 18 lateral, 16 medial, 1 bilateral) a mean of 40 months (range, 24 to 69 months) postoperatively. There were 18 males and 17 females whose mean age at surgery was 30 years (range, 14 to 49 years). A mean of 139 months (range, 12 to 372 months) had elapsed between the knee injury and the meniscus allograft procedure. A total of 128 prior operative procedures had been done, including 61 partial or total meniscectomies, 13 ACL reconstructions, four PCL reconstructions, one lateral collateral ligament reconstruction, five high tibial osteotomies, and three osteochondral autograft transfer procedures.

TABLE 11-1. Rehabilitation after Meniscus Transplant

	Postop Weeks					Postop Months			
	1–2	3–4	5–6	7–8	9–12	4	5	6	7–12
Brace: long-leg postoperative	X	X	X	X					
ROM minimum goals:									
0–90 degrees	X								
0–120 degrees		X							
0–135 degrees			X						
Weight bearing:									
Toe touch—1/4 body weight	X								
1/2 to 3/4 body weight		X							
Full				X					
Patellar mobilization	X	X	X						
Modalities:									
Electrical muscle stimulation	X	X	X						
Pain/edema cryotherapy	X	X	X	X	X	X	X	X	X
Flexibility: hamstring, gastrocsoleus, iliotibial band, quadriceps	X	X	X	X	X	X	X	X	X
Strengthening:									
Quad iso, SLR, active knee exten	X	X	X	X	X				
Closed-chain				X	X	X	X	X	
Knee flexion hamstring curls (90 degrees)					X	X	X	X	X
Knee extension quads (90–30 degrees)		X	X	X	X	X	X	X	
Hip abduction-adduction, multi-hip			X	X	X	X	X	X	X
Leg press (70–10 degrees)					X	X	X	X	X
Balance/proprioceptive training			X	X	X	X	X	X	
Conditioning:									
Upper body ergometer		X	X	X					
Bike (stationary)					X	X	X	X	X
Aquatic program					X	X	X	X	X
Swimming (kicking)						X	X	X	X
Walking					X	X	X	X	X
Stair climbing machine									X
Ski machine								X	X
Light recreational sports									X

Iso, isometrics; ROM, range of motion; SLR, straight leg raises.
Closed chain: gait retraining, toe raises, wall sits, mini-squats
Balance/proprioceptive training: weight-shifting, mini-trampoline, Biomechanical Ankle Platform System (BAPS, Camp, Jackson, MI), Kinesthetic Awareness Trainer (KAT, Breg, Inc., Vista, CA), plyometrics.
(Reprinted with permission from Noyes FR, Barber-Westin SD. Meniscus transplantation: indications, techniques, clinical outcomes. In: Pellegrini VD, ed: *Instructional course lectures*, vol. 54. Rosemont, IL: American Academy of Orthopaedic Surgeons; 2005:341–353.)

At the time of the lateral meniscus transplant, a concurrent osteochondral autograft transfer of the lateral femoral condyle was done in 13 knees for full-thickness articular cartilage defects. Knee ligament reconstructions were done before the meniscus allograft in four knees and at the same time as the transplant in four knees. In six knees, ACL reconstructions were done using either bone-patellar tendon-bone or semitendinosus-gracilis autografts. A PCL 2-strand quadriceps tendon autograft reconstruction (13) was done in one knee. Both the PCL and ACL were reconstructed in one knee.

Abnormal articular cartilage surfaces (lesion >15 mm in diameter with fissuring and fragmentation extending greater than one half of the depth of the cartilage, or subchondral bone exposed) were detected in the meniscectomized tibiofemoral compartment in 31 (88%) knees at the time of meniscus transplantation. Subchondral bone exposure was found in 18 knees and extensive fissuring and fragmentation was noted in 13 other knees.

Twenty-nine (73%) meniscus allografts were analyzed with MRI using our research protocol previously described in detail (15,21) an average of 35 months (range, 12 to 27 months) postoperatively. The radiographs were reviewed and measured by independent orthopaedic surgeons blinded to patient information. The height, width, and displacement of the transplant were determined during full or partial weight-bearing (loaded) conditions.

The subjective and functional results were assessed with the Cincinnati Knee Rating System. A classification system of meniscus transplant characteristics was developed on the basis of MRI, clinical examination, follow-up arthroscopy (when performed), and tibiofemoral symptoms (Table 11-2). The International Knee Documentations Committee (IKDC) classification system was used to determine knee ligament graft function.

Before surgery, 27 patients (77%) had moderate to severe pain with daily activities; but at follow-up, only two (6%) had pain with daily activities (Fig. 11-12, $p < 0.0001$). All patients had pain in the meniscectomized tibiofemoral compartment preoperatively; but at follow-up, only 10 (29%) had some component of tibiofemoral pain. Thirty-three of 35 (94%) patients stated their knee condition had improved on self-assessment ratings (Fig. 11-13). The mean preoperative patient perception score (scale, 1 to 10) of 3.1 points (range, 1 to 6 points) improved to a mean of 6.2 points (range, 1 to 9 points) at follow-up ($p < 0.0001$). Preoperatively, only one patient was able to participate in sports without problems. At follow-up, 27 patients (77%) were participating in light low-impact sports without problems, and one patient was participating with symptoms against advice.

One patient had signs of a meniscus tear at follow-up. One patient had tibiofemoral joint line pain and increased palpable crepitation compared with the preoperative examination. All patients had a normal range of knee motion. All knees that had an ACL reconstruction had normal or nearly normal anterior stability restored except one in which the reconstruction failed. The PCL reconstructions restored nearly normal function in both knees at 20 and 90 degrees of flexion, except for one knee in which partial function was restored at 90 degrees of flexion.

Five patients had follow-up arthroscopy for allograft-related symptoms. In three patients, tears in the periphery of the meniscus allograft at the capsular junction were successfully repaired. In two patients, small tears in the allograft were resected. None of these patients had further complaints. One other patient had a total knee replacement 35 months following the meniscus allograft for unresolved knee pain and a failed meniscus allograft. With the six patients described previously, and the four meniscus transplants that required removal early postoperatively, the reoperation rate for meniscal allograft symptoms was 25% (10 of 40 meniscus allografts).

The mean displacement of the 29 meniscus allografts examined with MRI was 2.2 ± 1.5 mm (range, 0 to 5 mm) in the coronal plane. Seventeen allografts (59%) had no displacement, 11 had minor displacement, and one could not be evaluated due to artifacts from other operative procedures.

In the sagittal plane, the mean displacement of the posterior horn of the allografts was 1.1 ± 2.0 mm (range, 0 to 9 mm). Twenty-five allografts (86%) had no displacement of the posterior horn, three had minor displacement, and one had major displacement (9 mm). The mean displacement of

TABLE 11-2. Meniscus Allograft Classification*

Allograft Classification	MRI Evaluation (N = 17)			Clinical Exam: Tibiofemoral (N = 28)		Follow-up Arthroscopy (N = 8)
	Peripheral Attachment	Position in Joint†	Signal Intensity	Meniscus Signs	Pain, Clinical Symptoms	Meniscus Tears
Normal	Healed	Normal (0%–25% of meniscus width)	None, Grade 1, 2	None	None	None
Altered		Displacement (26%–50% of meniscus width)			Mild pain, improved over preop	Partial meniscectomy (less than 1/3 removed)
Failed	Not Healed	Major displacement (>50% of meniscus width)	Grade 3 (tearing, signal intensity extended to articular surface)	Obvious signs meniscus tear	Definite return pain, not improved over preop	Partial or total meniscectomy (more than 1/3 removed)

*One abnormal result = failed.
†Coronal and sagittal planes, percent displacement posterior or medial plateau margin perpendicular to the joint line.
N = number of meniscus allografts.
(Adapted from Noyes FR, Barber-Westin SD, Rankin M. Meniscal transplantation in symptomatic patients less than fifty years old. *J Bone Joint Surg* 2004;86A:1392–1404.)

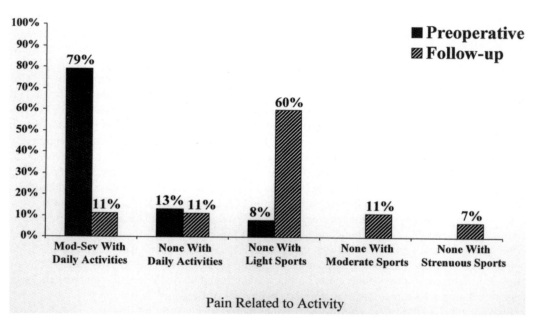

FIGURE 11-12

The pain scale shows the highest level of activity possible without the patient experiencing knee pain. The difference between preoperative and follow-up was statistically significant ($p < 0.0001$). Mod = moderate; Sev = severe. (Adapted from Noyes FR, Barber-Westin SD, Rankin, M. Meniscus transplantation in symptomatic patients less than fifty years old. *J Bone Joint Surg Am.* 2004;86:1392–1404, with permission.)

the anterior horn of the allografts was 1.2 ± 1.7 mm (range, 0 to 6 mm). Twenty-five allografts had no displacement of the anterior horn, three had minor displacement, and one had major displacement (6 mm). Intrameniscal signal intensity was normal in one, grade 1 in 13, grade 2 in 11, grade 3 in three, and could not be evaluated in one.

Seventeen (42.5%) of the meniscus transplants had normal characteristics (Fig. 11-14, Table 11-2), 12 (30%) had altered characteristics, and 11 (27.5%) failed. Of the 20 lateral menisci transplants, nine had normal characteristics, seven had altered characteristics, and four failed. Of the 20 medial meniscus allografts, eight had normal characteristics, five had altered characteristics, and seven failed. There was a correlation between the arthrosis rating on MRI and the allograft characteristics ($p = 0.01$). Of the 16 allografts in knees with mild arthrosis, 10 had normal characteristics and six had altered characteristics. Of the 12 allografts in knees with moderate arthrosis, three had normal characteristics, four had altered characteristics, and five failed.

All patients had a normal range of knee motion. All seven knees that had an ACL reconstruction had normal or nearly normal anterior stability restored, except one in which the reconstruction failed. The PCL reconstructions restored nearly normal stability in the two knees that had this operation at 20 and 90 degrees of flexion, except for one knee in which partial stability was restored at 90 degrees of flexion. A comparison of preoperative and follow-up weight-bearing posteroanterior radiographs revealed that three knees had further deterioration and narrowing of the tibiofemoral joint space in the involved compartment.

We previously described the results of 96 consecutive irradiated meniscus allografts implanted into 82 patients (14). Twenty-nine menisci in 28 patients were removed prior to the minimum 2-year follow-up; this left 67 meniscus allografts that were followed 22 to 58 months postoperatively with MRI and clinical examination. The overall rating of all 96 meniscus allografts was nine grafts (9%), normal; 19 grafts (20%), altered; 67 grafts (70%), failed; and one, unknown. Of the 67 meniscal allografts that survived at least 2 years postoperatively, the rating was nine grafts (13%), normal; 19 grafts (29%), altered; 38 grafts (57%), failed; and one, unknown.

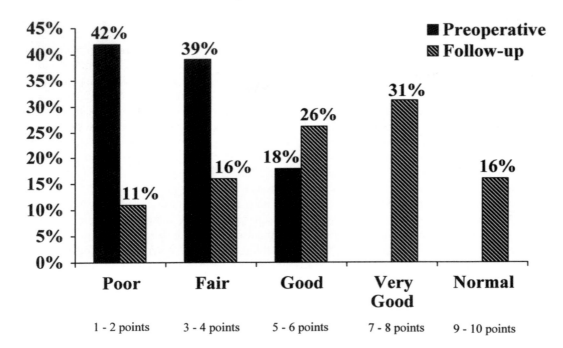

Patient Perception Knee Condition

FIGURE 11-13

Distribution of patient perception of the overall knee condition. The difference between preoperative and follow-up was statistically significant ($p < 0.0001$). (Adapted from Noyes FR, Barber-Westin SD, Rankin M. Meniscus transplantation in symptomatic patients under fifty years of age. *J Bone Joint Surg Am.* 2004;86: 392–1404, with permission.)

In this study, the meniscus transplant failure rate was 6% (1 of 18 knees) in knees with normal or only mild arthrosis on MRI, 45% (14 of 31 knees) in knees with moderate arthrosis, and 80% (12 of 15 knees) in knees with advanced arthrosis. The relationship between the meniscus allograft failure rate and increasing severity of joint arthrosis was significant ($p < 0.001$). The role of low-dose irra-

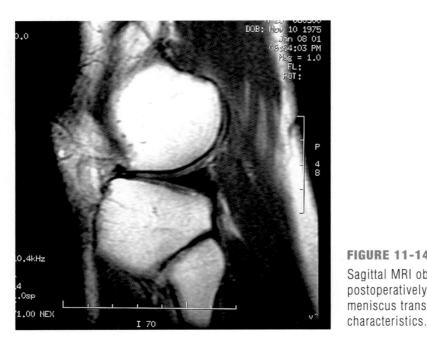

FIGURE 11-14

Sagittal MRI obtained 42 months postoperatively demonstrates a meniscus transplant with normal characteristics.

diation (2.0–2.5 Mrads) in terms of increasing the failure rate in any soft tissue graft is not scientifically known at this time.

The biology of meniscus healing and remodeling after implantation determines the final outcome regarding potential load-bearing function and chondroprotective effects. The meniscus transplant heals to the peripheral allograft–host rim junction in our experience within a short period of time, usually 4 to 6 weeks, providing initial stability of the transplant in the knee joint. In animal studies (2) and our analysis of failed meniscus transplants (14), there is an incomplete and disordered remodeling process including the minimal cellular repopulation of the allograft, disorganized collagen tissue lacking the normal collagen orientation required for load sharing, and a predominant fibrocyte cellular structure. Authors have reported an increase in water content and decrease in proteoglycan concentration (9).

In our experience, MRI done immediately after meniscus transplantation demonstrates uniform low signal intensity throughout the transplant tissue. Increased signal intensity at the capsular attachments of the transplant to the host meniscus rim is believed to be due to progressive healing. The low signal intensity within the body of the meniscus remains until remodeling of the transplant occurs. It is possible to see retention of the native meniscus low intensity signal for up to 2 to 3 years after implantation, indicating a delayed remodeling response. When remodeling occurs, MRI demonstrates an increased signal intensity that represents an ingrowth of cells into the transplant, removal of portions of the dense well-formed collagen framework, and replacement with randomized and disorganized collagenous tissues. During this stage, alterations in mechanical properties and decreased load-sharing capabilities of the transplant occur. With further remodeling, grade 3 signal intensity commonly appears, indicating early degeneration and tears in the transplant. We hypothesize that all meniscus allografts will undergo this deleterious remodeling process at different time periods postimplantation, resulting in altered mechanical properties and potential for tearing, fragmentation, and degeneration under joint-loading conditions.

CONCLUSIONS

On the basis of our investigations, we believe that the results of meniscus transplantation are more favorable when the operation is done before the onset of moderate tibiofemoral joint arthrosis. Several studies have documented a correlation between the final rating of the meniscus transplant and knee joint arthrosis, as success rate increases in knees with only mild arthrosis. This procedure is acceptable for younger patients, especially those who have symptoms with daily activities, as there are few if any other available treatment options. The short-term results are encouraging, as the majority of patients demonstrate improvement in knee function and pain in the affected compartment. However, no clinical study to date has determined if meniscus transplantation provides a chondroprotective effect.

Abnormal limb alignment and ligament instability require simultaneous or staged corrections to warrant meniscus transplantation. The long-term function of meniscus transplants remains questionable. The transplant undergoes limited remodeling, which results in alterations in meniscus collagen fiber micro-architecture, matrix, and cellular function required for load sharing and long-term survival. Patients are advised that the procedure is not curative in the long-term and additional surgery will probably be required. We believe the meniscus implant will eventually fail, requiring replacement in younger patients.

There are several important research areas that may improve the success rates of meniscus transplantation. These include issues related to transplant remodeling; collagen fiber restoration of micro-architecture to resist tensile, compressive, and shear forces; implant collagen matrix changes with altered material and structural properties; cellular repopulation and function in maintaining implant homeostasis; role of fresh transplants with viable cells; and the role of meniscus scaffolds and tissue engineering.

REFERENCES

1. Alhalki MM, Hull ML, Howell SM. Contact mechanics of the medial tibial plateau after implantation of a medial meniscal allograft. A human cadaveric study. *Am J Sports Med.* 2000;28(3):370–376.
2. Arnoczky SP, DiCarlo EF, O'Brien SJ, et al. Cellular repopulation of deep-frozen meniscal autografts: an experimental study in the dog. *Arthroscopy.* 1992;8(4):428–436.

3. Barber-Westin SD, Noyes FR, McCloskey JW. Rigorous statistical reliability, validity, and responsiveness testing of the Cincinnati knee rating system in 350 subjects with uninjured, injured, or anterior cruciate ligament–reconstructed knees. *Am J Sports Med.* 1999;27(4):402–416.

4. Barbour SA, King W. The safe and effective use of allograft tissue—an update. *Am J Sports Med.* 2003;31(5):791–797.

5. Berlet GC, Fowler PJ. The anterior horn of the medial meniscus. An anatomic study of its insertion. *Am J Sports Med.* 1998;26(4):540–543.

6. Cameron JC, Saha S. Meniscal allograft transplantation for unicompartmental arthritis of the knee. *Clin Orthop Relat Res.* 1997;337:164–171.

7. Cole BJ, Carter TR, Rodeo SA. Allograft meniscal transplantation. Background, techniques, and results. *J Bone Joint Surg Am.* 2002;84-A(7):1236–1250.

8. Farr J, Meneghini RM, Cole BJ. Allograft interference screw fixation in meniscus transplantation. *Arthroscopy.* 2004;20(3):322–327.

9. Jackson DW, Simon TM. Biology of meniscal allograft. In: Mow VC, Arnoczky SP, Jackson DW, eds. *Knee meniscus: basic and clinical foundations.* New York: Raven; 1992:141–152.

10. McLaughlin JR, Noyes FR. Arthroscopic meniscus repair: recommended surgical techniques for complex meniscal tears. *Techniques in Orthopaedics.* 1993;8(2):129–136.

11. Noyes FR, Barber-Westin SD. A comparison of results in acute and chronic anterior cruciate ligament ruptures of arthroscopically assisted autogenous patellar tendon reconstruction. *Am J Sports Med.* 1997;25(4):460–471.

12. Noyes FR, Barber-Westin SD. Meniscus transplantation: indications, techniques, clinical outcomes. *Instr Course Lect.* 2005;54:341–353.

13. Noyes FR, Barber-Westin SD. Posterior cruciate ligament replacement with a two-strand quadriceps tendon-patellar bone autograft and a tibial inlay technique. *J Bone Joint Surg Am.* 2005;87(6):1241–1252.

14. Noyes FR, Barber-Westin SD, Butler DL, et al. The role of allografts in repair and reconstruction of knee joint ligaments and menisci. *Instr Course Lect.* 1998;47:379–396.

15. Noyes FR, Barber-Westin SD, Rankin M. Meniscal transplantation in symptomatic patients less than fifty years old. *J Bone Joint Surg Am.* 2004;86-A(7):1392–1404.

16. Noyes FR, Berrios-Torres S, Barber-Westin SD, et al. Prevention of permanent arthrofibrosis after anterior cruciate ligament reconstruction alone or combined with associated procedures: a prospective study in 443 knees. *Knee Surg Sports Traumatol Arthrosc.* 2000;8(4):196–206.

17. Noyes FR, Mooar PA, Matthews DS, et al. The symptomatic anterior cruciate-deficient knee. Part I: the long-term functional disability in athletically active individuals. *J Bone Joint Surg Am.* 1983;65(2):154–162.

18. Pollard ME, Kang Q, Berg EE. Radiographic sizing for meniscal transplantation. *Arthroscopy.* 1995;11(6):684–687.

19. Potter HG, Foo LF. Magnetic resonance imaging of articular cartilage: trauma, degeneration, and repair. *Am J Sports Med.* 2006;34(4):661–677.

20. Potter HG, Linklater JM, Allen AA, et al. Magnetic resonance imaging of articular cartilage in the knee. An evaluation with use of fast-spin-echo imaging. *J Bone Joint Surg Am.* 1998;80(9):1276–1284.

21. Rankin M, Noyes FR, Barber-Westin SD, et al. Human meniscus allografts' in vivo size and motion characteristics: magnetic resonance imaging assessment under weightbearing conditions. *Am J Sports Med.* 2006;34(1):98–107.

22. Rosenberg TD, Paulos LE, Parker RD, et al. The forty-five-degree posteroanterior flexion weight-bearing radiograph of the knee. *J Bone Joint Surg.* 1988;70A:1479–1483.

23. Rubman MH, Noyes FR, Barber-Westin SD. Arthroscopic repair of meniscal tears that extend into the avascular zone. A review of 198 single and complex tears. *Am J Sports Med.* 1998;26(1):87–95.

24. Rubman MH, Noyes FR, Barber-Westin SD. Technical considerations in the management of complex meniscus tears. *Clin Sports Med.* 1996;15(3):511–530.

25. Stone KR, Walgenbach AW, Turek TJ, et al. Meniscus allograft survival in patients with moderate to severe unicompartmental arthritis: a 2- to 7-year follow-up. *Arthroscopy.* 2006;22(5):469–478.

26. Vangsness CT Jr, Garcia IA, Mills CR, et al. Allograft transplantation in the knee: tissue regulation, procurement, processing, and sterilization. *Am J Sports Med.* 2003;31(3):474–481.

27. Verdonk PC, Demurie A, Almqvist KF, et al. Transplantation of viable meniscal allograft. Survivorship analysis and clinical outcome of one hundred cases. *J Bone Joint Surg Am.* 2005;87-A(4):715–724.

PART THREE

LIGAMENT INJURIES AND INSTABILITY

12 Anterior Cruciate Ligament Reconstruction

Douglas W. Jackson and Peter R. Kurzweil

INDICATIONS

The treatment for a patient with an acutely torn anterior cruciate ligament (ACL) is individualized by factors such as age, occupation, level of sports participation, and associated intra-articular and ligament injuries. An important consideration in the discussion with the patient is the patient's willingness to modify high-risk activities in the future. We usually recommend anterior ligament reconstruction in the more physically active individuals of all ages who want to pursue activities that involve lateral movement, sudden stopping, and change of direction. We also suggest reconstruction of the ruptured ACL when there are significant associated meniscus tear(s) and/or a concomitant ligament injury. The decision to perform reconstructive surgery in someone with symptomatic knee instability due to chronic ACL deficiency is less controversial. Patients with an anterior cruciate deficient knee have had a chance to experience the limitations it imposes on their lifestyle. Usually the reason they have made the appointment with the surgeon is because they no longer want to live with the limitations if something can be done to correct the knee.

CONTRAINDICATIONS

The contraindications to ACL reconstruction have diminished over the past decade. The procedure is now done on an outpatient basis, with an increasing number of surgeons doing it technically well. The time taken from everyday activities for recovery following an acute ACL rupture can take a few weeks up to 2 months. The recovery time from the surgery to return to light work and/or school is about the same. There are several considerations that should be discussed with the patient who is considering a reconstruction:

- Not every ACL rupture needs to be reconstructed. Many individuals live with an ACL-deficient knee quite successfully.
- There is no urgency to reconstruct an ACL immediately after the injury. The patient can recover from the acute phase and determine if he or she wants to live with the deficient knee or have it reconstructed at a later date.
- The results from delayed reconstructions (>6 weeks or even months and years later) appear to be almost equivalent to those reconstructions done shortly after the acute injury. This is true as long as the patient does not sustain repeated subluxations with effusions, additional meniscal tears, additional bone contusions, and associated articular cartilage damage.

PREOPERATIVE PREPARATION

The first step in assessing the pathology of the injured knee with an ACL rupture is to perform a thorough history and physical examination. The history is often diagnostic in most acute ACL ruptures. The patient often describes hearing or feeling a pop within the knee which was associated with a cutting motion or sudden change in direction. The individual may report that the injury occurred as the result of a noncontact or contact injury. In many instances, the patient was unable to continue participating in that particular activity. The injured knee usually develops an effusion within a few hours following the injury.

Imaging of the knee includes routine radiographs to rule out fractures, evaluate pre-existing degenerative changes, and assess the overall alignment of the lower extremity. A magnetic resonance imaging (MRI) scan is not always necessary, but is an excellent independent method to confirm a torn ACL. In addition, it is helpful in documenting meniscal tears, the extent of bone contusions (Fig. 12-1), and other ligament injuries. However, other than bone contusions, the MRI may not offer much more information than an experienced clinician will find with a thorough preoperative evaluation, examination under anesthesia, and arthroscopic assessment at the time of reconstruction. If a decision is made to treat the knee operatively, the associated intra-articular pathology can be evaluated, documented, and treated during the surgical procedure.

When the patient with an acute injury arrives for evaluation, the knee is usually swollen (hemarthrosis) with restricted range of motion. If surgery is recommended, we prefer waiting for the acute inflammatory phase, with its associated pain and swelling, to subside. Waiting for the motion to improve has been associated with less difficulty re-establishing the range of motion of the knee after surgery. Patients typically take 2 or 3 weeks to re-establish their knee motion following an ACL tear. A displaced bucket handle tear causing a locked knee may be a consideration for shortening the waiting period for surgical reconstruction.

The planned incisions and graft options are discussed with each patient. During the 1990s, we preferred to use a patellar tendon autograft almost exclusively; and although it is still one of our primary choices, hamstrings and allografts are now used more commonly. This is particularly true if the patient has a pre-existing patellofemoral disorder, a history of anterior knee pain, or is particularly concerned about the cosmetics of an incision. We prefer to avoid incisions around the patellar tendon in workers who kneel and crawl as part of their occupation. With improved soft tissue graft aperture fixation and reported results, our use of hamstring grafts has increased significantly. We have used allografts in ACL reconstructions in a larger number of cases over a 20-year period and prefer them in certain revisions, older and less active patients, and those patients in whom the knee requires multiligament reconstruction.

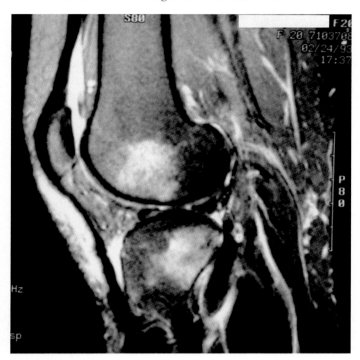

FIGURE 12-1

If the patient has had an MRI before surgery, we have the important films on the view box at the time of surgery. The MRI following an acute ACL rupture confirms the disrupted ACL, and quite accurately demonstrates associated torn menisci. The typical anterolateral femoral and posterolateral tibial kissing bone contusions are demonstrated in this figure.

SURGERY

The patient is placed in the supine position with both legs resting straight on the operating table. Our patients and anesthesiologists usually elect general anesthesia, although some choose an epidural block. A tourniquet is placed on the proximal thigh but is infrequently inflated during the procedure. A lateral thigh post clamped to the table allows a valgus stress to be applied to the knee, enhancing visualization and access to the medial meniscus.

Most of our patients receive a single-injection femoral nerve block. We believe this has significantly reduced the level of pain and need for narcotic analgesics in the immediate postoperative period. Most patients who have the block go home with very little discomfort. The femoral nerve block does shut down the quadriceps muscle temporarily, so all weight bearing on the operated knee is delayed for at least 1 day. Prophylactic antiobiotics—typically 1 g of a first-generation cephalosporin (Cefazolin)—are given 30 to 60 minutes prior to surgey.

After adequate anesthesia, we perform a ligament examination and document the preoperative arthrometric evaluation of both knees with the KT-1000. We look at the manual maximum displacement numbers and do not use the test at 20 and 30 pounds of force. A KT-1000 evaluation is also performed immediately following surgery, while the patient is still under anesthesia. These values are used to help confirm that the graft tensioning and fixation are satisfactory. The vast majority (98%) of the knees we reconstruct have a preoperative side-to-side difference of 5 mm or more under anesthesia and a positive pivot shift. If it is obvious that the ACL is nonfunctional, the autograft is routinely harvested before the arthroscopic portion of the procedure. When an allograft is used, it is not opened until we are certain that we will proceed with the ACL reconstruction. The graft is then prepared at a side table during the arthroscopy. However, when there is an equivocal pivot shift or a side-to-side difference of less than 5 mm with the KT-1000, the knee is first evaluated arthroscopically.

We make a concerted effort not to inflate a tourniquet during the procedure. Three techniques help control hemostasis and maintain our visual field. First, the pressure of the irrigation solution from gravity is maintained by the height of the irrigation bags. We have chosen not to use a pressurized inflow system (a pump) and prefer gravity irrigation. Second, the joint is injected with 25 mL of 0.50% Marcaine with 1:200,000 epinephrine immediately after draping the knee. Third, we selectively use intra-articular hemostasis with an insulated electrocuatery tip to control localized bleeding.

If the patellar tendon is being used as the graft, the skin over the patellar tendon is injected with 10 mL of the same anesthetic solution before harvesting the autograft. We believe this also helps reduce postoperative pain.

The surgery is performed in a stepwise fashion as follows: (a) evaluation under anesthesia, (b) graft harvesting and preparation, (c) notch preparation, (d) positioning and preparing the osseous tunnels, (e) graft implantation and fixation, (f) closure and postoperative assessment of stability, and (g) postoperative management and rehabilitation.

Technique

While under direct observation of the nurses in the preoperative area before sedation is given, the patient writes a "yes" on the ACL deficient knee. Once in the operating room, a "time out" is called to confirm the correct patient, procedure, and site. This "time out" requires the agreement of the circulator, scrub assistant, surgeon, and anesthesiologist . Our method of harvesting the patellar tendon is described later in this chapter when we elect to use it as our graft. Chapter 15 demonstrates another technique for patellar tendon bone-bone harvesting. When a patella tendon autograft is chosen, we prefer a vertical incision along the medial border of the patellar tendon. The incision starts at the level of the inferior pole of the patella and extends to the level of the tibial tubercle (Fig. 12-2). The peritenon is carefully dissected away from the tendon. We do not harvest more than one third of the total width of the tendon. If the width is at least 30 mm, a double-bladed scalpel (Fig. 12-3) with the blades set 10 mm apart is used to cut a central strip of tendon. In smaller individuals, a 9-mm strip of tendon is harvested.

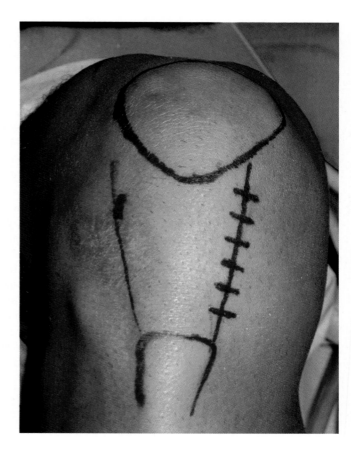

FIGURE 12-2

The skin incision to harvest the patella tendon autograft is vertical as depicted in this right knee. It extends from the inferior pole of the patella to a point approximately 1 cm medial to the tibial tubercle. Through this incision the anteromedial arthroscopy portal is placed as is the accessory anteromedial portal for the passage of the femoral interference screw. This incision allows the medially located tibial tunnel to be drilled with less skin retraction.

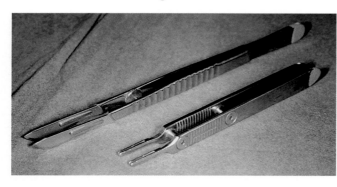

FIGURE 12-3

A double-handle scalpel (either 9 or 10 mm between the blades) ensures a parallel cut when harvesting the central third of the patellar tendon.

The tendon's bony attachments are outlined with electrocautery (Fig. 12-4A). The dimension of the patellar bone plug is typically 10×25 mm. The bone plug from the tibial side usually measures 10×25 mm. We use circular oscillating saws (Stryker, Kalamazoo, MI) with diameters of 9, 10, or 11 mm to harvest the bone plugs (Fig. 12-4B). Leaving a smooth, semicylindrical defect in the patella reduces stress risers and the potential for patella fracture postoperatively. This technique also allows for simple bone grafting of the created defects by using the cylindrical core of bone obtained from creating the the tibial tunnel. When split in half, the semicylindrical pieces of bone sit perfectly in the defects in the patella and tibial.

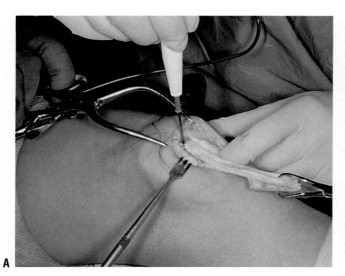

A

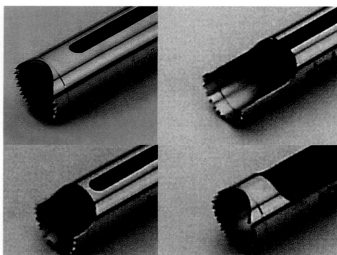

B

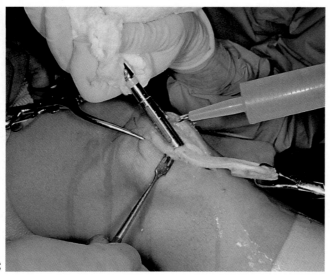

C

FIGURE 12-4

A: The tendon's bony attachments are outlined with electrocautery. **B:** The circular oscillating (Stryker, Kalamazoo, MI) saw used to harvest the bone plugs is smooth and recessed on top to prevent soft-tissue laceration when harvesting the bone plug. **C:** By pulling the mobile extensor mechanism distally and retracting the skin proximally, the incision can be shortened by 2 or 3 cm. The saw cuts better when the bone is kept moist, which also helps minimize thermal necrosis.

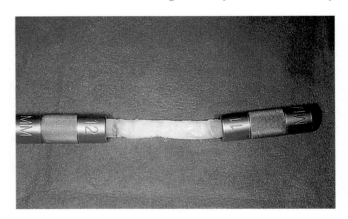

FIGURE 12-5

The tibial bone plug was harvested with a 10-mm circular saw and slides through an 11-mm spacer with minimal trimming. The patellar end of the graft was taken with a 10-mm harvester and easily slides through a 10-mm spacer. The spacers represent the diameter of the bone tunnels to be drilled.

The tibial plug is harvested first, typically with a 10-mm circular saw blade. Once the tibial bone plug is harvested, a towel clip is attached and used to pull the extensor mechanism distally, drawing the patella into the wound. Retracting the loose tissue over the patella proximally permits a shorter skin incision to be used. The patellar bone plug is then harvested with the same blade (Fig. 12-4C). To avoid burning the bone, saline drops are added to help dissipate the heat generated by the oscillating harvesting blade.

The graft is taken to a side table and prepared for implantation by the assistant surgeon. With minimal trimming, each bone plug should easily slide through a spacer matching the diameter of the osseous tunnel through which it will eventually pass (Fig. 12-5). The tibial plug, intended for the femoral side, is trimmed to slide through a 9-mm tunnel spacer (Fig. 12-6). The patellar plug, which will be fixed in an 10-mm diameter tibial tunnel, usually requires only minimal trimming. Three drill holes (using a 3/32-inch bit) are made in the patella bone plug and threaded with No. 5 Tevdek or Ticron sutures. The holes are oriented at right angles to each other to minimize the chance of suture laceration by the interference screw, and hence loosing tension on the graft during tibial screw insertion. A single drill hole is made in the tibial bone plug, which is threaded with a 30-inch No. 2 nylon suture. The graft is mounted on a tension board (8-lb load), which also facilitates final soft-tissue trimming. The bone–tendon junction is marked with a sterile pen. A line is drawn longitudi-

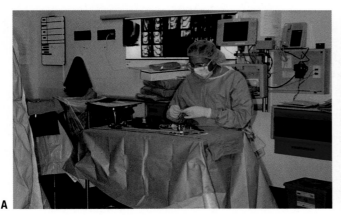
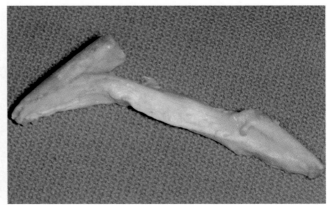

A   B

FIGURE 12-6

A: One surgeon shapes, sizes, and prepares the graft at a side table for passage through the knee and into the desired positions in the bone tunnels. Two surgeons working simultaneously shorten the operative time. **B:** A typical harvested graft before shaping, sizing, and preparation for passage. Note the different collagen insertions into the tibia and patella bone plugs. These different orientations to the collagen insertions can be used to position the collagen in the desired portion of the osseous tunnels.

nally along the center of the femoral plug to help orient its rotation as it is pulled into the femoral tunnel (Fig. 12-7). Once preparation of the graft is complete, it is left under tension and covered with an antibiotic-soaked sponge (Fig. 12-8). Using an assistant to prepare the graft while the surgeon works on the knee can save 15 to 30 minutes per case and can keep the surgical time for an isolated ACL reconstruction to less than 1 hour.

Regardless of graft choice, the intra-articular portion of the procedure begins by introducing the arthroscope into the anterolateral portal. When a patellar tendon autograft is harvested, the antero-medial portal is made by retracting the incision to expose the medial border of the patellar tendon (Fig. 12-9). A thorough diagnostic arthroscopy is performed through a separate anterolateral portal to confirm the torn ACL (Fig. 12-10) and determine the status of the menisci and articular cartilage. We prefer to debride the soft tissue from the lateral wall of the notch with a full-radius resector. Our

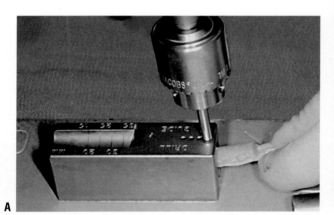

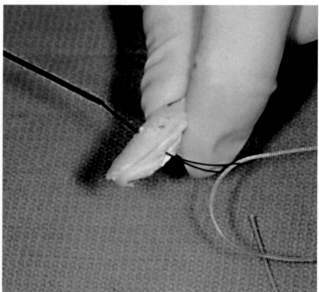

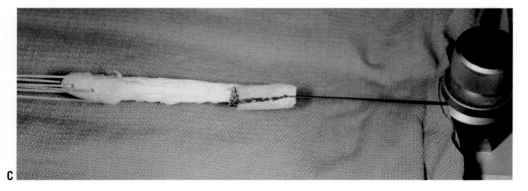

FIGURE 12-7

A: Three drill holes (using a 3/32-inch bit) are made in the harvested patella bone plug and threaded with No. 5 Tevdek sutures. The holes are oriented at right angles to each other to minimize the chance of suture laceration by the interference screw. We pass the sutures through the bone plugs with a Hewson suture passer **(B)**. There are no needles on the back table. This eliminates the possibility of a needle puncture wound to the surgeon preparing the graft. A single drill hole is made in the harvested tibial plug, which is threaded with a 30-inch No. 2 nylon suture. The graft is mounted on a tension board (8-lb load), which also facilitates final soft-tissue trimming **(C)**. The bone–tendon junction is marked with a sterile pen. A line is drawn longitudinally along the center of the femoral plug to help orient its rotation as it is pulled into the femoral tunnel. The prepared graft is mounted on a tensioning board, which facilitates final trimming.

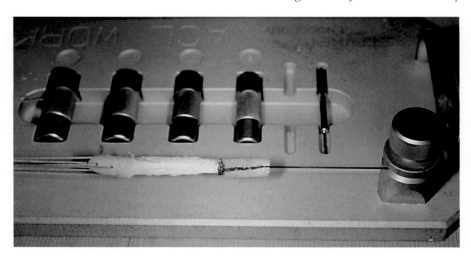

FIGURE 12-8

The larger bone plug has three No. 5 Tevdek sutures oriented at right angles, while the smaller bone plug has a single long (30 inches) suture passed through the cortical surface. The bone–tendon junction is marked with a sterile pen for orientation during passage.

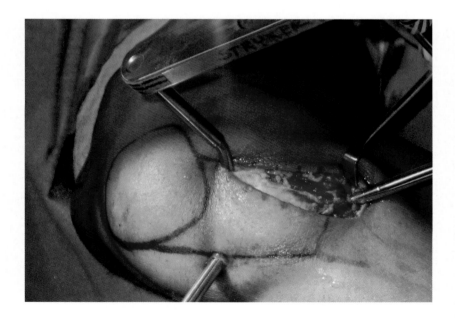

FIGURE 12-9

Because of the medially placed skin incision, a separate stab wound is used for the anterolateral arthroscopic portal. We place it close to the lateral border of the patellar tendon and approximately 1.5 cm above the tibial plateau as depicted in this figure. The extra-articular "starting point" determines the length and obliquity of the tibial tunnel. To facilitate placing the femoral tunnel toward the 10 o'clock postion in a right knee, the guide used for drilling is positioned at a point about 2 cm medial to the tibial tubercle. The distance of the starting position distal to the joint line determines the angle of the graft in the saggital plane. Starting too distal may create a tibial tunnel that is too steep.

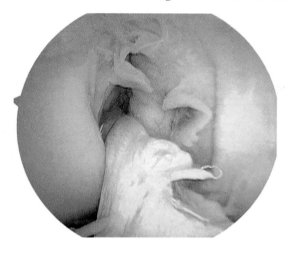

FIGURE 12-10

An acutely torn ACL. It has been disrupted near its femoral insertion.

goal is to visualize the "over-the-top" position. The center of the femoral tunnel is selected after preparing the notch. An endoscopic "over-the-top" guide is used to mark a point that will leave a thin shell of cortical bone posteriorly after the femoral tunnel is drilled. Guides are available for creating tunnel diameters from 6 to 11 mm (Fig. 12-11). When a 10-mm tunnel is planned with the typical patellar tendon autograft, we use a guide (Stryker, Kalamazoo, MI) that is designed to mark a point 6 to 7.0 mm anterior to the over-the-top position (Fig. 12-12). A 10-mm tunnel (5-mm radius) with 7-mm placement will leave a 2.0-mm posterior rim. The guide is inserted through an accessory anteromedial portal made just over the joint line and along the medial border of the patellar tendon. The desired site in the notch is drilled through the cannulated guide. The location of the femoral tunnel has changed slightly to avoid a more vertical graft. We prefer placing the center of the femoral tunnel at the 10:00 AM or 2:00 PM site. (See Chapter 14 for more in-depth discussion on tunnel placement.)

Attention is turned to preparation of the tibial tunnel. The length of the tunnel varies with the graft length. Although the intra-articular opening for the osseous tunnel is fixed, the position of the extra-articular opening of the tunnel can be varied. The preferred length of the tibial tunnel is calculated as explained in Figures 12-13 and 12-14. The total graft length (in millimeters) minus 50 mm esti-

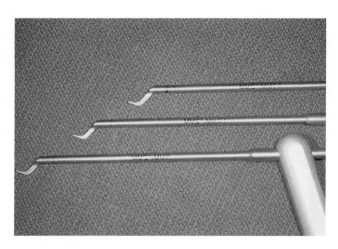

FIGURE 12-11

Over-the-top endoscopic guides for marking the site of the center of the femoral tunnel. Each is designed to leave a 2-mm rim of posterior cortical bone when drilling a 9-, 10-, or 11-mm femoral tunnel.

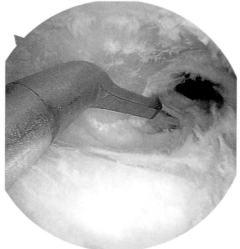

FIGURE 12-12

Intra-articular view of the femoral guide. The "prong" has hooked over the top. The guides are cannulated so that a drill will mark the desired location, in this case 6.5 mm anterior to the over-the-top position.

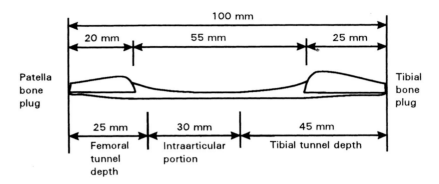

FIGURE 12-13

The calculation of tibial tunnel length. A typical graft has bone plugs of 20 and 25 mm, and is 100 mm long. Assuming a femoral tunnel of 25 mm and an intra-articular distance of 30 mm (the average length of an ACL), the tibial tunnel must be at least 45 mm long to accommodate the graft. Another 5 mm should be added to the calculated length, since drilling a 10- or 11-mm-diameter tibial tunnel effectively shortens the tunnel length by its radius.

mates the desired tibial tunnel length. This will prevent the tunnel from being too short, avoiding graft-tunnel mismatch. The tibial tunnel needs to be started medially to allow access to the lower femoral tunnel site. (See Chapter 14 for more detail on tunnel site selection.)

The intra-articular point for the tunnel opening is referenced from the posterior cruciate ligament (PCL), lateral meniscus, and tibial spines. The arc made by the posterior rim of the anterior horn of the lateral meniscus is followed to the medial tibial spine. This is about 7 mm anterior to the PCL (Figs. 12-15 and 12-16). The tip of the tibial drill guide is inserted through the anteromedial portal and placed on this spot. The angle of this calibrated guide is adjusted until the desired tunnel length is achieved (Fig. 12-17). The angle of the tunnel should place the graft in appropriate relationship to the slope of the intercondylar notch. The guide pin is then inserted (Fig. 12-18), with attention given to prevent it from "walking up" the tibia and shortening the tibial tunnel.

When a patella tendon bone autograft is harvested, we use a cannulated core drill, which removes a cylinder of bone, to create the tibial tunnel. This allows a clean removal of the tibial ACL stump (Fig. 12-19) and the acquisition of a solid piece of bone for grafting into the defects in the patella and tibial tubercle, as described previously (Fig. 12-20).

FIGURE 12-14

The probe is seated in the debrided stump of the ACL. This position is parallel with the posterior rim of the anterior horn of the lateral meniscus and 7 mm anterior to the PCL. It is at the level of the midportion of the medial tibial spine.

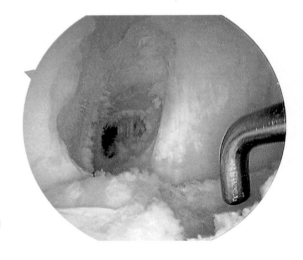

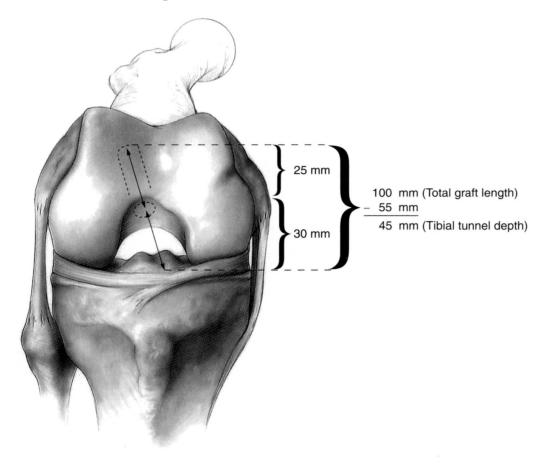

25 mm

30 mm

100 mm (Total graft length)
– 55 mm
45 mm (Tibial tunnel depth)

FIGURE 12-15

The length of the tibial tunnel is calculated by subtracting the total graft length from the sum of the length of the femoral tunnel (25 mm) and the intra-articular distance between the tunnel openings (30 mm). Another 5 mm is added to the difference, as described in Figure 12-13.

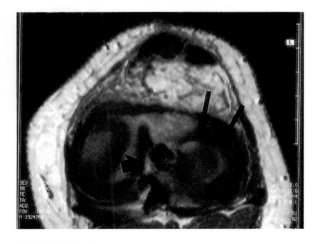

FIGURE 12-16

Magnetic resonance image of the tibial plateau taken after reconstruction. This demonstrates the posterior location of the tibial tunnel (*thick arrowhead*) and its relationship to the lateral meniscus (*thin arrows*).

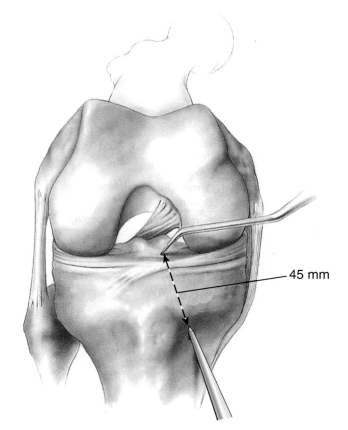

45 mm

FIGURE 12-17

Drilling the tibial tunnel. The tibial guide is set to drill a tunnel of a predetermined length, in this case 45 mm. The length should generally not exceed 55 mm, or the obliquity of the tibial tunnel will be too steep. Note the starting position of the tibial tunnel is halfway between the tubercle and medial border of the tibia.

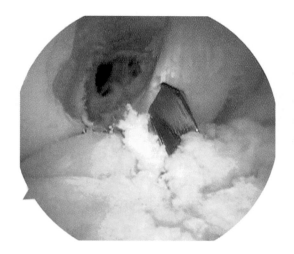

FIGURE 12-18

The guide pin has emerged in the joint in the desired location (as described in Fig. 12-16). The lateral meniscus can be seen in the lower-right-hand corner.

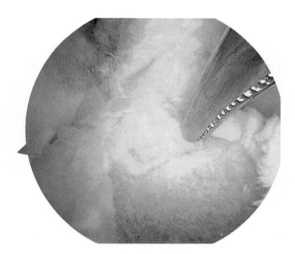

FIGURE 12-19

Removing a core of bone, rather than simply drilling the tibial tunnel, leaves an intra-articular opening with smooth margins. The articular cartilage and ligament stump have been cleanly removed rather than pushed aside.

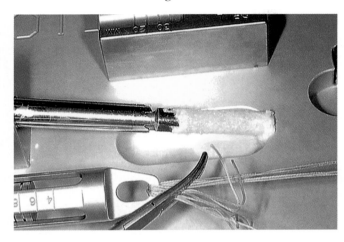

FIGURE 12-20

A core of bone is obtained when making the tibial tunnel. It is split in half and trimmed to fit the patellar defect at the time of closure.

The femoral tunnel is drilled through the tibial tunnel. The guide pin is retrograded through the tibial tunnel to the previously selected point in the notch. We recommend that this be done with at least 70 degrees of knee flexion, which reduces the chances of blowing out the posterior wall of the femoral tunnel and potential for vascular and/or nerve injury. Once the pin is inserted, the position of the knee should not vary, or the pin may bend or break during drilling. Sometimes the guide pin retrograded through the tibial tunnel cannot "hit" the previously marked center of the femoral tunnel. In these occasions, we will drill the tunnel through the anteriormedial poprtal in 120° of flexion.

A cannulated, acorn-shaped drill bit (usually 10-mm diameter) is manually passed over the guide pin and through the tibial tunnel. Care is taken in passing the tip past the PCL. When the bit touches the femoral wall, it is drilled to a depth of 25 to 30 mm (Fig. 12-21). The calibrated measurement at the distal opening of the tibial tunnel should be the same or slightly greater than the total graft length (Fig. 12-22), or the graft will protrude. The tibial tunnel is plugged and a suction device is passed into the notch area and femoral tunnel to remove extraneous morsels of bone from the joint. The integrity of the posterior cortical rim of the tunnel is arthroscopically confirmed (Fig. 12-23).

A small notch is made at the aperture of the femoral tunnel at 2 o'clock (in a left knee) into which the interference screw guidewire will later be placed. This helps prevent the screw from rotating around the plug as it is inserted in the tunnel. The knee is now ready for graft implantation. A Beath pin with an eyelet proximally is retrograded through the tibial and femoral tunnels and out the anterolateral thigh, with the knee flexed approximately 90 degrees. The graft is removed from the tension board and the nylon suture is threaded through the eyelet. The pin is grasped and pulled out

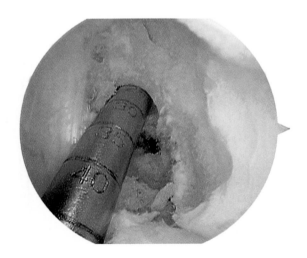

FIGURE 12-21

A calibrated drill allows the depth of the femoral tunnel to be visualized. We prefer 25 to 30 mm in length for the femoral osseous tunnel. These tunnel lengths are modified if the length of the graft bone plugs is shorter than usual.

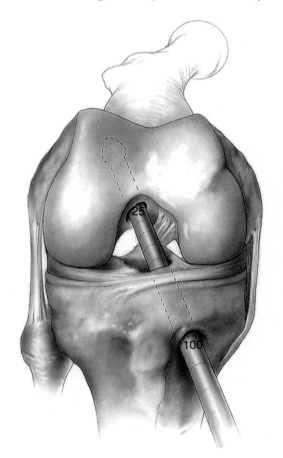

FIGURE 12-22

The calibrated drill used for making the femoral tunnel also provides the overall end-to-end length between the tunnels. The measurement at the distal opening of the tibial tunnel should match (or be slightly greater than) the length of the graft.

proximally, bringing with it the suture, which is then used to pull the graft into the joint. The bone plug is oriented so that the tendon is located posterior. The pen markings on the plug are helpful in achieving proper rotation. A clamp inserted through the anteromedial portal is often helpful in controlling the orientation of the plug as it is seated into the femoral tunnel (Fig. 12-24).

The bone plug in the femoral tunnel is fixed first. A guidewire for the cannulated interference screw is inserted through the accessory medial portal. It is placed into the notch of the femoral tunnel so that it is between the cancellous surface of the bone plug and the wall of the tunnel. Ideally, it is parallel to the longitudinal pen marking on the plug (Fig. 12-25). With the knee flexed 80 to 90 degrees, we prefer to use a 7-mm tap in the site for the interference screw. We then place a cannulated 8 × 23-mm interference screw over the wire (Fig. 12-26). It is advanced, giving secure inter-

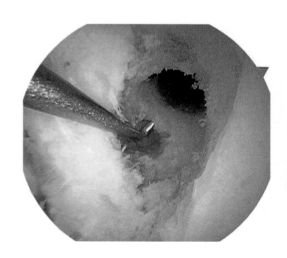

FIGURE 12-23

After drilling the femoral tunnel, the integrity of the posterior cortical rim should be assessed. If the drill has blown out the back wall, a second incision over the distal femur can be used to drill another tunnel from outside into the other tunnel, and interference fixation can still be used.

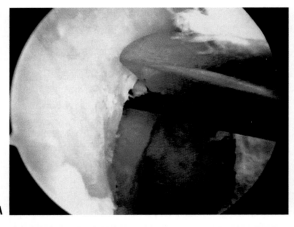

A

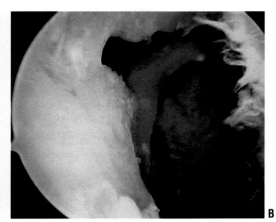

B

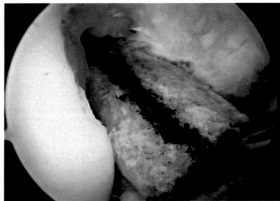

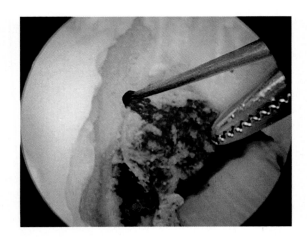

C

FIGURE 12-24

A–C: The opening to the femoral tunnel is notched for placement of the guide pin for the interference screw. As the graft is pulled into the joint, the bone plug rotation is controlled and oriented in relation to the notch and markings on the bone plug. The marked graft aids the surgeon in obtaining the desired rotation depth for seating the graft.

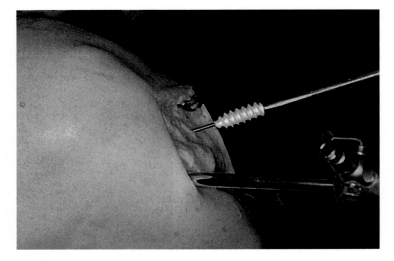

FIGURE 12-25
The guidewire for the cannulated femoral interference screw should be directed between the cancellous surface of the bone plug and the tunnel wall. We then use a cannulated pretap 7 mm in diameter passed over the guide pin. The tap is removed and an 8-mm-diameter bioabsorbable screw is passed over the guide pin.

FIGURE 12-26
The screw is inserted into the joint over the guidewire.

ference fixation. We have been using bioabsorbable screws routinely since 1998. The screw is inserted flush with the marked bone–tendon junction, which is also flush with the aperture of the femoral tunnel (Fig. 12-27).

The femoral fixation of the graft is tested by firmly pulling on the Tevdek sutures in the tibial bone plug. The surgeon should be able to pull hard enough to gently rock the patient without the fixation failing. It is important to keep the knee in flexion when assessing the fixation so that the pull is directly parallel to the femoral tunnel and screw. The knee is cycled several times while palpating for movement of the bone plug in the tibial tunnel. Lack of movement does not necessarily mean that the graft is perfectly isometric. Rather, it may indicate that the tibial bone plug is catching in the tunnel, in which case pulling on the sutures may not allow the graft to be properly tensioned. More than a few millimeters of bone-plug excursion is also undesirable and may indicate improperly placed tunnels. As the knee is ranged, the position at which the tibial plug is most distal in the tunnel is noted. This is usually close to full extension. The graft is tensioned in this position while pulling on the Tevdek sutures. A 9 or 10 × 28-mm bioabsorbable interference screw is then inserted for tibial fixation. A posteriorly applied force on the tibia helps ensure joint reduction during screw fixation. After the graft has been fixed, the knee is placed through a full range of motion. If a audible loud click or pop is heard at this time, it may indicate failure of fixation (usually at the femur). The pivot shift and Lachman test are performed, and if they are unacceptable, the graft is retensioned. We find ourselves retensioning less than 5% of reconstructions each year. The patient should not leave the operating room until we have achieved the desired stability.

The core of bone from the tibial tunnel is split in half and trimmed to fit the bony defect in the patella and tibial tubercle. The overlying tissue is sutured to hold the graft in place. The patellar tendon is loosely reapproximated to prevent any palpable gaps without shortening the patella tendon. The peritenon, subcutaneous tissue, and skin are closed in separate layers. Steri-strips are applied. The joint is injected with 25 mL of 0.50% Marcaine with 1:200,000 epinephrine and 5 mg of Duramorph.

After the wound is closed, sterile gauze and steri-drape are used to temporarily cover the wound to allow evaluation with KT-1000 (Fig. 12-28A). A postoperative side-to-side comparison is made in each patient (Fig. 12-28B). If the difference in the measurements is equal to or less than 2 mm in anterior translation, this is acceptable. A fresh sterile dressing is placed over the incision, and a TEDS stocking and knee immobilizer are applied (Fig. 12-29A–C). The patient is then taken to the recovery room. The reconstruction is performed as an outpatient procedure and patients are discharged home with oral pain medication.

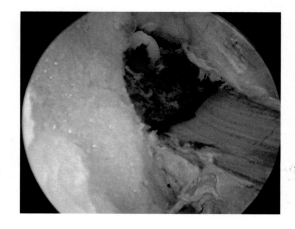

FIGURE 12-27

Advancement of the screw should be visualized to ensure the screw does not rotate around the graft as it is placed in its interference position. The screw is inserted to a depth that makes it flush with the end of the bone plug, which was highlighted with a marking pen. The location of the screw superolaterally pushes the collagen posteriorly and toward the PCL. It also minimizes contact with the collagen to prevent tendon abrasion.

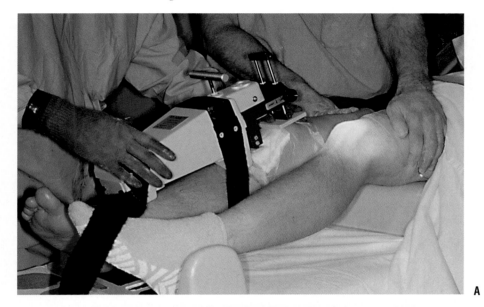

A

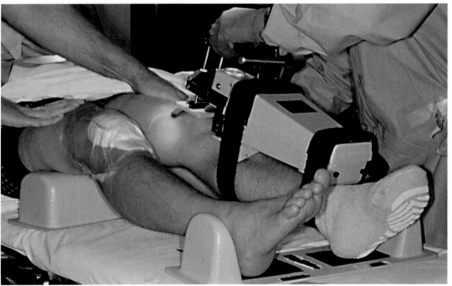

B

FIGURE 12-28

A,B: Manual maximum displacement KT-1000 readings are taken to confirm fixation. A temporary dressing is applied to maintain wound sterility. The uninvolved knee is also retested at the conclusion of the case. If there is more than 2 mm of side-to-side laxity in the reconstructed knee, the graft is retensioned. The ideal is to have symmetry side to side.

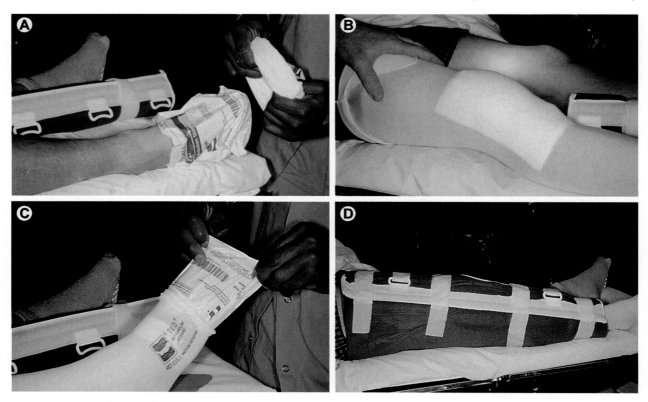

FIGURE 12-29

A–D: The sterile dressing is held in place with a thigh-high TEDS stocking rather than tape. Our nurses like to use a plastic bag over the foot to help slide on the stocking.

Pearls and Pitfalls

Graft Protrusion   Excessive tibial plug protrusion from the tibial tunnel precludes interference fixation. Graft tunnel mismatch (as described previously) is avoided by not drilling a tibial tunnel that is too short (see Figs. 12-13 and 12-14). Protrusions of a few millimeters can be handled with minor adjustments. The simplest is to shorten the protruding end of the bone plugs by 3 to 5 mm with a bone rongeur. If this is not enough, the femoral tunnel can be deepened by 5 mm. These two measures should compensate for 10 mm of graft protrusion. If necessary, distal fixation can be accomplished by tying the sutures in the tibial plug around a screw (post) and washer.

Problems with the Tibial Interference Screw   Two problems with the tibial interference screw may result in graft laxity. First, the screw can push the tibial plug into the tunnel when inserted, resulting in loss of tension on the graft. This is best avoided by maintaining a firm pull on the Tevdek sutures and watching the position of the plug as the screw is inserted. Second, the soft medullary bone and space of the tibia may result in inadequate interference fixation. A feeling for adequate interference fixation can be ascertained by noting the resistance when turning the screwdriver and by carrying out a full range of motion, Lachman, and pivot shift testing once fixation is felt to be adequate. If back-up tibial fixation is desired, we tie the traction sutures through small tunnels in the adjacent bony defect where the tibial bone was harvested.

Problems with the Interference Screw Guidewire   If the guidewire for the femoral or tibial screw is inserted too deeply, it can be difficult to extract after screw insertion. If the guide pin bends distal to the screw, there is the potential that it may break off. This should be suspected if the guidewire requires much force to extract. Be certain to examine the tip when the pin is extracted to be certain some has not broken off and remains in the osseous tunnel or knee. The chance of this problem occurring can be reduced by placing the guidewire directly between the bone plug and osseous tunnel wall and not advancing it too far beyond the place where the tip of the cannulated interference screw will be.

Difficulties in Harvesting the Graft   In attempting to harvest the patellar tendon graft, the circular saw may advance too deeply and lacerate the tendon. If this is recognized, it can be corrected by gently redirecting the saw. However, sudden changes in direction can fracture the plug. Switching to a larger-diameter saw blade or using an osteotome to complete the harvest may be helpful if this problem is recognized.

Blowout of the Posterior Wall of the Femoral Tunnel   It is important to check for blowout of the posterior wall of the femoral tunnel, since it would preclude endoscopic femoral interference fixation. If blowout does occur, the procedure could be salvaged by using an Endobutton or converting to the two-incision technique. Of course, prevention is the best way of avoiding this situation. The risk of blowout can be minimized by flexing the knee 70 degrees or more while drilling the femoral tunnel.

It is important in preparing the femoral tunnel that the knee be flexed at 70 degrees or greater. If the knee is in more extension during the drilling of the femora tunnel through the tibia tunnel and the drill goes out the back of the posterior cortex, there is the potential for nerve and/or vascular injury.

POSTOPERATIVE MANAGEMENT

We routinely perform ACL reconstructions on an outpatient basis. The femoral nerve block has helped with pain control. Patients are sent home with Norco 7.5 mg as an oral analgesic. They are allowed to shower the day after surgery with the wound covered. Treatment with ice is continued intermittently for 3 or 4 days. A knee immobilizer is worn for approximately 2 to 4 weeks during ambulation and sleeping. It is removed for therapy and when the patient is sitting. Weight bearing in the knee immobilizer is allowed as tolerated and dictated by swelling. Crutches are recommended outside the home for 2 to 4 weeks or until adequate muscular control of the lower extremity is regained. Patients are told to emphasize knee extension and muscle strengthening on their own and in therapy.

Rehabilitation

Exercises are started the day after surgery. We prefer the patient be involved in their recovery and re-etablishment of knee motion and strengthening. Many patients prefer a close working relationship with a physical therapist. The therapist should communicate and alert the surgeon if problems are developing. The surgeon and therapists guide the return to various activities. Table 12-1 shows our standard rehabilitation protocol. Our goal is to re-establish full knee range of motion and eliminate effusions by 2 months postoperatively. Some patients meet these goals before 2 months. In the uncomplicated recovery, cycling can usually begin by 1 month, and jogging can be initiatd by 3 months. Unrestricted activity is usually delayed until 6 to 12 months following ACL reconstruction and needs to be individualized for each patient.

COMPLICATIONS

Decreased Motion

Failure to regain motion is usually associated with (a) technical problems related to the surgery, (b) cyclops formation and adhesions, or (c) inadequate postoperative exercising and initiative.

Failure to regain knee extension is the most common range-of-motion complication. Loss of extension may be due to graft impingement. It is usually from anterior placement of the tibial tunnel. (See Chapter 14 for more details.) We prefer our patients to have full extension within a few weeks of their ACL reconstruction. Attention to extension is stressed and occasionally specific braces are prescribed if flexion contractures are not improving. Failure to regain full motion by 2 months may need to be addressed with aggressive treatment, such as arthroscopic lysis of adhesions, debridement of soft tissue anterior to the graft, roof notchplasty, and/or manipulation. Figure 12-30 demonstrates a well-placed ACL graft in relationship to the intercondylar notch. Note the extension of the knee in this MRI and the uniform signal within the graft. Graft impingement against the intercondylar roof most commonly results from anterior placement of the tibial tunnel. (See Chapter 14, where graft impingement in flexion and extension are discussed further.)

TABLE 12-1.   ACL Reconstruction and Rehabilitation Protocol

Phase I—The Acute Phase (1–10 days)
- ROM
  - 0–90 degrees; emphasize full extension with prone hangs or pillow under ankle
  - Active ROM exercises 5/day
  - Heel slides, assisted with belt as needed
  - Hip and ankle ROM
- Strength/Cardio
  - Straight leg raise cocontractions 5/day (10 reps)
  - Hamstring sets with good leg
- Gait
  - PWB with crutches
  - Knee immobilizer for ambulation and sleep
    - Remove for ROM exercises and periodically
- Other
  - Minimize swelling
  - Emphasize patellar mobilization for B-PT-B autografts

Phase II (10 days–3 weeks)
- ROM
  - 0–120 degrees; continue ROM exercises
- Strength/Cardio
  - Begin quadriceps and hamstring sets
  - Emphasize VMO
  - Continue ankle and knee exercises
  - Stationary bike: 1/2 to full revolutions
  - Pool exercises optional—when wounds healed
- Gait
  - Braced discontinued once quadriceps control regained
  - Wean off crutches
- Other
  - Balance and proprioception exercises

Phase III (3–6 weeks)
- ROM
  - Push full PROM
- Strength/Cardio
  - Stationary bike as tolerated
  - Stair Master
  - Hamstring curls—concentric and eccentric
- Gait
  - Emphasize normal gait without brace or crutches

Phase IV—The Normalization phase (6–12 weeks)
- ROM—Full active and PROM
- Strength/Cardio
  - Stair Master
  - Partial squats
  - Single leg squats
  - Wall sits
  - Open- and closed-chain exercises
- Gait—Normal
- Other
  - Most can return to jobs that require prolonged standing
  - Increase intensity of exercises as tolerated

Phase V—The Cardio phase (3–6 months)
- ROM—should be normal
- Strength/Cardio
  - Full, unrestricted low-impact workouts with Stair Master, elliptical trainer
  - Quadriceps sets, low weights for leg presses and hamstring curls
  - Strengthen hips, calves, ankles
  - Jump rope
- Gait
  - No limp
  - Increase walking distances (can use treadmill)
  - Begin jogging straight ahead and increase as tolerated
- Other
  - Can begin sport-specific training
  - Box drill
  - Gentle figure-8s

Phase VI—The Sport-Specific Phase (6–9 months)
- Strength/Cardio
  - Increase weights and intensity from last phase
  - Progress from jogging to running and sprinting
  - Continue figure-8s and box drills
  - Jump and hop drills
- Other
  - Return to sports when strength is within 90% of good leg, and ROM is normal
  - Completed sport-specific training
  - Intensity and duration of sports participation increases as tolerated

PROM, passive range of motion; PWB, partial weight bearing; ROM, range of motion; VMO, vastus medialis obliquus.

Neurologic Complications

The most commonly injured nerve in harvesting the patellar tendon graft is the infrapatellar branch of the saphenous nerve. It frequently produces a small area of numbness along the anterolateral aspect of the knee. This is usually not a significant problem unless a painful neuroma develops.

Hemarthrosis

Hemarthrosis results in an uncomfortable swelling immediately after surgery. It usually resolves spontaneously but may increase postoperative pain, decrease mobility, slow progress in physical therapy, and increase the risk of infection. Meticulous hemostasis during surgery, with use of the intra-articular electrocautery, can be helpful in controlling persistent bleeding. We have not found it necessary or helpful to insert a drain postoperatively in our ACL reconstructions.

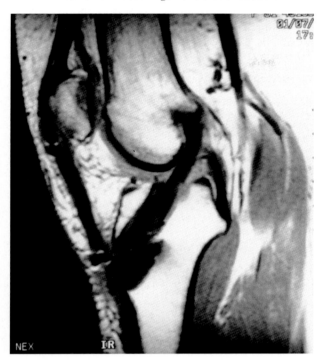

FIGURE 12-30
This MRI obtained 2 months after the ACL reconstruction demonstrates extension of the knee with no graft impingement against the intercondylar notch and uniform signal throughout the graft.

Effusions

Effusions can be a problem in the first few weeks after surgery and can retard progress in rehabilitation, particularly flexion and quadriceps control. The management of effusions includes aspiration (when necessary), anti-inflammatory medication, and decreased activity. Persistent effusions after 2 months are indicative of an intra-articular problem (i.e., articular cartilage surface particulate shedding) or a technical aspect related to tunnel placement and graft position from the surgery.

Postoperative Infections

Intra-articular infections following ACL reconstruction are a quite infrequent occurrence. Those that do occur have the best chance of successful treatment if recognized early. We would prefer, if recognized early, to immediately perform an arthroscopic lavage, debridement with graft retention, and to obtain cultures. Further treatment continues with the desired administration and duration of appropriate antibiotics. Those that respond as expected can be followed until all the infection is eliminated. If the infection does not respond in a reasonable time, the graft and fixation may need to be removed.

RESULTS

It has been our experience that 90% of our patients are pleased with their stabilty following ACL reconstruction. Our results in patients over age 40 are comparable to those in younger patients. Although stablization of the ACL deficient knee is quite successful, it is the associated injuries and pathology that often limit outcomes. Those who do not regain full symmetrical knee motion or have meniscal pathology, underlying degenerative articular disease, associated ligament injury, and malalignment of the lower extremity may not have as good long-term functional outcomes.

RECOMMENDED READING

Chhabra A, Starman JS, Ferretti M, et al. Anatomic, radiographic, biomechanical, and kinematic evaluation of the ACL and its two functional bundles. *J Bone Joint Surg*, 2006;88:2–10.

Frank CB, Jackson DW. Current concepts review. The science of reconstruction of the anterior cruciate ligament. *J Bone Joint Surg.* 1997;79A(10):1556–1576.

Jackson DW, ed. *The anterior cruciate ligament: current and future concepts.* New York: Raven Press; 1993.

Matsumoto A, Howell SM. Avoiding posterior cruciate ligament and roof impingement with transtibial anterior cruciate ligament reconstruction: keys to correct tunnel placement. *Techniques in Orthopaedics.* 2005;20(3):211–217.

Schaefer RK, Jackson DW. Cyclops syndrome: loss of extension following intra-articular ACL reconstruction. *Arthroscopy* 1990;6:171–178.

Scranton PE, Beynnon BD, Johnson RJ, et al. Outcomes of different autografts and grafting techniques in anterior cruciate ligament replacement. *J Bone Joint Surg Am.* 2003;85(7):1397–1399.

13 Anatomic Anterior Cruciate Ligament Double-Bundle Reconstruction

Mario Ferretti, Wei Shen, Hanno Steckel, and Freddie H. Fu

INDICATIONS/CONTRAINDICATIONS

Anterior cruciate ligament (ACL) tear is a common injury in orthopaedic sports medicine. Surgical reconstruction is the preferred choice in management to restore knee stability and prevent intra-articular injuries. Current techniques in ACL surgery have been associated with satisfactory long-term results in the majority of patients; however, there remains a considerable subset of patients with unsatisfactory outcomes. Specifically, patients report difficulties relating to rotational instability and return to previous level of activity. The anatomic ACL double-bundle (DB) reconstruction aims to restore the original anatomy and footprints of the ACL by reconstructing the anteromedial (AM) and posterolateral (PL) bundle to achieve a better functional outcome, which is in contrast to single-bundle (SB) reconstruction, which attempts to restore the fibers of the AM bundle. The indications for a reconstruction of a torn ACL applying the anatomic ACL DB reconstruction are like the traditional SB reconstruction and are influenced by several factors. Universally accepted indications for ACL reconstruction are heavy work occupation, high-risk lifestyle, demanding level of sports activity, instability in spite of rehabilitation, and associated injuries like meniscal tears or severe injuries to other ligament structures in the knee. Age is also an important parameter to take into account; however, it is not so much the biologic age, but the status of the knee and the individual lifestyle which have to be considered.

Contraindications for the anatomic ACL DB reconstruction include advanced osteoarthritis of the knee, patients who are unable to comply with the postoperative rehabilitation protocol, and acute intra-articular sepsis. Open physes are not an absolute contraindication for the DB reconstruction, since several authors have described satisfactory results with reconstruction of the ACL using soft tissue grafts passed through the transphysial drill holes. However, extra attention should be paid to patients with large open physes or patients with potential to grow.

PREOPERATIVE PLANNING

Planning the surgical procedure includes taking the patient's history as well as a physical examination. For outcome evaluation, clinical parameters such as range of motion (ROM), Lachman grade, anterior drawer grade, pivot-shift grade, objective measurements of knee laxity as obtained with KT-1000 arthrometer, and scores such as the International Knee Documentation Committee Subjective Knee Form (IKDC) and Lysholm are important and are routinely applied. Especially validated outcome instruments like 36-Item Short Form Health Survey (SF-36), Activities of Daily Living (ADLS), Knee Injury and Osteoarthritis Outcome Score (KOOS), and Sports Activities Scales (SAS) are also needed for future evaluation of the DB reconstruction. Imaging of the knee is performed with routine radiographs to determine fractures, osteoarthritis, and the alignment of the lower extremity (Fig. 13-1). Magnetic resonance imaging is always done to assess further intra- and extra-articular injury and to confirm the rupture of the ACL (Fig. 13-2). The time interval from injury to reconstruction is not as important as the condition of the knee at the time of surgery. The knee should have minimal effusion and full range of motion. The patient must be physically and mentally prepared for surgery and free of pain when determining the date of reconstruction.

SURGERY

The patient and the limb to be operated on are identified by the surgeon in the preoperative holding area. In the operating room, the patient is placed in a supine position. Either general or spinal anesthesia is performed according to the preference of the patient and anesthesiologist. Examination under anesthesia is executed with the Lachman test and pivot shift. Special attention is given to the laxity of the knee joint. Under anesthesia, when the pivot shift is grade 1 or graded as a gliding pivot and the side-to-side difference using KT 1000 is less than 5 mm, a possible partial tear of the ACL is considered as a differential diagnosis and further arthroscopic evaluation will elucidate the correct diagnosis. It is important to note that in the case of a complete ACL tear, an anatomic ACL DB reconstruction will be performed. Rarely, when a partial tear of the ACL is diagnosed, an augmentation of the torn bundle, AM or PL bundle, may be a logical approach.

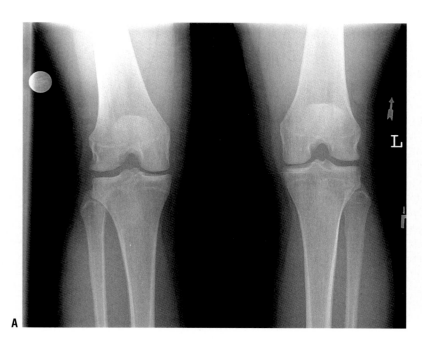 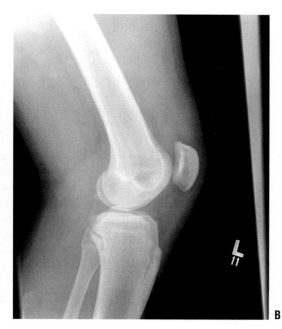

A   **B**

FIGURE 13-1

Anteroposterior **(A)** and lateral **(B)** views of radiographs are taken at the patient's initial visit. Possible injures like fractures and osteoarthritis, and the alignment of the lower extremity, are examined.

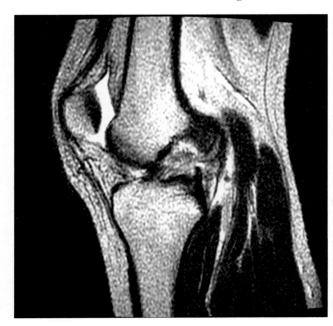

FIGURE 13-2

A sagittal view of MRI confirms a torn ACL.

The procedure is performed with the patient in supine position with the nonoperative leg placed in a well-leg holder in the abducted position. The operative leg is exsanguinated by elevation for 3 minutes; a pneumatic tourniquet is applied around the upper thigh and insufflated to 350 or 400 mmHg depending on the patient's size. Finally, the operative leg is placed in an arthroscopic leg holder, which allows good range of motion (Fig. 13-3), sterile preparation, and draping. The surgery is performed in a stepwise fashion as follows: (a) evaluation under anesthesia, (b) patient set-up, (c) graft preparation, (d) evaluation of the ACL rupture pattern and marking of the footprints of the ACL, (e) positioning and preparation of the tunnels, (f) graft passage and fixation, (g) closure and postoperative assessment of stability, and (h) postoperative management and rehabilitation.

Technique

Arthroscopy is performed for diagnosis and treatment of associated injuries. The portals are critical to obtain optimal intra-articular visualization and management of the arthroscopic instruments. We use the standard anterolateral (AL) and anteromedial (AM) portal; an accessory anteromedial portal (AAM) is also used (Fig. 13-4). To establish the AAM portal, the arthroscope is placed into the standard AL or AM portal and an 18-gauge spinal needle is inserted medially and distally to this portal just above the meniscus to reach the center of the femoral footprint of the PL bundle (Fig. 13-5). Once the needle is placed correctly, the AAM portal is performed with a #11 blade. While the arthroscopy is being performed, the grafts are being prepared in a back table by another surgeon. We prefer the use of two separate tibialis anterior or tibialis posterior tendon allografts. These allografts are usually 24 to 30 cm in length, and we fold each tendon graft to obtain 12 to 15 cm double-stranded grafts (Fig. 13-6). First, the tendon allografts are trimmed and the diameters of the double-stranded grafts are adjusted. Usually, the AM tendon graft is trimmed such that the diameter of the double-stranded graft is 8 mm; the PL graft is trimmed such that the diameter of the double-stranded graft is 7 mm. However, the diameters of the graft should be smaller in a small patient. The ends of the grafts are sutured using a baseball stitch fashion with 2-0 Ticron sutures. An EndoButton CL (Smith & Nephew, Andover, MA) is used to loop each graft and obtain a double-stranded graft. The length of the EndoButton loop is chosen according to the measured length of the femoral tunnels.

During the arthroscopy, it is important to observe the rupture pattern of the ACL (Fig. 13-7). This step definitively diagnoses the total tear of the ACL and shows us the original footprint of the AM and PL bundles on the lateral wall of the intercondylar notch and on the tibial side (Fig. 13-8). When

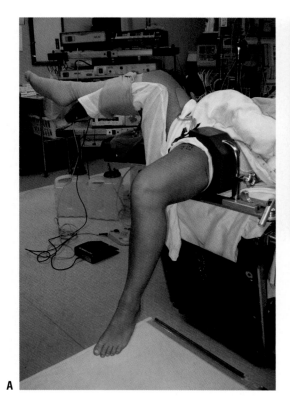

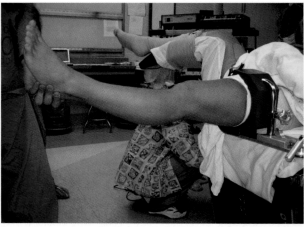

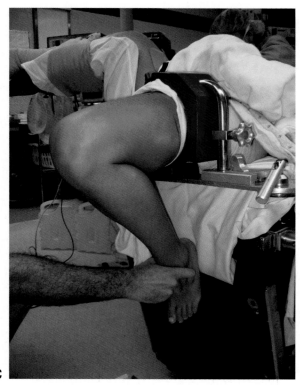

FIGURE 13-3

A knee holder is used to keep the surgery knee stable during the surgery **(A)**. It also allows a good range of motion, both extension **(B)** and flexion **(C)**, during the surgery.

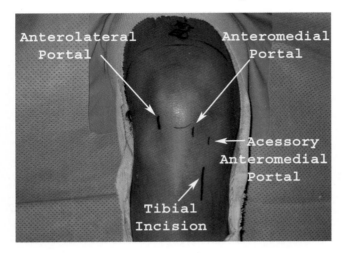

FIGURE 13-4

Standard anterolateral and anteromedial portal are used. In addition, an accessory anteromedial portal is used to provide better view of the lateral wall of the femoral notch. Tibial incision is made at the medial aspect of tibia, and it is anterior to the tibial attachment of MCL.

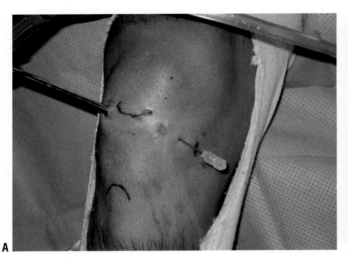

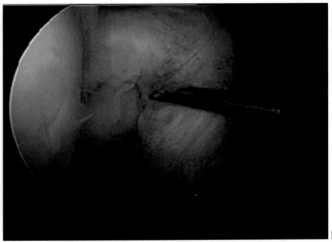

FIGURE 13-5

A spinal needle is inserted to decide the position of the accessory anteromedial portal. **A:** Outside and **(B)** inside.

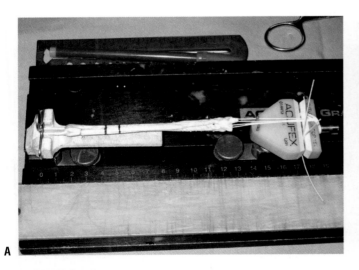

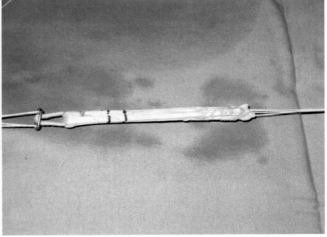

FIGURE 13-6

A,B: The graft is prepared on a back table by an assistant surgeon. The length of the femoral tunnels is measured, and the length of the grafts is adjusted accordingly.

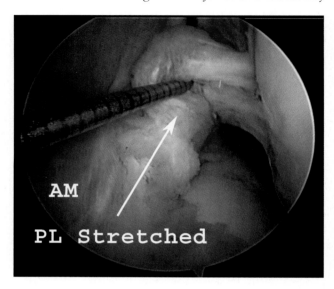

FIGURE 13-7

A thermal device is used to investigate the injury pattern of ACL. One example shows that the AM bundle is intact, whereas the PL bundle is stretched.

identified, the footprints of each bundle are marked by a thermal device (Artrocare Corporation, Sunnyvale, CA). A small hole in the center of the femoral AM and PL footprint is created by Steadman awl to facilitate further guidewire placement to create the femoral tunnels (Fig. 13-9). After marked by a thermal device, the remaining tibial footprint fibers are left intact due to their proprioceptive and vascular contributions. It is important to note that in acute cases, the rupture pattern and original anatomy are more easily observed than in chronic cases, in which you may not find the ACL footprints as well. A good understanding of the double-bundle ACL anatomy is essential to identify and mark the correct footprints.

The PL femoral tunnel is the first tunnel to be drilled. The PL femoral tunnel is drilled through the AAM portal, and a 3.2-mm guidewire is inserted through the portal. The tip of the guidewire is placed on the small hole created previously by Steadman awl on the center of the femoral footprint of the PL bundle. Once the tip of the guidewire is malleted in the correct position, the femoral PL tunnel is drilled with an acorn drill that is inserted over the guidewire. The PL femoral tunnel is drilled to a depth of 25 to 30 mm (Fig. 13-10). The far cortex is breached with a 4.5-mm EndoButton drill (Smith & Nephew, Andover, MA) and the depth gauge is used to measure the distance to the far cortex. It is important to note that during the drilling of the PL bundle tunnel, the arthroscopy

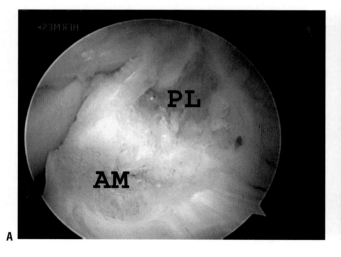
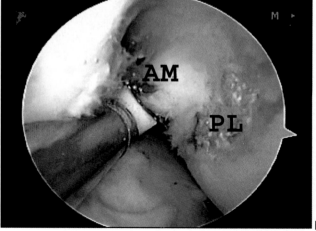

FIGURE 13-8

The insertion sites of AM and PL on both tibial side **(A)** and femoral side **(B)** are marked by a thermal device.

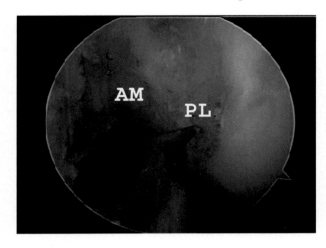

FIGURE 13-9

A Steadman awl is used to mark the desired femoral AM and PL positions for guide pins. It also makes it easier for the guide pins to stick to the chosen spot.

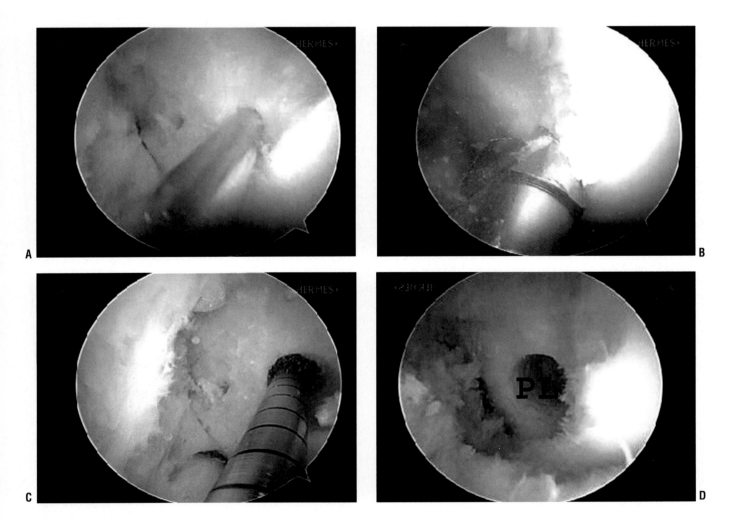

FIGURE 13-10

A guide pin is used first **(A)**, followed by an acorn drill **(B)**. The EndoButton drill is then used to drill a narrower tunnel for the EndoButton **(C)**. The finished PL femoral tunnel is shown **(D)**.

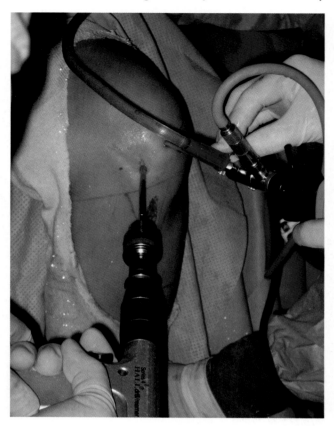

FIGURE 13-11

The PL femoral tunnel is drilled through the accessory anteromedial portal.

is placed through the anteromedial portal and the tunnel is drilled through the accessory anteromedial portal (Fig. 13-11). It is also important to note that during the entire procedure to create a PL femoral tunnel the knee is positioned at 110 degrees of flexion, which brings the PL bundle footprint anteriorly.

To create the two tibial tunnels, a 4-cm skin incision is made over the anteromedial surface of the tibia at the level of the tibial tubercle. The PL tibial tunnel is the first one to be drilled. The elbow ACL tibial drill guide is set up at 45 degrees and the tip of the drill guide is placed intra-articularly on the tibial footprints of the PL bundle. Another way to locate the tip of the tibial guide intra-articularly, is to place it just in front of the posterior root of the lateral menisci, and posterolateral to the AM bundle of the ACL (Fig. 13-12). On the tibial cortex, the tibial drill starts just anterior to the superficial medial collateral ligament fibers. Once the tibial drill guide is set up intra-articularly and on the tibial cortex, a 3.2-mm guidewire is passed into the stump of the PL tibial footprint (Fig. 13-13). The AM tibial tunnel is drilled with the elbow ACL tibial drill guide set at 45 degrees, and the

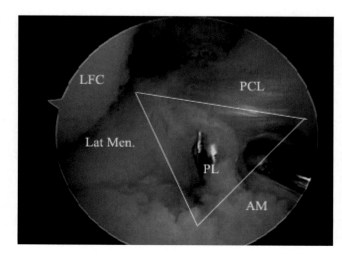

FIGURE 13-12

The tibial PL insertion site is located posterolaterally to the tibial AM insertion site. It is also located 2 to 4 mm in front of the posterior root of lateral meniscus. The PL triangle is formed by PCL, posterior root of lateral meniscus, and the AM insertion site.

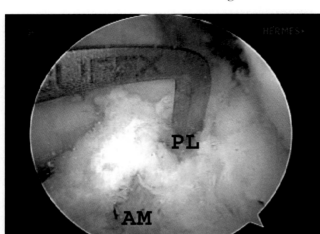

FIGURE 13-13

The tibial insertion sites of AM and PL bundles are shown. The ACUFEX aiming elbow is used to guide the direction of the guide pin.

tip of the drill guide is placed on the tibial footprint of the AM tunnel already marked with the thermal device, and anteromedial to the PL guidewire. On the tibial cortex the starting point for the AM bundle is placed anterior, central, and proximal than the PL starting point. Once the elbow ACL tibial drill guide is placed in the desired position, a 3.2-mm guidewire is passed into the stump of the AM tibial footprint (Fig. 13-14). After passing the tibial guidewire into an adequate position, the two tibial tunnels are drilled using a cannulated drill. A curette is used for protection (Fig. 13-15). Finally, a dilator is used to enlarge the tunnels to the desired diameters (Fig. 13-16).

The femoral AM tunnel is the last tunnel to be drilled. We use three methods to drill the AM femoral tunnel. A transtibial AM technique in a similar fashion for a single-bundle ACL reconstruction is our first choice to create the AM femoral tunnel. However, in some cases, the transtibial AM technique cannot reach the center of the AM bundle marked previously. Then, we can try to reach the center of the AM femoral footprint through the PL tibial tunnel. If the center of the AM femoral footprint is also not reached through the PL tibial tunnel, we use the AAM portal to reach the center of the AM bundle. The AM tunnel is drilled in a similar fashion that the PL femoral tunnel was drilled (Fig. 13-17). Once the tip of the guidewire is placed in a correct position, the

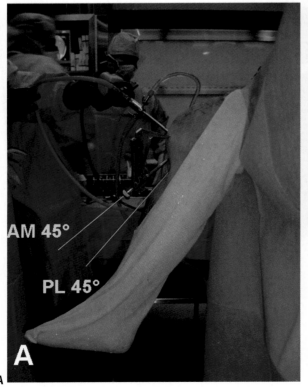

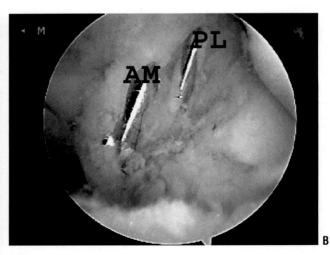

FIGURE 13-14

The AM and PL guide pins are inserted at 45 and 45 degrees, respectively (A). A scope picture shows that AM and PL guide pins are inserted, and PL insertion site is posterolateral to AM insertion site (B).

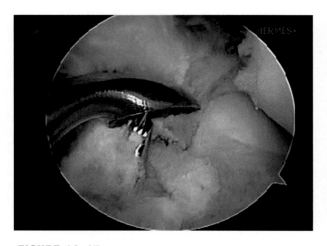

FIGURE 13-15

A curette is used for protection when a cannulated drill is used to enlarge the tibial tunnels.

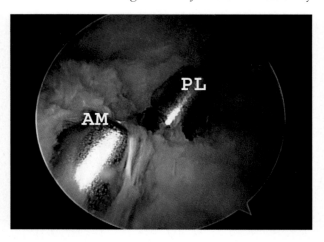

FIGURE 13-16

Dilators are used to enlarge the tibial tunnels.

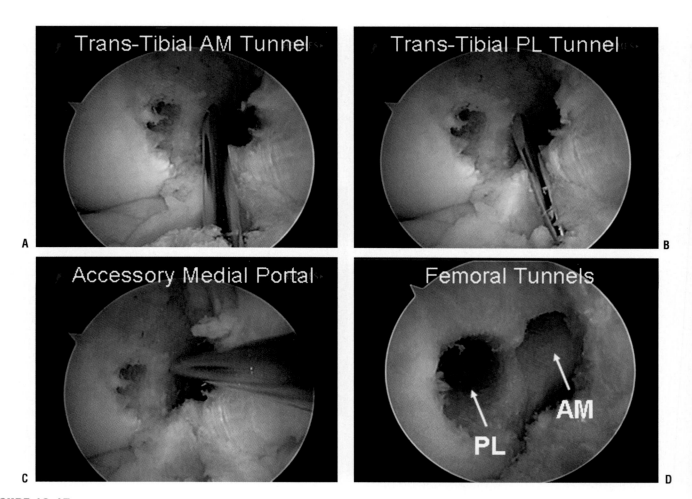

FIGURE 13-17

The femoral AM insertion site can be reached by different routes. By transtibial AM tunnel **(A)**, transtibial PL tunnel **(B)**, or accessory anteromedial portal **(C)**, the femoral AM tunnel can be drilled. The finished femoral AM and PL tunnels are shown **(D)**.

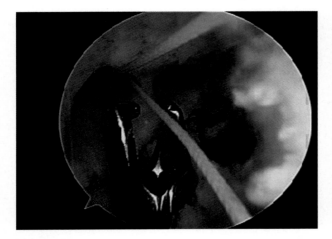

FIGURE 13-18

The looped suture is visualized and retrieved with an arthroscopic suture grasper through the PL tibial tunnel.

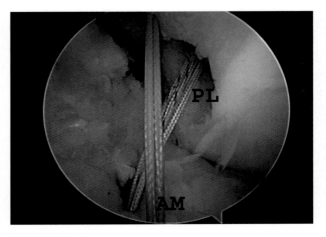

FIGURE 13-19

When in flexion, the AM and PL graft sutures show a crossing pattern, which is also true in intact ACL.

guidewire is malleted, an acorn drill is inserted over the guidewire, and the AM femoral tunnel is drilled to a depth of 35 to 40 mm when it is done transtibially either through AM tibial tunnel or PL tibial tunnel. If the AM femoral tunnel is performed through the AAM portal, it is drilled to a depth of 30 mm to avoid breaking cortex. The far cortex of the AM femoral tunnel is breached with a 4.5 mm EndoButton drill, and the depth gauge is used to measure the distance to the far cortex. The first graft to be passed is the PL graft. A Beath pin with a long looped suture attached to the eyelet is passed through the AAM portal and out through the PL femoral tunnel. The looped suture is visualized within the joint and retrieved with an arthroscopic suture grasper through the PL tibial tunnel (Fig. 13-18). A crossing pattern of the AM and PL graft is clearly seen after passing both looped sutures through the tunnels (Fig. 13-19). The graft is passed and the EndoButton is flipped to establish cortex fixation of the PL bundle graft (Fig. 13-20). The AM is passed using the transtibial technique when the tunnel was created transtibially or through the AAM portal when the tunnel was created through the AAM portal, using the same technique as in the PL bundle graft passage. The En-

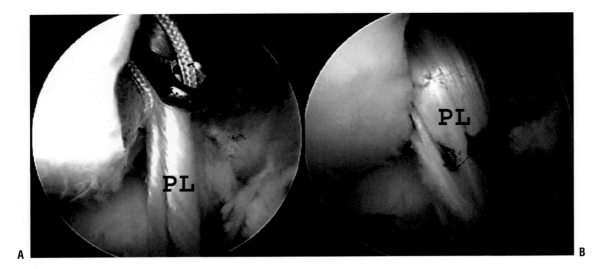

FIGURE 13-20

The PL graft is passed first. An EndoButton fixation is used to fix on the femoral side **(A)**. The graft will be pulled through **(B)** and the EndoButton will be flipped on the femoral cortex.

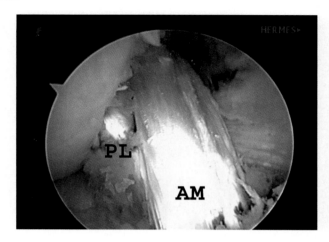

FIGURE 13-21

The AM graft is pulled through after PL graft. The reconstruction product restores the normal anatomy of ACL very closely.

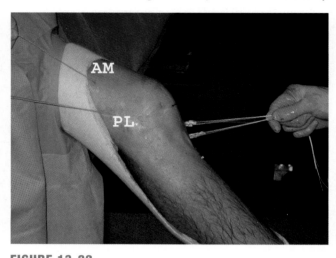

FIGURE 13-22

The grafts are conditioned by repetitive flexion and extension motion. This figure also shows the exits of AM and PL sutures on the femoral side.

doButton is flipped in a standard fashion for AM bundle graft to establish AM bundle femoral cortex fixation (Fig. 13-21). Preconditioning of the grafts is performed by flexing and extending the knee through a range of motion from 0 to 120 degrees approximately 20 to 30 times (Fig. 13-22). On the tibial side, we prefer to use bioabsorbable screws (Fig. 13-23). The graft fixation is important for the tensioning of the grafts. The tensioning is performed manually by the surgeon and fixed during the tibial fixation. The PL graft is fixed at 0 to 10 degrees of flexion. The AM graft is fixed at 60 degrees of flexion. After tibial fixation, a final arthroscopic inspection is performed to confirm the status of the graft, the absence of anterior impingement, and posterior cruciate ligament (PCL) impingement (Fig. 13-24). Subcutaneous tissue and skin are closed in a standard fashion. A Cryo Cuff (Aircast, Vista, CA) is used for cold therapy and compression. A brace is used to keep the knee locked in full extension (Fig. 13-25). A radiograph is taken to make sure the hardware is in place

FIGURE 13-23

On the tibial side, the AM and PL grafts are fixed by biodegradable screws.

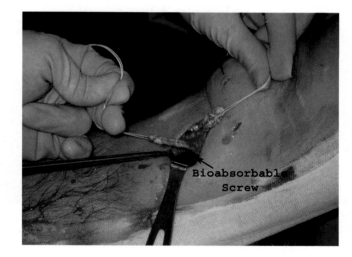

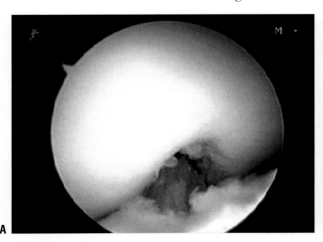
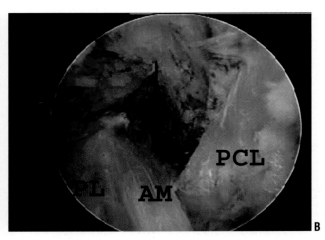

FIGURE 13-24

By anatomic double-bundle reconstruction, anterior **(A)** and PCL **(B)** impingements are usually avoided. The arrow shows that there are still spaces.

(Fig 13-26). A magnetic resonance image is not routinely taken. However, it can show the anatomic double-bundle graft (Fig. 13-27).

Pearls and Pitfalls

- The accessory AM portal is established using an 18-gauge needle under direct visualization. The portal location is medial and inferior to the standard AM portal (see Fig. 13-4). Placement is critical in obtaining the correct trajectory and entry point for the PL femoral tunnel, and to avoid injury to the medial femoral condyle surface and medial meniscus during drilling. The accessory anteromedial portal offers a complete view of both the AM and PL femoral origins.
- It is essential to position the leg to allow for a range of motion between full extension and 120 degrees of flexion intraoperatively. This position is needed to fully appreciate the anatomy of the ACL since the relative positions of the femoral insertions of the AM and PL bundles change with the flexion angle.
- Anatomic landmarks for the PL femoral tunnel pin are as follows: 5 to 7 mm from the anterior lateral femoral condyle (LFC) cartilage, and 3 mm from the inferior LFC cartilage. The knee

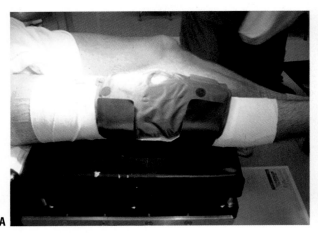
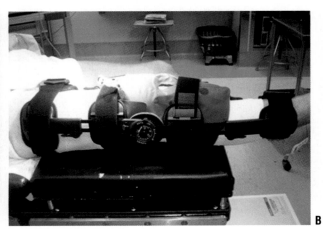

FIGURE 13-25

In addition to standard dressing, the knee is wrapped up by cryocuff for cold therapy and compression **(A)**. A knee brace is used to lock and protect the knee in extension **(B)**.

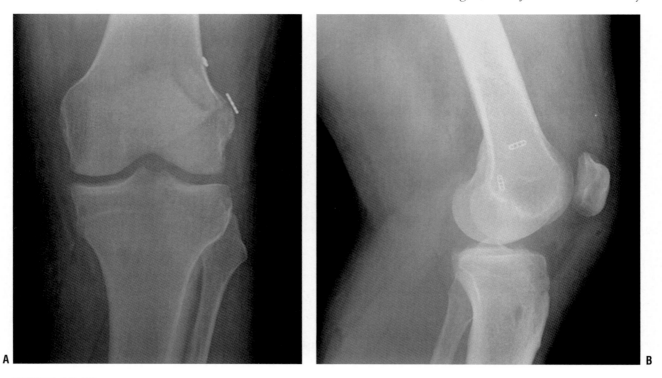

FIGURE 13-26

Anteroposterior **(A)** and lateral **(B)** views of radiographs are taken after the surgery to check the position of hardwares.

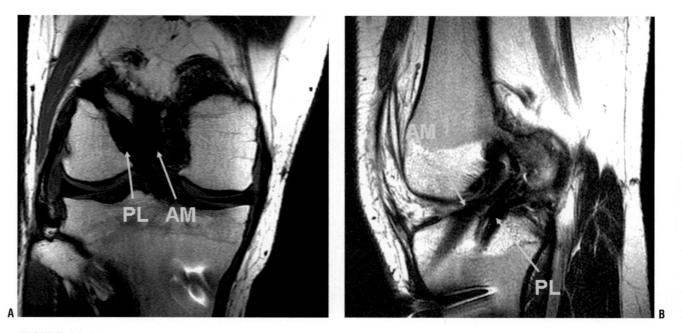

FIGURE 13-27

Coronal **(A)** and sagittal **(B)** views of MRI show the AM and PL grafts.

is flexed to 110 degrees to protect the peroneal nerve and to ensure adequate EndoButton tunnel length.

- The PL tibial insertion is located anterior and medial to the posterior root of the lateral meniscus. It is lateral and anterior to the PCL, and posterolateral to the AM bundle insertion site. Thus, the PL tibial insertion site is located within the triangle formed by the AM, the PCL, and the posterior root of the lateral meniscus. A proximal medial tibial incision is made. A tibial drill guide is set at 45 and 45 degrees for the PL and AM bundles, respectively, and placed on the tibial PL and AM insertion marked previously.
- The AM femoral tunnel placement is referenced 2 to 3 mm posterior to the PL tunnel posterior rim, with the knee held at 90 degrees. The guidewire may be placed using either transtibial approaches or accessory anteromedial portal approach, to achieve correct position relative to the PL tunnel. Transtibial is preferred to achieve more divergent tunnels; however, accurate tunnel position is the most important factor.
- Prior to fixation, each graft is cycled through a full range of motion 25 to30 times using maximal manual tension.The AM graft is tensioned and fixed in 60 degrees of flexion.The PL graft is tensioned and fixed in 0 to 10 degrees of flexion.
- Caution is warranted when using the AAM portal to drill the femoral tunnel. The tunnel tends to be short, and the femoral cortex may be more easily broken for this reason. If the cortex is broken, the EndoButton fixation is not feasible. A lateral incision is made to change the EndoButton femoral fixation to a femoral post fixation.
- By using an allograft, we can decide the exact diameter of the tunnels and grafts. It is important to note that our standard tunnels sizes are 8 mm for the AM bundle and 7 mm for the PL bundle. However, in smaller patients the standard tunnels may be too large and may cause problems such as blowout of the posterior wall of the femoral tunnel as well as blowout of the bridge between AM and PL femoral tunnels. In addition, excessive grafts may cause anterior impingement. Thus, the tunnel and graft size should be adjusted for small patients.
- The cortex of the lateral femoral condyle becomes thinner as it comes distally. For this reason we should be careful when placing the PL tunnel and sometimes even the AM tunnel, especially when it is drilled through the AAM portal. When using EndoButton fixation, the EndoButton is flipped and fixed in the distal part of the thin cortex. When pulling the graft for tensioning and confirming the fixation, a large traction force is applied to the graft and the EndoButton puts a large pressure on the thin cortex. The cortex may be broken by the hardware and the EndoButton is pulled into the tunnel, leading to failure of the fixation.

POSTOPERATIVE MANAGEMENT

The double-bundle ACL reconstruction is performed on an outpatient basis. Patients will be taken to the recovery room when the operation is over and will remain there for up to 2 hours. Their vital signs will be monitored, and they are usually sent to home when they are fully awake and have recovered from the anesthesia, unless they have significant discomfort from anesthesia or pain. The patient is prescribed pain medication that is taken every 4 hours during the first 2 postoperative days, and as needed after that. In addition, we recommend that patients take pain medication 1/2 hour before exercise or using the continuous passive motion (CPM) machine. Ice or cryocuff is suggested, as well as elevation of the knee, especially 20 to 30 minutes after physical therapy or other activities. The patients are taught to change their dressing 2 days after surgery and keep their incision site clean and dry. A brace is prescribed after the surgery. During the first week the brace should be locked straight except while performing exercises or using a CPM machine. Crutches are used for 4 to 6 weeks after surgery, depending on the recovery of the patient. Weight bearing is permitted as long as the patient tolerates it.

Rehabilitation

Rehabilitative therapy is begun the day after surgery. The important issues in rehabilitation of double-bundle ACL reconstruction include minimizing inflammation, restoring motion and muscle strength, enhancing proprioception and dynamic stability, returning to function, and preventing recurrence. In the immediate postoperative period, our goal is to reduce pain and swelling of the knee, increase range of motion, and strengthen the quadriceps and hamstring muscles. The weight bearing should progress from a partial level to full. At 1 to 3 months postoperatively, the work on range of motion and muscle strength should be continued. Closed chain and functional exercises should be incorporated, as well as activities to enhance balance and neuromuscular control. After 3 months postoperatively, rehabilitation should continue to improve strength and neuromuscular control. At this time plyometric and sports-specific exercises should be added. In terms of returning to sports, we believe that the individual has to have no pain or swelling, 80% to 90% quadriceps strength, a normal hop test, and adequate proprioception and neuromuscular control. Our rehabilitation protocol is outlined in Table 13-1.

TABLE 13-1.   ACL Reconstruction and Rehabilitation Protocol

Stage 1: Begins immediately postoperatively through approximately 6 weeks
- **Goals:**
  1. Protect graft fixation
  2. Minimize effects of immobilization
  3. Control inflammation
  4. Full extension and flexion range of motion
  5. Educate patient on rehabilitation progression
- **Therapeutic exercises:**
  1. Heel slides
  2. Quadriceps sets
  3. Patellar immobilization
  4. Non–weight-bearing gastro/soleus stretches, begin hamstring stretches at 4 weeks
  5. Straight leg raises in all planes with brace in full extension until quadriceps strength is sufficient to prevent extension lag
  6. Quadriceps isometrics at 60 and 90 degrees

Stage 2: Begins immediately 6 weeks postoperatively and extends to approximately 8 weeks
- **Goals:**
  1. Restore normal gait
  2. Maintain full extension, progress flexion range of motion
  3. Protect graft fixation
- **Therapeutic exercise**
  1. Wall slides 0 to 45 degrees
  2. 4-way hip machine
  3. Stationary bike
  4. Closed-chain terminal extension with resistance tubing or weight machine
  5. Toe raises
  6. Balance exercises
  7. Hamstring curls
  8. Aquatic therapy with emphasis on normalization of gait
  9. Continue hamstring stretches, progress to weight-bearing gastro/soleus stretches

Stage 3: Begins approximately 8 weeks and extends through approximately 6 months
- **Goals:**
  1. Full range of motion
  2. Improve strength, endurance, and proprioception of the lower extremity to prepare for functional activities

- **Therapeutic exercises:**
  1. Continue flexibility exercises as appropriate for patient
  2. Stair Master (begin with short steps, avoid hyperextension)
  3. NordicTrack
  4. Advanced closed-chain strengthening (one-leg squats, leg press 0 to 50 degrees, step-ups, etc.)
  5. Progress proprioception activities (slide board, use of ball with balance activities, etc.)
  6. Progress aquatic therapy to include pool running, swimming (no breaststroke)

Stage 4: Begins approximately 6 months and extends through approximately 9 months
- **Goals:**
  1. Progress strength, power, proprioception to prepare for return to functional activities
- **Therapeutic exercises:**
  1. Continue to progress flexibility and strengthening program
  2. Initiate plyometric program as appropriate for patient's functional goals
  3. Functional progression including, but not limited to, walk/jog progression, forward/backward running at 1/2, 3/4, full speed, cutting, crossover, carioca, etc.
  4. Initiate sport-specific drills as appropriate for patient

Stage 5: Begins approximately 9 months postoperatively
- **Goals:**
  1. Safe return to athletics
  2. Maintenance of strength, endurance, proprioception
  3. Patient education with regard to any possible limitations
- **Therapeutic exercises:**
  1. Gradual return to sports participation
  2. Maintenance program for strength and endurance

COMPLICATIONS

When considering double-bundle reconstruction, it is important to address potential complications. General complications after knee surgery include hemarthrosis, effusions, and wound infection, which are treated according to the common postoperative procedures. Tunnel widening and sclerosis, tibial and femoral fractures, and notch or posterior cruciate ligament impingement following ACL reconstruction are known to occur in a single-bundle reconstruction, but can also occur when applying the anatomic ACL DB reconstruction. When performing the tibial incision, the infrapatellar branch of the saphenous nerve can be damaged, leaving a small numb area along the anterolateral aspect of the knee and, rarely, a painful neuroma.

RESULTS

From November 2003 to September 2006, the senior author has performed 340 anatomic ACL reconstructions. In a total of 275 primary cases, 261 patients (95%) had primary double-bundle reconstruction and 14 patients (5%) had primary one-bundle augmentation. In a total of 65 revision cases, 44 patients (68%) had double-bundle revision and 21 patients (32%) had secondary one-bundle augmentation. In the primary augmentation patients, we found in surgery that either the AM or the PL bundle was still functional, so that only the torn bundle was reconstructed and the functional bundle was left intact. In the 21 patients who underwent secondary augmentation, 19 patients had previous single-bundle reconstruction. They were unstable and had positive pivot shift test, despite good range of motion and minimal side-to-side difference of KT-2000 score. The original graft was found functionally intact or savable during the surgery, and only PL bundle reconstruction was performed. The other two secondary augmentation patients had previous double-bundle reconstruction. They were found to have a failed AM graft and a functional PL graft. Only the AM graft was reconstructed, and the PL graft was left intact. With primary or secondary one-bundle augmentation, the double-bundle anatomy of ACL and the stability of the knee were restored.

A prospective study was designed to evaluate the outcomes of all these patients. Outcome measurements included the Lachman and pivot shift tests, KT-2000, range of motion, and overall IKDC rating. Short-term results demonstrated that the range of motion after primary double-bundle ACL reconstruction is better than primary single-bundle ACL reconstruction at 1, 4, and 12 weeks postoperatively following the same rehabilitation protocol. To determine if this technique offers advantages over single-bundle reconstruction in the long term, these patients are being continuously followed. The initial 100 consecutive patients who underwent primary double-bundle ACL reconstruction have been followed for an average of nearly 2 years. Lachman test, pivot shift test, and KT-2000 results demonstrated that anteroposterior stability was effectively restored by double-bundle ACL reconstruction. Approximately 94% of patients had an excellent or good IKDC rating. There were four failures in our initial 100 patients, three of whom required double-bundle revision surgery. For the augmentation and the double-bundle revision cases, preliminary results are currently being reviewed and appear promising.

Rotational stability should be an important portion of outcome evaluation after ACL reconstruction. In an in vivo laboratory study, Tashman et al. have suggested the superiority of double-bundle ACL reconstruction in restoring the rotational stability when compared to single-bundle ACL reconstruction. In the near future, an ACL surgery navigation system may also be used as a tool for clinical measurement of rotational stability in our study.

RECOMMENDED READING

Amis AA, Dawkins GPC. Functional anatomy of the anterior cruciate ligament. Fiber bundle actions and related to ligament replacement and injuries. *J Bone Joint Surg Br*. 1991;73:260–267.

Girgis FG, Marshall JL, Monajem A. The cruciate ligaments of the knee joint. Anatomical, functional, and experimental analysis. *Clin Orthop*. 1975;106:216–231.

Tashman S, Collon D, Anderson K, et al. Abnormal rotational knee motion during running after anterior cruciate ligament reconstruction. *Am J Sports Med*. 2004;32:975–983.

Yagi M, Wong EK, Kanamori A, et al. Biomechanical analysis of an anatomic anterior cruciate ligament reconstruction. *Am J Sports Med*. 2002;30:660–666.

14 Avoiding ACL Graft Impingement: Principles for Tunnel Placement Using the Transtibial Tunnel Technique

Keith W. Lawhorn and Stephen M. Howell

INDICATIONS/CONTRAINDICATIONS

The transtibial tunnel technique in which the femoral tunnel is drilled through the tibial tunnel is a common technique for tunnel placement. This technique can be used regardless of the type of graft material and fixation. The transtibial technique can be used in all patients requiring a primary anterior cruciate ligament (ACL) reconstruction both acute and chronic, revision ACL surgery, and ACL reconstruction in the setting of the multiligament knee injury. There are no absolute contraindications to use of the transtibial tunnel technique for ACL reconstruction. Correct tunnel placement for ACL reconstruction is imperative to the success of the procedure. Graft sources, fixation methods, and rehabilitation cannot overcome the adverse consequences of poor tunnel placement.

There are three criteria of correctly placed tibial and femoral tunnels for ACL reconstruction: (a) the avoidance of roof impingement, (b) avoidance of posterior cruciate ligament (PCL) impingement, and (c) the establishment of the tensile behavior in the ACL graft similar to the native ACL. All three criteria are required for a successful ACL reconstruction.

Roof impingement occurs when the ACL graft prematurely makes contact with the intercondylar roof of the notch before the knee reaches terminal extension, which causes loss of extension and anterior laxity. The cause of roof impingement is positioning the tibial tunnel too anterior in the sagittal plane.

PCL impingement occurs when the ACL graft makes contact with the leading edge of the PCL before the knee reaches terminal flexion, which causes loss of flexion and anterior laxity. The cause of PCL impingement in the transtibial technique is positioning the tibial tunnel too vertical and medial in the coronal plane.

Finally, correct femoral tunnel position in both the sagittal and coronal planes is required to establish the tensile behavior in the ACL graft similar to the native ACL. Because the femoral tunnel is drilled through the tibial tunnel using size-specific aimers, the position of the tibial tunnel determines the position of the femoral tunnel with the transtibial technique. Therefore, the tibial tunnel sets up the position of the femoral tunnel, which means that the key tunnel in the transtibial tunnel technique is the tibial tunnel.

PREOPERATIVE PLANNING

Once the decision has been made by the patient to undergo surgical treatment of the ACL deficient knee, the surgeon must decide on the technique for placing the tunnels, graft choice, and fixation. All tunnel placement techniques including the transtibial, transportal, and two-incision technique can be used with any type of graft and fixation. Scientific studies by a variety of authors support the use of the transtibial tunnel technique and the use of the 65-degree tibial guide (Arthrotek, Warsaw, IN) that references the intercondylar roof with the knee in full extension for placing the tibial tunnel (Fig. 14-1).

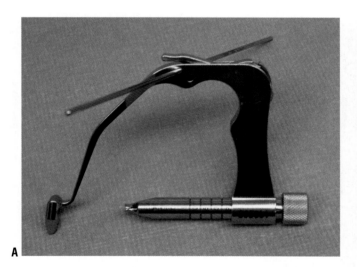

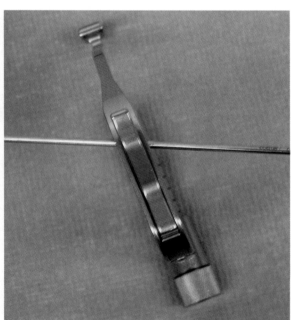

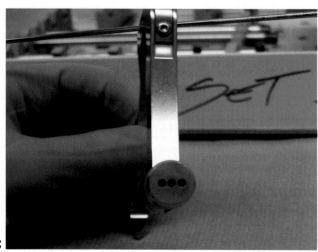

FIGURE 14-1

A: Lateral view of 65-degree tibial guide with coronal alignment rod. **B:** Superior view of 65-degree tibial guide with coronal alignment rod. **C:** Axial view of 65-degree tibial guide demonstrating bullet with multiple holes for guidewire placement.

An advantage of the transtibial technique with the 65-degree tibial guide is that the tunnel placement is accurate and customized without the need for tedious preoperative planning or time-consuming intraoperative imaging. Customization begins with the use of the 9.5-mm wide tip of the 65-degree tibial guide to gauge the width of the space between the lateral edge of the PCL and the lateral femoral condyle. Generally, the space between the PCL and the lateral femoral condyle is substantially smaller than the width of the ACL graft. The portion of the notch allocated to the ACL graft varies among patients as evidenced by some notches being narrower than others, and by the cross-sectional area of some notches being dominated by the PCL, leaving little room for the ACL graft. We advocate widening the notch by removing bone from the medial edge of the lateral femoral condyle (i.e., wallplasty) until the space between the PCL and lateral femoral condyle exceeds the width of the ACL graft by 1 mm. Since most grafts range from 8 to 10 mm, the free insertion of the 9.5-mm wide tip of the guide between the PCL and lateral femoral condyle indicates that the notch is sufficiently wide. Customizing the width of the notch to accommodate the width of the ACL minimizes PCL impingement by moving the tibial tunnel, femoral tunnel, and ACL graft lateral away from the PCL, which minimizes PCL impingement improving flexion and anterior stability.

A second step of customization is that the 65-degree tibial guide accounts for the anatomic variability in the angle of the intercondylar roof and knee extension that exists between patients and consistently positions the tibial tunnel in the posterior half of the native ACL tibial footprint and avoids roof impingement without a roofplasty. The roof angle (23 to 60 degrees) and knee extension (− to 30 degrees) both vary widely among patients. The correlation between the two is weak, so that patients with the same roof angle often have a different knee extension and patients with the same knee extension often have a different roof angle. Surgeons need to account for these two independent variables simultaneously. By drilling the tibial tunnel with the knee in full extension while referencing the intercondylar roof with the 65-degree tibial guide, the sagittal placement of the tibial tunnel has simultaneously accounted for the patient's unique combination of roof angle and knee extension. Magnetic resonance imaging studies have demonstrated the native ACL is located posterior and parallel to the intercondylar roof with the knee in terminal extension. The tibial tunnel is positioned posterior and parallel to the intercondylar roof and prevents roof impingement of the ACL graft without performing a roofplasty, which improves knee extension and anterior stability.

A third step of customization is that the 65-degree tibial guide incorporates the use of a coronal alignment rod, which improves the accuracy of setting the angle of the tibial tunnel in the coronal plane, further minimizing the risk of PCL impingement. Setting the angle of the tibial tunnel at 65 ± 5 degrees in the coronal plane avoids PCL impingement. The use of the transtibial technique and a tibial tunnel at 65 ± 5 degrees in the coronal plane positions the femoral tunnel so that the tensile behavior of the ACL graft is similar to the native ACL while improving knee flexion and anterior stability.

The last step in customization is the use of size-specific femoral aimers through a tibial tunnel placed to create a femoral tunnel with a 1-mm back-wall for any diameter ACL graft. The use of the size-specific femoral aimers in a knee in which the notch has been sufficiently widened, without roof impingement and without PCL impingement, ensures correct placement of the femoral tunnel. The remnants of the ACL origin in the over-the-top position must be removed so that the femoral aimer rests on bone. Resting the femoral aimer directly on bone creates a femoral tunnel with a thin 1-mm back-wall and eliminates "blowingout" the posterior wall of the femoral tunnel. Therefore, the advantage of the transtibial technique is that the surgeon needs to focus on the meticulous placement of only one tunnel, the tibial tunnel, reducing the error associated by placing the femoral and tibial tunnels independently.

For surgeons, choosing to use a point-and-shoot guide, preoperative lateral radiographs taken with the knee in full extension, helps determine the intercondylar roof angles and knee extension and aids them intraoperatively when positioning the tibial tunnel in the sagittal plane. Surgeons must estimate coronal plane positioning with these guides since there are no coronal alignment devices on these guides. The standard is to use intraoperative fluoroscopy to check the position of the tibial guidewire in both the sagittal and coronal planes before drilling the tibial tunnel.

SURGERY

Patient Positioning

Position the patient supine on the operating table. After induction of anesthesia, perform an examination under anesthesia. Place a tourniquet around the proximal thigh of the operative leg. Position the operative leg in a standard knee arthroscopy leg holder with the foot of the operating table flexed completely. Alternatively, surgeons may decide to use a lateral post instead of a leg holder. Position the contralateral leg in a gynecologic leg holder with the hip flexed and abducted with mild external rotation. Ensure there is no pressure on the peroneal nerve and calf (Fig. 14-2). Alternatively, surgeons can position the operative leg flexed over the side of the table using a lateral post and maintaining the contralateral leg extended on the operating table.

Technique

After sterile prep and drape, exsanguinate the leg and inflate the tourniquet. Establish inferolateral and inferomedial portals touching the edges of the patella tendon starting 1 cm distal to the inferior pole of the patella. Alternatively, a transpatellar inferolateral portal can be used with a medical portal placed along the medial border of the patella tendon (Fig. 14-3). The medial portal must touch the edge of the patella tendon because if it is placed more medial, the tibial guide may not stay seated in the intercondylar notch with the knee in full extension. An optional outflow portal can be established superiorly.

Perform a diagnostic arthroscopy. Treat meniscal or articular cartilage injuries. Identify and remove the torn remnant ACL stump (Fig. 14-4). It is not necessary to denude the tibial insertion of the native ACL tissue. In fact, retaining the insertion of the native ACL helps seal the edges of the ACL graft at the joint line and does not result in roof impingement if the tibial tunnel has been appropriately positioned. Remove the synovium and soft tissue in the notch to expose the lateral edge of the PCL (Fig. 14-5). Remove any of the ACL origin from the over-the-top position using an angled curette and shaver (Fig. 14-6).

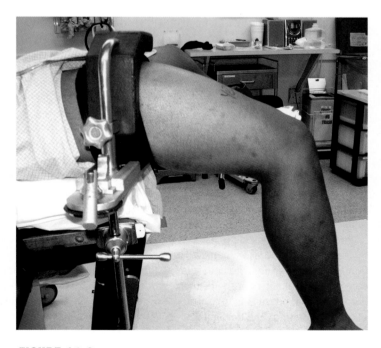

FIGURE 14-2

Patient set-up.

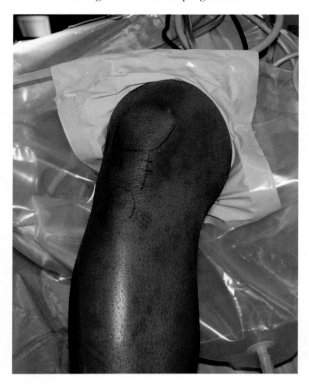

FIGURE 14-3
Portal placement for use of 65-degree tibial guide.

Insert the tibial guide through the medial portal. Advance the guide into the intercondylar notch (Fig. 14-7). The tip of the guide is 9.5 mm wide. If the guide makes contact and deforms the PCL as it enters the intercondylar notch, perform a lateral wallplasty. Remove bone in 1- to 2-mm-wide slivers from the lateral wall until the tip of the guide passes into the notch without deforming the PCL, which creates a wide enough area for an 8- to 10-mm-wide graft (Fig. 14-8). Do not remove any bone from the intercondylar roof since the roof anatomy is crucial for proper positioning of the tibial guide-pin in the sagittal plane using the 65-degree tibial guide (Fig. 14-9). Remove the lateral wallplasty fragments (Fig. 14-10).

Insert the 65-degree tibial guide through the anteromedial portal that touches the medial edge of the patella tendon into the intercondylar notch between the PCL and lateral femoral condyle to ensure adequate width of the notch for the ACL graft (Fig. 14-11). Fully extend the knee. Visualize that the tip of the guide is captured inside the notch and that the arm of the 65-degree tibial guide contacts the trochlea groove (Fig. 14-12). Place the heel of the patient on a Mayo stand to maintain

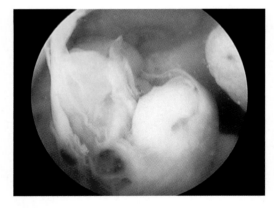

FIGURE 14-4
Torn ACL stump.

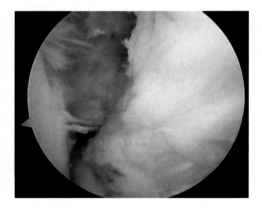

FIGURE 14-5
Identify the leading superior border of the PCL.

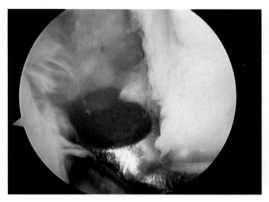

FIGURE 14-6

Clean the over-the-top position using an angled curette.

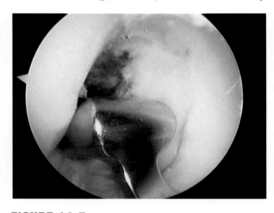

FIGURE 14-7

The 9.5-mm-wide tip of the 65-degree tibial guide demonstrates notch stenosis with deformation of PCL.

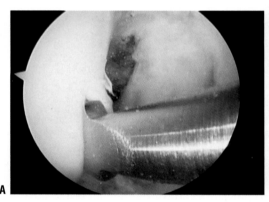

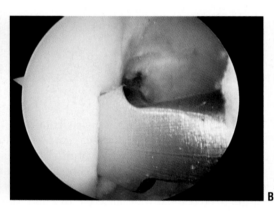

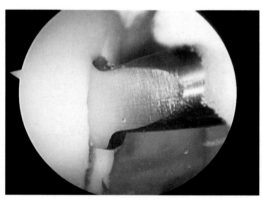

FIGURE 14-8

A–C: Lateral wallplasty performed using angled osteotome.

FIGURE 14-9

Angled osteotome prevents extension of wallplasty into roof of intercondylar notch.

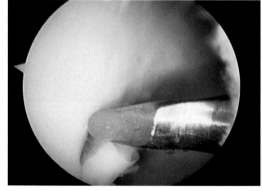

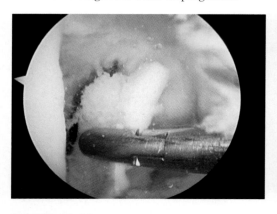

FIGURE 14-10
Removal of lateral wallplasty fragments.

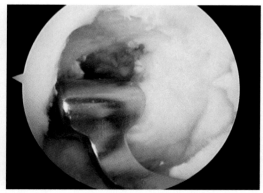

FIGURE 14-11
Sixty-five-degree tibial guide tip ensures
adequate notch width.

the knee in maximum hyperextension. Stand on the lateral side of the leg and insert the coronal alignment rod through the proximal hole in the guide. Rotate the 65-degree guide in varus and valgus until the coronal alignment rod is parallel to the joint and perpendicular to the long axis of the tibia (Fig. 14-13). Insert the combination bullet guide/hole changer into the 65-degree guide and advance the bullet until seated against the anteromedial cortex of the tibia. Drill the tibial guide-pin through the lateral hole in the bullet until it strikes the guide intra-articularly (see Fig. 14-13). Remove the bullet from the tibial guide and remove the guide from the notch. Tap the guide-pin into the notch and assess its position.

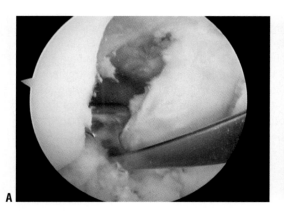

A

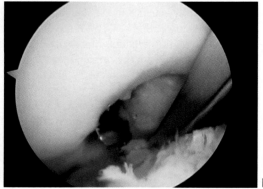

B

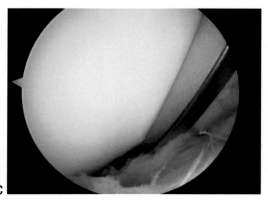

C

FIGURE 14-12
A: Sixty-five-degree tibial guide tip positioned in the intercondylar notch. **B:** Extend the knee maintaining 65-degree tibial guide tip in the intercondylar notch. **C:** Position of the 65-degree tibial guide arm against the trochlea groove with the knee in terminal extension.

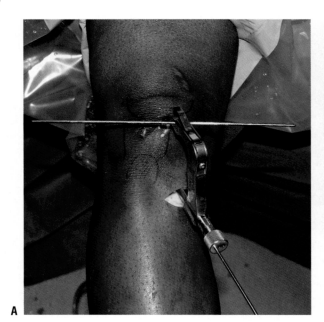

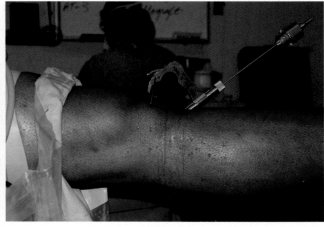

A

B

FIGURE 14-13
A: Tibial guidewire drilled through lateral hole in bullet with the knee in full extension and coronal alignment rod positioned parallel to the knee joint. **B:** Lateral view.

The tibial guide-pin is properly positioned in the coronal plane when it enters the notch midway between the lateral edge of the PCL and the lateral femoral condyle. The guide-pin should not touch the PCL (Fig. 14-14). The tibial guide-pin is properly positioned in the sagittal plane when there is 2 to 3 mm of space between the guide-pin and intercondylar roof with the knee in full extension. The space can be assessed by manipulating a 2-mm-wide nerve hook probe between the between the guide-pin and intercondylar roof in the fully extended knee.

Prepare the tibial tunnel. Ream the tibial cortex with a reamer with the same diameter as the prepared ACL graft. Harvest a bone dowel from the tibial tunnel by inserting an 8-mm-in-diameter bone dowel harvester and centering rod over the tibial guide-pin. Use a mallet and drive the bone dowel harvester until it reaches the subchondral bone (Fig. 14-15). Remove the dowel harvester with cancellous bone dowel (Fig. 14-16). If the tibial guide-pin is removed with the bone dowel, then replace it by inserting it through an 8-mm reamer that has been reinserted into the tunnel created by the bone dowel harvester. Ream the remainder of the tibial tunnel with the appropriate diameter reamer.

Check for PCL impingement by placing the knee in 90 degrees of flexion and inserting the impingement rod into the notch. A triangular space at the apex of the notch and no contact at the base of the notch between the PCL and impingement rod confirms the absence of PCL impingement (Fig. 14-17). Check for roof impingement by placing the knee in full extension and inserting an impinge-

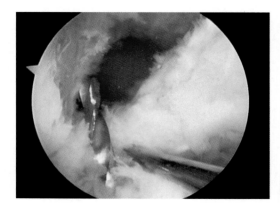

FIGURE 14-14
Guide-pin position in the intercondylar notch.

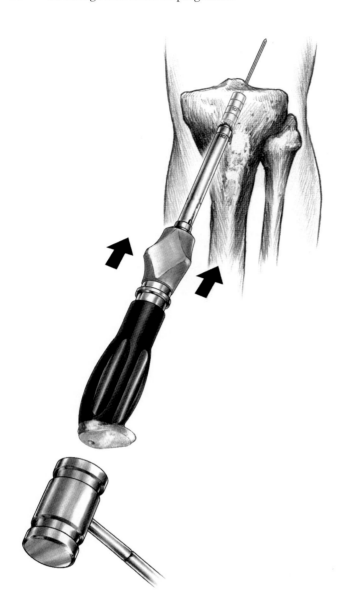

FIGURE 14-15
Impact bone dowel harvester
over guide-pin.

ment rod the same diameter as the tibial tunnel into the intercondylar notch (Fig. 14-18). Free pistoning of the impingement rod in and out of the notch with the knee in full extension confirms the absence of roof impingement.

Place the femoral tunnel using the transtibial technique. Insert the size-specific femoral aimer through the tibial tunnel with the knee in flexion. The size of the "off-set" of the femoral aimer is based on the diameter of the ACL graft and is designed to create a femoral tunnel with a 1-mm backwall. Extend the knee and hook the tip of the femoral aimer in the over-the-top position. Allow gravity to flex the knee until the femoral guide seats on the femur. Rotate the femoral aimer a quarter turn lateral away from the PCL, which positions the femoral guide-pin farther down the lateral wall of the notch minimizing PCL impingement (Fig. 14-19). Drill a pilot hole in the femur through the aimer and remove both the guide-pin and femoral aimer.

Redirect the femoral guide-pin to shorten the femoral tunnel from 35 to 50 mm in length with use of the following technique. Reinsert the femoral guide-pin into the pilot hole and flex the knee to 90

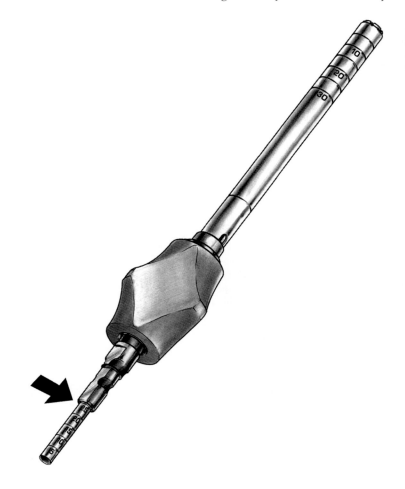

FIGURE 14-16
Remove harvester with cancellous graft inside of harvester tube.

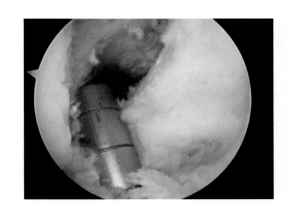

FIGURE 14-17
Impingement rod in notch.

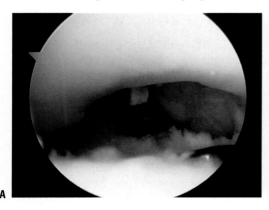
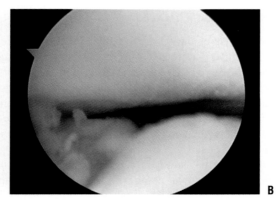

A   **B**

FIGURE 14-18

A: Extend knee and assess for roof impingement. **B:** Roof impingement not seen with knee in full extension.

to 100 degrees. Drill the guide-pin through the anterolateral femoral cortex. Pass a cannulated 1-in reamer the same diameter as the ACL graft over the guide-pin. Ream the femoral tunnel. Confirm the back wall of the femoral aimer is only 1 mm thick (Fig. 14-20). Confirm the center of the femoral tunnel is midway between the apex and base of the lateral half of the notch (Fig. 14-21). A femoral tunnel placed correctly down the sidewall does not allow room for a second posterolateral tunnel.

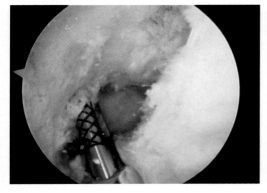
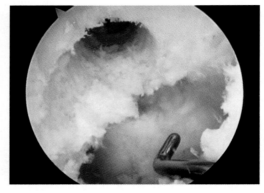

FIGURE 14-19
Femoral guide-pin position using femoral aimer through tibial tunnel.

FIGURE 14-20
Back wall thickness of femoral tunnel.

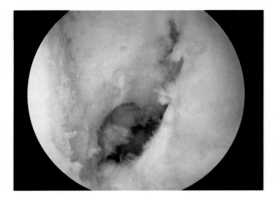

FIGURE 14-21
Femoral tunnel position assessed through lateral portal.

Pearls and Pitfalls

Proper use of the 65-degree tibial guide minimizes the complications of impingement associated with tunnel placement for ACL reconstruction surgery. Pitfalls typically stem from improper use of the 65-degree tibial guide. First, it is important not to alter the anatomy of the intercondylar roof when performing the lateral wallplasty should a wallplasty be required. A significant roofplasty at the time of wallplasty can change the sagittal plane position of the tibial tunnel. In revision cases where the intercondylar notch anatomy may be distorted, the use of intraoperative fluoroscopy or radiography may help to further ensure satisfactory tunnel position (Fig. 14-22). A second pitfall is improper position of the medial portal. The 65-degree tibial guide requires medial portal placement adjacent to the medial border of the patella tendon to ensure the 65-degree tibial guide seats centrally in the intercondylar notch with the knee in full extension. Too medial placement of the medial portal will position the 65-degree tibial guide medial in the notch. Too medial placement of the tibial tunnel in the notch using the transtibial tunnel technique will result in PCL impingement of the graft. Finally, it is important to clean the over-the-top position using the angled curette. Because the sized-specific femoral aimers position the femoral tunnel with only a 1- to 2-mm-thick posterior wall, any soft tissue remaining in the over-the-top position will lead to further posterior positioning of the femoral tunnel with possible blowout of the posterior wall.

POSTOPERATIVE MANAGEMENT

Postoperative management of ACL reconstruction depends on (a) the use of slippage resistance, stiffness, and strength of the femoral and tibial fixation devices; (b) placement of the tibial and femoral tunnels so that roof impingement is prevented, PCL impingement is prevented, and the tension pattern in the ACL graft matches the tension of the native ACL; and (c) the rapidity of tendon-tunnel healing. Brace-free, self-administered, aggressive rehabilitation of an impingement-free graft is safe when slippage-resistant, high-strength, and high-stiffness fixation devices are used. Placing the ACL graft without roof and PCL impingement eliminates the concern that the graft might be injured by knee extension and flexion exercises. The addition of the bone dowel in the tibial tunnel eliminates tunnel widening, increases stiffness, and snugs the fit in the tunnel, which speeds tendon-tunnel healing.

COMPLICATIONS

Poor tibial and femoral tunnel placement causes catastrophic complications, including loss of extension and anterior instability from roof impingement and loss of flexion and anterior instability from PCL impingement. Because there are few salvage options available to improve the success of ACL reconstruction in the setting of poorly placed tibial and femoral tunnels, prevention is the best treatment for avoiding complications associated with poor ACL tunnel placement. In the case of loss of extension in a stable knee caused by mild roof impingement, a roofplasty may help regain extension and reduce injury to the ACL graft from abrasion against the roof. Loss of flexion due to PCL impingement is not treatable unless the ACL graft is removed. The use of cross-pin fixation devices, not widening the notch, and the drilling of the femoral tunnel through the anteromedial portal, all tend to place the femoral tunnel too vertical causing PCL impingement and a loss of knee flexion and increased instability.

When using a transtibial tunnel technique, the 65-degree tibial guide prevents impingement complications associated with poor tunnel placement by allowing surgeons to consistently customize sagittal plane position of the tibial tunnel for all patients regardless of the differences in roof angle anatomy and knee extension. The use of a coronal alignment rod with the 65-degree tibial guide improves the accuracy of tibial tunnel position in the coronal plane, thereby effectively avoiding PCL impingement and improving rotational stability of the knee. The femoral tunnel position is automatic with the transtibial tunnel technique. Therefore, consistent anatomic placement of tibial tunnel in both the sagittal and coronal planes avoiding both roof and PCL impingement results in proper femoral tunnel placement that establishes graft tension behavior similar to the native ACL and increases the long-term success of ACL reconstruction (Fig. 14-23).

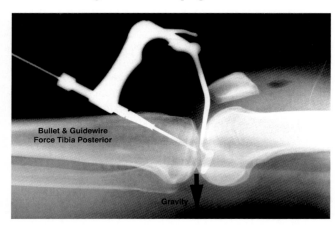

Bullet & Guidewire
Force Tibia Posterior

Gravity

FIGURE 14-22

Lateral radiograph with knee in full extension demonstrating knee joint and guide-pin position with the 65-degree tibial guide in place.

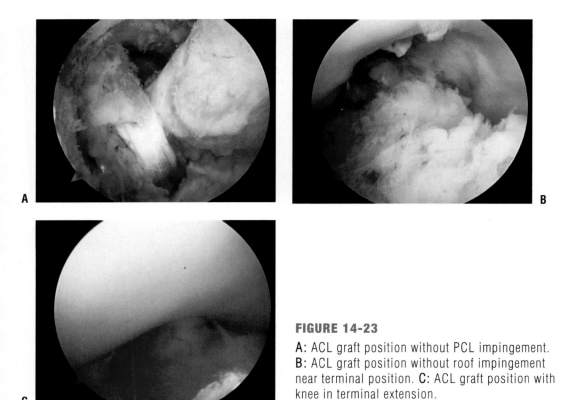

A

B

C

FIGURE 14-23

A: ACL graft position without PCL impingement.
B: ACL graft position without roof impingement near terminal position. **C:** ACL graft position with knee in terminal extension.

RESULTS

The use of the 65-degree tibial guide with coronal alignment rod increases the accuracy of tibial tunnel placement in both the sagittal and coronal planes. The increased accuracy of tibial tunnel placement avoids the complications of graft impingement leading to better knee range of motion and stability. In addition, because the 65-degree tibial guide was designed to reference the patient's anatomy, a roofplasty is not required when the guide is properly used. Minimizing the notchplasty required to position an impingement-free graft decreases the amount of graft pretensioning required to stabilize the ACL-deficient knee and is favorable for graft remodeling and long-term function.

RECOMMENDED READING

Cuomo P, Edwards A, Giron F, et al. Validation of the 65 degrees Howell guide for anterior cruciate ligament reconstruction. *Arthroscopy.* 2006;22:70–75.

Giron F, Cuomo P, Aglietti P, et al. Femoral attachment of the anterior cruciate ligament. *Knee Surg Sports Traumatol Arthrosc.* 2006;14:250–256.

Hame SL, Markolf KL, Hunter DM, et al. Effects of notchplasty and femoral tunnel position on excursion patterns of an anterior cruciate ligament graft. *Arthroscopy.* 2003;19:340–345.

Howell SM. Principles for placing the tibial tunnel and avoiding roof impingement during reconstruction of a torn anterior cruciate ligament. *Knee Surg Sports Traumatol Arthrosc.* 1998;6(suppl 1):S49–S55.

Howell SM, Barad SJ. Knee extension and its relationship to the slope of the intercondylar roof. Implications for positioning the tibial tunnel in anterior cruciate ligament reconstructions. *Am J Sports Med.* 1995;23:288–294.

Howell SM, Berns GS, Farley TE. Unimpinged and impinged anterior cruciate ligament grafts: MR signal intensity measurements. *Radiology.* 1991a;179:639–643.

Howell SM, Clark JA. Tibial tunnel placement in anterior cruciate ligament reconstructions and graft impingement. *Clin Orthop.* 1992:187–195.

Howell SM, Clark JA, Farley TE. A rationale for predicting anterior cruciate graft impingement by the intercondylar roof. A magnetic resonance imaging study. *Am J Sports Med.* 1991b;19:276–282.

Howell SM, Gittins ME, Gottlieb JE, et al. The relationship between the angle of the tibial tunnel in the coronal plane and loss of flexion and anterior laxity after anterior cruciate ligament reconstruction. *Am J Sports Med.* 2001;29:567–574.

Howell SM, Lawhorn KW. Gravity Reduces the Tibia When Using a Tibial Guide that Targets the Intercondylar Roof. *Am J Sports Med.* 2004;32:1702–1710.

Howell SM, Roos P, Hull ML. Compaction of a bone dowel in the tibial tunnel improves the fixation stiffness of a soft tissue anterior cruciate ligament graft: an in vitro study in calf tibia. *Am J Sports Med.* 2005;33:719–725.

Karchin A, Hull ML, Howell SM. Initial tension and anterior load-displacement behavior of high-stiffness anterior cruciate ligament graft constructs. *J Bone Joint Surg Am.* 2004;86-A:1675–1683.

Khalfayan EE, Sharkey PF, Alexander AH, et al. The relationship between tunnel placement and clinical results after anterior cruciate ligament reconstruction. *Am J Sports Med.* 1996;24:335–341.

Lawhorn KW, Howell SM. Scientific justification and technique for anterior cruciate ligament reconstruction using autogenous and allogeneic soft-tissue grafts. *Orthop Clin North Am.* 2003;34:19–30

Loh JC, Fukuda Y, Tsuda E, et al. Knee stability and graft function following anterior cruciate ligament reconstruction: comparison between 11 o'clock and 10 o'clock femoral tunnel placement. 2002 Richard O'Connor Award paper. *Arthroscopy.* 2003;19:297–304.

Matsumoto A, Howell SM, Liu-Barba D. Time-related changes in the cross-sectional area of the tibial tunnel after compaction of an autograft bone dowel alongside a hamstring graft. *Arthroscopy.* 2006;22:855–860.

Simmons R, Howell SM, Hull ML. Effect of the angle of the femoral and tibial tunnels in the coronal plane and incremental excision of the posterior cruciate ligament on tension of an anterior cruciate ligament graft: an in vitro study. *J Bone Joint Surg Am.* 2003;85-A:1018–1029.

Singhatat W, Lawhorn KW, Howell SM, et al. How four weeks of implantation affect the strength and stiffness of a tendon graft in a bone tunnel: a study of two fixation devices in an extra-articular model in ovine. *Am J Sports Med.* 2002;30:506–513.

15 Patellar Tendon Graft Harvesting

David A. McGuire and Stephen D. Hendricks

INDICATIONS/CONTRAINDICATIONS

The patellar tendon graft is indicated in most patients undergoing reconstruction of a torn anterior cruciate ligament (ACL). Situations in which an autogenous patellar tendon may be contraindicated include the multiply operated knee where reharvest of previously harvested patellar tendon would be needed, patients with an arthritic patellofemoral joint, or patients with previous patellar trauma such as a fracture. In addition, individuals whose occupation requires repetitive kneeling or working on their hands and knees may pose a relative contraindication. In these patients, other graft sources such as hamstring tendons or allografts should be considered.

PREOPERATIVE PLANNING

Certain preoperative steps should be taken when an autogenous patellar tendon graft is considered. Radiologic imaging will help identify those patients with a degenerative patellofemoral joint or significant patellar baja or alta. If patella alta is identified, there are several techniques available to deal with a graft that is longer than required. The knee also should be examined for any signs of patella maltracking or instability. A suitable graft table and required instrumentation should be available to prepare the graft efficiently for fit and insertion ease.

SURGERY

Patient Positioning

The patient is positioned supine with the leg hung free. A standard arthroscopy prep and drape of the knee is used. A tourniquet is placed around the thigh, and a leg holder is placed at the level of the tourniquet. Anesthesia is typically general, although an epidural is an alternative.

Technique

The bone patellar tendon bone (BTB) graft can be harvested through two small vertical incisions (Fig. 15-1). The vertical incisions are cosmetic, and may lead to less morbidity and pain than a single long incision. Because the tibial drill guide will be positioned through the tibial harvest incision, the location of this incision is important to the placement of the tibial tunnel. With this in mind, the tibial incision begins 2 cm distal to the joint line and 1 cm medial to the tibial tubercle and extends 2.5 cm distally. The patellar incision begins at the distal pole of the patella and extends 2.5 cm proximally over the midline of the patella. Although we prefer the two-incision technique, a single skin incision can be used.

The tibial bone plug is harvested first. Lateral retraction of the skin will allow clear visualization of the tendon attachment site. The central 10 mm of the patellar tendon attachment is measured, and the medial/lateral borders are marked with electrocautery (Fig. 15-2). Using a stoppered plunge blade (Plunge Blade, Linvatec, Largo, FL), the tibial bone plug is created (Fig. 15-3). With the saw blade angled to approximately 45 degrees, the cuts are made to a depth of 8 mm (Fig. 15-4). The stoppered plunge blade will limit the cut depth to 8 mm and therefore eliminate the risk of overpenetration. Us-

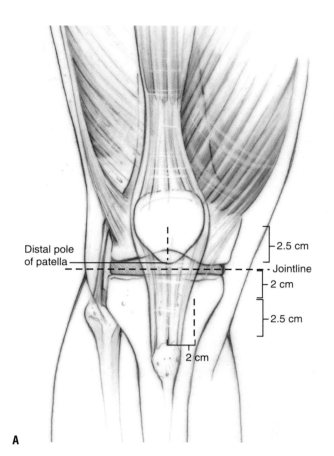

Distal pole of patella —

- - - Jointline

2.5 cm

2 cm

2.5 cm

2 cm

A

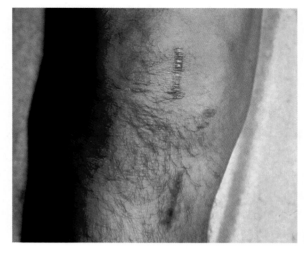

B

FIGURE 15-1

A: The BTB tendon can be harvested through two 1-in incisions. The two small incisions are more cosmetic than one large one. **B:** Incisions closed and healed.

FIGURE 15-2

The medial and lateral borders of the patellar tendon tibial attachment are measured and marked with electrocautery. We prefer electrocautery over a pen because pen marks can become smeared and difficult to read.

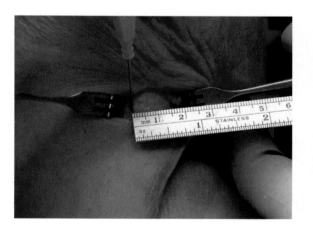

FIGURE 15-3

The plunge blade has a stopper 8 mm from the saw blade teeth, preventing penetration of the saw blade beyond that depth.

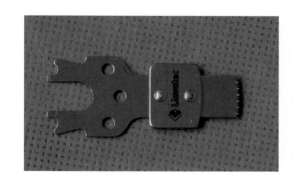

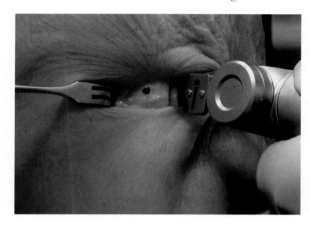

FIGURE 15-4

Angling the saw blade during harvest will produce a trapezoidal bone plug.

ing a side-to-side rocking motion, the side cuts are carried distally for 2.5 cm. A horizontal saw cut is made to connect the distal ends of the parallel side cuts.

Beginning distally at the tibial bone plug and working proximally toward the patella, a double-bladed tendon harvester (Parasmillie meniscotome, Linvatec, Largo, FL) is used to incise both sides of the graft simultaneously (Fig. 15-5). The fixed width of the blades (10 mm) helps maintain a constant graft width throughout tendon harvest. The tendon harvester is advanced proximally until the harvester tips make contact with the distal pole of the patella. The tips of the harvester should be visible through the patellar incision.

Using the tips of the harvester as a guide, the medial and lateral margins of the patellar bone plug are marked with electrocautery (Fig. 15-6), generating a patellar bone plug width of 11 mm. Beginning distally at the marked sites, use the stoppered plunge blade to create the side cuts for the patellar bone plug. With the blade angled to 45 to 60 degrees, the saw cuts are made to a depth of 8 mm (Fig. 15-7). Advance the cuts proximally until a bone plug length of 25 mm is obtained. Using a horizontal saw cut, connect the proximal termination of the two side cuts (Fig. 15-8).

Attention is directed to the tibial bone plug. Using a ¼-inch osteotome, remove the tibial bone plug from the tibia (Fig. 15-9). Scissors may be needed to cut any remaining soft tissue connections.

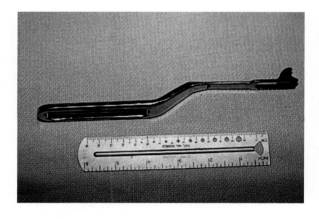

FIGURE 15-5

The Parasmillie meniscotome cleaves both the medial and lateral borders of the patellar tendon simultaneously, ensuring a constant graft width along the entire length of the harvest.

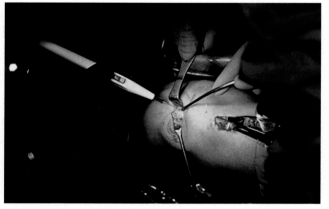

FIGURE 15-6

The medial and lateral borders of the patellar bone plug are measured from the tips of the harvester. Marking bone plug borders in this manner ensures that all tendon fibers attached to the tibial bone plug are also attached to the patellar bone plug.

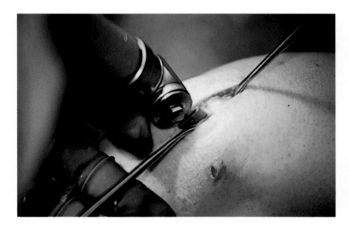

FIGURE 15-7

When in use, the stopper prevents the blade from producing cuts with variable depths. A bone plug defect with varying cut depths may lead to stress risers and patellar fracture.

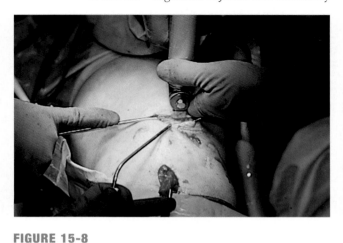

FIGURE 15-8

The proximal ends of medial and lateral saw cuts are connected with a short horizontal saw cut. To avoid creating stress risers, do not allow the horizontal cut to extend beyond and therefore intersect either of the two side cuts.

Grasp the tibial bone plug with a Kocher, and advance the bone plug proximally through the tibial incision and out the patellar incision (Fig. 15-10). Using an osteotome, remove the patellar bone plug. Again, scissors may be needed to remove any remaining soft tissue connections and completely free the graft. Carefully transfer the graft to a back table for preparation.

Using a motorized burr, contour the corners of the patellar defect (Fig. 15-11). The bone plug is trimmed to approximate a trapezoid shape and sharp edges are contoured (Fig. 15-12). Save the bone chips created during sizing. The bone plugs are sized with the aid of a sizing tube to ensure passage within the tunnels (Fig. 15-13). Typically, the bone plugs are sized to 10 and 11 mm. A single hole is drilled in each bone plug. A size 0 Ethibond suture is placed in the smaller bone plug (Fig. 15-14), which will eventually be positioned within the femur. A 24-gauge flexible wire suture is placed in the larger bone plug. Fill the patellar defect with the bone chips saved during graft preparation. The patella defect is closed.

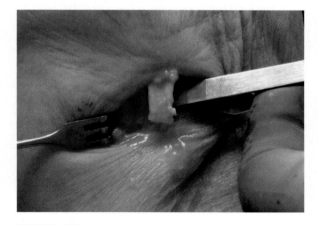

FIGURE 15-9

The tibial bone plug is pried loose with a ¼-in osteotome. Pry the bone plug loose by hand; do not use a mallet.

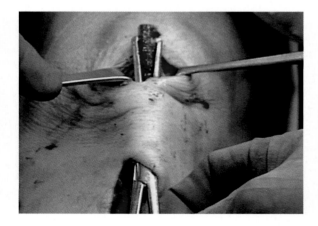

FIGURE 15-10

Once removed, the patellar bone plug is grasped with a Kocher and advanced proximally.

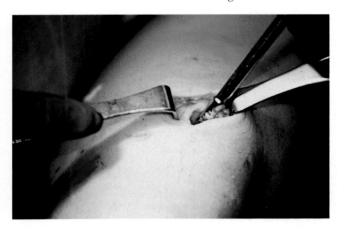

FIGURE 15-11

The sharp corners of the patella defect should be contoured with the aid of a motorized burr. Failure to contour the defect corners can increase the risk of postoperative patella fracture.

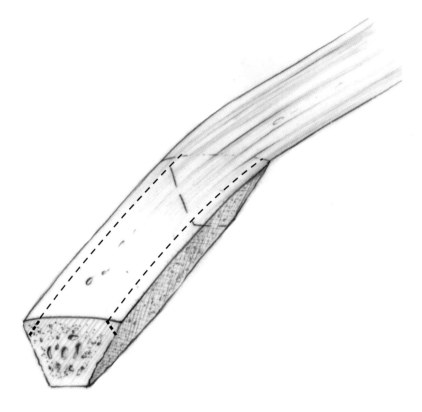

FIGURE 15-12

The bone plugs are trimmed into a trapezoidal shape. When inserted into the tunnel, a trapezoidal plug leaves space for the advancing interference screw.

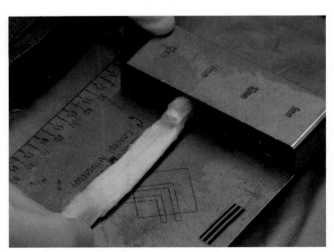

FIGURE 15-13

A graft table is useful when preparing the graft. Using the table, the graft can be sized, the length measured, and holes drilled for the sutures used during graft insertion and tensioning.

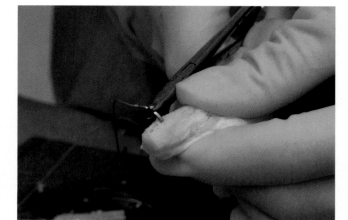

FIGURE 15-14

A size 0 Ethibond suture is placed in the smaller bone plug, and a wire suture is placed in the larger bone plug. The larger of the two bone plugs will be oriented within the tibial tunnel. The wire suture cannot be lacerated by the passing screw during fixation.

Pearls and Pitfalls

Pearls and pitfalls are outlined in Table 15-1.

TABLE 15-1. Pearls and Pitfalls of Patellar Tendon Graft Harvesting

Pitfall	Problem(s) Significance	Tips
Single long incision	Less cosmetic, increased difficulty healing, increased risk of infection, increased proprioception loss.	Use two small incisions. The proximal one at the distal portion of the patella and the distal one medial to the tibial tuberosity.
Excessive bone plug length	Increased risk of patellar fracture.	Use 25 mm maximum length; shorter lengths may be used and matched with shorter length interference screws.
Stress risers during bone plug creation	Increased risk of patellar fracture caused by saw cuts (kerfs) beyond the corners of the removed plug or kerfs of uneven depth.	Use plunge saw blade with depth stop and rocking technique to prevent stress riser creation.
Square corners in bone plug defects	Increased risk of patellar fracture.	Round corners with rotary shaver.
Empty patellar defect	Prolonged regrowth and associated pain and patellar weakness beyond the ACL remodeling interval.	Bone graft defect with tibial tuberosity chips or from cored bone removed from tibial tunnel with coring reamer (Trephine).
Tendon fibers to bone plug mismatch	Cross-cut or unattached fibers create reduction in connected width of fibers resulting in weaker graft with increased risk or graft failure.	Use a Parasmillie meniscotome that, once the distal plug is created, cleaves fibers and identifies connected region of patellar tendon bone plug harvest site.
Bone plug graft tunnel mismatch	Increased difficulty inserting graft to desired location.	Round ends with rongeur and confirm graft size with tunnel diameter–matched sizing tube.
Bone plug trapping from tilted insertion	Increased difficulty inserting graft to desired location because suture hole is too distal in the femoral plug.	Use graft table with drill guide to place to pull hole at ¼ to ⅛ distal to the proximal end of the femoral plug (Fig. 15-15).
Interference screw insertion torque is too high	Increased risk of fracture potential of bone plug or bioabsorbable screw and metal screw auguring of cancellous material during initial insertion.	Shape bone in trapezoid configuration by angling the plunge blade during insertion to 60 degrees from vertical during plug harvest. Notch the tunnel wall for screw insertion or tap it.
Interference screw insertion torque is too low	Increased risk of fixation failure.	Use next larger screw size or use a second screw of same size.
Patella baja	Distal bone plug hangs out of the tibial tunnel precluding secure interference screw fixation.	Keep T tunnel between 55 and 60 degrees. Drill the F tunnel 5 mm deeper to 30 mm for its 25-mm plug or fold the distal plug over onto itself to shorten the LOA (Fig. 15-16).

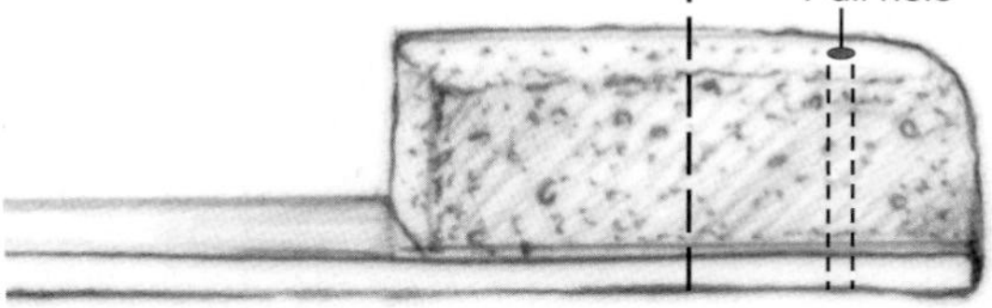

Midpoint   Pull hole

FIGURE 15-15

The proximal end of the bone plug should be rounded to facilitate ease of insertion and the draw tunnel placed less than one quarter the length of the plug toward the same end to prevent tilting-produced trapping at the femoral tunnel distal entrance during graft insertion.

POSTOPERATIVE MANAGEMENT

The patellar tendon harvest described here is part of an overall ACL reconstruction and, therefore, the postoperative management and rehabilitation program are primarily dictated by the circumstances of that procedure. However, some special management and rehabilitation considerations should be taken into account when using a patellar tendon autograft. Exercises that include kneeling, squatting, jumping, or extension against resistance should be avoided. The increased stress to the patella caused by these exercises may lead to patellar fracture.

COMPLICATIONS

There are several notable complications associated with BTB autograft harvest: infrapatellar contracture syndrome (2,4), patella infera, patellar tendon rupture (1), quadriceps insertion rupture, and patella fracture (2,3). Although these complications are significant and may be debilitating to the patients in the relatively few incidences reported, their occurrence can usually be avoided.

Patella fracture, although uncommon, can occur following autogenous patellar tendon harvest (Fig. 15-17). Fracture is typically the result of stress risers caused by saw cuts beyond the corners of the removed plug (Fig. 15-18), cuts made too deeply and unevenly into the patella (Fig. 15-19), or the sharp corners of the trapezoid-shaped bone plug defect. A lack of bone grafting also prolongs the risk of patellar fracture beyond the rehabilitation and remodeling period for the ACL graft.

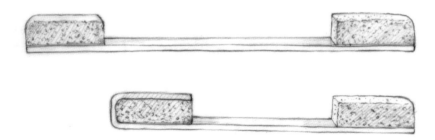

FIGURE 15-16

The distal plug of the BTB graft may be rolled over on itself to shorten the length between the plugs if it protrudes significantly distally. If this procedure is used, the distal bone plug may need resizing for it to fit properly in the tibial tunnel. Once sized, suturing the configuration together will ease graft insertion, tensioning, and fixation.

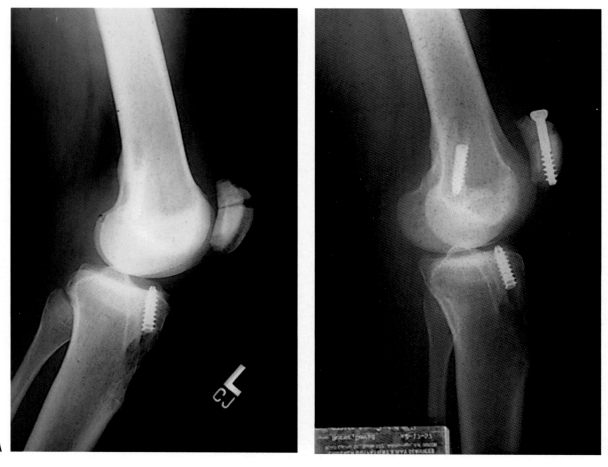

FIGURE 15-17

A: Patellar fracture postoperatively. B: Patellar fracture reduced with ASIF screw.

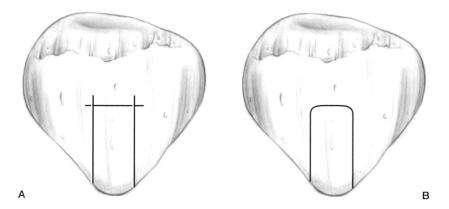

FIGURE 15-18

A: Failure to eliminate stress risers can increase the incidence of postoperative stress risers. Intersection of the saw kerfs is a common stress riser. B: If produced, these intersections should be rounded with the aid of a motorized burr.

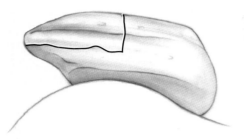

FIGURE 15-19

Cuts made too deeply risk damage to retropatellar surface and longitudinal fractures.

To reduce the risk of cutting too deeply into the patella, a stoppered plunge saw blade (Linvatec, Largo, FL) should be used. With such a stopper, cuts are limited to a depth of 8 mm and, as a result, stress risers from this source are moderated. In addition, kerfs are of uniform depth and stress risers from this source are eliminated. The kerfs must not extend beyond the ends of the graft, also helping avoid injury to the retropatellar surface. The use of these measures also avoids injury to the retropatellar surface and potential interruption of the quadriceps tendon insertion.

Another patellar tendon harvest pitfall arises when the tibial and patellar bone plugs are offset and as a result not all tendon fibers are attached to both bone fragments (Fig. 15-20). The width of the BTB graft is usually 10 mm, although 9 or 11 mm widths are feasible alternatives depending on patient size. With a 10-mm width, the corresponding bone plugs are 10 mm from the tibial tuberosity and 11 mm from the patella. This is a technical variation that simplifies insertion. The 10-mm "femoral" end of the graft slides easily through the 11-mm tibial tunnel. The graft is weaker if the fibers are offset and all fibers are not attached to both bone fragments (see Fig. 15-20A). It is possible to have a mismatch, even with the central one third of the patellar tendon completely exposed by

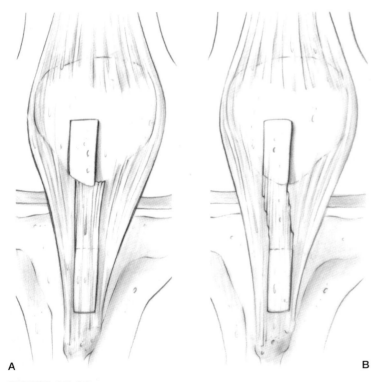

A   B

FIGURE 15-20

A: If the bone plugs are harvested prior to cleaving the tendon, any medial/lateral offset in the plugs will result in a portion of the graft fibers only being attached to one bone plug. **B:** This illustration of a cross-cut mismatch depicts the relative fiber width which is defined by those fibers attached to both plugs and in this case it is significantly less than the width of the bone plugs. To avoid these complications, the tibial bone plug should be harvested first, the graft second, and the patellar bone plug last.

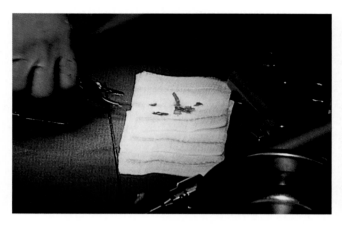

FIGURE 15-21
Bone chips removed from the tibial defect with a rongeur.

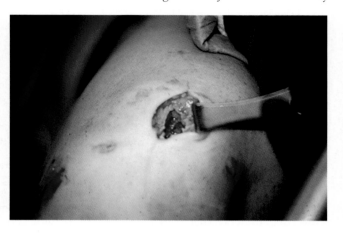

FIGURE 15-22
Bone grafting with chips inserted into the patellar defect.

a 4-inch incision. The mismatch can also occur if both of the bone plugs are harvested first and either of the plugs is offset medial or lateral to one another (see Fig. 15-20B). The solution to this problem is to harvest the tibial bone plug first, the tendon fibers second, and the patellar bone plug last. As long as the tibial bone plug is located centrally on the tibial tuberosity and the graft fibers are cleaved vertically, then simply matching the distal portion of the patellar tendon bone plug with the separated fibers will eliminate a mismatch. A double-bladed harvester (Parasmillie meniscotome, Linvatec, Largo, FL) that cleaves both sides of the patellar tendon simultaneously helps maintain evenly spaced and parallel cuts, which lead to better and more consistent grafts.

Bone grafting can be accomplished by filling the patellar defect with bone chips removed from the bone plugs on the end of the graft during the shaping and sizing or from the tibial defect area (Figs. 15-21 and 15-22). Since we have begun using a coring reamer (Trephine, Smith & Nephew, Andover, MA) to make the tibial tunnel, we extract a core of the patient's bone in every case (Fig. 15-23). The cored bone plug is an excellent source of bone graft material that may be shaped to fit the patellar and tibial defects exactly. These solid plugs seem to reduce the long-term pain in our recent patient population when compared with patients with no grafting or chip bone grafting.

FIGURE 15-23
Bone plug removed with coring reamer ready to be shaped into graft for patellar and tibial graft harvest defects.

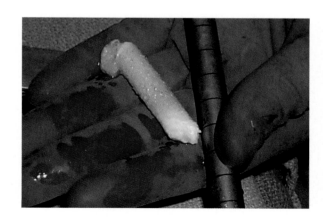

REFERENCES

1. Bonamo JJ, Krinick RM, Sporn RM. Rupture of the patellar ligament after use of its central third for anterior cruciate reconstruction: a report of two cases. *J Bone Joint Surg.* 1984;66-A:1294–1297.
2. Graf B, Uhr F. Complications of intra-articular anterior cruciate reconstruction. *Clin Sports Med.* 1988;7(4):835–848.
3. McCarroll JR. Fracture of the patella during a golf swing following reconstruction of the anterior cruciate ligament: a case report. *Am J Sports Med.* 1983;11(1):26–27.
4. Rosenberg TD, Franklin JL, Baldwin GN, et al. Extensor mechanism function after patellar tendon graft harvest for anterior cruciate ligament reconstruction. *Am J Sports Med.* 1992;20(5):519–526.

16 Anterior Cruciate Ligament Reconstruction with Autogenous Hamstring Tendon Autografts and EndoButton Femoral Fixation

Roger V. Larson

INDICATIONS/CONTRAINDICATIONS

Injuries to the anterior cruciate ligament (ACL) are common and appear to be increasing. The goal of treating an ACL-insufficient knee is to provide functional stability to prevent recurrent injuries that may lead to subsequent damage to the menisci and articular surfaces. Individuals of any age who wish to remain active in jumping and pivoting sports can become candidates for ACL reconstructive surgery. The success of ACL reconstruction depends on strict adherence to surgical principles, including the selection of a graft of adequate strength and stiffness, graft placement that avoids overstraining and bony impingement, and graft fixation that provides initial strength and stiffness to allow early rehabilitation (5).

Historically, many tissues have been used to serve as ACL substitutes, including autografts, allografts, and synthetic materials. The most common grafts currently used for ACL reconstruction include autogenous bone patellar tendon bone grafts as well as those of quadrupled hamstring tendons. Allografts are being used with increasing frequency. Both patellar tendon and hamstring autogenous grafts have been shown to be effective in restoring normal anterior knee laxity when used correctly. The use of hamstring tendons offers the advantage of avoiding the extensor mechanism for graft harvest. This is of particular importance in patients with pre-existing patellofemoral disease as well as in situations of revision surgery where the patellar tendon has been used previously. Hamstring tendon grafts are also indicated when cosmesis is of more than a casual concern. There are no absolute contraindications to the use of hamstring tendon autografts for ACL reconstructive surgery with the exception of their unavailability due to previous harvest.

The use of semitendinosus and gracilis tendon autografts for reconstruction of the ACL has been well established (3,8,19). When both the semitendinosus and gracilis tendons are harvested and doubled, the combined four-stranded graft offers several potential advantages over other commonly used autografts such as patellar tendons. The potential advantages of hamstring tendon autografts include increased strength, stiffness characteristics more similar to a normal ACL, a large surface area for graft revascularization or nutrient diffusion, a predictable means of tensioning, and adaptability to precise positioning (15).

When the semitendinosus and gracilis tendons are both doubled and used as an ACL graft, they provide a large-diameter, strong ACL substitute with a significantly greater cross-sectional area of collagen than a 10-mm-wide patellar tendon autograft. The ability to place a hamstring tendon graft precisely is enhanced over that of a patellar tendon, since bone tunnels can be created in the desired locations and then completely filled with collagen tissue. When using patellar tendon grafts with bone blocks on each end, it is necessary to overdrill bone tunnels to fit the bone block. Interference fit screws are frequently used for fixing patellar tendon grafts, and the use of interference fit screws can distort the position of the collagen portion of the graft. The ability of a multistranded graft to obtain nutrition by either diffusion or vascular ingrowth is enhanced over that of a solid graft due to the increased surface area and smaller depth of penetration needed for either revascularization or nutrient diffusion.

Another potential advantage of using hamstring tendons for ACL reconstruction is that the resulting graft tissue has stiffness characteristics that are more similar to a normal ACL, particularly when compared with a patellar tendon autograft (20). The stiffness characteristics at the time of implantation, however, depend on the type of fixation used (9,27,29). Newer techniques of fixing hamstring tendon autografts have alleviated what was once considered a weak link providing initial fixation comparable to or superior to the fixation of bone tendon bone grafts (17,20,32). Soft-tissue grafts such as hamstring tendons also allow for more precise tensioning of the grafts, making overconstraint of the joint less likely. It has also been shown that the process of tendon healing in a bone tunnel occurs relatively early, and thus with improved initial fixation rehabilitation protocols do not need to be significantly different from those used with bone tendon bone grafts (25). It also has been shown by histology and biochemical analysis that post implantation, semitendinosus grafts undergo changes in collagen crimp pattern, cell type, glycosaminoglycan composition, and collagen crosslinking, which suggest a structural change toward that of a normal ACL (14).

The most compelling reason to consider hamstring tendon autografts for ACL reconstruction, however, is the decreased surgical morbidity associated with this procedure. With the use of hamstring tendon autografts, problems of motion and patellofemoral arthrosis are rare (26,28). Several investigators have demonstrated equal success rates when using this technique compared with the use of patellar tendon autografts (1,18,21). These studies, when taken in combination, tend to show increased patient satisfaction with the use of hamstring tendons and slightly, although not significantly, tighter knees when reconstructed with patellar tendon grafts (4,6,7,13,22,24).

PREOPERATIVE PLANNING

Before embarking on surgical treatment of ACL insufficiency, it is imperative to document the abnormal laxity and to obtain radiographs that clearly demonstrate the bony anatomy. The diagnosis of ACL insufficiency can usually be suspected by taking a careful history of the injury and the subsequent symptomatology of the knee. The diagnosis can usually be confirmed by physical examination. In the acute situation, physical examination may be difficult and subsequent examinations to confirm the diagnosis must be planned. The most sensitive test for determining ACL laxity is the Lachman test, in which an anterior force is applied to the tibia with the knee flexed approximately 25 degrees. This examination when compared with the normal knee can be diagnostic in up to 95% of cases, including acute injuries. Tests that elicit the "pivot shift phenomenon" are helpful in grading the ACL laxity, but can seldom be performed adequately in the acute situation.

An arthrometer can be helpful in demonstrating ACL laxity and documenting the extent of abnormal laxity. It has been shown that in normal individuals there is a 95% chance that there will be a side-to-side difference of less than 2 mm in ACL laxity. If 3 mm or greater of side-to-side difference can be demonstrated with an arthrometer, it can be assumed that the ACL has been injured.

Magnetic resonance imaging (MRI) when performed in the proper plane can be very accurate in diagnosing an injury of the ACL. With careful study of MRI images, partial tears of the ACL can also be identified when either the posterolateral or anteromedial band of the ACL may remain intact. The MRI may also show a typical bone bruising pattern involving the posterior aspect of the lateral tibial plateau and the mid anterior portion of the lateral femoral condyle. This bruising pattern in the "impact zone" is highly suggestive of a torn ACL. The MRI is also important in delineating associated pathology which may influence whether surgical intervention is undertaken or the timing of such intervention.

It is also necessary before embarking on surgical intervention to review the technical points that are important to a successful outcome. As with any surgical procedure, several technical points must be respected to predictably obtain a successful outcome when using hamstring tendon grafts. These include the successful harvest and preparation of the grafts, correct tunnel placement, secure graft fixation, and rehabilitation appropriate for the procedure performed.

SURGERY

Principles

Graft Harvest and Preparation: Technical Points   The potential difficulties in harvesting the hamstring tendons and the variability in tissue obtained were once major detriments to the routine use of these grafts. It was also once necessary to obtain considerable graft length to directly fix grafts extraosseously. With newer endoscopic techniques, it is usually only necessary to harvest 22 to 24 cm of tendon, and this amount of tendon can be consistently harvested. The quadrupled graft is generally from 7 to 9 mm in diameter, which is adequate for ACL substitution. It is important to be aware of the anatomy of the semitendinosus and gracilis tendons, particularly of the routinely encountered bands of tissue that extend from the inferior surfaces of each tendon to the medial head of the gastrocnemius (16, 23) (Fig. 16-1). These bands must be identified and sectioned before passing a tendon stripper to ensure that the stripper follows a direct course to the muscle

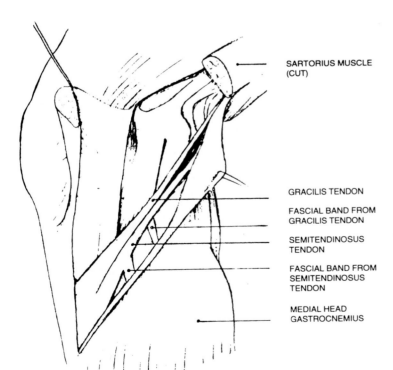

SARTORIUS MUSCLE
(CUT)

GRACILIS TENDON

FASCIAL BAND FROM
GRACILIS TENDON

SEMITENDINOSUS
TENDON

FASCIAL BAND FROM
SEMITENDINOSUS
TENDON

MEDIAL HEAD
GASTROCNEMIUS

FIGURE 16-1

The semitendinosus and gracilis tendons must be isolated and separated before harvesting. Extraneous bands of tissue that often connect to the medial head of the gastrocnemius must be identified and released before passing a tendon stripper to avoid deflecting the stripper and cutting the tendon short of its maximal length.

belly. In cases in which the semitendinosus tendon is of exceptionally high quality and length or where a gracilis tendon is inadequate, a quadrupled semitendinosus tendon graft can be used with some modification of fixation technique (2).

Once the tendons have been harvested and sized, it is important to remove muscle tissue from each graft and secure each end of each graft with a nonabsorbable suture. The use of a supplemental suture technique allows for the fixation of every fiber of the graft and for important secondary fixation. It has been shown that slippage under washers, or against interference fit screws, can be considerably reduced by adding a suture technique to the primary source of fixation.

Tunnel Placement   For a successful ACL reconstruction with hamstring tendons or any other graft, the graft must be placed so that it does not overstrain as the knee passes through a full range of motion and so that it does not impinge against the bony anatomy of the intercondylar notch, particularly in terminal extension. This can usually be accomplished by placing the tibial tunnel in a central position and the femoral tunnel at the extreme back of the intercondylar notch at approximately the 10:30 or 1:30 position (30) (Fig. 16-2A). This is at the point where the sidewall and roof of the notch meet. When properly positioned, this provides for a graft that deviates from the vertical position of the posterior cruciate ligament (PCL) at an angle of approximately 25 to 30 degrees. This placement requires careful attention to the start point of the tibial tunnel, particularly when the femoral tunnel is to be created through the tibial tunnel (12). When ideally placed, the ACL graft will avoid contact with the lateral wall of the intercondylar notch and will barely touch the roof of the intercondylar notch at full terminal extension. The proper placement will also avoid excessive impingement with the PCL, particularly in hyperflexion. The femoral tunnel should extend to or near the "over-the-top" area. It is acceptable to blow out the back wall of the notch when creating the femoral tunnel, and in fact this would ensure that the tunnel is far enough to the back of the notch.

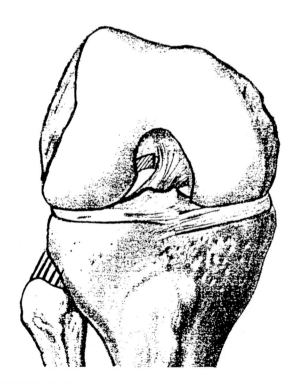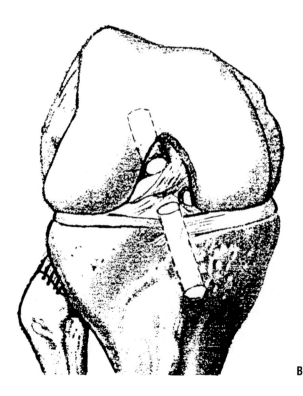

FIGURE 16-2

The position of a femoral tunnel that corresponds to a central tibial tunnel at 10:30 or 1:30 o'clock and to the extreme back of the intercondylar notch. The cross-hatched area noted in **(A)** shows the area that strains less than 5% through a full range of motion. It is located at the extreme back of the intercondylar notch. This area can be accessed through a tibial tunnel if the start point of the tibial tunnel is correctly positioned **(B)**.

With EndoButton (EndoButton™, Smith and Nephew, Corp., Boston, MA) fixation on the femur, blowing out of the back wall of the tunnel does not compromise fixation strength. The leading edge of the femoral tunnel should be chamfered to avoid a sharp corner that could traumatize the ACL substitute (21). The proper position of the femoral tunnel is demonstrated in Figure 16-2B.

The tibial tunnel should be created far enough posterior in the notch so that at full terminal extension the graft will barely graze the superior notch but will not be impinged or "guillotined" by it. It has been shown that impinged grafts remain inflamed and their MRI signals do not return to normal (10). With extreme impingement knee extension can be blocked and anterior graft fibers can be broken, creating a "cyclops" lesion (11). The tibial tunnel should also be placed in a position that avoids lateral notch impingement. If the femoral tunnel is to be drilled through the tibial tunnel, the start point must be medial enough to allow drilling of the femoral tunnel at the appropriate position. This usually requires starting the tibial tunnel within the fibers of the medial collateral ligament. It is appropriate when possible to fit the tunnels to the anatomic notch. Routine notchplasty should be discouraged, since with notchplasty the exposed cancellous surfaces often form fibrocartilage and eventual reformation of the anatomic notch.

Graft Fixation Options   The goal of ACL reconstruction is to provide an ACL substitute that will reproduce as nearly as possible the functional properties of the native ACL. For the graft to perform this function it must be placed in a near isometric or "physiometric" position, and it must have the strength and stiffness to mimic ACL function. During the first 6 to 12 weeks, before biologic healing of the grafts to the bone tunnels, the behavior of the graft depends not only on the material properties of the graft being used but also on the method of graft fixation used. The graft/fixation construct must be strong enough to avoid failure with tensile loading, and it must be stiff enough to restore the load displacement response of a normal ACL and secure enough to resist slippage with cyclic loading.

The important parameter to consider in fixation strength is yield load. This is the point at which plastic deformation begins and functional failure occurs (17). Most fixation devices used for the femoral fixation of hamstring tendon grafts have yield loads of between 350 to 800 newtons (N). The newer-generation fixation devices may increase this strength to 1,200 N. Techniques of femoral fixation that involve rigid cross-pin fixation provide the greatest initial strength.

Tibial fixation of hamstring tendon grafts is a more problematic consideration than femoral fixation. Initial fixation yield strength ranges from approximately 350 N for an interference fit screw to 1,160 N for tandem screws and washers. Graft slippage is an additional consideration, particularly with tibial fixation methods.

The initial stiffness of an ACL substitute is highly dependent on the fixation method used. Howell has pointed out that the stiffness of fixation methods is from four to 40 times less than that of grafts used. Increasing the stiffness of an ACL replacement would best be achieved, therefore, by selecting fixation methods with higher stiffness and not by shortening or increasing the cross-sectional area of the grafts used (33). The stiffness of a doubled semitendinosus and gracilis tendon complex alone is approximately 1,000 N/mm. The stiffness of various fixation devices of hamstring tendons varies from approximately 25 to 230 N/mm. A normal ACL has a stiffness of approximately 200 N/mm.

Slippage of grafts from their point of fixation during cyclic loading is a major early problem that can compromise results (31). The slippage around interference fit screws is considerably greater than that which occurs with a cross-pin technique. The slippage around an interference fit screw during cyclic loading is also quite dependent on bone quality, which can be extremely variable in a patient population. When using screw and washer fixation of soft-tissue grafts, slippage can be considerably reduced by utilizing an additional suture technique to secure the graft beneath the soft-tissue washer. Supplemental suture fixation for grafts fixed with interference fit screws is highly recommended.

Hamstring Graft Fixation   It is important in fixing hamstring tendon grafts to fix every fiber of the graft. This cannot be done with devices such as interference fit screws alone. It is also important to be able to tension all limbs of the graft to a desired level. To fix every fiber of the graft on the femur it is important to cross-pin the looped end of the graft. This can be done by a rigid cross-pin fixation or by a device such as an EndoButton. The second-generation EndoButton with attached heavy-duty continuous loop provides the ability to loop each fiber of the graft and gives strength and stiffness adequate to withstand early rehabilitation techniques.

The preferred method for tibial fixation of hamstring tendon grafts is to use a suture technique through each end of each graft. The sutures are then tied around a post, before direct fixation of the grafts, by a soft-tissue washer. To better stabilize the graft within the tibial tunnel and closer to the joint line and to increase construct stiffness, an accessory bioabsorbable screw is used in the tibial tunnel anterior to the grafts. The interference fit screw is placed after tensioning and fixation have been accomplished extraosseously by sutures and washer.

Technique: ACL Reconstruction with Hamstring Tendon Autografts

Setup   The setup for this procedure includes a tourniquet placed as proximal as possible on the thigh. The thigh holder should be low profile, particularly anteriorly, so as not to interfere with the passage of a guide pin through the anterior thigh (Fig. 16-3). It is our current practice to exsanguinate the limb and inflate the tourniquet at the beginning of the case; however, diagnostic arthroscopy and any meniscal work as well as hamstring tendon harvest could be accomplished before inflation of the tourniquet, if desired. The operating table should have a break at the level of the knee joint so that the knee can be easily flexed to 90 degrees.

Diagnostic Arthroscopy   At the beginning of the case, diagnostic arthroscopy can be performed if necessary for precise diagnosis. Any meniscal work or joint debridement can be done at that time. It is important to make anteromedial and anterolateral portals as close as possible to the patellar tendon to allow easy and direct access to the intercondylar notch (Fig. 16-4). If the diagnosis of ACL insufficiency is obvious with preoperative planning, the graft preparation can be completed prior to starting the arthroscopic portion of the case.

Graft Harvest   A skin incision is next made vertically overlying the insertion of the pes anserinus (see Fig. 16-4). This same incision is used as a start point to create a tibial tunnel. The incision starts approximately 3 cm distal to the anteromedial portal and slightly medial to it. The incision needs to extend only approximately 2 to 3 cm. Once the semitendinosus and gracilis tendons have been identified, they are isolated and released together from their tibial insertion (Fig. 16-5A). The grafts are then flipped over; and from the under surface, the interface between the two tendons can be identified, allowing separation. Each tendon is then separately clamped with a Kocher clamp. The semitendinosus tendon is usually harvested first. Extraneous bands along the inferior surface are identified and released. It is helpful to cross-clamp the tendon and pull quite strongly on it to break up some adhesions and to deliver any extraneous bands into the wound for sectioning under direct vision. It is usually possible to pass a fingertip up the tendon to the level of the muscle belly to ensure that all bands have been sectioned. It is also helpful to feel a "bounce" from the muscle belly when pulling on the tendon. The medial calf can also be observed while pulling on the tendon to be sure the medial gastrocnemius is not being "dimpled."

An arthroscopic grabber is then passed through a closed-end tendon stripper to deliver the graft through the tendon stripper. The graft is then cross-clamped and held under tension while the tendon stripper is passed in line with the direction of the tendon to the muscle belly for harvesting (see Fig. 16-5B). The gracilis tendon is then similarly harvested.

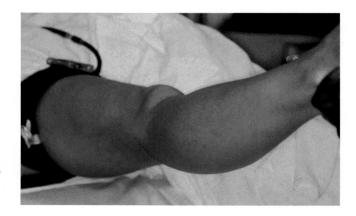

FIGURE 16-3

Proper setup requires a proximal tourniquet, a low-bulk thigh holder, and a table that bends at the knee to allow flexion to 90 degrees.

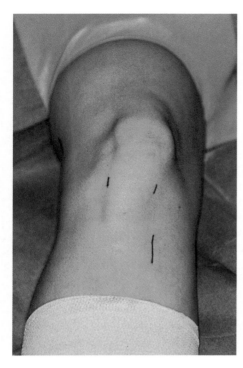

FIGURE 16-4

The incisions necessary to perform this procedure include anterolateral and anteromedial arthroscopy portals adjacent to the patellar tendon. A tibial incision begins approximately 3 cm distal to the anteromedial portal and extends 2 or 3 cm. This incision allows for harvesting of the semitendinosus and gracilis tendons and for creation of the tibial tunnel.

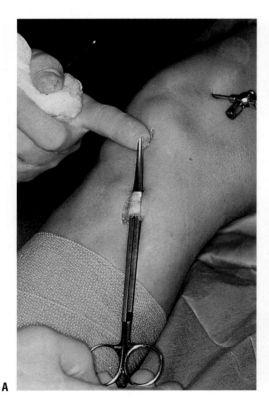

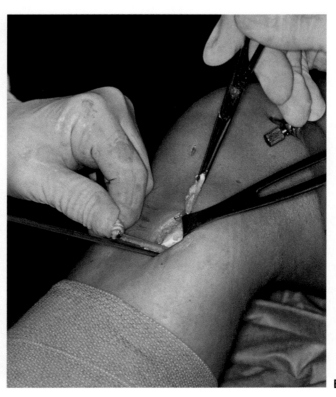

A   B

FIGURE 16-5

The semitendinosus and gracilis tendon harvest begins by first isolating the two combined tendons **(A)**. The tendons are then released from their tibial attachments and inverted to facilitate separation. Harvesting is performed with a closed-end tendon stripper **(B)**.

Graft Preparation   Once the tendons have been harvested, they are shortened to approximately 22 to 24 cm in length, depending on the size of the patient's bones. It is almost always possible to obtain this length of tendon. Muscle tissue is then scraped from the graft with either a curette or a scalpel, and each end of each graft is then tagged with a Bunnell or whipstitch of No. 2 nonabsorbable suture (Fig. 16-6A). The looped grafts are then passed through a sizing tube to determine the size of tunnels to be created (see Fig. 16-6B). The prepared grafts are then soaked in an antibiotic solution until used.

Notch Preparation   The intercondylar notch is prepared by first removing a significant portion of the anterior fat pad to allow proper visualization. This allows for the arthroscope to be "backed out" enough to get a perspective on the notch and ACL. The stump of the ACL is generally removed; however, if either the anteromedial or posterolateral band of the ACL is intact, that intact portion can be maintained and a reconstruction performed of the damaged band. The notch debridement is usually performed using a basket forceps, a curette, and a motorized shaver. The intercondylar notch debridement needs to extend to the extreme posterior aspect of the notch so that the "over-the-top" area can be clearly defined with a nerve hook. It is usually not necessary or advisable to perform a bony notchplasty. This is especially true in the case of acute disruption of the ACL, where osteophytic spurring has not occurred. When a notchplasty is created it is not uncommon for the cancellous surfaces that are created to rescar and reform the notch to the size that was present before notchplasty. This often can cause problems postoperatively with graft impingement that was not present at the completion of surgery. It is therefore best, when possible, to adjust tunnel position to fit the anatomic intercondylar notch.

Creation of Tibial Tunnel   A tibial guide is next used to pass a guide pin from the anteromedial tibia to a point corresponding to a central tibial attachment site (Fig. 16-7A). The intra-articular site is just medial to the medial tibial spine and approximately 7 mm anterior to the anterior edge of the PCL. Once the initial guide pin has been placed, it is essential to check the position and modify it if indicated (see Fig. 16-7B). When the knee is extended with the guide pin in place, the guide pin should move directly toward the apex of the intercondylar notch, and at full extension it should be approximately 4 to 5 mm short of touching the superior notch (see Fig. 16-7C). If the position is not correct, it should be modified with the use of a guide that will allow placement of a parallel pin at the desired location (see Fig. 16-7D).

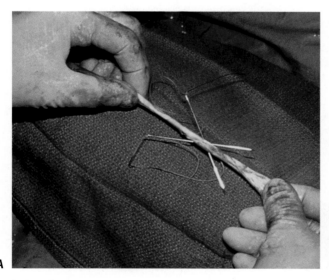
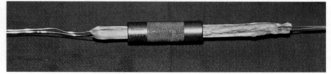

A   **B**

FIGURE 16-6

The hamstring tendons are cut to approximately 22 to 24 cm in length, and muscle tissue is removed from each graft. Each end of each graft is then tagged with a Bunnell or whipstitch of No. 2 nonabsorbable suture **(A)**. The combined double-looped tendons are then passed through a sizing tube **(B)** so that tunnels can be created to fit the grafts as tightly as possible.

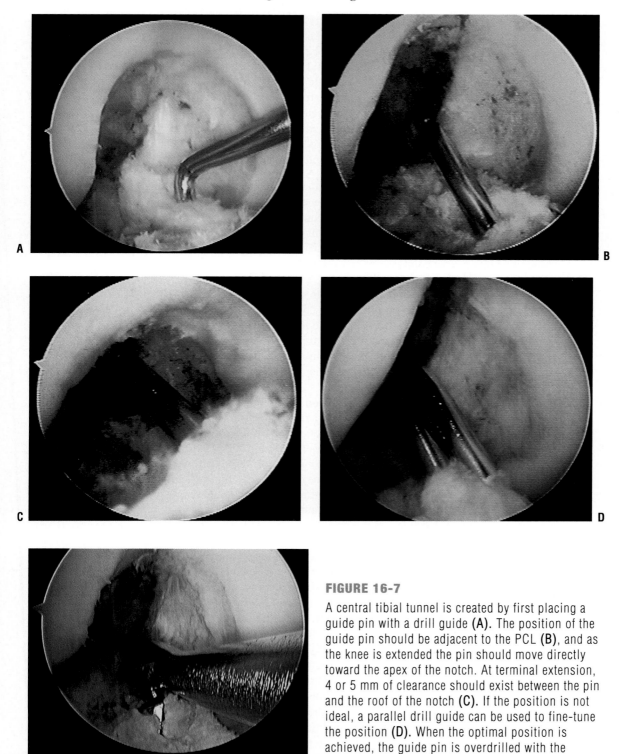

FIGURE 16-7

A central tibial tunnel is created by first placing a guide pin with a drill guide (A). The position of the guide pin should be adjacent to the PCL (B), and as the knee is extended the pin should move directly toward the apex of the notch. At terminal extension, 4 or 5 mm of clearance should exist between the pin and the roof of the notch (C). If the position is not ideal, a parallel drill guide can be used to fine-tune the position (D). When the optimal position is achieved, the guide pin is overdrilled with the appropriately sized cannulated drill (E).

The start point of the tibial tunnel is critical since the direction of the tunnel will limit access to the femur for preparation of the femoral socket (7). The start point must be medial enough to provide access to the correct femoral position. This usually involves moving the start point into the anterior fibers of the superficial medial collateral ligament (see Fig. 16-2B). The guide should be adjusted to provide a tunnel angle of approximately 45 degrees when viewed laterally, and it should be angled approximately 25 to 30 degrees in the frontal plane. Once the position of the tibial guide pin has been optimized, it is overdrilled with a cannulated drill of 7 mm. The initial tibial tunnel is always created with a 7-mm drill and is enlarged to the final size by the acorn drill used to create the femoral socket. We have found that this step reduces the over enlargement of the tibial tunnel, which can potentially occur when drilling the femoral tunnel through it.

Preparation of Femoral Socket   A socket is next created in the femur to accept the looped end of the hamstring tendon grafts. This socket needs to be placed at approximately the 10:30 or 1:30 position and to the extreme back of the intercondylar notch. It can be created through a properly positioned tibial tunnel. It is essential that the direction of the tibial tunnel allow access to the extreme back of the intercondylar notch and to the 10:30 or 1:30 position. It is generally possible to do this if the tibial tunnel start point is correctly placed.

An "over-the-top" referencing drill guide is used to place the guide pin for the femoral socket (Fig. 16-8A). It is best to use a femoral offset of no more than 5 mm to ensure that the graft is to the extreme back of the intercondylar notch. It may be preferable to use a 3-mm offset. This would often cause a "blowout" of the posterior wall of the femoral socket, which is acceptable.

The guide pin is placed through the tibial tunnel and into the femur at the desired location. This must be done with the knee flexed to approximately 90 degrees to ensure that the guide pin can exit the exposed anterior thigh distal to the tourniquet and drapes. The guide pin is initially passed until it engages the anterolateral femoral cortex.

An acorn drill of the diameter predetermined to be required to accept the tendon graft is then used to create a femoral socket from inside out to a depth of 35 mm (see Fig. 16-8B). The 35-mm socket allows pulling the graft 25 mm into the socket and also allows room to pull the graft initially an extra 10 mm into the socket during the "flipping" of the EndoButton. During the creation of the femoral socket, the tibial tunnel is enlarged by the acorn drill to the required diameter. A 4.5-mm passing channel is next created over the guide pin from the base of the socket to the anterolateral femoral cortex (see Fig. 16-8C). The length of the entire tunnel is next measured (see Fig. 16-8D). The final position of the femoral tunnel is shown in Figure 16-8E.

A continuous-loop EndoButton is next selected that will allow the looped end of the graft to penetrate the femoral socket approximately 25 mm (Fig. 16-9). The loop length of Endobutton is determined by subtracting 25 mm from the measured total length of the femoral socket and passing channel. Most commonly, the continuous-loop EndoButton selected ranges from 25 to 45 mm.

The semitendinosus and gracilis tendons are next looped through the continuous loop of the EndoButton. Passing sutures are next attached to the EndoButton. Two sizes of passing sutures are used, No. 5 and No. 2. This allows for pulling of the EndoButton with the No. 5 sutures and flipping the EndoButton with the No. 2 suture (Fig. 16-10).

The knee is again flexed to the angle that was used for drilling the femoral tunnel. The guide pin is passed through the tibial tunnel across the joint and into the femoral tunnel and passing channel and exits through the quadriceps on the anterolateral thigh. The passing sutures are passed through the eye of the passing pin with the EndoButton oriented so that the No. 5 sutures enter the tunnel first. The passing sutures are then pulled through the tibial tunnel, across the joint, and into the femoral tunnel and out to the anterolateral thigh. The EndoButton is next pulled by the No. 5 sutures through the tunnels to the anterolateral femoral cortex (Fig. 16-11A,B). It is pulled until the graft "bottoms out" into the femoral socket. The flipping sutures are then used to "set" the EndoButton.

The free ends of the tendons are then pulled to secure the Endobutton on the anterolateral femoral cortex. The "passing" and "flipping" sutures are then removed by releasing one end of each and pulling them through the thigh. If the graft length has been properly selected there should be approximately 1 cm of each end of each graft exiting the tibial tunnel.

Tibial Fixation   The grafts are next tensioned and fixed to the tibia by placing a low-profile screw and washer at the distal ends of the grafts near the exit point of the tibial tunnel. Each of the two grafts is separately tied as tightly as possible around the shaft of the tibial screw (Fig. 16-12A). The grafts are then tensioned separately while the knee is cycled approximately 10 times to ensure

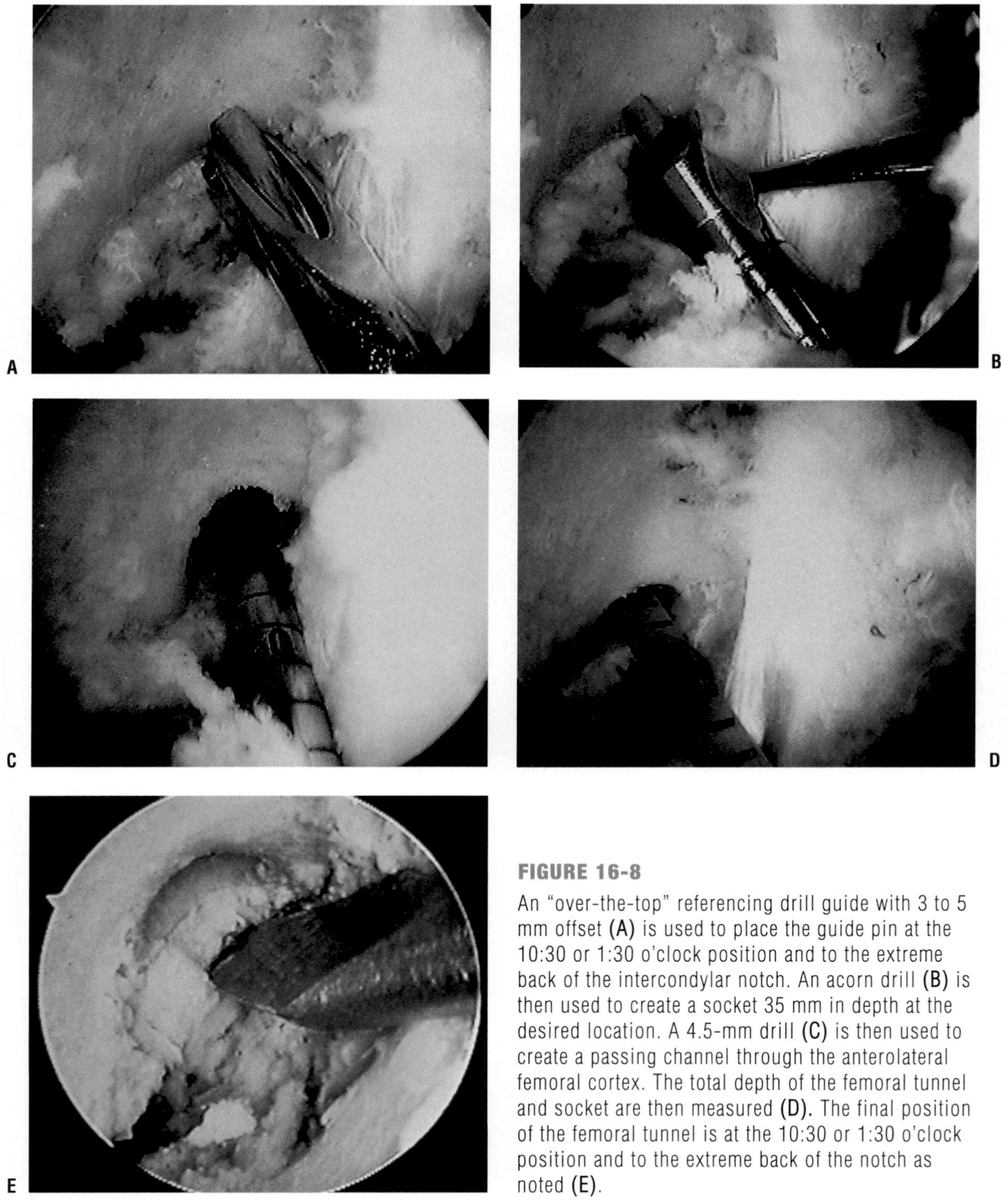

FIGURE 16-8

An "over-the-top" referencing drill guide with 3 to 5 mm offset (A) is used to place the guide pin at the 10:30 or 1:30 o'clock position and to the extreme back of the intercondylar notch. An acorn drill (B) is then used to create a socket 35 mm in depth at the desired location. A 4.5-mm drill (C) is then used to create a passing channel through the anterolateral femoral cortex. The total depth of the femoral tunnel and socket are then measured (D). The final position of the femoral tunnel is at the 10:30 or 1:30 o'clock position and to the extreme back of the notch as noted (E).

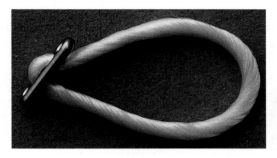

FIGURE 16-9

The continuous-loop EndoButton provides increased strength and stiffness of the femoral fixation when compared with the conventional EndoButton, which uses tape and knots.

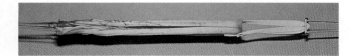

FIGURE 16-10

The completed construct (with conventional EndoButton and tape). Passing sutures are of No. 5 for pulling and No. 2 for flipping the EndoButton.

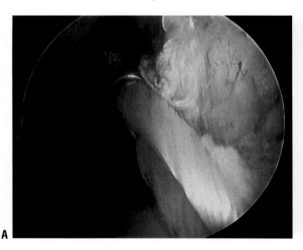
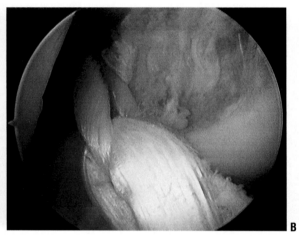

A   B

FIGURE 16-11

The EndoButton is pulled into the femoral tunnel by the No. 5 pulling sutures, which have been passed to the anterior thigh (**A**). The closed loop then delivers the looped ends of the tendons into the femoral socket (**B**).

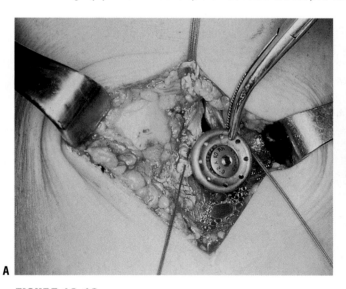
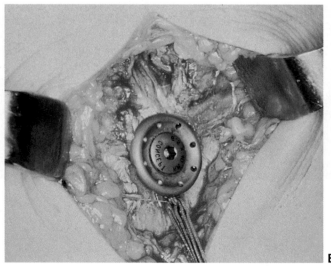

A   B

FIGURE 16-12

Tibial fixation is accomplished by placing the screw at the distal ends of the grafts (**A**). The graft sutures are then tied to the post and the grafts, sutures, and knots are directly fixed by the soft-tissue washer after final tensioning (**B**). To augment tibial fixation and to increase stiffness and reduce micromotion in the tibial tunnel, a bioabsorbable screw is next passed up the tibial tunnel anterior to the grafts, and advanced to just short of entry into the joint.

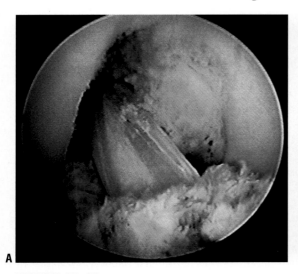
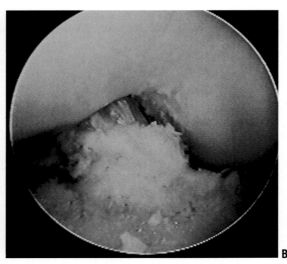

FIGURE 16-13

The final position of the graft (**A**). It is adjacent to the PCL, has excellent clearance with the lateral wall of the intercondylar notch, and just grazes the superior notch at terminal extension (**B**).

that there is no slack within the tunnels. The grafts, sutures, and knots are then directly fixed with a soft-tissue washer (see Fig. 16-12B). Some fine tuning of graft tension can be done at this point since the soft tissue washer directly fixes the graft, sutures, and knots. This is usually done with the knee at approximately 20 degrees of flexion.

To better stabilize the grafts within the tibial tunnel, and to increase the stiffness of the tibial fixation, a bioabsorbable interference fit screw is next selected and used in the tibial tunnel. A screw sized 1 mm greater than the tibial tunnel drilled is passed up the tibial tunnel anterior to the grafts and advanced to just short of entry into the joint. The final position of the grafts is demonstrated in Figure 16-13A. The graft avoids the lateral wall of the intercondylar notch and barely grazes the superior notch at full terminal extension (see Fig. 16-13B).

Closure and Bracing   The tourniquet is next deflated and hemostasis is secured. The joint and wound are both copiously irrigated. Closure is accomplished with subcutaneous and subcuticular stitches followed by Steri-strips. Sterile dressings are applied to the wound followed by a compressive stocking and a cold therapy device. The patient is then placed into a hinged knee brace that is initially locked at 10 degrees of flexion. The patient will remain in the locked knee brace for the first 6 days following surgery. No drains are used. Prophylactic antibiotics are routinely prescribed, giving one dose when the patient enters the operating room and one before the patient leaves the recovery suite. In most instances further antibiotics are not administered. The patient is taken from the operating room to recovery and in most instances is discharged to home within 2 to 3 hours of the procedure's completion.

Pearls and Pitfalls

Setup
- Proximal low-profile thigh holder
- Table break at knee to allow flexion

Graft Harvest
- Isolate semitendinosus and gracilis as a pair.
- Invert tendons to isolate and separate.
- Cross clamp and pull each tendon to expose extraneous bands.
- Section all extraneous bands before advancing stripper.

Tibial Tunnel
- Start medial enough to allow access to desired femoral site.
- Pass provisional guide pin and observe position as knee is extended.

- Modify pin position if needed with parallel drill guide.
- Drill initial tunnel 7 mm diameter. Enlarge if needed when creating femoral socket.

Femoral Tunnel
- Place guide pin at 10:30 or 1:30 position and near extreme back of notch.
- Drill femoral socket to 35 mm.

Femoral Fixation
- Feel EndoButton "bounce" on femur to ensure position.

Tibial Fixation
- Tie sutures for each graft separately around post.
- Cycle knee before "pulling" final tension.
- Secure graft, sutures, and knots with soft tissue washer.
- Place bioscrew in tunnel anterior to graft. Use size 1 mm greater than tibial tunnel diameter.

POSTOPERATIVE MANAGEMENT

The patients are kept in a locked knee brace for the first 6 days following surgery. They can use crutches with weight bearing as tolerated and discontinue the use of crutches when comfortable. In general, crutches are used for the first 10 to 14 days. At the end of 1 week, the knee brace is opened to allow motion from 10 degrees to unlimited flexion. Generally, at that time patients have full extension of their knee and can easily flex to 90 degrees. The 10-degree extension block is used when weight bearing to prevent hyperextension. The knee brace can be removed when non–weight bearing.

The patients are generally seen in physical therapy two or three times a week for the first 12 weeks. When other facilities are available for the patient's rehabilitation and when no problems are encountered, formal physical therapy can be considerably reduced. After the first week, patients can begin low-resistance stationary bicycling out of the brace. The patients also can perform quadriceps sets, straight leg raises, early hamstring resistance exercises, and closed-chain exercises with an elastic cord. Bracing is discontinued at 6 weeks after surgery, when patients generally have excellent muscle control about the knee. Other functional activities such as stair-climbing machines and elliptical trainers are started at 6 weeks following surgery. When the patient has reached 12 weeks postoperatively, he or she is cleared for all activities except for running on hard surfaces, terminal knee extensions with resistance, and sports that involve jumping and pivoting. At 6 months postoperatively, the restrictions are removed for running and terminal knee extensions with weights. A return to full, unrestricted sport is generally delayed until approximately 8 months following surgery, and then begun only if the patient has regained approximately 90% of hamstring and quadriceps strength. We continue to encourage the use of a functional knee brace for participation in jumping and pivoting sports until 18 months following surgery. The complete postoperative protocol is detailed in Tables 16-1 through 16-4.

TABLE 16-1. Phase I-A: Physical Therapy Following Arthroscopic Anterior Cruciate Ligament Surgery (0 to 6 Weeks)	
Therapy	**Goals**
Range of motion—limiting brace locked first 6 days, then 10 degrees to unlimited flexion	Demonstrated independent home exercise program
Weight bearing as tolerated with crutches and brace; discontinue crutches as tolerated	Passive range of motion between 0 and 5 degrees of extension and between 115 and 125 degrees of flexion
Physical therapy will work for full passive range of motion and patellar mobility	Normal gait at 6 weeks without a brace on level ground
Daily stretching out of brace for full passive extension	Stationary bike at 80 rpm for 20 minutes
Electrical muscle stimulator used as needed	
Daily low-resistance stationary biking when range of motion allows (out of brace); resistance as tolerated	
Exercises performed in brace include quadriceps sets, straight leg raises, hamstrings, abductors, adductors, and gluteals; add weights as tolerated, with the exception of no weights on straight leg raises	
Stretching of hamstrings and heel cords	

TABLE 16-2.   Phase I-B: Physical Therapy Following Arthroscopic Anterior Cruciate Ligament Surgery (6 to 12 Weeks)

Therapy	Goals
Off crutches	At 8 weeks, bike with resistance for 20 minutes
Brace worn when away from home	At 12 weeks, 0-pound straight leg raise without a
Range of motion in brace 10 degrees to unlimited flexion	quadriceps lag
Full active extension out of brace, no resistance	Able to walk 15 to 20 minutes with a limp
Full active flexion with resistance	Stair-climbing machine, 20 minutes
Stationary biking with increasing resistance as tolerated	Normal gait without a brace
Swimming kicking from the hip only, no wall push-offs	Upstairs step-over-step two flights
Physical therapy continued at least on a limited basis	Sit-to-stand transfer normal
Gym weights equipment or ankle weights used for	Full passive range of motion
strengthening exercises. Precaution: straight leg raise	
must be limited to 5 lbs and resisted knee extension	
range from 90 to 45 degrees only	
Stair-climbing machine and closed kinetic chain exercises	
Sport cord	

TABLE 16-3.   Phase II: Physical Therapy Following Arthroscopic Anterior Cruciate Ligament Surgery (12 to 24 Weeks)

Therapy	Goals
No brace or crutches	At 16 weeks, 5-lb straight leg raise without a
Full passive and active range of motion	quadriceps lag
More aggressive strengthening via cycling, stairs,	At 16 weeks, stairs step-over-step for two flights
closed kinetic chain activities as tolerated	ascending and descending
Patient monitors pain and swelling and reports this	Unlimited walking without a limp
to physical therapist	At 24 weeks, or 6 months, 10-lb straight leg raise
Progressive resistive exercises continued, straight leg	without a quadriceps lag
raise weights increased to 10 lbs	Stair climbing for exercise
No resisted knee extension through full range of motion	At 24 weeks, balance on one leg for 2 minutes
until 6 months postoperatively	
Begin proprioception-balance training	

COMPLICATIONS

Serious complications specifically related to the harvest of hamstring tendon autografts are uncommon. Complications, however, can be associated with the technical harvest of the hamstring tendons and also at the donor site (16). Also, as with any ACL substitute, if tunnel placement and graft fixation are not adequate, early failure of grafts due to overzealous rehabilitation can be encountered.

During the actual harvest of hamstring tendons, it is imperative to release all attachments to the medial head of the gastrocnemius to ensure clear passage of the tendon stripper to the muscle belly. If this precaution is not taken, it is possible to obtain grafts of inadequate length to serve as an adequate ACL substitute. It is also not uncommon to create sensory abnormalities in the distribution of the saphenous nerve or its branches. This is usually a temporary neuroproxia, but it may take several months for areas of decreased sensation to resolve, and it is advisable to inform the patients of this possibility before surgery. On rare occasions patients will develop adhesions of the posterior thigh to the healing muscle bellies. This can result in a dimpling of the skin with knee flexion. This potential complication has been markedly reduced with the use of tendon strippers to harvest the hamstring tendons when compared with open harvest techniques.

TABLE 16-4.   Phase III: Physical Therapy Following Arthroscopic Anterior Cruciate Ligament Surgery (6 Months to 1 Year)

Therapy	Goals
Aggressive strengthening exercises and return-activity exercises (straight-line running) are initiated	Able to run without a limp
Aggressive contact, pivoting, and quick acceleration–deceleration movements avoided until 9 months following surgery	Quads and hamstrings at 90% of uninvolved leg on a Cybex test with quad-to-hamstring ratio at a minimum of 3 to 2
If deemed appropriate, patient is measured for a derotation brace before starting jumping or pivoting	Full muscle mass for brace fitting
	Return to unrestricted activity including sports
	Derotation bracing as indicated

RESULTS

The use of hamstring tendon autografts with the described technique has been used successfully to consistently restore normal anterior laxity in ACL-insufficient knees in both acute and chronic situations. There are several studies in the literature that compare hamstring tendon autografts to patellar tendon autografts and demonstrate that they are of equivalent efficacy (4,6,7,13,22,24). The use of hamstring tendon autografts has been effective in avoiding complications, particularly motion problems or patellofemoral pain complaints. Figure 16-14 shows the appearance of a double-looped semitendinosus and gracilis tendon 1 year after implantation. The depicted graft is well synovialized, and both the tibial and femoral attachments have a "splayed" appearance similar to a normal ACL. The described procedure is also cosmetically acceptable, particularly since it avoids an incision over the patellar tendon where the skin needs to adapt to considerable motion. The incision location below the joint line more medially on the tibia is a region of very little skin motion; thus, the incision generally does not tend to spread. Figure 16-15 is an example of an incision approximately 1 year following surgery in a young woman.

The importance of adhering to technical detail when performing this or any other procedure for ACL reconstruction cannot be overemphasized. Attention to graft preparation, tunnel placement, avoidance of notch impingement, fixation, and rehabilitation are much more important factors in the success of ACL reconstruction than is the origin of the autogenous graft. Although the described technique is applicable in almost all situations of ACL insufficiency, it is particularly applicable to those patients in whom a patellar tendon ACL reconstruction has failed, in those with pre-existing patellofemoral disease, in skeletally immature patients, or in any other situation in which avoidance of the extensor mechanism is desirable. The procedure is also appropriate when cosmesis is of more than casual concern.

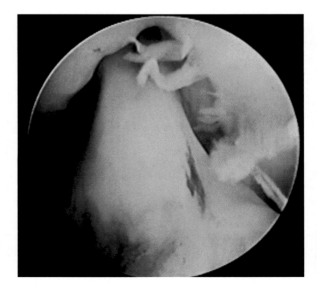

FIGURE 16-14

Semitendinosus and gracilis grafts 1 year after implantation. The grafts are well synovialized. The attachment site on the tibia has a normal "splayed" appearance.

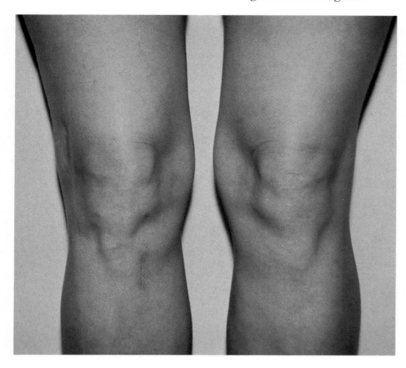

FIGURE 16-15

The skin incision 1 year after surgery. The skin incision is in an area of minimal skin motion, and spreading of the incision is unusual. A good cosmetic result is usually obtained.

REFERENCES

1. Aglietti P, Buzzi R, Zaccherotti G, et al. Patellar tendon versus doubled semitendinosus and gracilis tendons for anterior cruciate ligament reconstruction. *Am J Sports Med.* 1994;22:211–218.
2. Barrett GR, Papendick L, Miller C. EndoButton button endoscopic fixation technique in anterior cruciate ligament reconstruction. *Arthroscopy.* 1995;11:340–343.
3. Cho KO. Reconstruction of the anterior cruciate ligament by semitendinosus tenodesis. *J Bone Joint Surg.* 1975;57A:608–612.
4. Feller JA, Webster KE. A randomized comparison of patellar tendon and hamstring tendon anterior cruciate ligament reconstruction. *Am J Sports Med.* 2003;31:564–573.
5. Frank CB, Jackson DW. The science of reconstruction of the anterior cruciate ligament (current concepts review). *J Bone Joint Surg* 1997;79A:1556–1576.
6. Freedman KB, D'Amato MJ, Nedeff DD, et al. Arthroscopic anterior cruciate ligament reconstruction: a meta-analysis comparing patellar tendon and hamstring tendon autografts. *Am J Sports Med.* 2003;31:2–11.
7. Gobbi A, Sanjeev M, Zanazzo M, et al. Patellar tendon versus quadrupled bone-semitendinosus anterior cruciate ligament reconstruction: a prospective clinical investigation in athletes. *Arthroscopy.* 2003;19:592–601.
8. Gomes JLE, Marczyk LRS. Anterior cruciate ligament reconstruction with a loop or double thickness of semitendinosus tendon. *Am J Sports Med.* 1984;12:199–203.
9. Hamner DL, Brown CH, Steiner ME, et al. Hamstring tendon grafts for reconstruction of the anterior cruciate ligament: biomechanical evaluation of the use of multiple strands and tensioning techniques. *J Bone Joint Surg.* 1999;4:549–557.
10. Howell SM, Berns GS, Farley TE. Unimpinged and impinged anterior cruciate ligament grafts: MR signal intensity measurements. *Radiology.* 1991;179:639–643.
11. Howell SM, Taylor MA. Failure of reconstruction of the anterior cruciate ligament due to impingement by the intercondylar roof. *J Bone Joint Surg Am.* 1993;75:1044–1055.
12. Howell SM, Wallace MP, Hull ML. Evaluation of the single-incision arthroscopic technique for anterior cruciate ligament replacement (a study of tibial tunnel placement, intraoperative graft tension, and stability). *Am J Sports Med.* 1999;27:284–293.
13. Jansson KA, Linko E, Sandelin J, et al. A prospective randomized study of patellar versus hamstring tendon autografts for anterior cruciate ligament reconstruction. *Am J Sport Med.* 2003;31:12–18.
14. Lane JG, McFadden P, Bowden L, et al. The ligamentization process: a four-year case study following ACL reconstruction with a semitendinosus graft. *J Arthros Rec Surg.* 1993;9:149–153.
15. Larson RV. The use of hamstring tendons in anterior cruciate ligament surgery. In: *Current techniques in arthroscopy,* 2nd ed. New York: Thieme 1998.
16. Larson RV, Ericksen D. Complications in the use of hamstring tendons for anterior cruciate ligament reconstruction. *Sports Med Arthroscopy Rev.* 1997;5:83–90.
17. Magen HE, Howell SM, Hull ML. Structural properties of six tibial fixation methods for anterior cruciate ligament soft tissue grafts. *Am J Sports Med.* 1999;27:35–43.
18. Marder RA, Raskind JR, Carroll M. Prospective evaluation of arthroscopically assisted anterior cruciate ligament reconstruction: patellar tendon versus semitendinosus and gracilis tendons. *Am J Sports Med.* 1991;19:478–484.
19. Mott HW. Semitendinosus anatomic reconstruction for cruciate ligament insufficiency. *Clin Orthop.* 1983;172:90–92.
20. Noyes FR, Butler DL, Grood ES, et al. Biomechanical analysis of human ligament grafts used in knee-ligament repairs and reconstructions. *J Bone Joint Surg.* 1984;66A:344–352.
21. O'Neill DB. Arthroscopically assisted reconstruction of the anterior cruciate ligament: a prospective randomized analysis of three techniques. *J Bone Joint Surg Am.* 1996;78:803–813.

22. Otero AL, Hutcheson L. A comparison of the doubled semitendinosus/gracilis and central third of the patellar tendon autografts in arhtroscopic anterior cruciate ligament reconstruction. *Arthroscopy.* 1993;9:143–148.
23. Pagnani MJ, Warner JJP, O'Brien SJ, et al. Anatomic considerations in harvesting the semitendinosus and gracilis tendons and a technique for harvest. *Am J Sports Med.* 1993;21:565–571.
24. Pinczewski LA, Deeham DJ, Salmon LJ, et al. A five-year comparison of patellar tendon versus four-strand hamstring tendon autograft for arthroscopic reconstruction of the anterior cruciate ligament. *Am J Sport Med.* 2002;30:523–536.
25. Rodeo SA, Arnoczky SP, Torzilli PA, et al. Tendon-healing in a bone tunnel: a biomechanical and histological study in the dog. *J Bone Joint Surg.* 1993;75A:1795–1803.
26. Rosenberg TD, Deffner KT. ACL reconstruction: semitendinosus tendon is the graft of choice. *Orthopedics.* 1997;20:396–398.
27. Rowden NJ, Sher D, Rogers GJ, et al. Anterior cruciate ligament graft fixation: initial comparison of patellar tendon and semitendinosus autografts in young fresh cadavers. *Am J Sports Med.* 1997;25:472–478.
28. Shino K, Nakagawa S, Inoue M, et al. Deterioration of patellofemoral articular surfaces after anterior cruciate ligament reconstruction. *Am J Sports Med.* 1993;21:206–211.
29. Sidles JA, Clark JM, Garbini JL. A geometric theory of equilibrium mechanics of fibers in ligaments and tendons. *J Biomech.* 1991;29:943–949.
30. Sidles JA, Larson RV, Garbini JL, et al. Ligament length relationships in the moving knee. *J Orthop Res.* 1988;6:593–610.
31. Simonian PT, Williams RJ, Deng XH, et al. Hamstring and patellar tendon graft response to cyclical loading. *Am J Knee Surg.* 1998;11:101–105.
32. Steiner ME, Hecker AT, Brown CH Jr, et al. Anterior cruciate ligament graft fixation: comparison of hamstring and patellar tendon grafts. *Am J Sports Med.* 1994;22:240–246.
33. To JT, Howell SM, Hull ML. Contributions of fixation methods to the stiffness of anterior cruciate ligament replacements at implantation. *Arthroscopy.* 1999;15:379–387.

17 Allograft Preparation for ACL Reconstruction

William H. Warden III

INDICATIONS/CONTRAINDICATIONS

Allograft is an attractive option for anterior cruciate ligament (ACL) reconstruction, as there is no donor site morbidity and therefore less discomfort in the early postoperative period. In my experience, patients with allograft ACL reconstructions are clearly more comfortable immediately after surgery than patients who have received autograft. The most striking example I can recall is a patient who walked into the office, did a deep knee bend, and jumped into the air 1 week after a bilateral ACL reconstruction with no formal physical therapy.

One of the few strict contraindications to allograft reconstruction is a patient who is unwilling to accept the risk of disease transmission. Although there are few strict indications or contraindications, there are a number of advantages and disadvantages to consider.

Advantages

- No donor site morbidity, therefore useful for:
  - Revision
  - Multiple ligament injuries
  - Early return to light work
- Decreased anesthesia, operating room, tourniquet time
- Cosmesis

Disadvantages

- Risk of disease transmission
- Cost
  - Patellar tendon, $1,800
  - Achilles tendon, $1,200
  - Soft tissue, $800
  - Offset by decreased operating room time
- Potential for delayed incorporation

Although not entirely scientific, my personal bias is to avoid allograft in children and women of childbearing age, and lean toward allograft in patients who are age 50 or older.

PREOPERATIVE PLANNING

An early step involves a discussion with the patient of the risk of viral transmission.

Use tissue from a well-established tissue bank certified by the American Association of Tissue Banks (AATB) from donors under age 40. Ideally, grafts are obtained with sterile harvest, antibiotic soaks, low-dose radiation, and freezing. Higher dose irradiation in a radioprotectant solution is an emerging technique.

There are a number of allograft options including bone-patellar tendon-bone (BTB), Achilles tendon, quadriceps tendon, hamstring, and tibialis anterior. The choice is mainly surgeon preference. BTB is an excellent choice for a surgeon who prefers bone fixation, but this allograft can potentially carry more antigens. Preoperative planning is critical for BTB, to avoid graft-tunnel mismatch. This is not an issue with a large patient; for a small patient, request collagen lengths of 45 mm or less. If you cannot obtain a short graft, consider a soft tissue or single bone plug graft.

Always have a back-up graft. Occasionally, an allograft will appear discolored or macerated. A degenerative Achilles tendon may not be evident until the graft is sectioned. In case of the dreaded drop, one can potentially scrub an autograft, but it's difficult to justify scrubbing an allograft that can simply be replaced by a backup.

SURGERY

Patient Positioning

Position the graft preparation table so that it does not interfere with entry into the room, draping, or setup of arthroscopy equipment. Ideally, you should have a good view of the arthroscopy monitor.

Technique

If it is certain that a graft will be required, graft preparation can begin before the patient is in the room. Thaw time ranges from 5 to 30 minutes including a soak in saline with "double antibiotic" (bacitracin and polymyxin B) solution. Grafts prepared with radioprotectant typically require three separate soaks over a total of 30 minutes. Inspect the graft for discoloration or signs of structural compromise. Trim excess fatty or loose connective tissue from the graft.

Achilles Tendon   Achilles tendon grafts have two unique features to address during graft preparation: the collagen insertion into the bone plug is angular and the tendinous portion is fan shaped. Although Achilles tendon grafts come with ample bone blocks, the nature of the tendinous insertion is such that the bone plug length is always short. Therefore, bone should not be removed from the distal end of the bone block unless necessary during final preparation (Fig. 17-1). A prominent pump bump at the posterior aspect of the plug may need to be trimmed along with a small amount of tendinous tissue (Fig. 17-2). The bone plug should be fashioned to fit easily through the sizing tube. We typically use a 10-mm bone plug. Next, shorten the graft to a length of approximately 120 mm and trim excess collagen from the sides (Fig. 17-3A). A No. 2 nylon passing suture is placed through the bone plug. Next, suture the distal portion of the graft by placing a No. 2 Ethibond suture 40 to 50 mm distal to the bone block. Distal interference screws seem to get better purchase on the graft if they are placed adjacent to a sutured graft; suturing can begin more distally if interference fixation is not used. The first suture placed should be used to tubularize the graft (see Fig. 17-3B). A second arm of the suture is run down opposite this and then a second suture is placed rotated 90 degrees to the initial suture. With each strand of the suture place one or two locked passes and then run distally.

Soft Tissue   Although soft tissue allows a tighter fit in the sizing tubes compared with bone plugs, avoid the tendency to make a collagen graft that is too large. A 10-mm bundle of collagen may not fit well in the knee of a petite gymnast.

Most femoral-sided soft tissue fixation devices require a folded graft. Fold the graft over a passing suture (No. 2 nylon) or fixation device and shorten if longer than 120 mm, optimizing thicker collagen sections. This should be ample length for even the largest patient and allow extra graft if backup fixation with a post and soft tissue washer is required on the tibial side. For a tight soft tis-

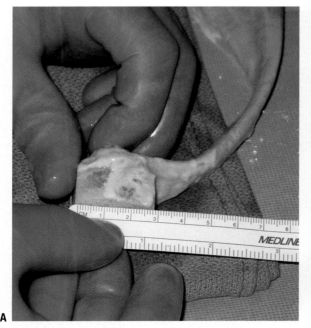

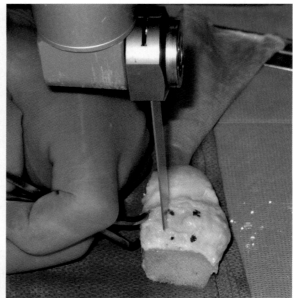

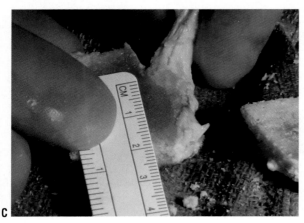

FIGURE 17-1

The uncut Achilles bone block is 30 mm in length **(A)**. However, after 10-mm wide coronal cuts are completed **(B)**, it becomes clear that there are only 20 mm of bone distal to the tendinous insertion **(C)**. Attempts to include bone proximal to the tendinous insertion will leave a graft that is too thick or compromise the tendinous insertion.

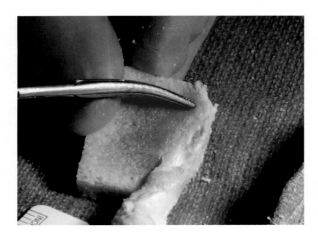

FIGURE 17-2

Some grafts may have a prominent "pump bump" that must be trimmed.

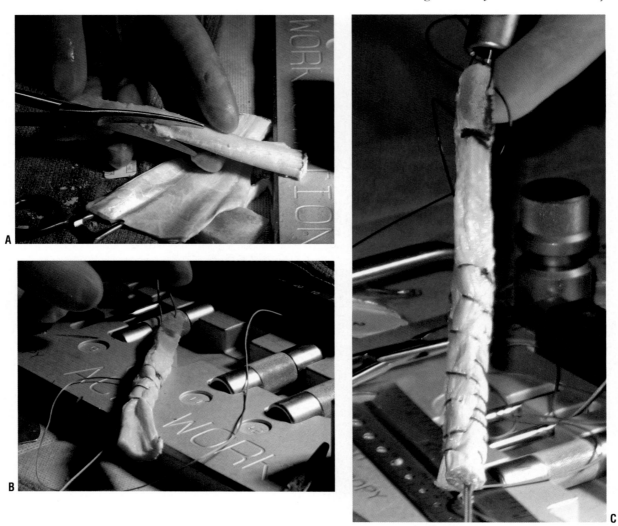

FIGURE 17-3

After the graft is shortened to 120 mm and the distal sides are trimmed down **(A)**, distal sutures are passed tubularizing the Achilles graft **(B)**. Final graft **(C)**.

sue graft, trim the corners of the folded section slightly to allow easy entrance into bone tunnels (Fig. 17-4A).

Although some prefer suturing each distal strand independently to optimize graft tension, I find it is more time consuming and makes a bulky graft. However, some fixation devices such as the Intrafix require independent suturing, whereas others such as the EndoButton are easier to use with independent suturing.

Holding distal ends in a clamp, suture the proximal portion of the graft together using a 0-vicryl whip stitch. Start 5 to 10 mm distal to the fold (closer than this tends to bunch up the leading edge of the graft) to a distance of approximately 25 mm from the leading edge of your graft (this may vary depending on your fixation technique). Be sure to mark the graft at the appropriate distance from the proximal end (usually 25 mm) so that passage to the appropriate depth can be confirmed arthroscopically. Unless your fixation device requires independent graft ends, suture the distal ends together using two No. 2 Ethibond sutures and a tapered needle. Start 40 to 50 mm distal to the mark in the proximal end (more distal if interference screws are not used), throw one or two locking passes attempting to incorporate all strands, and then run distally with a whipstitch, including at least two strands with every bight. The other limb of the suture is run down the graft on the opposite side. The second suture is then placed in a similar fashion rotated 90 degrees from the initial suture. Be sure to confirm that your graft fits through the appropriate sizing tube after suturing. If there is a portion of the graft that is slightly snug, trim the appropriate section or keep the snug area in the sizing tube until passage (see Fig. 17-4B,C).

Patellar Tendon   The main concern with patellar tendon allograft is a graft that is too long for the patient, even with an appropriate length tibial tunnel (see Preoperative Planning). Be sure to center the patellar bone plug at the tip of the inferior pole of the patella to minimize graft length (Fig. 17-5). A 10 mm wide section is cut from the patellar block and then a similar plug is cut directly distal to this in the tibial plug. The 10 mm wide strip of collagen between them is isolated from surrounding tissue. Note that larger bone blocks may be required for revision cases. Graft preparation proceeds as with a typical patellar tendon graft. The blocks are trimmed with a rongeur to fit the appropriate sizing tube (9 to 11 mm) and to a length of 22 to 25 mm (Fig. 17-6). Some find special compaction pliers helpful for contouring bone plugs. Undersize the bone plugs slightly and taper the leading edge (Fig. 17-7) so that they pass easily through the appropriate sizing tube, as bone plugs tend to jam in bone tunnels. Passing sutures are inserted through drill holes, a 30-in No. 2 nylon in the lead plug, and three No. 2 Ethibonds in the distal plug at 45-degree angles to each other to minimize the risk of suture laceration during interference screw placement.

The prepared graft is irrigated with antibiotic saline, kept under 10 to 20 lb of tension, and covered with gauze until required (Fig. 17-8).

Pearls and Pitfalls

- Undersized bone plugs slightly and taper the leading end for easy passage (see Fig. 17-7).
- Soft tissue grafts can be slightly snug in the sizing tube, but avoid too much collagen for the patient.

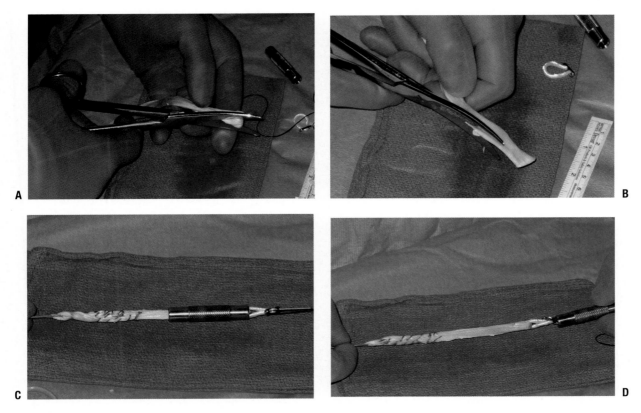

FIGURE 17-4

For a tight soft tissue graft, trim the corners of the leading fold slightly to allow easy entrance into bone tunnels (**A**). A very large graft such as a tibialis anterior may require trimming along the entire length (**B**). If a portion of the final graft is still slightly too tight, keep the sizing tube over that area until passage (**C**). Final graft (**D**).

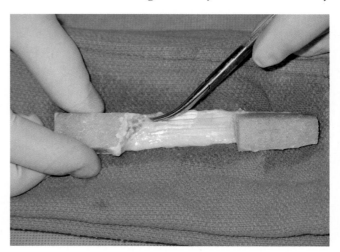

FIGURE 17-5

Center the patellar bone plug at the tip of the inferior pole of the patella to minimize graft length, especially when using a hemipatella graft.

- Trim and tubularize wide soft tissue grafts (see Fig. 17-3B).
- Trim the entering corners of a tight folded soft tissue graft (see Fig. 17-4A).
- Keep a tight section of a soft tissue graft (usually the leading loop) in a sizing tube until required (see Fig. 17-4C).
- Avoid BTB graft-tunnel mismatch (see previous discussion) with preoperative graft length selection and appropriate tibial tunnel length.
- Don't miss the "nose" of the patella (see Fig. 17-5).
- Trim the "pump bump" from the calcaneal bone plug (see Fig. 17-2).
- Always have a back-up graft.

POSTOPERATIVE MANAGEMENT

Although there are concerns regarding delayed incorporation of allograft compared with autograft we use the same accelerated early rehabilitation regardless of graft choice. Consider more vigilance regarding late effusions when allograft is used.

COMPLICATIONS

Although rare, infection can be devastating. The AATB now requires nucleic acid testing of grafts for HIV-1 and HCV. Furthermore, emerging techniques for soft tissue graft sterilization show promise. Nevertheless, reports of compromised acquisition/preparation of allograft requiring recall

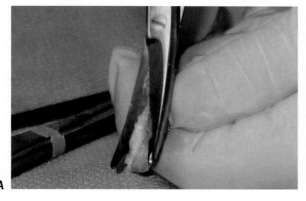
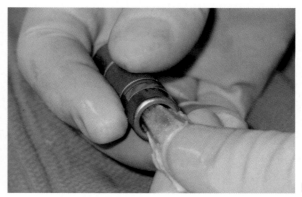

A   **B**

FIGURE 17-6

With a rongeur, trim the corners and fashion the plug to fit easily in a 12-mm sizing tube. Excess soft tissue and bone is trimmed from the cortical sides of the bone plugs **(A)**. Use progressively smaller sizing tubes to locate raised areas to trim **(B)**. Compression with pliers may help final contouring.

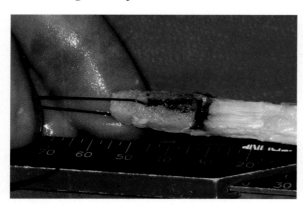

FIGURE 17-7

Taper the leading edge of the bone plug for easy passage.

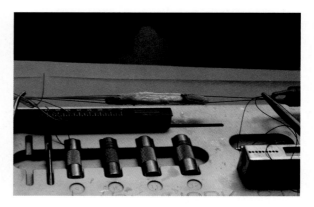

FIGURE 17-8

Final patellar tendon graft. The femoral plug is marked to facilitate arthroscopic evaluation of graft passage and orientation.

continue. An important consideration is follow-up with your tissue bank in cases of suspected infection. Delayed incorporation leading to early failure is a theoretical complication that is difficult to assess clinically. As yet unrecognized immune responses are another potential concern.

RESULTS

Please see Chapters 13 and 18 for discussions of ligament reconstruction results.

RECOMMENDED READING

Jackson DW, Corsetti J, Simon TM. Biologic incorporation of allograft anterior cruciate ligament replacements. *Clin Orthop*. 1996;324:126–133.

Jackson DW, Grood ES, Goldstein JD, et al. A comparison of patellar tendon autograft and allograft used for anterior cruciate ligament reconstruction in the goat model. *Am J Sports Med*. 1993;21:176–185.

Joyce MJ. Safety and FDA regulations for musculoskeletal allografts: perspective of an orthopaedic surgeon. *Clin Orthop Relat Res*. 2005;435:22–30.

Vangsness CT, Jr Garcia IA, Mills CR, et al. Allograft transplantation in the knee: tissue regulation, procurement, processing, and sterilization. *Am J Sports Med*. 2003;May(31):474–481.

18 Arthroscopically Assisted Posterior Cruciate Ligament Reconstruction

Gregory C. Fanelli, Craig J. Edson, and Kristin N. Reinheimer

The incidence of posterior cruciate ligament (PCL) injuries is reported to be from 1% to 40% of acute knee injuries. This range depends on the patient population reported, and is approximately 3% in the general population and 38% in reports from regional trauma centers (1,6,13). Our practice at a regional trauma center has a 38.3% incidence of PCL tears in acute knee injuries, and 56.5% of these PCL injuries occur in multiple trauma patients. Of these, 45.9% are combined anterior cruciate ligament (ACL)/PCL tears, whereas 41.2% are PCL/posterolateral corner tears. Only 3% of acute PCL injuries seen in our practice are isolated.

This chapter illustrates the senior author's surgical techniques for the arthroscopic single-bundle–single-femoral tunnel, and double-bundle–double-femoral tunnel, transtibial PCL reconstruction surgical procedure. We will also present the Fanelli Sports Injury Clinic 2-to 10-year results of PCL reconstruction using these surgical techniques. The information presented in this chapter has also been presented elsewhere, and the reader is referred to these sources for additional information regarding this topic (2–5,7–20,22,23).

The single-bundle–single-femoral tunnel transtibial tunnel PCL reconstruction is an anatomic reconstruction of the anterolateral bundle of the PCL. The anterolateral bundle tightens in flexion, and this reconstruction reproduces that biomechanical function. While the single-bundle–single-femoral tunnel transtibial tunnel PCL reconstruction does not reproduce the broad anatomic insertion site of the normal PCL, there are certain factors that lead to success with this surgical technique:

- Identification and treatment all pathology (especially posterolateral and posteromedial instability)
- Accurate tunnel placement
- Anatomic graft insertion sites
- Strong graft material
- Minimal graft bending
- Final tensioning at 70 to 90 degrees of knee flexion

- Graft tensioning
- Arthrotek mechanical tensioning device
- Primary and back-up fixation
- Appropriate rehabilitation program

INDICATIONS/CONTRAINDICATIONS

Indications

Our indications for surgical treatment of acute PCL injuries include insertion site avulsions, tibial step-off decreased 6 to10 mm or greater, and PCL tears combined with other structural injuries. Our indications for surgical treatment of chronic PCL injuries are when an isolated PCL tear becomes symptomatic demonstrated by progressive functional instability.

Contraindications

There are no significant contraindications.

PREOPERATIVE PLANNING

History and Physical Examination

The typical history of a patient with a PCL injury includes a direct blow to the proximal tibia with the knee in 90 degrees of flexion. Hyperflexion, hyperextension, and a direct blow to the proximal medial or lateral tibia in varying degrees of knee flexion, as well as a forced varus or valgus force, will induce PCL-based multiple ligament knee injuries.

Physical examination of the injured knee compared with the noninjured knee reveals decreased tibial step-offs, and a positive posterior drawer test. Since isolated PCL tears are rare, collateral ligament injury is common (posterolateral and posteromedial corner injuries), and posterolateral and posteromedial drawer tests, dial tests, external rotation recurvatum tests, varus and valgus laxity, and even anterior laxity may be present.

Isolated Posterior Cruciate Ligament Injury Diagnostic Features
- Abnormal posterior laxity less than 5 mm
- Abnormal posterior laxity decreases with tibial internal rotation
- No abnormal varus
- Abnormal external rotation of the tibia on the femur less than 5 degrees compared with the un-involved side tested with the knee at 30 and 90 degrees knee flexion.

Posterior Cruciate Ligament/PLC Injury Diagnostic Features
- Abnormal posterior laxity greater than 5 to 10 mm
- Abnormal varus rotation at 30 degrees knee flexion is variable and depends on the posterolateral instability grade.
- Abnormal external rotation thigh foot angle test greater than 10 degrees compared with the normal lower extremity tested at 30 and 90 degrees of knee flexion. (If you can see the difference, then PLI exists.)
- Posterolateral drawer–positive

Combined Anterior Cruciate Ligament/Posterior Cruciate Ligament Injuries Diagnostic Features
- Grossly abnormal anterior-posterior tibial-femoral laxity at both 25 and 90 degrees of knee flexion
- Positive Lachman and pseudo-Lachman tests
- Positive pivot-shifting phenomenon
- Negative tibial step-off (posterior sag)
- Increased varus-valgus laxity in full extension

Imaging Studies

Plain radiographs used to evaluate PCL injuries include the following views: anterior-posterior weight bearing both knees, 30-degree flexion lateral, intercondylar notch, 30-degree axial of the patellas, and stress views at 90 degrees of knee flexion of both knees. Magnetic resonance imaging (MRI) is helpful in acute cases; however, we have found MRI to be less beneficial in chronic PCL injuries. Bone scan is used in chronic cases of PCL instability presenting with pain to define early degenerative joint disease.

SURGERY

Patient Positioning and Initial Setup

The patient is positioned on the operating table in the supine position, and the surgical and nonsurgical knees are examined under general or regional anesthesia. A tourniquet is applied to the operative extremity, and the surgical leg is prepped and draped in a sterile fashion. Allograft tissue is prepared before beginning the surgical procedure, and autograft tissue is harvested prior to beginning the arthroscopic portion of the procedure. The arthroscopic instruments are inserted with the inflow through the superior lateral patellar portal, the arthroscope in the inferior lateral patellar portal, and the instruments in the inferior medial patellar portal. The portals are interchanged as necessary. The joint is thoroughly evaluated arthroscopically, and the PCL is evaluated using the three-zone arthroscopic technique (17). The PCL tear is identified, and the residual stump of the PCL is debrided with hand tools and the synovial shaver.

Initial Incision

An extra capsular posteromedial safety incision approximately 1.5 to 2.0 cm long is created (Fig. 18-1). The crural fascia is incised longitudinally, taking precautions to protect the neurovascular structures. The interval is developed between the medial head of the gastrocnemius muscle and the posterior capsule of the knee joint, which is anterior. The surgeon's gloved finger is positioned so that the neurovascular structures are posterior to the finger, and the posterior aspect of the joint capsule is anterior to the surgeon's finger. This technique enables the surgeon to monitor surgical instruments, such as the over-the-top PCL instruments and the PCL/ACL drill guide, as they are positioned in the posterior aspect of the knee. The surgeon's finger in the posteromedial safety incision also confirms accurate placement of the guidewire prior to tibial tunnel drilling in the medial-lateral and proximal-distal directions (Fig. 18-2). This is the same anatomic surgical interval that is used in the tibial inlay posterior approach.

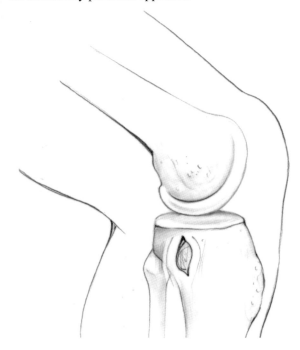

FIGURE 18-1

Posteromedial extra-articular extracapsular safety incision. (Redrawn from Arthrotek, Inc., Warsaw, Indiana, with permission.)

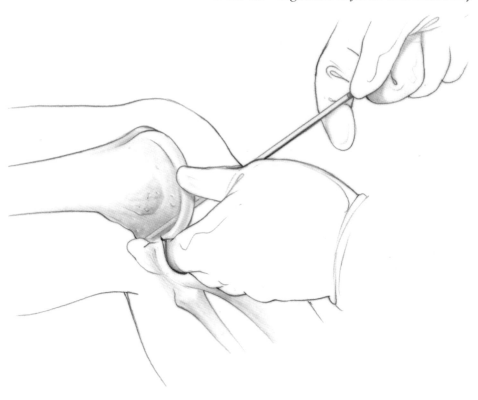

FIGURE 18-2

The surgeon is able to palpate the posterior aspect of the tibia through the extracapsular extra-articular posteromedial safety incision. This enables the surgeon to accurately position guidewires, create the tibial tunnel, and protect the neurovascular structures. (Redrawn from Arthrotek, Inc., Warsaw, Indiana, with permission.)

Elevating the Posterior Capsule

The curved over-the-top PCL instruments are used to carefully lyse adhesions in the posterior aspect of the knee, and to elevate the posterior knee joint capsule away from the tibial ridge on the posterior aspect of the tibia. This capsular elevation enhances correct drill guide and tibial tunnel placement (Fig. 18-3).

Drill Guide Positioning

The arm of the Arthrotek Fanelli PCL-ACL Drill Guide is inserted into the knee through the inferior medial patellar portal and positioned in the PCL fossa on the posterior tibia (Fig. 18-4). The bullet portion of the drill guide contacts the anterior medial aspect of the proximal tibia approximately 1 cm below the tibial tubercle, at a point midway between the tibial crest anteriorly and the posterior medial border of the tibia. This drill guide positioning creates a tibial tunnel that is relatively vertically oriented and has its posterior exit point in the inferior and lateral aspect of the PCL tibial anatomic insertion site. This positioning creates an angle of graft orientation such that the graft will turn two very smooth 45-degree angles on the posterior aspect of the tibia, eliminating the "killer turn" of 90-degree graft angle bending (Fig. 18-5).

The tip of the guide in the posterior aspect of the tibia is confirmed with the surgeon's finger through the extra capsular posteromedial safety incision (see Fig. 18-2). Intraoperative anteroposterior and lateral radiographs may also be used, as well as arthroscopic visualization to confirm drill guide and guide pin placement. A blunt spade-tipped guidewire is drilled from anterior to posterior and can be visualized with the arthroscope, in addition to being palpated with the finger in the posteromedial safety incision. We consider the finger in the posteromedial safety incision the most important step for accuracy and safety.

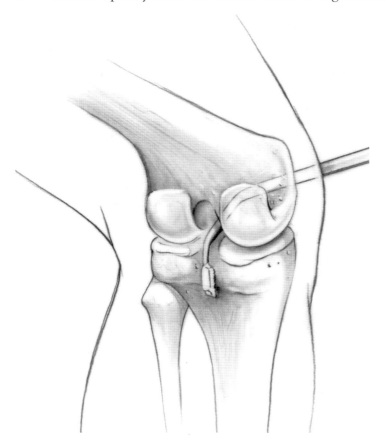

FIGURE 18-3
Posterior capsular elevation using the Arthrotek PCL instruments. (Redrawn from Arthrotek, Inc., Warsaw, Indiana, with permission.)

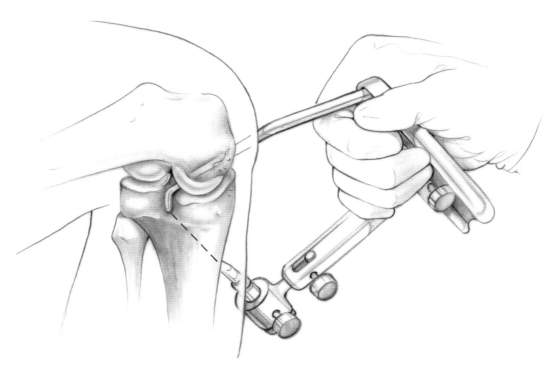

FIGURE 18-4
Arthrotek Fanelli PCL-ACL drill guide positioned to place guidewire in preparation for creation of the transtibial PCL tibial tunnel. (Redrawn from Arthrotek, Inc., Warsaw, Indiana, with permission.)

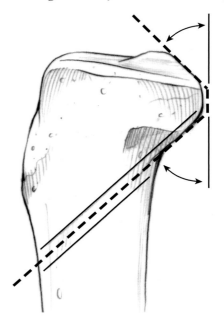

FIGURE 18-5

Drawing demonstrating the desired turning angles the PCL graft will make after the creation of the tibial tunnel. (Redrawn from Arthrotek, Inc., Warsaw, Indiana, with permission.)

Tibial Tunnel Drilling

The appropriately sized standard cannulated reamer is used to create the tibial tunnel. The closed curved PCL curette may be positioned to cup the tip of the guidewire (Fig. 18-6). The arthroscope, when positioned in the posteromedial portal, visualizes the guidewire being captured by the curette and protecting the neurovascular structures in addition to the surgeon's finger in the posteromedial safety incision. The surgeon's finger in the posteromedial safety incision is monitoring the position of the guidewire. The standard cannulated drill is advanced to the posterior cortex of the tibia. The

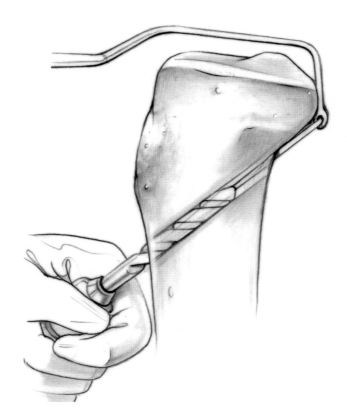

FIGURE 18-6

The Arthrotek PCL closed curette may be used to cap the guidewire during tibial tunnel drilling. (Redrawn from Arthrotek, Inc., Warsaw, Indiana, with permission.)

drill chuck is then disengaged from the drill, and completion of the tibial tunnel reaming is performed by hand. This gives an additional margin of safety for completion of the tibial tunnel. The tunnel edges are chamfered and rasped with the PCL/ACL system rasp (Fig. 18-7).

Drilling the Femoral Tunnel Outside In: Single- and Double-Bundle Posterior Cruciate Ligament Reconstruction

The Arthrotek Fanelli PCL/ACL drill guide is positioned to create the femoral tunnel. The arm of the guide is introduced through the inferomedial patellar portal and is positioned such that the guidewire will exit through the center of the stump of the anterior lateral bundle of the PCL (Fig. 18-8). The blunt spade-tipped guidewire is drilled through the guide, and just as it begins to emerge through the center of the stump of the PCL anterior lateral bundle, the drill guide is disengaged. The accuracy of the placement of the wire is confirmed arthroscopically with probing and visualization. Care must be taken to ensure the patellofemoral joint has not been violated by arthroscopically examining the patellofemoral joint prior to drilling, and that there is adequate distance between the femoral tunnel and the medial femoral condyle articular surface. The appropriately sized standard cannulated reamer is used to create the femoral tunnel. A curette is used to cap the tip of the guidewire so there is no inadvertent advancement of the guidewire, which may damage the ACL or articular surface. As the reamer is about to penetrate interiorly, the reamer is disengaged from the drill and the final reaming is completed by hand (Fig. 18-9). This adds an additional margin of safety. The reaming debris is evacuated with a synovial shaver to minimize fat pad inflammatory response with subsequent risk of arthrofibrosis. The tunnel edges are chamfered and rasped.

When the double-bundle PCL reconstruction is performed, the Arthrotek Fanelli PCL/ACL drill guide is positioned to create the second femoral tunnel. The arm of the guide is introduced through the inferior medial patellar portal and is positioned such that the guidewire will exit through the center of the stump of the posterior medial bundle of the PCL (Fig. 18-10). The blunt spade-tipped guidewire is drilled through the guide, and just as it begins to emerge through the center of the stump of the PCL posterior medial bundle, the drill guide is disengaged. The accuracy of the placement of the wire is confirmed arthroscopically with probing and visualization. Care must be taken to ensure that there will be an adequate bone bridge (approximately 5 mm) between the two femoral tunnels prior to drilling. This is accomplished using the calibrated probe and direct arthroscopic visualization. The appropriately sized standard cannulated reamer is used to create the posterior medial bundle femoral tunnel. A curette is used to cap the tip of the guidewire so there is no inadvertent advancement of the guidewire, which may damage the anterior cruciate ligament or articular surface. As the reamer is about to penetrate interiorly, the reamer is disengaged from the drill and the final reaming is completed by hand (Fig. 18-11). This adds an additional margin of safety. The reaming

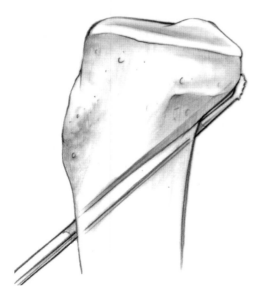

FIGURE 18-7

The tunnel edges are chamfered after drilling to smooth any rough edges. (Redrawn from Arthrotek, Inc., Warsaw, Indiana, with permission.)

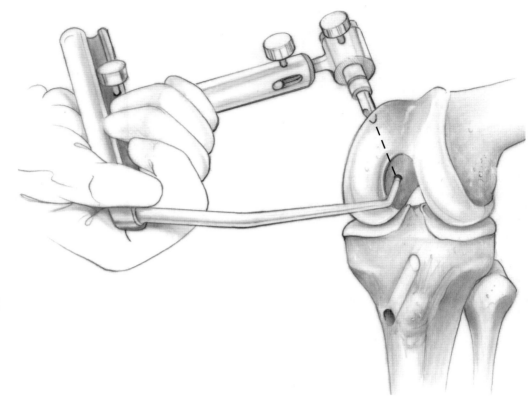

FIGURE 18-8

The Arthrotek Fanelli PCL-ACL drill guide is positioned to drill the guidewire from outside in. The guidewire begins at a point halfway between the medial femoral epicondyle and the medial femoral condyle trochlea articular margin, approximately 2 to 3 cm proximal to the medial femoral condyle distal articular margin, and exits through the center of the stump of the anterolateral bundle of the PCL stump. (Redrawn from Arthrotek, Inc., Warsaw, Indiana, with permission.)

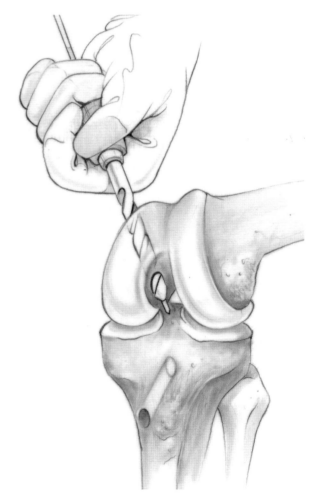

FIGURE 18-9

Completion of anterolateral bundle femoral tunnel reaming by hand for an additional margin of safety. (Redrawn from Arthrotek, Inc., Warsaw, Indiana, with permission.)

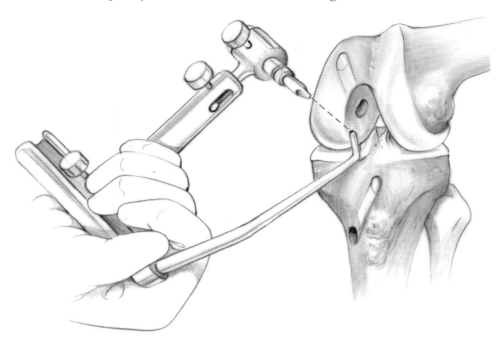

FIGURE 18-10

The Arthrotek Fanelli PCL-ACL drill guide is positioned to drill the guidewire from outside in for creation of the posteromedial bundle PCL femoral tunnel. (Redrawn from Arthrotek, Inc., Warsaw, Indiana, with permission.)

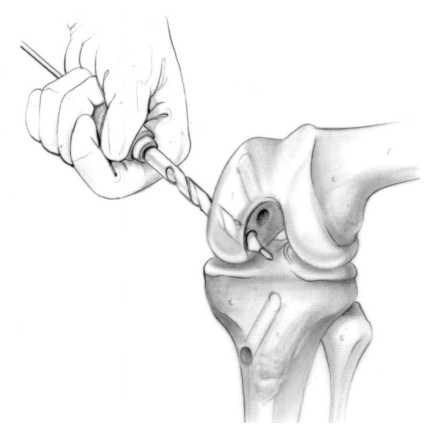

FIGURE 18-11

Completion of femoral tunnel reaming by hand for an additional margin of safety. (Redrawn from Arthrotek, Inc., Warsaw, Indiana, with permission.)

debris is evacuated with a synovial shaver to minimize fat pad inflammatory response with subsequent risk of arthrofibrosis. The tunnel edges are chamfered and rasped.

Drilling the Femoral Tunnel Inside Out: Single- and Double-Bundle Posterior Cruciate Ligament Reconstruction

The PCL single-bundle or double-bundle femoral tunnels can be made from inside out using the Arthrotek Fanelli Double-Bundle Aimers. Inserting the appropriately sized Arthrotek Fanelli double-bundle aimer through a low anterior lateral patellar arthroscopic portal creates the PCL anterior lateral bundle femoral tunnel. The double-bundle aimer is positioned directly on the footprint of the femoral anterior lateral bundle PCL insertion site (Fig. 18-12). The appropriately sized guidewire is drilled through the aimer, through the bone, and out a small skin incision. Care is taken to ensure there is no compromise of the articular surface. The double-bundle aimer is removed, and an acorn reamer is used to endoscopically drill from inside out the anterior lateral PCL femoral tunnel (Fig. 18-13). The tunnel edges are chamfered and rasped. The reaming debris is evacuated with a synovial shaver to minimize fat pad inflammatory response with subsequent risk of arthrofibrosis. When the

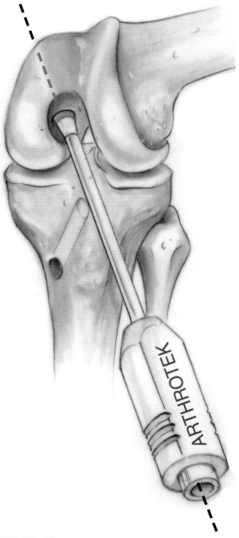

FIGURE 18-12

Arthrotek Fanelli double-bundle aimer positioned to drill a guidewire for creation of the PCL anterolateral bundle tunnel. (Redrawn from Arthrotek, Inc., Warsaw, Indiana, with permission.)

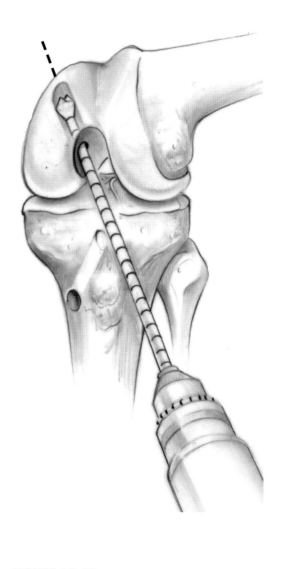

FIGURE 18-13

Endoscopic acorn reamer is used to create the PCL anterolateral bundle femoral tunnel through the low anterolateral patellar portal. (Redrawn from Arthrotek, Inc., Warsaw, Indiana, with permission.)

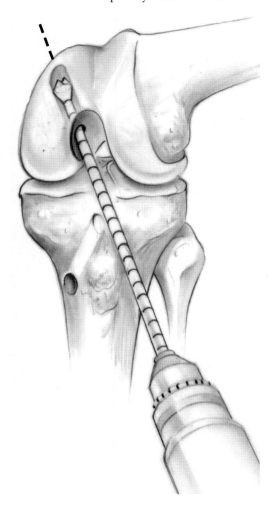

FIGURE 18-14

Arthrotek Fanelli double-bundle aimer positioned to drill a guidewire for creation of the PCL posteromedial bundle femoral tunnel through the low anterolateral patellar portal. (Redrawn from Arthrotek, Inc., Warsaw, Indiana, with permission.)

surgeon chooses to perform a double-bundle double femoral tunnel PCL reconstruction, the same process is repeated for the posterior medial bundle of the PCL (Figs. 18-14 and 18-15). Care must be taken to ensure that there will be an adequate bone bridge (approximately 5 mm) between the two femoral tunnels prior to drilling. This is accomplished using the calibrated probe and direct arthroscopic visualization (Fig. 18-16).

Tunnel Preparation and Graft Passage

The Arthrotek Magellan suture-passing device is introduced through the tibial tunnel and into the knee joint, and is retrieved through the femoral tunnel with an arthroscopic grasping tool (Fig. 18-17). The traction sutures of the graft material are attached to the loop of the Arthrotek Magellan suture-passing device, and the PCL graft material is pulled into position.

Graft Tensioning and Fixation

Fixation of the PCL substitute is accomplished with primary and backup fixation on both the femoral and tibial sides. Our most commonly used graft source for PCL reconstruction is the Achilles tendon allograft alone for single-bundle reconstructions, and Achilles tendon and tibialis anterior allografts for double-bundle reconstructions, although other allografts and autografts may be used as preferred by an individual surgeon. Femoral fixation is accomplished with cortical suspensory backup fixation using polyethylene ligament fixation buttons, and aperture opening fixation using the Arthrotek Bio-Core bioabsorbable interference screws. The Arthrotek Graft Tensioning Boot is applied to the traction sutures of the graft material on its distal end, and tensioned to restore the anatomic tibial step-off. The knee is cycled through several sets of 25 full flexion–extension cycles for graft pretensioning and set-

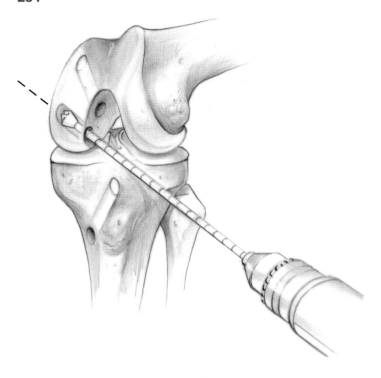

FIGURE 18-15

Endoscopic acorn reamer is used to create the PCL posteromedial bundle through the low anterolateral patellar portal. (Redrawn from Arthrotek, Inc., Warsaw, Indiana, with permission.)

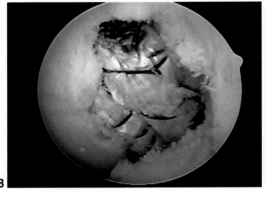

FIGURE 18-16

A: Tunnel placement for double-bundle PCL reconstruction. **B:** Double-bundle PCL reconstruction using Achilles tendon allograft for the anterolateral bundle, and tibialis anterior allograft for the posteromedial bundle.

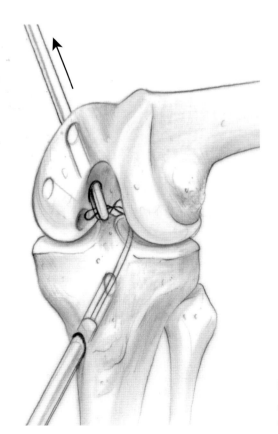

FIGURE 18-17

Arthrotek Magellan suture-passing device. (Redrawn from Arthrotek, Inc., Warsaw, Indiana, with permission.)

tling (Fig. 18-18). The PCL reconstruction graft is tensioned in approximately 70 degrees of knee flexion. Graft fixation is achieved with primary aperture opening fixation using the Arthrotek Bio-Core bioabsorbable interference screw, and back-up fixation with a ligament fixation button, or screw and post, or screw and spiked ligament washer assembly (Fig. 18-19).

Pearls and Pitfalls

The posteromedial safety incision protects the neurovascular structures, confirms accurate tibial tunnel placement, and allows the surgical procedure to be done at an accelerated pace (see Fig. 18-1). It is important to be aware of the two tibial and femoral tunnel directions, and to have an adequate bone bridge between the PCL and ACL tibial and femoral tunnels. This will reduce the possibility of fracture. We have found it useful to use primary and back-up fixation. Primary fixation is with Arthrotek BioCore interference screws, and back-up fixation is performed with a screw and spiked ligament washer, and Arthrotek ligament fixation buttons. Secure fixation is critical to the success of this surgical procedure (Fig. 18-19). Restoration of the normal tibial step-off at 70 degrees of flexion has provided the most reproducible method of establishing the neutral point of the tibia-femoral relationship in our experience. Full range of motion is confirmed on the operating table to ensure the knee is not "captured" by the reconstruction. When multiple ligament surgeries are performed at the same operative session, the PCL reconstruction is performed first, followed by the ACL reconstruction, followed by the collateral ligament surgery.

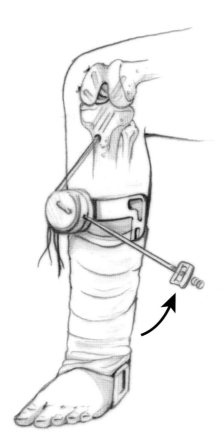

FIGURE 18-18

Arthrotek knee ligament graft-tensioning boot. This mechanical tensioning device uses a ratcheted torque wrench device to assist the surgeon during graft tensioning. (Redrawn from Arthrotek, Inc., Warsaw, Indiana, with permission.)

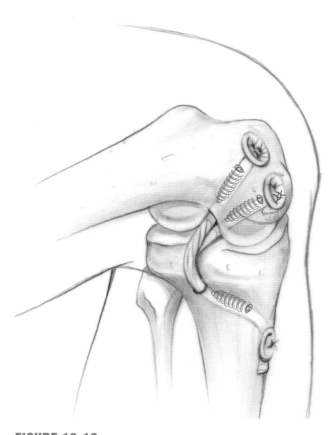

FIGURE 18-19

Final graft fixation using primary and back-up fixation. (Redrawn from Arthrotek, Inc., Warsaw, Indiana, with permission.)

POSTOPERATIVE MANAGEMENT

The knee is immobilized in a long leg brace in full extension for 6 weeks, non–weight bearing using crutches. Progressive range of motion occurs during weeks 4 through 6. The brace is unlocked between weeks 3 and 6, and progressive weight bearing at 25% body weight per week is allowed during postoperative weeks 7 through 10. The crutches are discontinued at the end of postoperative week 10. Progressive strength training and range-of-motion exercises are performed. Return to sports and heavy labor occurs after the sixth to ninth postoperative month, when sufficient strength, range of motion, and proprioceptive skills have returned.

COMPLICATIONS

Posterior cruciate ligament reconstruction is a technically demanding surgery. Complications encountered with this surgical procedure include failure to recognize associated ligament injuries, neurovascular complications, persistent posterior sag, osteonecrosis, knee motion loss, anterior knee pain, and fractures (5,18,19). A comprehensive preoperative evaluation, including an accurate diagnosis, a well-planned and carefully executed surgical procedure, and a supervised postoperative rehabilitation program will help to reduce the incidence of these complications.

RESULTS

We have previously published the results of our arthroscopically assisted combined ACL/PCL and PCL/posterolateral complex reconstructions using the reconstructive technique described in this chapter (7,10,11,14–16). Our most recently published 2- to 10-year results of combined ACL-PCL reconstructions without the Arthrotek Graft Tensioning Boot are presented here (10).

This study presented the 2- to10-year (24 to 120 month) results of 35 arthroscopically assisted combined ACL/PCL reconstructions evaluated pre- and postoperatively using Lysholm, Tegner, and Hospital for Special Surgery knee ligament rating scales, KT 1000 arthrometer testing, stress radiography, and physical examination.

This study population included 26 males, 9 females, 19 acute, and 16 chronic knee injuries. Ligament injuries included 19 ACL/PCL/posterolateral instabilities, 9 ACL/PCL/MCL instabilities, 6 ACL/PCL/posterolateral/MCL instabilities, and 1 ACL/PCL instability. All knees had grade III preoperative ACL/PCL laxity, and were assessed pre- and postoperatively with arthrometer testing, three different knee ligament rating scales, stress radiography, and physical examination. Arthroscopically assisted combined ACL/PCL reconstructions were performed using the single incision endoscopic ACL technique, and the single femoral tunnel–single-bundle transtibial tunnel PCL technique. Posterior cruciate ligaments were reconstructed with allograft Achilles tendon (26 knees), autograft BTB (7 knees), and autograft semitendinosus/gracilis (2 knees). Anterior Cruciate ligaments were reconstructed with autograft BTB (16 knees), allograft BTB (12 knees), Achilles tendon allograft (6 knees), and autograft semitendinosus/gracilis (1 knee). MCL injuries were treated with bracing or open reconstruction. Posterolateral instability was treated with biceps femoris tendon transfer, with or without primary repair, and posterolateral capsular shift procedures as indicated. No Arthrotek graft tensioning boot was used in this series of patients.

Postoperative physical examination results revealed normal posterior drawer/tibial step-off in 16/35 (46%) of knees. Normal Lachman and pivot shift tests were found in 33/35 (94%) of knees. Posterolateral stability was restored to normal in 6/25 (24%) of knees, and tighter than the normal knee in 19/25 (76%) of knees evaluated with the external rotation thigh foot angle test. Thirty-degree varus stress testing was normal in 22/25 (88%) of knees, and grade 1 laxity in 3/25 (12%) of knees. Thirty-degree valgus stress testing was normal in 7/7 (100%) of surgically treated MCL tears, and normal in 7/8 (87.5%) of brace treated knees. Postoperative KT 1000 arthrometer testing mean side-to-side difference measurements were 2.7 mm (PCL screen), 2.6 mm (corrected posterior), and 1.0 mm (corrected anterior) measurements, a statistically significant improvement from preoperative status ($p = 0.001$). Postoperative stress radiographic side-to-side difference measurements measured at 90 degrees of knee flexion, and 32 lbs of posteriorly directed proximal force were 0 to 3 mm in 11/21 (52.3%), 4 to 5 mm in 5/21 (23.8%), and 6 to 10 mm in 4/21 (19%) of knees. Postoperative Lysholm, Tegner, and Hospital for Special Surgery knee ligament rating scale mean values were 91.2, 5.3, and 86.8, respectively, demonstrating a statistically significant improvement from preoperative status ($p = 0.001$). No Arthrotek graft-tensioning boot was used in this series of patients.

The conclusions drawn from the study were that combined ACL/PCL instabilities could be successfully treated with arthroscopic reconstruction and the appropriate collateral ligament surgery. Statistically significant improvement was noted from the preoperative condition at 2- to 10-year follow-up using objective parameters of knee ligament rating scales, arthrometer testing, stress radiography, and physical examination. Postoperatively, these knees are not normal, but they are functionally stable. Continuing technical improvements will most likely improve future results.

A more recent study presents the 2-year follow-up results of 15 arthroscopic assisted ACL/PCL reconstructions using the Arthrotek graft-tensioning boot (14). This study group consists of 11 chronic and four acute injuries. These injury patterns included six ACL/PCL/PLC injuries, four ACL/PCL/MCL injuries, and five ACL/PCL/PLC/MCL injuries. The Arthrotek tensioning boot was used during the procedures as in the surgical technique described previously. All knees had grade III preoperative ACL/PCL laxity, and were assessed pre- and postoperatively using Lysholm, Tegner, and Hospital for Special Surgery knee ligament rating scales, KT 1000 arthrometer testing, stress radiography, and physical examination.

Arthroscopically assisted combined ACL/PCL reconstructions were performed using the single-incision endoscopic ACL technique, and the single femoral tunnel–single-bundle transtibial tunnel PCL technique. Posterior cruciate ligaments were reconstructed with allograft Achilles tendon in all 15 knees. Anterior cruciate ligaments were reconstructed with Achilles tendon allograft in all 15 knees. MCL injuries were treated surgically using primary repair, posteromedial capsular shift, and allograft augmentation as indicated. Posterolateral instability was treated with allograft semitendinosus free graft, with or without primary repair, and posterolateral capsular shift procedures as indicated. The Arthrotek graft-tensioning boot was used in this series of patients.

Post reconstruction physical examination results revealed normal posterior drawer/tibial step-off in 13/15 (86.6%) of knees. Normal Lachman test in 13/15 (86.6%) knees, and normal pivot shift tests in 14/15 (93.3%) knees. Posterolateral stability was restored to normal in all knees with posterolateral instability when evaluated with the external rotation thigh foot angle test (9 knees equal to the normal knee, and 2 knees tighter than the normal knee). Thirty-degree varus stress testing was restored to normal in all 11 knees with posterolateral lateral instability. Thirty- and zero-degree valgus stress testing was restored to normal in all nine knees with medial side laxity. Postoperative KT-1000 arthrometer testing mean side-to-side difference measurements were 1.6 mm (range, 3 to 7 mm) for the PCL screen, 1.6 mm (range, 4.5 to 9 mm) for the corrected posterior, and 0.5 mm (range, 2.5 to 6 mm) for the corrected anterior measurements, a significant improvement from preoperative status. Postoperative stress radiographic side-to-side difference measurements measured at 90 degrees of knee flexion and 32 lbs of posteriorly directed proximal force using the Telos stress radiography device were 0 to 3 mm in 10/15 knees (66.7%), 4 mm in 4/15 knees (26.7%), and 7 mm in 1/15 knees (6.67%). Postoperative Lysholm, Tegner, and Hospital for Special Surgery knee ligament rating scale mean values were 86.7 (range, 69 to 95), 4.5 (range, 2 to 7), and 85.3 (range, 65 to 93), respectively, demonstrating a significant improvement from preoperative status.

The study group demonstrates the efficacy and success of using a mechanical graft-tensioning device (Arthrotek graft-tensioning boot) in single-bundle–single femoral tunnel arthroscopic PCL reconstruction.

Another group of PCL-based ligament reconstructions of interest are our 2- to 10-year results of combined PCL-posterolateral reconstruction (11). This study presented the 2- to 10-year (24 to 120 month) results of 41 chronic arthroscopically assisted combined PCL/posterolateral reconstructions evaluated pre- and postoperatively using Lysholm, Tegner, and Hospital for Special Surgery knee ligament rating scales, KT 1000 arthrometer testing, stress radiography, and physical examination.

This study population included 31 males, 10 females, 24 left, and 17 right chronic PCL/posterolateral knee injuries with functional instability. The knees were assessed pre- and postoperatively with arthrometer testing, three different knee ligament rating scales, stress radiography, and physical examination. Posterior cruciate ligament reconstructions were performed using the arthroscopically assisted single femoral tunnel–single-bundle transtibial tunnel PCL reconstruction technique using fresh frozen Achilles tendon allografts in all 41 cases. In all 41 cases, posterolateral instability reconstruction was performed with combined biceps femoris tendon tenodesis, and posterolateral capsular shift procedures. The paired t-test and power analysis were the statistical tests used. Ninety-five percent confidence intervals were used throughout the analysis.

Postoperative physical examination revealed normal posterior drawer/tibial step-off in 29/41 (70%) of knees for the overall group, and 11/12 (91.7%) normal posterior drawer and tibial step-off in the knees tensioned with the Arthrotek tensioning boot. Posterolateral stability was restored to normal in 11/41 (27%) of knees, and tighter than the normal knee was achieved in 29/41(71%) of knees evaluated with the external rotation thigh foot angle test. Thirty-degree varus stress testing was normal in 40/41 (97%) of knees, and grade 1 laxity was found in 1/41 (3%) of knees. Postoperative KT 1000 arthrometer testing mean side-to-side difference measurements were 1.80 mm (PCL screen), 2.11 mm (corrected posterior), and 0.63 mm (corrected anterior). This is a statistically significant improvement from preoperative status for the PCL screen and the corrected posterior measurements ($p = 0.001$). The postoperative stress radiographic mean side-to-side difference measurement with 90 degrees of knee flexion and 32 lbs of posterior directed force applied to the proximal tibia using the Telos device was 2.26 mm. This is a statistically significant improvement from preoperative measurements ($p = 0.001$). Postoperative Lysholm, Tegner, and Hospital for Special Surgery knee ligament rating scale mean values were 91.7, 4.92, and 88.7, respectively, demonstrating a statistically significant improvement from preoperative status ($p = 0.001$).

Conclusions drawn from this study were that chronic combined PCL/posterolateral instabilities could be successfully treated with arthroscopic PCL reconstruction, using fresh frozen Achilles tendon allograft combined with posterolateral corner reconstruction, using biceps tendon transfer combined with posterolateral capsular shift procedure. Statistically significant improvement is noted ($p = 0.001$) from the preoperative condition at 2- to10-year follow-up using objective parameters of knee ligament rating scales, arthrometer testing, stress radiography, and physical examination. Use of the Arthrotek Graft-Tensioning Boot is advised since postoperative physical examination revealed normal posterior drawer/tibial step-off in 29/41 (70%) of knees for the overall group, and 11/12 (91.7%) normal posterior drawer and tibial step-off in the knees tensioned with the Arthrotek tensioning boot.

FUTURE DIRECTIONS

We have chosen to perform the double-bundle–double-femoral tunnel PCL reconstruction surgical technique since there are convincing basic science data supporting the efficacy of this procedure (21). This double-bundle–double femoral tunnel technique more closely approximates the anatomic insertion site of the native PCL, and should theoretically provide improved results. Our early clinical results are encouraging; however, there are no long-term clinical results available as of this writing.

Another area of interest is the incorporation of autologous platelet-rich fibrin matrix into the grafts used in the cruciate and collateral ligament reconstructive procedures (Fig. 18-20). There are several studies indicating favorable effects on the ligament graft tissue and the clinical results (24,25,26). We have demonstrated favorable initial clinical results with respect to graft incorporation, wound healing, and early stability; however, there is no long-term follow-up as of this writing.

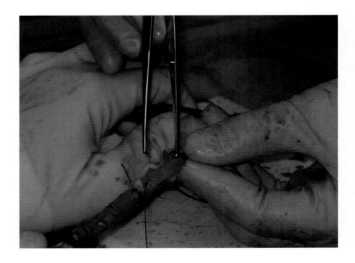

FIGURE 18-20

A platelet-rich fibrin matrix clot created by the Musculoskeletal Transplant Foundation Cascade System is incorporated into the graft during the tubularization process to potentially enhance graft incorporation in the tunnels.

CONCLUSIONS

The arthroscopically assisted single-bundle–transtibial PCL reconstruction technique is a reproducible surgical procedure. There are documented results demonstrating statistically significant improvements from preoperative to postoperative status evaluated by physical examination, knee ligament rating scales, arthrometer measurements, and stress radiography. Factors contributing to the success of this surgical technique include identification and treatment of all pathology (especially posterolateral and posteromedial instability), accurate tunnel placement, placement of strong graft material at anatomic graft insertion sites, minimizing graft bending, performing final graft tensioning at 70 to 90 degrees of knee flexion using the Arthrotek graft-tensioning boot, using primary and back-up fixation, and the appropriate postoperative rehabilitation program. Due to a more anatomic reconstruction, double-bundle reconstruction may provide better results. This will need to be demonstrated in long-term clinical studies.

REFERENCES

1. Daniel DM, Akeson W, O'Conner J, eds. *Knee ligaments—structure, function, injury, and repair.* New York: Raven Press; 1990.
2. Fanelli GC. Arthroscopic evaluation of the PCL. In: Fanelli GC, ed. *Posterior cruciate ligament injuries. A guide to practical management.* New York: Springer-Verlag; 2001.
3. Fanelli GC. Arthroscopic PCL reconstruction: transtibial technique. In: Fanelli GC, ed. *Posterior cruciate ligament injuries. A guide to practical management.* New York: Springer-Verlag; 2001.
4. Fanelli GC. Arthrotek PCL reconstruction surgical technique guide. Fanelli PCL-ACL drill guide system. Arthrotek, Inc. Warsaw, Indiana; 1998.
5. Fanelli GC. Complications in PCL surgery. In: Fanelli GC, ed. *Posterior cruciate ligament injuries. A guide to practical management.* New York: Springer-Verlag; 2001.
6. Fanelli GC. PCL injuries in trauma patients. *Arthroscopy* 1993;9(3):291–294.
7. Fanelli GC. Point counter point. Arthroscopic posterior cruciate ligament reconstruction: single bundle/single femoral tunnel. *Arthroscopy.* 2000;16(7):725–731.
8. Fanelli GC. Rationale and surgical technique for PCL and multiple knee ligament reconstruction. Surgical technique guide. Arthrotek, Inc.; 2006.
9. Fanelli GC. Surgical treatment of ACL-PCL-medial side-lateral side injuries of the knee. *Operative techniques in sports medicine.* 2003;11(4):263–274.
10. Fanelli GC, Edson CJ. Arthroscopically assisted combined ACL/PCL reconstruction. 2–10 year follow-up. *Arthroscopy.* 2002;18(7):703–714.
11. Fanelli GC, Edson CJ. Combined posterior cruciate ligament–posterolateral reconstruction with Achilles tendon allograft and biceps femoris tendon tenodesis: 2–10 year follow-up. *Arthroscopy.* 2004;20(4):339–345.
12. Fanelli GC, Edson CJ. Management of posterior cruciate ligament and posterolateral instability of the knee. In: Chow J, ed. *Advanced Arthroplasty.* New York: Springer-Verlag; 2001.
13. Fanelli GC, Edson CJ. PCL injuries in trauma patients. Part II. *Arthroscopy.* 1995;11:526–529.
14. Fanelli GC, Edson CJ, Orcutt DR, et al. Treatment of combined ACL–PCL medial lateral side injuries of the knee. *Journal of Knee Surgery.* 2005;28 (3):240–248.
15. Fanelli GC, Giannotti BF, Edson CJ. Arthroscopically assisted combined anterior and posterior cruciate ligament reconstruction. *Arthroscopy.* 1996;12(1):5–14.
16. Fanelli GC, Giannotti B, Edson CJ. Arthroscopically assisted PCL/posterior lateral complex reconstruction. *Arthroscopy.* 1996;12(5).
17. Fanelli GC, Giannotti B, Edson CJ. Current concepts review. The posterior cruciate ligament: arthroscopic evaluation and treatment. *Arthroscopy.* 1994;10(6):673–688.
18. Fanelli GC, Monahan TJ. Complications and pitfalls in posterior cruciate ligament reconstruction. In: Malek MM, ed. *Knee Surgery: complications, pitfalls, and salvage.* New York: Springer-Verlag; 2001.
19. Fanelli GC, Monahan TJ. Complications of posterior cruciate ligament reconstruction. *Sports Medicine and Arthroscopy Review.* 1999;7(4):296–302.
20. Fanelli GC, Orcutt DR, Edson CJ. Current concepts: the multiple ligament injured knee. *Arthroscopy.* 2005;21(4): 471–486.
21. Harner CD, Janaushek MA, Kanamori A, et al. Biomechanical analysis of a double-bundle posterior cruciate ligament reconstruction. *Am J Sports Med.* 2000;28:144–151.
22. Malek MM, Fanelli GC. Technique of arthroscopically PCL reconstruction. *Orthopaedics.* 1993;16(9):961–966.
23. Miller MD, Cooper DE, Fanelli GC, et al. Posterior cruciate ligament: current concepts. In: Beaty JH, ed. American Academy of Orthopaedic Surgeons Instructional Course Lectures. 2002;51:347–351. Available from the American Academy of Orthopaedic Surgeons, Rosemont, IL.
24. Sanchez M, Azofra J, Aizpurua B, et al. Application of growth factor rich autologous plasma in arthroscopic surgery. *Cuadernos de Arthroscopia.* 2003;10:12–19.
25. Weiler A, Forster C, Hunt P, et al. The influence of locally applied platelet-derived growth factor BB on free tendon graft remodeling after anterior cruciate ligament reconstruction. *Am J Sports Med.* 2004;4:881–891.
26. Yasuda K, Tomita F, Yamazaki S, et al. The effect of growth factors on biomechanical properties of the bone patellar tendon bone graft after anterior cruciate ligament reconstruction. *Am J Sports Med.* 2004;4:870–880.

19 Double-Bundle Posterior Cruciate Ligament Reconstruction

Anthony M. Buoncristiani, Fotios P. Tjoumakaris, and Christopher D. Harner

INDICATIONS/CONTRAINDICATIONS

Posterior cruciate ligament (PCL) injuries are rare and infrequently occur in isolation. Although we have an increased knowledge of the anatomy and mechanism of injury, PCL reconstruction has not obtained the success of anterior cruciate ligament (ACL) reconstruction. In addition, frustrating to the surgeon is the lack of consensus regarding the optimal management of PCL injuries. Isolated PCL injuries (grades I and II) can be treated nonoperatively with protected weight-bearing and quadriceps muscle rehabilitation. However, some studies have demonstrated degenerative changes and poor objective outcomes associated with conservative treatment of PCL injuries.

The absolute indications for reconstruction of an isolated PCL tear would be for persistent instability (grade III) or a boney avulsion. However, some authors dispute the existence of an isolated PCL injury. Regardless, most PCL reconstructions occur in conjunction with a knee dislocation. Advances in the understanding of the anatomy and biomechanics of the PCL have led to an increased interest in arthroscopic reconstruction of the PCL. Anatomic studies have delineated separate characteristics of the anterolateral (AL) and posteromedial (PM) bundles within the PCL. The larger AL bundle has increased tension in flexion, whereas the PM bundle becomes more taut in extension. In addition, the smaller meniscofemoral ligaments also contribute to the overall strength of the PCL. The timing of PCL reconstruction is controversial, but an acute reconstruction is generally accepted for boney avulsion injuries or while addressing combined ligamentous injuries—especially a posterolateral corner injury. The double-bundle PCL reconstruction technique is most commonly performed in the chronic setting, when very little native ligament remains available for augmentation.

Contraindications to an acute PCL reconstruction would be in the setting of a traumatic knee arthrotomy or with a stiff knee. The double-bundle technique is not recommended if any bundle remains intact. In this scenario, we prefer a single-bundle augmentation, which is the most likely clinical presentation. We always attempt to preserve any remnant tissue whenever possible unless located directly at the insertion site of the target bundle. The grafts are passed around the meniscofemoral ligaments, which does increase the complexity of the reconstruction.

PREOPERATIVE PLANNING

A thorough history and physical examination are obtained preoperatively in a clinic setting. It is important to determine the chronicity of the injury. Acutely, there is usually a history of a direct blow to the anterior lower leg or a hyperextension injury with concomitant mild swelling. A PCL injury may also occur in the setting of a knee dislocation with involvement of the posterolateral structures (approximately 60%). Chronically, instability may be the only complaint.

On physical examination, it is important to assess the neurovascular status of the injured limb. This is especially important if there is a history of a knee dislocation, which has a higher risk of such an injury. Inspect and palpate for an effusion followed by assessing the range of motion. With the knee in a flexed position, palpate for the natural tibial step-off and evaluate the anterior border of tibial plateau in relation to the femoral condyles. In addition, a Godfrey test can be performed whereby the lower leg is elevated with the knee flexed approximately 90 degrees to assess for the presence of a "sag." A posterior drawer with the knee in 90 degrees of flexion is also performed to evaluate the amount of posterior tibial translation (Fig. 19-1). It is important to recognize the presence of a posterolateral corner knee injury, which will accentuate the posterior drawer. The gait pattern is inspected for any varus thrust. If a posterolateral corner injury is suspected, the physical examination should include a reverse pivot shift test, a dial test, a posterolateral drawer, and varus stress testing at both 30 and 90 degrees.

Radiographs of the knee should be performed to inspect for any fracture in the acute setting or for any medial or patellofemoral compartmental arthrosis in the chronic setting. Long-leg cassette films should be obtained if any coronal instability is suspected. Posterior tibial subluxation can possibly be seen on the lateral radiograph. Otherwise, a comparative stress lateral radiograph can also be obtained. A bone scan may be useful in chronic PCL insufficiency to identify degenerative changes. A magnetic resonance image (MRI) is essential not only to confirm a PCL injury, but more importantly to assess for any concomitant posterolateral corner injury or meniscal pathology that will affect the operative plan.

SURGERY

Patient Positioning

The patient is identified in the preoperative holding area and the operative site is signed. Sciatic and femoral nerve blocks are performed by the anesthesiology staff. The patient is taken to the operating room, where spinal or general anesthesia is induced. The patient is positioned supine on the operating room table. A padded bump is taped to the operating room table at the foot with the knee flexed to 90 degrees to hold the leg flexed during the case. A side post is placed on the operative side just distal to the greater trochanter to support the proximal leg with the knee in flexion. Padded cush-

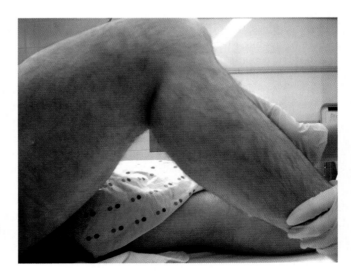

FIGURE 19-1

The posterior drawer test is demonstrated. With a posteriorly directed force, the anterior tibia can be subluxed beyond the medial femoral condyles.

ions are placed under the nonoperative leg. We do not routinely use a tourniquet so that the vascular status of the extremity can be checked intraoperatively (Fig. 19-2).

Examination under Anesthesia

An examination under anesthesia (EUA) is then performed. The nonoperative knee is examined followed by the operative knee. The alignment and range of motion are assessed with specific attention to terminal extension and flexion. A thorough ligamentous examination as previously described is then performed to confirm our preoperative diagnosis and assess for any other pathology. Lower grades of posterior drawer and reverse pivot shift tests may represent an intact AL or PM bundle of the PCL. Fluoroscopy is used after the EUA. Lateral views are obtained with the tibia displaced posteriorly and then reduced with an anterior force. The sloped posterior tibial fossa is identified for later tibial tunnel placement.

Surface Anatomy and Skin Incisions

The knee is flexed to 90 degrees and the vertical arthroscopy portals are delineated. The anterolateral portal is placed just lateral to the lateral border of the patellar tendon and adjacent to the inferior pole of the patella. The anteromedial portal is positioned approximately 1 cm medial to the medial border of the superior aspect of the patellar tendon (Fig. 19-3). An accessory posteromedial portal is created just proximal to the joint line and posterior to the medial collateral ligament under direct arthroscopic guidance. If meniscal repair or other surgical procedures are expected, these incisions are marked as well. The proposed incisions are then cleansed with sterile Betadine paint and injected with a local anesthetic and epinephrine. The leg is cleansed with an alcohol solution and Betadine, with care taken to preserve the incision marks. The operative leg is draped using a sterile technique. A hole is cut in the stockinette for access to the dorsalis pedis pulse throughout the case. After draping, the arthroscopy equipment is prepared and the fluoroscopy machine is later draped (Fig. 19-4).

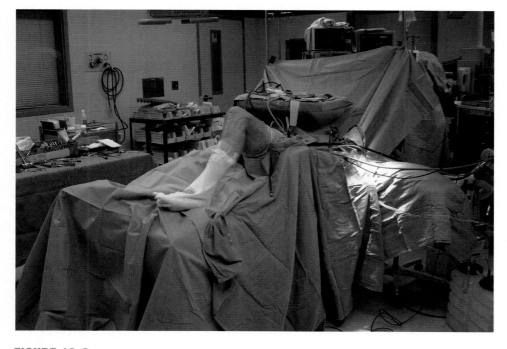

FIGURE 19-2

The positioning and preparation are demonstrated. The knee rests comfortably at 90 degrees of flexion without the use of assistants.

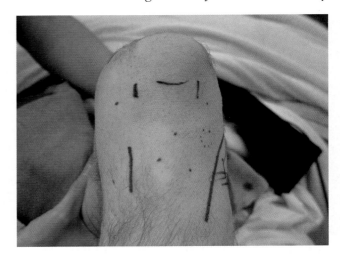

FIGURE 19-3

The landmarks are drawn on the skin. In this figure, the portal sites are marked as well as the medial tibial incision for later tibial tunnel placement.

Graft Preparation

In general, two long (approximately 24 cm in length) tibialis anterior allografts are preferred over a split allograft. The soft tissue allografts are thawed in sterile saline solution. A whipstitch is placed in each of the free ends of the graft. A closed Endoloop of 30 to 40 mm in length is used without the EndoButton (Smith & Nephew, Inc., Andover, MA) (Fig. 19-5). With the standard EndoButton technique, a significant portion of the tunnel will contain only the Endoloop suture, with some graft left outside the tibial tunnel. The EndoButton is carefully removed using a wire cutter to avoid damage to the loop. This is done to minimize the amount of Endoloop and maximize the amount of graft within the femoral tunnel.

The allograft is passed through and doubled over the Endoloop, halving its length to 12 cm. A No. 5 braided suture is placed through the Endoloop and the graft is tensioned. The graft is marked 25 mm from the Endoloop end for later referencing when passing the graft into the femoral tunnel and 50 mm from this mark to represent the intra-articular portion of the graft. The width of the graft is measured on the tibial and femoral ends. The desired AL allograft width is 9 to 10 mm versus 7 mm for the PM allograft. The graft is kept in a damp sponge until needed for graft passage.

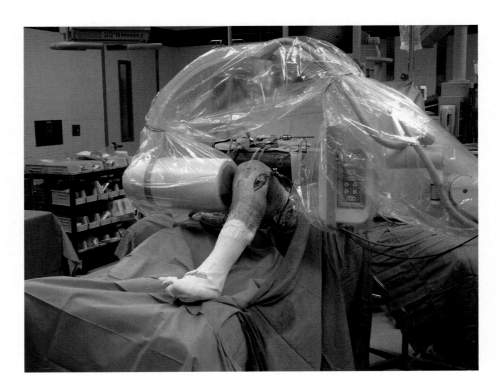

FIGURE 19-4

Fluoroscopy is used for proper placement of the tibial tunnel. The knee can be easily visualized in this setting when placed at 90 degrees.

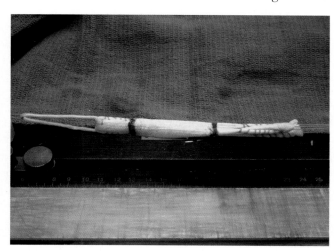

FIGURE 19-5

A tibialis anterior allograft is prepared with an Endoloop attached. Two marks are placed, one at 25 mm of graft and the other at 75 mm. Between the designated marks lies the intra-articular portion of the allograft. Both grafts are marked in similar fashion.

Arthroscopy

A thorough diagnostic arthroscopy is performed to assess the cruciate ligaments and evaluate for other cartilage or meniscal derangements. The notch is examined for any remaining intact PCL fibers of the AL or PM bundles. If specific fibers from either bundle or the meniscofemoral ligaments are left, care should be taken to preserve these fibers during the case for augmentation. Frequently, the AL bundle is ruptured and the PM bundle remains intact.

Overlying synovium and ruptured PCL fibers are debrided. An arthroscopic electrocautery device and shaver are used to define the superior interval between the ACL and PCL. A 70-degree arthroscope is routinely used when viewing through the notch. The arthroscope is placed between the PCL remnants and the medial femoral condyle (Gillquist view) to assess the posterior horn of the medial meniscus. This view is also used for spinal needle localization of the posteromedial portal. The Gillquist view and the interval between the intact ACL and torn PCL remnants (transseptal view) are routinely used throughout the case to view the tibial footprint. The 30-degree arthroscope is used when viewing via the posteromedial portal. A switching stick may be placed into the posteromedial portal to facilitate exchange of the arthroscope.

The 70-degree arthroscope is placed into the anterolateral portal, and a commercially available PCL curette is introduced through the anteromedial portal. The PCL curette (and later the PCL drill guide) is placed in proper relationship to the preserved PCL bundle footprints. Once the curette is in place, a lateral fluoroscopic image may be obtained to confirm its position. The 30-degree arthroscope is introduced through the posteromedial portal. The soft tissue on the posterior aspect of the tibia is carefully elevated centrally and slightly lateral. A transseptal portal is created for access to the tibial PCL insertion. A shaver may be placed from the anterolateral portal to debride some of the surrounding synovium with care taken to preserve the PCL origin. The camera should be switched to the 70-degree arthroscope in the anterolateral portal and the shaver placed in the posteromedial portal for further debridement. Adequate preparation of the posterior tibia can be technically demanding and tedious, but it is essential for proper exposure and safety in drilling the tunnel.

Tunnel Location and Preparation

Tibial Tunnel Preparation   To begin tunnel location and preparation (Figs. 19-6 and 19-7), a commercially available PCL tibial drill guide is placed through the anteromedial portal. The guide is set to 50 degrees, and its position is checked with a lateral fluoroscopic view and via the posteromedial arthroscopic view (Fig. 19-8). The superior tibial insertion site of the PCL begins in a fossa located between the two palpable prominences of the medial and lateral plateaus of the tibia. The recommended landmark for placement of this guide is approximately 1.5 cm distal to the articular edge of the posterior plateau, which corresponds to the junction of the middle and distal 1/3 of the posterior tibial slope (Fig. 19-9).

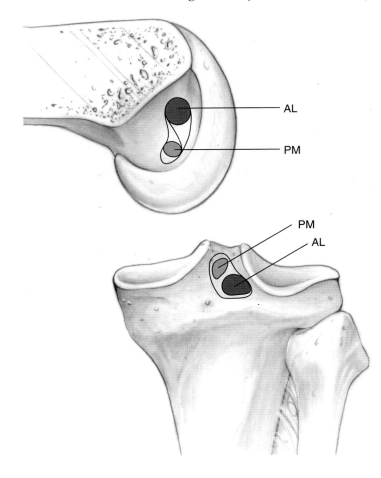

FIGURE 19-6

Schematic representation of the femoral and tibial insertion sites of the two bundles of the PCL. AL, anterolateral; PM, posteromedial.

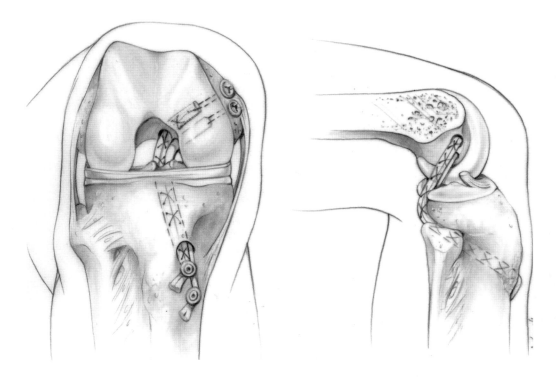

FIGURE 19-7

Schematic representation of the two bundles after graft passage.

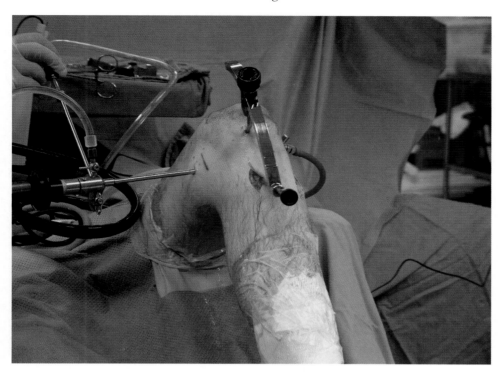

FIGURE 19-8

With the arthroscope placed in the posteromedial portal as shown, the tibial footprint can be visualized and the tibial guide correctly placed.

The guide is aligned on the anteromedial aspect of the tibia and an incision is made. Dissection is performed through periosteum down to bone. In contrast, a small incision on the anterolateral surface of the tibia can be used for placement of the tibial AL tunnel to provide tunnel separation from the PM tibial tunnel. Otherwise, if both tunnels are going to be made on the anteromedial aspect of the tibia, care is taken to avoid tunnel convergence and ensure that adequate separation with a bony bridge exists between the two tibial tunnels. The PCL guide is reset in the lateral aspect of the PCL tibial footprint and its position is again confirmed with fluoroscopy and arthroscopy. The guide is then clamped down onto the anterior tibial surface. A guidewire is drilled up to but not through the posterior cortex. Another fluoroscopic image is obtained to confirm the path of the guidewire, and the drill guide is removed (Fig. 19-10). The PCL curette is introduced through the anteromedial portal, and the 30-degree arthroscope is placed in the posteromedial portal. The curette is used to protect the posterior knee structures as the guidewire is carefully advanced through the posterior cortex

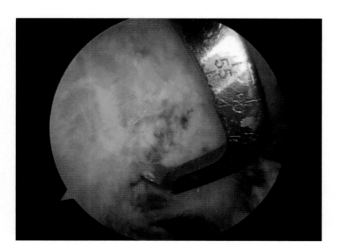

FIGURE 19-9

View from the posteromedial portal demonstrating the guide being placed for the anterolateral tibial tunnel.

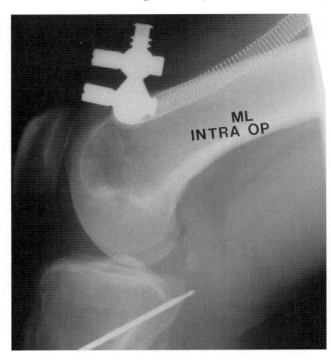

FIGURE 19-10

Fluoroscopic image demonstrating tibial guide pin placement for the anterolateral tibial tunnel.

under arthroscopic visualization. A parallel pin guide can be used to make small pin placement corrections if necessary. The same steps and precautions are repeated for placement of the PM tibial guidewire. However, it is placed more medial and slightly proximal to the AL tibial guidewire (Fig. 19-11). Once again, it is important to ensure that adequate separation between the two guide pins exists to accommodate both tunnels with a bony bridge separation. Once the guidewire positions are satisfactory, a cannulated compaction reamer is used to drill the AL tibial tunnel first. Drill advancement is performed under fluoroscopic guidance, but the posterior tibial cortex is cautiously perforated by hand reaming under arthroscopic visualization. The tunnel is irrigated and increasing serial dilators are used under arthroscopic visualization up to the graft size (Fig. 19-12). The steps are repeated for drilling the PM tibial tunnel with a 7-mm cannulated compaction reamer.

Femoral Tunnel Preparation   The shaver is used to debride any soft tissue off of the lateral wall of the medial femoral condyle, with care taken to preserve any remnant PCL bundle tissue. An angled awl is used to create a starting hole at the appropriate position for the bundle being reconstructed. For the AL bundle, the starting hole is placed at the 1:00 or 11:00 position for right and left knees, respectively. This will place the superior edge of the tunnel at the 12:00 position. The anteroposterior distance from the articular cartilage of the medial femoral condyle depends on the size

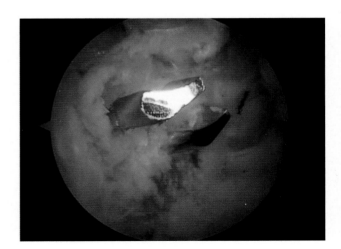

FIGURE 19-11

View from the posteromedial portal demonstrating the placement of both the AL and PM guide pins within the tibial footprint. In this figure, the AL guide pin is on the right side and distal.

of the graft, but the tunnel edge should be located at the junction with the articular cartilage. A 3/32 guidewire is placed via the anterolateral portal and impacted into the starting hole.

The appropriately sized cannulated acorn reamer is passed over the guidewire. The reamer should be passed carefully given the close proximity of the patellar articular surface. The tunnel is drilled to a depth of approximately 30 mm, with care taken to avoid penetration of the outer cortex of the medial femoral condyle. Increasing serial dilators are passed to match the size of the graft. A smaller EndoButton drill is used to perforate the outer cortex of the medial femoral condyle.

This inside-out femoral tunnel preparation technique is then repeated for the PM tunnel. The angled awl is used again to create the starting hole at the 3:00 or 9:00 position for right and left knees, respectively. The PM tunnel is placed parallel or slightly posterior to the AL tunnel. The 3/32 guide pin is then placed via the anterolateral portal and impacted into the starting hole. A 7-mm acorn reamer is passed over the guidewire and drilled to a depth of approximately 30 mm. The medial femoral condylar cortex is perforated with the EndoButton drill (Fig. 19-13).

The anterolateral portal may require a larger incision to ensure passage of the graft. Arthroscopic graspers are placed via the anterolateral portal through the notch under direct visualization with the 30-degree arthroscope in the anteromedial portal. The 30-degree arthroscope is then placed in the posteromedial portal. The AL graft is passed first. A long 18-gauge bent wire loop is passed retrograde through the AL tibial tunnel with the loop bent upward. The previously placed arthroscopic graspers are used to retrieve the bent wire loop. The wire loop is advanced out the anterolateral portal. Leading sutures from the free ends (tibial side) of the graft are placed through the wire loop and the wire is pulled back through the tibial tunnel with the sutures in an anterograde fashion. The free ends of the graft can be visualized passing through the notch and into the tibial tunnel, with the femoral-sided leading suture remaining in the anterolateral portal. A small scooped malleable is introduced through the anterolateral portal and placed just posterior to the AL tunnel to retract the fat pad and provide an unobstructed path for the beath pin. The beath pin is inserted through the anterolateral portal and through the AL femoral tunnel and exits the skin on the medial thigh. Care is taken to avoid penetrating soft tissue with the beath pin while passing through the anterolateral portal because this will cause the graft to be entangled in the soft tissue. The lead suture limbs from the Endoloop side are threaded through the eye of the Beath pin, and the pin with the suture limbs is pulled proximally. Traction on the suture limbs pulls the graft into the femoral tunnel to the marked line, which is confirmed arthroscopically (Fig. 19-14). Tag the suture ends of the graft together. This process is then repeated for the PM graft. It can be cumbersome passing the second graft. Always keep traction on the AL graft suture ends when passing the PM graft to ensure that the AL graft does not inadvertently get pulled into the joint (Fig. 19-15).

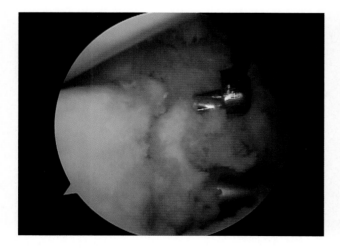

FIGURE 19-12

A dilator can be seen penetrating the AL tibial tunnel. The PM tibial tunnel is drilled and a curette is placed over the tip of the pin when reaming to protect the neurovascular structures.

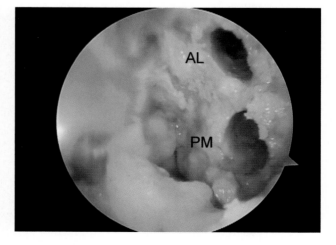

FIGURE 19-13

The AL and PM femoral tunnels have been drilled on the face of the medial femoral condyle.

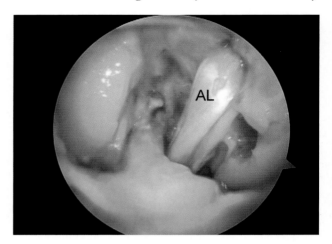

FIGURE 19-14

The AL graft has been passed, and the PM tunnel can be visualized inferior to the graft on the medial femoral condyle.

Next, an incision is made parallel to Langer's lines over the anteromedial aspect of the distal medial femoral condyle, at the estimated exit of the graft suture ends from the cortex. The vastus medialis obliquus fascia and muscle are identified and either elevated and retracted en masse or split in line with their fibers depending where the sutures are located. The muscle and periosteum are elevated off of the anteromedial distal femur and the drill holes are exposed.

Graft Fixation

The closed Endoloop is placed in position along the medial femur with a tonsil to estimate its most proximal extent. Because this is frequently positioned on a sloped surface and bicortical purchase may not be possible, a 3.2-mm drill bit is used to drill a unicortical hole at the most proximal extent of the Endoloop. After measuring the length and using a 6.5-mm tap, a commercially available 6.5-mm cancellous screw and washer are placed through the Endoloop into the femur as the graft is pulled tight distally. The fixation is palpated to ensure the Endoloop limbs are tight distal to the screw and washer. This process is repeated for the second graft. Ensure enough separation exists between the two screws and washers to prevent overlap.

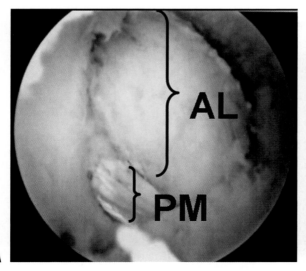
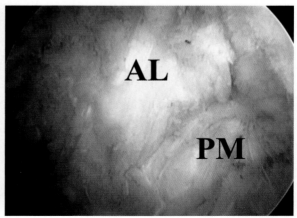

FIGURE 19-15

A: After femoral and tibial fixation, the final placement is visualized from the lateral portal in a left knee. The anterolateral graft almost completely obstructs the view of the PM graft from this view. **B:** Final view of a double-bundle PCL reconstruction in a right knee.

An anterior tibial force is applied to reduce the tibia before and during final tibial fixation. In similar fashion to the femoral side, two bicortical 4.5-mm cortical screws and washers are placed from anteromedial to posterolateral within the proximal tibia. The amount of knee flexion at final fixation depends on which PCL bundle is being secured. The AL graft is secured first at 90 degrees flexion followed by the PM bundle at approximately 15 degrees of flexion. Before the screw advances to the second cortex, the suture limbs from the tibial side of the graft are tied with tension over the post, and then the screw is tightened. The arthroscope is inserted to confirm adequate position, tension, and fixation of the grafts.

Closure

Both incisions are irrigated, and the fascia in the anterolateral femoral incision is closed with 0 vicryl suture. The subcutaneous layer is approximated with interrupted, inverted 3-0 vicryl suture and the skin is closed with a running 4-0 absorbable suture. The portals are closed with 3-0 nylon suture. The dorsalis pedis and posterior tibialis pulses are assessed by palpation and a Doppler ultrasound if necessary. The incisions are covered with adaptic gauze and sterile gauze then wrapped in cast padding and bias wrap. Assess knee motion to ensure that it is not captured. The anterior tibial step-off should be re-established. A hinged knee brace is applied and locked in extension. Maintain an anterior drawer at all times when handling the leg. The patient is awakened and taken to the recovery room, where the patient's pain and neurovascular status are re-evaluated.

Pearls and Pitfalls

- It is important to assess for concomitant posterolateral corner (PLC) injury on the EUA and following PCL reconstruction. Deficiency of these structures may lead to graft failure.
- Exposure of the posterior tibia is essential for the success of this technique. This can be tedious but the surgeon should be careful and patient. Both aggressive debridement and inadequate exposure can lead to neurovascular injury.
- A parallel pin guide can be used to make small corrections for placement of the tunnels.
- Perforate the posterior tibial cortex with the guide pins or reamers in a controlled fashion under direct arthroscopic visualization by hand to avoid neurovascular injury.
- If resistance is met when attempting to place the acorn reamer over the guide pin in the femur, it is most likely the patella. A smaller sized acorn reamer can be used in this situation to make a starting hole. Then larger sized reamers can be placed freehanded to dilate the tunnel to the appropriate size.
- An arthroscopic switching rod can be placed via the posteromedial portal between the graft and the posterior tibial cortex to help facilitate graft passage by decreasing the friction.
- Fluid extravasation during arthroscopy is also a concern. Lower extremity compartments should be monitored throughout the procedure.

POSTOPERATIVE MANAGEMENT

Patients are kept overnight for pain management and to monitor their neurovascular status. Patients are given instructions for exercises (quadriceps sets, straight-leg raises, and calf pumps) and crutch use before discharge the next day. Patients are instructed to maintain a touchdown weight-bearing status for 1 week. Partial weight bearing (30%) is initiated after the first postoperative visit. All dressing changes are performed with an anterior tibial force applied.

The knee is locked in extension for the first week. Symmetric full hyperextension is achieved and passive prone knee flexion, quadriceps sets, and patellar mobilization exercises are performed with the assistance of a physical therapist for the first month. Mini-squats are performed from 0 to 60 degrees after the first week, and increased to 90 degrees for weeks 3 to 4. The brace is unlocked at 4 weeks postoperatively and usually discontinued at 8 weeks. Closed-chain terminal knee extension exercises may begin at 8 weeks. Once full, pain-free range of motion is achieved, strengthening is addressed.

COMPLICATIONS

Complications are rare, but can happen. Failure to carefully position the extremity with adequate padding can lead to neurapraxia. Loss of motion (usually decreased flexion) can result from errors in graft positioning and excessive tensioning during graft fixation or from inadequate range-of-motion exercises during postoperative rehabilitation. Residual laxity can also occur. Injury to the popliteal vessels is an infrequent but very serious complication. With the transtibial technique, great care must be taken to ensure overpenetration of the posterior tibial cortex does not occur. The surgeon should regularly palpate the vessels about the ankle for any diminished pulses. In addition, the thigh and calf should be routinely palpated to ensure no compartmental syndrome develops from fluid extravasation into the soft tissues. Avascular necrosis of the medial femoral condyle can be avoided by placing the femoral tunnel entry-exit points proximal enough to allow preservation of the subchondral bone.

RESULTS

Recent biomechanical in vitro cadaveric studies have documented the advantage of a double bundle PCL construct. Race and Amis demonstrated that anatomic double bundle PCL reconstruction with a bone-patellar tendon-bone graft more closely approximated normal knee kinematics in a cadaver model compared with single bundle reconstruction (2). In addition, Harner et al. published a paper supporting double bundle PCL reconstruction with a transtibial Achilles allograft (1). Furthermore, a biomechanical cadaveric study noted no difference regarding a transtibial versus a tibial inlay technique for PCL reconstruction.

Clinical double-bundle PCL reconstruction studies are in evolution. Wang et al. is the only group to publish a randomized prospective study (3). Thirty-five patients underwent either single or double-bundle transtibial PCL reconstruction with an Achilles allograft. No statistically significant clinical or radiographic differences were demonstrated.

RECOMMENDED READING

Ahn JH, Chung YS, Oh I. Arthroscopic posterior cruciate ligament reconstruction using the posterior transseptal portal. *Arthroscopy.* 2003;19(1):101–107.
Fox RJ, Harner CD, Sakane M, et al. Determination of the in situ forces in the human posterior cruciate ligament using robotic technology—a cadaveric study. *Am J Sports Med.* 1998;26(3):395–401.
Giffin JR, Haemmerle MJ, Vogrin TM, et al. Single- versus double-bundle PCL reconstruction: a biomechanical analysis. *J Knee Surg.* 2002;15(2):114–120.
Harner CD, Janaushek MA, Kanamori A, et al. Biomechanical analysis of a double-bundle posterior cruciate ligament reconstruction. *Am J Sports Med.* 2000;28(2):144–151.
Margheritini F, Mauro CS, Rihn JA, et al. Biomechanical comparison of tibial inlay versus transtibial techniques for posterior cruciate ligament reconstruction: analysis of knee kinematics and graft in situ forces. *Am J Sports Med.* 2004;32(3):587–593.
Margheritini F, Rihn JA, Mauro CS, et al. Biomechanics of initial tibial fixation in posterior cruciate ligament reconstruction. *Arthroscopy.* 2005;21(10):1164–1171.
Noyes FR, Barber-Westin S. Posterior cruciate ligament replacement with a two-strand quadriceps tendon-patellar bone autograft and a tibial inlay technique. *J Bone Joint Surg Am.* 2005;87(6):1241–1252.
Sekiya JK, Haemmerle MJ, Stabile KJ, et al. Biomechanical analysis of a combined double-bundle posterior cruciate ligament and posterolateral corner knee reconstruction. *Am J Sports Med.* 2005;33(3):360–369.
Sekiya JK, West RV, Ong BC, et al. Clinical outcomes after isolated arthroscopic single-bundle posterior cruciate ligament reconstruction. *Arthroscopy.* 2005;21(9):1042–1050.
Shelbourne KD, Davis TJ, Patel DV. The natural history of acute, isolated, nonoperatively treated posterior cruciate ligament injuries. A prospective study. *Am J Sports Med.* 1999;27:276–283.
Shelbourne KD, Gray T. Natural history of acute posterior cruciate ligament tears. *J Knee Surg.* 2002;15(2):103–107.
Sheps DM, Otto D, Fernhout M. The anatomic characteristics of the tibial insertion of the posterior cruciate ligament. *Arthroscopy.* 2005;21(7):820–825.
Torg JS, Barton TM, Pavlov H, et al. Natural history of the posterior cruciate ligament-deficient knee. *Clin Orthop Relat Res.* 1989;(246):208–216.
Yoon KH, Bae DK, Song SJ, et al. Arthroscopic double-bundle augmentation of posterior cruciate ligament using split Achilles allograft. *Arthroscopy.* 2005;21(12):1436–1442.

REFERENCES

1. Harner CD, Vogrin TM, Hoher J, et al. Biomechanical analysis of a double-bundle posterior cruciate ligament reconstruction. Deficiency of the posterolateral structures as a cause of graft failure. *Am J Sports Med.* 2000;28(1):32–39.
2. Race A, Amis AA. PCL reconstruction—in vitro biomechanical comparison of "isometric" versus single- and double-bundle "anatomic" grafts. *J Bone Joint Surg Br.* 1998;80(1):173–179.
3. Wang JC, Weng LH, Hsu CC, et al. Arthroscopic single- versus double-bundle posterior cruciate ligament reconstructions using hamstring autograft. *Injury.* 2004;35(12):1293–1299.

20 Inlay Posterior Cruciate Ligament Reconstruction

Michael A. Rauh, John A. Bergfeld, William M. Wind, and Richard D. Parker

Treatment for posterior cruciate ligament (PCL) injuries has improved recently due in part to greater understanding of the biomechanics and pathophysiology. However, current understanding of this condition continues to lag behind that of the anterior cruciate ligament (ACL) due in part to the relative infrequency with which this injury is encountered. A ruptured PCL, either isolated or combined, is rare compared with other ligamentous injuries of the knee, and accounts for only 5% to 20% of ligamentous disruptions in the knee.

In addition, focused examination on the PCL with the "dial" test, posterior drawer test, and the quadriceps active test along with the development of improved imaging techniques has greatly improved the physician's ability to provide a reliable diagnosis differentiating between an isolated PCL injury and combined injury to the PCL and other capsuloligamentous structures. Knowledge of the correct diagnosis and observation of natural history of these injuries has allowed for the development of improved treatment recommendations.

Most would agree that isolated injuries to the PCL are best treated nonoperatively with adequate results. However, the natural history of isolated injury to the PCL is still debated in the sports community. Definite episodes of instability are uncommon with chronic PCL deficiency as opposed to that feature which is commonly seen after ACL disruption. Our experience has shown a small percentage of patients with PCL deficiency is reported to experience chronic pain and may exhibit degenerative changes in the patellofemoral and medial compartments with time. Furthermore, operative treatment of isolated PCL injuries has had inconsistent results.

Nonetheless, there is a subset of patients for which reconstruction of the PCL is indicated: chronic, isolated grade 3 abnormal laxity of the PCL that has failed nonoperative treatment, as well as acute or chronic PCL injury with combined ligamentous injury. Identifying this subset of patients is the key to a successful outcome from reconstruction of the PCL.

In the past, there have been multiple surgical procedures designed to reconstruct the PCL, yet the literature reveals no long-term studies indicating normal stability following a reconstruction. Early experience with PCL surgery using a transtibial tunnel in a modified open procedure demonstrated that ligament reconstruction would result in an initially stable knee; however, there would be considerable laxity by 1-year follow-up.

Surgical options include the transtibial and posterior tibial inlay reconstructions. The transtibial method involves arthroscopic visualization of the tibial insertion of the PCL with graft passage beyond the acute or commonly referred to "killer turn" at the posterior aspect of the tibial plateau into the medial femoral condyle. With a single-bundle reconstruction, the anterolateral bundle is usually reconstructed since it is larger and stronger than the posteromedial bundle. The posterior inlay technique of PCL replacement has gained recent popularity, and it is currently the technique used for PCL reconstructions at our institutions. We feel that this technique is superior to the other methods for several reasons. First, it is believed to more closely duplicates the normal PCL anatomy. Second, it avoids the so-called "killer curve" found in the arthroscopic-assisted posterior tibial tunnel method. Biomechanical studies have demonstrated that the inlay reconstruction as well as the tibial tunnel reconstruction both provide immediate stability (11). However, these initial studies also demonstrated an area of thinning with the arthroscopic technique as the graft passed around the tibial "killer curve." Subsequent studies demonstrated failure at this location prior to completion of cyclic loading to 2,000 cycles (11,12). Third, the operative technique is considerably easier and safer to perform although it is not an all arthroscopic procedure.

INDICATIONS/CONTRAINDICATIONS

Indications

Optimal management of PCL injuries continues to be an area of debate among orthopaedic surgeons and health care professionals. Current treatment options can be clearly categorized as operative and nonoperative. Nonsurgical treatment is advocated for patients with acute isolated PCL injury, chronic isolated PCL injury in which the patient has not participated in a formal physical therapy regimen, and those injuries found in a patient who is unwilling or unable to participate in the postoperative rehabilitation program (Fig. 20-1).

Operative indications for PCL reconstruction include patients found to have "isolated" tears associated with functional disability, as well as patients with other ligamentous injuries combined with complete PCL injury (Fig. 20-2).

Some authors extend their indications to include what are termed "complete" PCL tears. Clancy and Shelbourne has classified a PCL tear as "complete" if the anterior tibial plateau recedes beyond the distal aspect of the femoral condyles on posterior drawer testing at 90 degrees of flexion. Bergfeld et al noted that if abnormal laxity with the posterior drawer test does not decrease with internal rotation of the tibia, the PCL injury is less likely to do well without surgery (2–4).

Two conditions which few would argue indicate for surgical intervention are:

- Acute and chronic PCL injuries in combination with other capsuloligamentous injuries
- Chronic grade III isolated PCL injuries that are symptomatic.

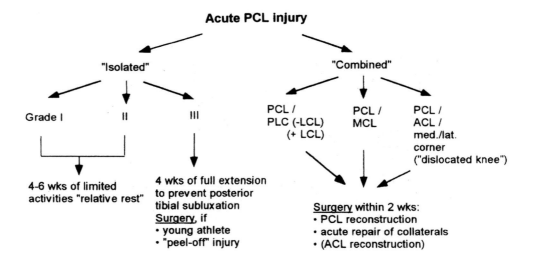

FIGURE 20-1

Treatment algorithm for acute PCL injuries.

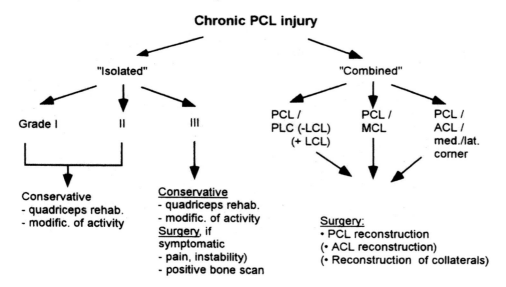

FIGURE 20-2

Treatment algorithm for chronic PCL injuries.

Ultimately, the decision for surgical reconstruction of the PCL is based on the activity level of the patient and whether the injury is isolated or in combination with other ligament injuries. If the posterior drawer test does not decrease with tibial internal rotation, suspicion of associated significant collateral ligament injury must be raised. Clearly, a full discussion of the injury, natural history, as well as the risks and benefits of operative and nonoperative treatment must occur with the patient before any treatment decision.

Contraindications

- An acute, isolated grade I or II PCL tear
- Posterior drawer test with less than 10 mm abnormal posterior laxity at 90 degrees of flexion
- Posterior drawer excursion decreasing with internal rotation of the tibia with less than approximately 5 mm of abnormal posterior laxity
- Less than 5 degrees of abnormal rotatory laxity
- No significant varus or valgus laxity
- Isolated rupture of the PCL in a patient who has not undergone a formal physical therapy program focusing on quadriceps strengthening
- Knee dislocation with arterial or venous injury resulting in limb compromise
- Flexion contracture greater than 10 degrees or extension contracture greater than 30 degrees
- Regional pain syndrome

PREOPERATIVE PLANNING

History

Complete medical history and physical examination are necessary. Orthopaedic examination begins with a history of previous knee injury. Often, an individual has sustained injuries to their knees which may go unnoticed or unremembered unless the patient is specifically asked. It is important to know if the patient had issues with patellar subluxation, meniscal symptoms, or had a prior ligamentous injury. This is important as it can point the physician toward associated injuries and conditions that may alter the treatment plan. Unfortunately, patients with PCL ruptures will infrequently report feeling or hearing a "pop" as is the case with an ACL rupture.

Motor vehicle accidents commonly induce PCL injuries. The knee is commonly flexed when the individual is seated in a car, and the knee is subjected to a posterior-directed force on the tibia. Similarly, the PCL can be ruptured during athletic participation through a fall on the flexed knee, with the foot plantar flexed (Fig. 20-3).

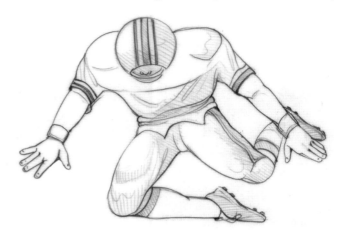

FIGURE 20-3

Mechanism of injury for an isolated PCL injury.

Physical Examination

The physical examination is crucial to identifying patients requiring reconstruction of the PCL. Patients with an acute isolated injury to the PCL usually present with mild to moderate effusion, and often have vague anterior or posterior soreness particularly with flexion. Patients with acute combined injuries may have a more tense effusion. Knee alignment should be noted. In cases of chronic PCL deficiency, attention to gait and lower extremity alignment is performed. Individuals demonstrating a varus alignment and varus thrust with ambulation suggest a combined PCL, posterolateral corner injury.

A complete neurovascular examination of the lower extremity is performed on all patients with suspected ligamentous injuries. Particular attention should be given to the peripheral pulses and the function of the peroneal nerve. Individuals with intact but diminished pulses or ankle-brachial indices less than 0.8 compared with the opposite extremity should undergo observation or further investigation with an angiogram based on vascular surgical consultation.

The integrity of the PCL is most accurately determined through the posterior drawer test, which is performed with the knee in 70 to 90 degrees of flexion and the tibia in neutral, external, and internal rotation. Before performing this test, the normal step-off of the anterior tibia in relation to the femur should be assessed by comparing the contralateral leg. Posterior subluxation of the tibia secondary to PCL insufficiency can give a false impression on the posterior drawer test. If this is the case, an anterior drawer should be performed first to reduce the tibia to its normal position followed by the posterior drawer. Key information is obtained by performing the posterior drawer test at 90 degrees in neutral, internal, and external rotation. An isolated injury to the PCL will show a substantial decrease in the posterior drawer with internal rotation (4). Ritchie et al found the drawer to decrease from 10 mm in neutral rotation to 4 mm with internal rotation in an isolated PCL injury. This decrease is not seen with most combined injuries. The posterior drawer test performed with external rotation, if positive, is suggestive of a combined PCL/posterolateral corner injury.

Knees with isolated Posterolateral Corner (PCL) injuries should also not exhibit increased varus or valgus laxity at 0 or 30 degrees of flexion. If present, this also suggests a combined posteromedial or posterolateral injury. Combination PCL and Posterolateral Corner (PLC) injuries are best determined by the tibial external rotation (dial) test with the knee in both 30 and 90 degrees of flexion.

Although we rely heavily on the posterior drawer test, other important tests include the quadriceps active test, posterior sag test, reverse pivot shift, external rotation recurvatum, and external tibial rotation at 0 and 30 degrees. Again, the key is to differentiate isolated from combined PCL injuries.

Radiographic Examination

Plain radiographs are the next step in evaluating PCL and knee injuries in general. We routinely include bilateral standing anteroposterior, 45-degree flexion weight bearing, Merchant patellar views, as well as a lateral view of the affected extremity. These views allow the orthopaedic physician to document pre-existing arthritis, fractures, joint spaces, knee alignment, as well as evaluate the slope of the proximal tibia. Stress radiographs can be used, with only the risk of radiation and minimal cost, to determine the sagittal translation between the injured and noninjured, presumably intact, knee.

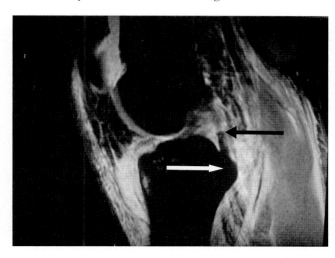

FIGURE 20-4

MRI demonstrating a disrupted PCL (*dark arrow*) with posterior sag (*white arrow*).

Magnetic resonance imaging is felt to be between 96% and 100% sensitive, accurate, and specific in determining PCL ruptures. Magnetic resonance imaging also provides additional necessary information on the status of the remainder of the knee structures such as the ACL, articular cartilage, and menisci (Fig. 20-4).

Graft Options

Graft options for PCL reconstruction include autografts such as bone-patellar-bone, hamstring, and quadriceps. Limitations of these grafts include but are not limited to donor site morbidity and increased operative duration. Allograft options such as Achilles tendon, patella, posterior tibialis, and anterior tibialis tendon are often used for the multiple ligament reconstructions; however, these are associated with a real risk of viral transmission and do rely on creeping substitution for graft incorporation. Despite these limitations, our present graft of choice is Achilles tendon allograft obtained from a reputable bone bank.

SURGERY

Special Items to Have

- Two operating room tables
- Thirty- and seventy-degree arthroscopes with a full arthroscopy setup
- Sterile tourniquet
- PCL femoral drill guide
- Graft passer (DePuy Graft Passer, Johnson & Johnson, New Brunswick, NJ)
- Osteotomes
- Standard 6.5-mm stainless steel cancellous screws with washer
- PCL (vaginal) retractors—blunt tipped with differential angles of retraction

Patient Positioning

- The patient is identified in the holding area and the operative extremity is marked.
- Preoperative prophylactic antibiotics (usually a first-generation cephalosporin) are administered within 30 minutes of incision.
- After induction of general anesthesia, an examination is performed of both knees, again looking for associated capsuloligamentous injuries. Specifically, the operating surgeon is responsible for determining the presence or absence of injury to the posterolateral and posteromedial structures in the operative extremity.
- A "time out" is performed and again the operative extremity is identified by the operating surgeon, the head circulating nurse, and the anesthesia team.
- The surgery begins with the patient supine on the operating table.
- Before the knee is prepped and draped, an intra-articular injection of 0.25% bupivicaine with 1:400,000 epinephrine and 2 mg of morphine sulfate is given into the operative knee.

- The opposite lower extremity is placed in a padded gynecologic stirrup that is widely abducted away from the operative extremity. A Mayo stand cover does well to provide a first sterile cover over the nonoperative leg.
- The operative leg is positioned hanging free to allow for full knee flexion during surgery. A lateral post is used to assist in arthroscopy treatment of associated intra-articular pathology.

Technique

Arthroscopic Evaluation and Debridement   The procedure begins with a diagnostic arthroscopy without elevating the tourniquet. Articular cartilage and meniscal pathology are addressed at this time. The PCL injury is documented as well as the status of the ACL and meniscofemoral ligaments. The ACL will usually appear lax secondary to the posterior tibial subluxation. An anterior drawer will restore its normal appearance. The PCL remnant on the medial wall of the intercondylar notch is debrided arthroscopically. Care is taken to preserve the intact meniscofemoral ligament. Exposure of the notch allows for identification of the femoral anatomic attachment site of the PCL complex—composed of the PCL, and the anterior and posterior meniscofemoral ligaments of Humphrey and Wrisberg, respectively (FAAS). The FAAS is located anterior and distal in the notch, approximately 8 to 10 mm from the articular margin at the 11 o'-clock position in a left knee and the 1 o'clock position in a right knee. The femoral footprint is identified, and remnants are left to provide an anatomic landmark for placement of the femoral tunnel guidewire. A curette is used to score the desired femoral tunnel site. The FAAS is only marked at this stage as it will be rechecked later through a small medial arthrotomy at the time of guide pin placement. Again, careful attention is paid to preservation of the meniscofemoral ligaments. In particular, the anterior meniscofemoral ligament of Humphrey remains intact and should remain so after debridement and tunnel drilling. Note that if concomitant ACL surgery is planned, the ACL femoral and tibial anatomic attachment sites are identified and drilled at this time.

Graft Preparation   If using an Achilles tendon allograft, prepare the calcaneal bone plug for anticipated implantation in the posterior tibial trough. Optimally, it should be 10 mm wide, 20 mm long, and approximately 5 mm thick. This is the bone that will ultimately fit into the trough to be created posteriorly. Using Krackow-type suture fixation, the tendinous end of the Achilles graft is made tubular to allow for later passage through the femoral tunnel and ultimate fixation. If using a bone-patellar tendon-bone autograft, the bone plug from the patella is usually 10 mm wide and 30 mm long, whereas the bone plug from the tibia should be 10 mm wide, 20 mm long, and approximately 5 mm thick. The patellar bone plug should pass easily through a 9-mm sizer, and is fashioned to fit in the femoral tunnel. The tibial bone plug should be fashioned to fit in a trough made at the tibial attachment site of the PCL. The trough will correspond to the size of the tibial bone plug. Once this is completed, use a 2-mm drill to make two holes in the patellar bone plug, 5 mm and 15 mm from the distal tip, respectively. A No. 5 nonabsorbable suture is passed through each hole for later graft passage and tensioning. The tibial plug should be fashioned into a rectangle 10 mm wide and 20 mm long. For either graft choice, a drill hole should be made with a 3.2-mm drill bit through the center of this bone plug. The hole should be angled slightly distal to make up for the slope of the posterior tibia, which will cause the screw to angle toward the joint otherwise. The hole should be drilled from the cancellous side to avoid injury to the soft tissue portion of the graft. The hole should be over-drilled with a 4.5-mm drill and tapped accordingly. Next, a 6.5-mm partially threaded screw, 35 mm in length, and washer should be inserted until it protrudes approximately 5 mm past the cancellous surface. Alternatively, two small-fragment cancellous screws may be used to fix the posterior bone plug. A cadaveric study in press performed by the lead author showed no difference in pull-out strength between the two techniques (13). The graft is now ready for implantation (Fig. 20-5).

Femoral Tunnel Creation

While the graft is being prepared by an assistant on the back table, the femoral tunnel is made through a medial arthrotomy. If autograft is being used, it can be done through the same incision as for graft harvest. A small medial arthrotomy is made adjacent to the patellar tendon, extending to the vastus medialis at the level of the adductor tubercle. The arthrotomy extends posteriorly along the inferior aspect of the muscle, which is elevated anteriorly, revealing the medial femoral condyle (1). The intercondylar notch is visualized by retracting the patella laterally. The previously marked FAAS is identified and checked for accurate placement. Through the arthrotomy the PCL femoral guide tip is

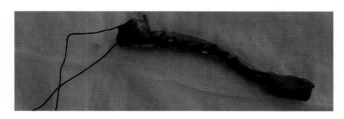

FIGURE 20-5
Prepared Achilles tendon allograft.

placed at the FAAS, approximately 8 mm proximal to the articular margin. This should leave the edge of the tunnel 2 to 3 mm from the articular edge after drilling. The tunnel should be angled proximally and posteriorly to decrease the obliquity of the femoral tunnel, which decreases the stress on the graft as it enters the tunnel. Using this aiming guide, the femoral guide pin is then drilled from the outside to the inside. As demonstrated by Handy et al, the PCL tracks at approximately 85 degrees. An inside-out technique makes reproduction of this angle difficult. The anterior/distal tunnel guide pin, reproducing the anterolateral bundle, should enter the intracondylar notch at the 11 or 1 o'clock position as noted previously and optimally should be approximately 8 to 10 mm proximal to the articular surface of the medial femoral condyle. The wire should be directed lateral, posterior, and proximal, duplicating the direction of the native PCL ligament (3). Ideally, graft preparation is occurring simultaneously as this step. The diameter of the femoral tunnel is determined by adding 1 mm to the size of the femoral/tendinous portion of the Achilles allograft. Usual tunnel size is 10 mm. Tunnel sizers are used to obtain this measurement. The edges are chamfered and smoothed with a rasp. A suture passing device is then placed within the tunnel (DePuy Graft Passer, Johnson & Johnson, New Brunswick, NJ). Next, an 18-gauge wire loop or commercially available graft passer is placed through the femoral tunnel and directed posteriorly into the notch. This is placed posterior within the notch so as to facilitate later graft passage through the posterior approach. The wound is loosely approximated, and the tourniquet deflated if employed. A sterile circumferential dressing is placed, and the entire leg is covered in a sterile bag (Mayo stand cover). This is overwrapped with a long ACE wrap.

First Patient Turn, Burk's Approach to the Posterior Tibia   After having placed the operative extremity in a sterile circumferential dressing, a second operating room table is positioned beside the patient. Under the direction of the surgeon and anesthetist, the patient is turned to the prone position. We have found the extra 10 to 15 minutes needed to perform this is well worth the effort. The previous operating table should be cleaned and prepared to place the patient back in the supine position after posterior dissection and graft placement. Ensure that all bony prominences have been padded adequately. Once the patient is in the prone position, the sterile dressing is removed. If there is any question of a break in sterile technique, then the entire leg is reprepped and draped. A modified Burk approach to the posterior tibia is performed (Fig. 20-6). The landmarks for the incision are the medial border of the medial head of the gastrocnemius, the lateral border of the semitendinosis, the popliteal crease, and the midline of the distal thigh (5). This portion of the procedure is performed without elevating the tourniquet to ensure adequate hemostasis is achieved. The skin is incised and the fascia exposed. The medial sural cutaneous nerve is vulnerable near the midline at this level and should be avoided if possible. The fascia is incised and the interval between the medial head of the gastrocnemius and semitendinosis is developed (Fig. 20-7). The fascia over the proximal popliteus muscle near the distal portion of the insertion of the PCL is incised to allow for distal retraction of the popliteus muscle if necessary. A broad blunt retractor is placed in this interval, and the medial head of the gastrocnemius is retracted laterally protecting the neurovascular bundle. A portion of the medial gastrocnemius origin can be released if extra exposure is needed, but we have usually found this unnecessary. The inferior medial geniculate artery and vein may be ligated as necessary. Next, the capsule is incised longitudinally and reflected medially and laterally. This exposes the tibial insertion of the PCL. The remaining scar tissue and PCL remnants are excised with care to avoid the meniscofemoral ligaments. To facilitate exposure, the knee may be flexed 15 to 20 degrees and the tibia externally rotated.

Creation of the Posterior Tibial Trough, Femoral Graft Passage, and Graft Fixation   Once the insertion site is marked, a cortical window is made with an osteotome. The window is approximately 11 × 20 mm and corresponds to the bone plug previously prepared (Fig. 20-8). The graft is now brought into the operative field. The femoral plug is passed through the

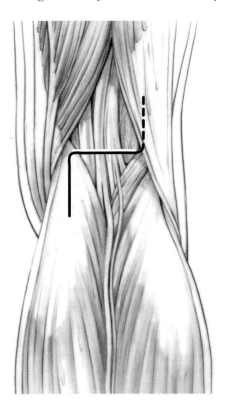

FIGURE 20-6

Modified Burk and Shaffer posterior exposure with the surgical incision (*solid line*) centered proximally on the medial head of the gastrocnemius. The incision can be extended (*dashed line*) proximally for further exposure

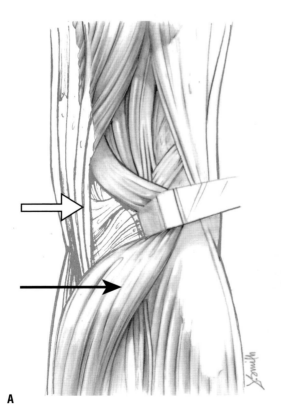

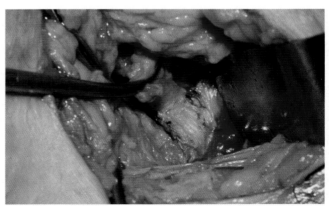

A   **B**

FIGURE 20-7

Drawing **(A)** and clinical photograph **(B)** of the interval between the medial gastrocnemius (*dark arrow*) and semimembranosus (*light arrow*).

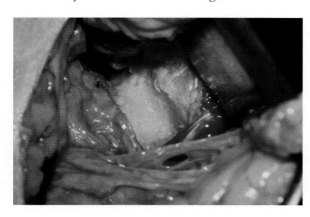

FIGURE 20-8
Bony trough created in the posterior tibia.

intercondylar notch and into the femoral tunnel using the previously placed graft passer. Next, the tibial bone plug is fitted into the prepared trough on the back of the tibia. The 6.5 screw is tightened securing the bone plug to the posterior tibia. It is not necessary to predrill the cancellous bone. Tension is then placed on the femoral end of the graft to ensure adequate fixation is present. Intraoperative radiographs can be used to check screw placement. Once adequate tibial fixation is achieved, the capsule is closed with No. 1 nonabsorbable suture, as well as the fascia. The subcutaneous tissue is closed with a 2-0 absorbable suture, and the skin is closed with a subcuticular closure. The leg is again covered with a sterile Mayo stand cover and the patient is placed supine on the original operating table.

Second Patient Turn and Femoral Graft Fixation   The sterile dressing is removed. If there is any concern of breakdown of sterile technique, the leg is reprepped and draped as described previously. With attention and care, this step is not frequently necessary. With the knee flexed to 80 degrees in neutral rotation, an anterior drawer is applied to the proximal tibia. The graft in the femoral tunnel is tensioned in this position by pulling on the sutures in the femoral bone plug. If using a bone-patellar tendon-bone graft, it is important to determine the amount of bone within the femoral tunnel. If 20 to 25 mm of bone is in the femoral tunnel, the graft is fixed with a 9×20 mm interference screw placed proximally to secure the bone plug distally in the tunnel (closest to the articular surface). If less than 20 mm of bone plug is within the femoral tunnel or an Achilles allograft is being used, a trough is made in the medial femoral condyle and fixation is achieved with either two spiked staples or by tying the sutures to a 6.5-mm post in the medial femoral condyle. Alternatively, one may choose to use an interference screw within the femoral tunnel with back-up staple fixation. After fixation, the knee is flexed and extended to ensure an adequate range of motion. A gentle posterior drawer at 90 degrees can be performed, and the anterior tibial step-off should be restored. Once the surgical team is satisfied with stability, the wounds are irrigated and a layered closure is performed.

Pearls and Pitfalls

- When using a bone patellar tendon bone graft, careful attention should be paid to the tibial fixation site because the graft is a fixed length. Once the graft is fixed on the posterior tibia, it is tensioned on the femoral side, and the position of the bone plug in the femoral tunnel is assessed. If 25 mm or more of the bone plug is within the femoral tunnel at this point, the tibial attachment site is accepted. On the other hand, if less than 25 mm of bone is within the femoral tunnel, the tibial attachment site can be adjusted distally. The tibial side of the graft can be distalized 10 mm without affecting the mechanical properties of the reconstruction. If it is felt that more than 10 mm of distalization is needed, do not move the tibial attachment site, and fix the femoral end in a trough as described previously.
- It may be necessary to divide a portion of the upper (proximal) aspect of the popliteus muscle to gain good exposure of the posterior tibia.
- As mentioned previously, when placing the 6.5-mm screw in the tibial bone plug, it is helpful to angle distally slightly. Otherwise, when the graft is placed on the posterior slope of the tibia, the screw will angle toward the articular surface.

- It is helpful, when identifying the FAAS of the PCL on the femur, to use an angled curet to mark the site. To locate a spot 8 to 10 mm from the articular margin, the tip of the curet is placed at the articular margin. Next, your thumb can be placed on the curet 8 to 10 mm from the edge of the skin where the curet enters the medial portal. Advance the curet until your thumb touches the skin. This will place the curet tip 8 to 10 mm off the articular margin, and this spot can be marked.

- If an ACL reconstruction is being performed in conjunction with a PCL reconstruction, care must be taken not to damage the tibial tunnel for the ACL. This can occur in the inlay technique if the 6.5 screw securing the bone plug to the tibia is directed into the ACL tibial tunnel. This can be avoided by directing the screw slightly lateral. With the tibial tunnel technique the starting point for the ACL and PCL tibial tunnels are close. Care should be taken that these do not intersect. To avoid this, a drill can be placed and left in one tunnel while the other is being drilled.

- As previously mentioned, excess penetration with a guide pin while drilling a tibial tunnel can cause injury to the posterior neurovascular structures. This can be avoided by locking the pin into the drill 1 cm shorter than the distance required to reach the guide tip. It can be advanced slowly the rest of the way by hand. Also, a curet can be placed over the tip of the pin through the posteromedial portal while reaming to avoid advancement of the pin.

POSTOPERATIVE MANAGEMENT

Following wound closure, a cryotherapy pad and compressive stocking are applied. The knee is immobilized in full extension. The postoperative regimen involves keeping the leg immobilized for 4 weeks. During this period of immobilization, we use a cast or a range of motion brace locked in extension and are careful not to allow posterior sag. If using a cast, it is changed at week 1, week 2, and week 4. At 4 weeks postoperatively, the patient begins gentle range of motion. Once the patient gains 90 degrees of motion, the knee immobilizer is discarded. Following this, a posterior stabilizing knee brace is applied. The patient wears the brace for all activities for the first 2 months. The patient then is started on isotonic quadriceps, extension exercises, and closed chain exercises to strengthen the hamstring muscles. We do not allow any isotonic hamstring muscle exercises. Once the patient is walking well, we progress to a "slideboard" activity, which usually occurs at approximately 3 months. Agility drills and sports-specific activities follow, with an anticipated return to play at approximately 9 to 12 months following surgery.

COMPLICATIONS

As with any surgical procedure, there is a constant risk of infection. Other than prophylactic antibiotics, attention to sterile technique, and appropriate soft tissue handling, not much more can be done to lessen this risk. The process of repositioning the patient for this surgery twice definitely increases the opportunity for contamination; however, the use of a sterile tourniquet and strict attention to detail by the surgeon and staff should limit patient exposure.

In addition, exposures that are unfamiliar to an operating surgeon can be filled with danger. Preoperative cadaveric dissection and anatomy review is essential to the posterior approach described herein. The surgeon needs to be aware of anomalous branches of the genicular arteries as well. Complications can also be related to the creation of tunnels and placement of hardware. The operating surgeon must be fully aware of the position of bony tunnels and the implications on the survival of the graft and the ability to perform other procedures.

RESULTS

Given the relative infrequency with which the PCL is reconstructed in the sports-injured patient, it is difficult to obtain the numbers necessary to create a randomized prospective study that definitively determines the optimal mode of reconstruction. The inlay technique has been compared with the all-arthroscopic technique and some have felt that there is no true difference in outcomes. However, our decision to use the inlay technique has been based on basic science research that has shown that avoidance of the "killer turn" can lead to decreased laxity at follow-up (1–4,8–11). Current outcomes following PCL reconstruction rely on retrospective studies and control groups. Two good studies with at least 2-year follow-up have shown satisfactory outcomes with significantly less posterior laxity at final followup (6,7). Certainly, the biomechanical studies create speculation regarding the long-term viability of the implanted graft, which, if failed, could lead to long-term instability and arthrosis.

CONCLUSION

Reconstructions of the PCL are uncommon compared to other knee procedures. This procedure is generally reserved for patients with acute or chronic combined PCL/capsuloligamentous injuries, as well as isolated PCL injuries that have failed nonoperative treatment. Isolated PCL injuries are not routinely operated on otherwise. Key components of the history, physical examination, and diagnostic studies are used to identify candidates for PCL reconstruction. There is a great deal of technical difficulty with this procedure and a relative lack of knowledge about the natural history and reconstructive biomechanics of PCL injuries compared with ACL injuries. In light of this, reconstruction of the PCL is currently an evolving process.

RECOMMENDED READING

Cosgarea AJ, Jay PR. Posterior cruciate ligament injuries: evaluation and management. *JAAOS*. 2001;9:297–307.

Oliviero J, Miller MD. Posterior cruciate ligament reconstruction: tibial inlay technique. *Tech in Knee Surg*. 2003;2(1): 63–72.

Wind WM, Bergfeld JA, Parker RD. Evaluation and treatment of posterior cruciate ligament injuries: revisited. *Am J Sports Med*. 2004;32(7):1765–1775.

REFERENCES

1. Bergfeld JA, Graham SM. Tibial inlay procedure for PCL reconstruction: one-tunnel and two-tunnel. *Op Tech Sports Med*. 2001;9(2):69–75.
2. Bergfeld JA, McAllister DR, Parker RD, et al. A biomechanical comparison of posterior cruciate ligament reconstruction techniques. *Am J Sports Med*. 2001;29(2):129–136.
3. Bergfeld JA, Graham SM, Parker RD, et al. A biomechanical comparison of posterior cruciate ligament reconstructions using single- and double-bundle tibial inlay techniques. *Am J Sports Med*. 2005 Jul;33(7):976–981.
4. Bergfeld JA, McAllister DR, Parker RD, et al. The effects of tibial rotation of posterior translation in knees in which the posterior cruciate ligament has been cut. *J Bone Joint Surg Am*. 2001;83:1339–1343.
5. Burks RT, Schaffer JJ. A simplified approach to the tibial attachment of the posterior cruciate ligament. *Clin Orthop Relat Res*. 1990;254:216–219.
6. Cooper DE, Stewart D. Posterior cruciate ligament reconstruction using single-bundle patella tendon graft with tibial inlay fixation: 2- to 10-year follow-up. *Am J Sports Med*. 2004 Mar;32(2):346–360.
7. Jung YB, Tae SK, Jung HJ, et al. Replacement of the torn posterior cruciate ligament with a mid-third patellar tendon graft with use of a modified tibial inlay method. *J Bone Joint Surg Am*. 2004 Sep;86-A(9):1878–1883.
8. Markolf K, Davies M, Zoric B, et al. Effects of bone block position and orientation within the tibial tunnel for posterior cruciate ligament graft reconstructions: a cyclic loading study of bone-patellar tendon-bone allografts. *Am J Sports Med*. 2003;31(5):673–679.
9. Markolf KL, O'Neill G, Jackson SR, et al. Reconstruction of knees with combined cruciate deficiencies: a biomechanical study. *J Bone Joint Surg Am*. 2003;85-A(9):1768–1774.
10. Markolf KL, Slauterbeck JR, Armstrong KL, et al. A biomechanical study of the replacement of the posterior cruciate ligament with a graft. *J Bone Joint Surg Am*. 1997;79(3):375–387.
11. Markolf KL, Zemanovic JR, McAllister DR. Cyclic loading of posterior cruciate ligament replacements fixed with tibial tunnel and tibial inlay methods. *J Bone Joint Surg Am*. 2002;84-A(4):518–524.
12. McAllister DR, Markolf KL, Oakes DA, et al. A biomechanical comparison of tibial inlay and tibial tunnel posterior cruciate ligament reconstruction techniques: graft pretension and knee laxity. *Am J Sports Med*. 2002;30(3):312–7.
13. Rauh MA, Munjal S, Carney K, et al. Fixation strength of tibial inlay graft with one versus two screws. A cadaveric study. *Orthopedics*. In Press.

21

Posterolateral Corner and Fibular Collateral Ligament Reconstruction

E. Lyle Cain, Jr., and William G. Clancy, Jr.

Posterolateral rotatory instability (PLRI), unlike anterior cruciate ligament (ACL) deficiency, is a relatively infrequently encountered instability pattern that has historically been under-diagnosed and poorly treated. Because this instability pattern is uncommon, it is frequently not diagnosed at the time of initial injury, often presenting as chronic disability. Posterolateral corner injury may result in the worst functional instability pattern of any type of knee ligament injury. These injuries produce excessive tibial external rotation, posterior tibial translation, and varus laxity. Excessive external rotation of the tibia allows for an unwinding moment on the cruciate ligaments, which enhances joint laxity and adversely affects the cruciate ligament reconstruction or the native ligament mechanics. External tibial rotation brings the ACL tibial insertion laterally toward its lateral femoral condyle origin, producing laxity in the ACL. Similarly, external tibial rotation brings the posterior cruciate ligament (PCL) tibial insertion medially toward the medial femoral condyle origin, producing laxity of the PCL.

INDICATIONS/CONTRAINDICATIONS

Posterolateral rotatory instability of the knee, defined has excessive external tibial rotation producing functional instability, can be one of the most disabling of all knee instability patterns. The posterolateral corner consists anatomically of one dynamic stabilizer and several static stabilizers that contribute to a functional stability of the knee. The popliteus muscle tendon complex is the primary dynamic stabilizer, and the popliteal fibular ligament has received added attention recently in the orthopaedic literature as a static stabilizer. The other static structures important for stability include the fibular collateral ligament (FCL) complex as well as the arcuate ligament, posterolateral capsule, and PCL. The importance of PLRI is that if not diagnosed and treated properly, it may lead to failure of other ligament reconstructions, particularly ACL or PCL reconstruction procedures. Harner and colleagues have found that sectioning of the posterolateral structures of the knee resulted in a 150% increase in PCL forces in cadaveric knees. Posterolateral rotatory instability can be classified into one of five types according to the etiology and associated instability patterns with or without varus laxity or thrust.

The first type of PLRI is traumatic. This often occurs secondary to a significant contact injury, most commonly a varus blow from the medial surface of the knee causing a lateral or posterolateral corner tear. The lateral stabilizing instructions of the knee are frequently torn concomitantly, including the fibular collateral ligament as well as other ligamentous structures including the ACL, PCL, or both. With traumatic PLRI, treatment of the other ligament injuries such as cruciate ligament injury will correct anterior and posterior translation of the knee; however, rotational instability may persist. Failure to address PLRI may ultimately lead to failure of ACL or PCL reconstruction. The second type PLRI is known as symptomatic physiologic instability. This type of PLRI is most commonly caused by relatively minor injury occurring in persons already having symmetric excessive external rotation in both knees. However, it may occur without history of even minor trauma, similar to the development of multidirectional instability of the shoulder. We believe that this type of PLRI may be due to electromechanical dissociation of the popliteus muscle, similar to that described by Rowe in the multidirectionally unstable shoulder. In this typem of PLRI, the cruciate ligaments are normal as is the fibular collateral ligament. Lateral (varus) laxity is similar to the ininvolved leg. This rotational instability produces clinical symptoms and history of giving way and instability, particularly with rotational maneuvers, because of excessive lateral tibial rotation with pivoting maneuvers. The diagnosis of symptomatic physiologic instability is often overlooked because of intact cruciate ligaments and a relatively minor trauma necessary to produce this clinical instability. We have observed physiologic asymptomatic excessive external tibial rotation in approximately 10% to 15% of normal knees. Cooper and others have reported excessive physiologic external tibial rotation in 35% of patients. It is important to note that this type of PLRI is typically bilateral and usually does not occur with any significant varus laxity.

The third type of PLRI is combined traumatic cruciate injury with physiologic posterolateral laxity. This occurs with isolated tearing of either the ACL or PCL with concomitant low-grade injury to the posterolateral corner in an individual already having excessive physiologic external rotation. We assume this injury to be the case whenever there is a 3+ posterior drawer present along with excessive tibial external rotation equal to the contralateral side with a PCL injury. Clinically, there is often no increased varus laxity nor is there any injury visible to the popliteus tendon or fibular collateral ligament seen on magnetic resonance imaging (MRI). With concomitant tearing of the ACL, the ACL deficiency and posterolateral rotatory instability often negate each other. Reconstruction of the ACL without attention to the posterolateral corner eliminates the anterior posterior instability but effectively increases the dysfunction of posterolateral excessive rotation of PLRI. Sometimes this occurs to such extent that the individual complains of symptoms with instability worse than was felt before ACL surgery. It is very difficult to determine whether the physiologic posterolateral laxity is pathologic and whether it should be addressed during ACL reconstruction. After the ACL graft has been fixed during reconstruction, the presence of a mild increase in Lachman or pivot glide strongly suggests that the PLRI is pathologic and should be corrected surgically.

In cases of isolated PCL injury with physiologic external rotation deformity, isolated reconstruction of the PCL without reconstruction of the posterolateral corner results in persistence of external rotation excess and posterior tibial sag. Increased external rotation causes the tibial insertion of the PCL to rotate medially and anteriorly, shortening the distance of insertion of the PCL on the medial femoral condyle, and producing functional laxity of the PCL although the PCL reconstruction may be intact. Therefore, symptoms may persist after PCL reconstruction if PLRI is not addressed.

The fourth type of PLRI includes posterolateral instability with varus alignment and varus thrust. This clinical situation occurs in the patient who has an injury to the posterolateral structures with or without fibular collateral ligament injury in a varus knee. When this patient is weightbearing, they have a significant varus thrust which leads to worsening of the PLRI and varus instability. With this situation, medial compartment degenerative changes and joint space narrowing are often present as well as the native varus alignment. We often perform valgus osteotomy in these patients to correct both the varus position as well as a varus thrust prior to, or in combination with, posterolateral reconstruction.

The fifth type of PLRI is posterolateral instability with medial and lateral laxity. This is a rare entity but is seen when the femur has a medial then lateral shift on the tibia during the stance phase of gait. This could be significant for posterolateral laxity with varus thrust; however, it is a straight medial-lateral instability pattern not associated posterolateral corner injury. Most likely, this represents musculoelectrical disassociation similar to pathology in some patients with multidirectional instability of the shoulder and will not benefit from present surgical techniques to reconstruct the posterolateral corner.

Our current indications for posterolateral cruciate reconstruction or fibular collateral ligament reconstruction include a symptomatic knee with any of the PLRI patterns classified previously. The most common patient in our practice presents with either ACL or PCL injury with combined traumatic posterolateral corner injury as well. Any findings on MRI or examination of ecchymosis or swelling along the posterolateral structures of the knee including popliteus, fibular collateral ligament, or posterolateral capsule should be assumed to have posterolateral rotatory instability until proven otherwise by appropriate examination. In the acute setting, we generally repair all the injured structures including the fibular collateral ligament, biceps femorus muscle tendon complex, iliotibial band, popliteus tendon complex, as well as the posterolateral capsule. In many acute cases, the popliteus muscle tendon complex has been damaged to the extent that is not reasonable to repair this structure. Injuries to the popliteus often occur in the muscle tendon junction and are not amenable to acute repair. In these acute settings with posterolateral corner instability and poor tissue quality or muscle tendon junction popliteus tear, we generally perform an acute posterolateral cruciate reconstruction using allograft Achilles tendon. In the chronic situation, we perform posterolateral cruciate reconstruction with or without fibular collateral ligament reconstruction using Achilles tendon allograft.

Several authors have described techniques for either reattaching, repairing, or reconstructing the posterolateral and fibular collateral structures. Hughston's posterolateral reconstruction, described as anterior and superior advancement of the lateral gastrocnemius tendon, superior posterolateral capsule, fibular collateral ligament, and popliteus tendon, is possible only with intact native structures and has not been met with much success in our experience. Jakob and associates have recommended recession of the popliteus tendon insertion on the femur, but this often fails to improve static or functional stability because of damage to the structures distal to that insertion site. Until 1996, biceps femoris tendon tenodesis and rerouting at the lateral femoral condyle was the senior author's (WCG) preference for correction of mild to moderate PLRI without the presence of varus thrust. Although this procedure led to predictable and satisfactory results in the mild and moderate cases, it required an intact biceps muscle tendon complex and often required hardware removal at a second surgical procedure. We have performed the posterolateral cruciate reconstruction in severe cases since 1979, and have employed it exclusively in mild, moderate, or severe PLRI since 1996.

Our current preference for acute augmentation or chronic injuries to the posterolateral corner is the posterolateral cruciate reconstruction (PLCR) with one-half Achilles tendon allograft as well as fibular collateral ligament reconstruction with the opposite half of the Achilles tendon allograft. Posterolateral cruciate reconstruction differs from the Hughston or Jakob reconstructions in that PLCR does not rely on healthy native tissues. Immediate knee motion is possible, and hardware removal is usually unnecessary. However, posterolateral cruciate reconstruction alone does not correct for straight lateral (varus) laxity. Therefore, if varus laxity is additionally present with PLRI, the fibular collateral ligament is reconstructed as well. Valgus tibial osteotomy may be considered in conjunction with PLCR or other cruciate ligament procedures in some cases. These patients typically have varus laxity with medial joint space narrowing and a varus thrust in the stance phase of gait. Failure to correct the varus alignment may cause stretching and eventual failure of the posterolateral structures, as suggested by Noyes. At the time of surgery, the osteotomy should be performed first followed by either concomitant or delayed posterolateral cruciate reconstruction and fibular collateral ligament reconstruction.

PREOPERATIVE PLANNING

A proper preoperative evaluation is essential to correctly evaluate the instability pattern for posterolateral rotatory instability.

History

The typical history of patients with acute PLRI is significant for a discrete injury with a blow to the medial side of the knee resulting in varus force, often combined with hyperextension (Fig. 21-1). The mechanism of injury should alert the examiner to look for disruption of the posterolateral structures, the lateral structures, especially the fibular collateral ligament, and associated ACL or PCL injury.

In the chronically disabled individual, the history of significant remote trauma is frequently elucidated but the mechanism is often unclear. More importantly, the individual expresses a very frequent sense of instability with minimal activities, causing giving way that may be associated with

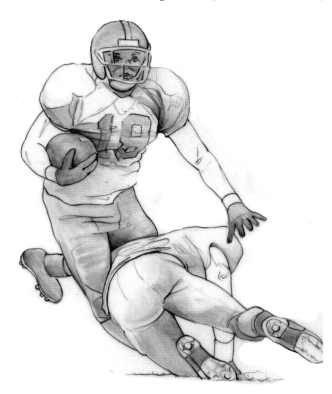

FIGURE 21-1

Typical mechanism for acute
posterolateral corner and ACL injury
by a blow to the anteromedial tibia
causing varus and hyperextension.

ACL instability. In addition, each episode of giving way is usually accompanied by pain along the posterolateral corner of the knee.

Physical Examination

In the acutely injured knee, findings often include marked rotational and varus instability at 30 degrees of flexion (with fibular collateral and posterolateral injury). If significant varus instability is present at full extension (0 degrees) or 90 degrees flexion, suspicion for disruption of one of the cruciate ligaments must be evaluated. The amount of excessive external rotation can be measured with the pateint supine with hips flexed 90 degrees and the knee flexed 30 degrees. The lower leg is externally rotated and heel and foot position is noted for both legs to determine the amount of relative side to side exernal rotation. The knee is then flexed to 90 degrees and similar external rotation is performed. Some believe that the amount of external rotation is best assessed in the prone position with foot external rotation at 30 and 90 degrees knee flexion. We believe that a more accurate method to measure excessive external rotation is done by placing the patient supine with the hips flexed 90 degrees and knees 30 degrees. The lateral femoral epicondyle and anterior and posterior borders of the fibular head are marked and both legs are externally rotated. The test is repeated at 90 degrees knee flexion. Excessive external rotation is present if the anterior border of the fibular head passes posterior to the mark on the lateral femoral epicondyle. Warren and Noyes have clearly demonstrated that excessive external rotation noted to increase between 30 and 90 degrees knee flexion indicates probable PCL injury.

Ecchymosis and soft tissue swelling may be present along the lateral and posterolateral side of the knee, and the fibular collateral ligament frequently is not palpable as a tight cord-like structure as is found in the normal knee. If the cruciate ligaments have also been damaged, a positive result on Lachman, anterior drawer, posterior drawer, pivot shift, or reverse pivot shift test may be present. As a rule, complete isolated tear of the PCL will not have more than a 2+ posterior drawer (i.e., the tibial plateau will be flush with the femoral condyles with the knee flexed at 90 degrees of flexion). Any further posterior sag of the tibia on the femur (3+ posterior drawer) is almost always indicative of concomitant posterolateral rotatory instability with posterolateral corner injury. In the awake patient, when the acute knee is examined, further evaluation is always difficult. One should, however, try to evaluate the amount of external rotation of the tibia at 30 and 90 degrees of knee flexion as well as attempt to perform a reverse pivot shift maneuver to test the posterolateral corner and PCL.

In the individual with chronic instability, determination of external rotation compared with the opposite knee at 30 and 90 degrees is essential. This maneuver should reproduce a sense of giving way as well as pain along the lateral side of the knee with PLRI. Varus alignment of the knee may or may not be present, and ambulation may bring out a significant varus thrust. Finally, while sitting with the knee flexed at 90 degrees and the affected foot on the floor, PLRI patients can often reproduce the sensation of dynamic instability by voluntarily firing the biceps femoris muscle, thereby producing marked external rotation and subluxation of lateral tibial plateau on the lateral femoral condyle. This may be considered a pathognomonic sign of posterolateral rotatory instability but must be distinguished from the performance of an anterior drawer in the case of isolated ACL or posterior drawer in the case of PCL deficiency.

Additional Testing

Routine radiographs including both supine and standing anteroposterior views of both knees should be performed to assess lower extremity alignment. In the acute setting, a fracture of the posterolateral tibial plateau should raise the suspicion of PLRI. In the knee with chronic PLRI, significant degeneration of the medial compartment and varus alignment may dictate the need for concomitant osteotomy. Magnetic resonance imaging is routinely ordered to confirm the status of the cruciates, the menisci, and the articular cartilage structures as well as assess any fibular collateral or posterolateral capsular injury.

SURGERY

Preoperatively, the patient is instructed on proper crutch ambulation. Information is also provided about the expected hospital course, which is typically a 24-hour observation stay after surgery. The patient is instructed on immediate postoperative rehabiltation activities including quadricep exercises and early range of motion.

General anesthesia is preferred in this procedure due to the potential length and complexity of multiligament reconstruction. Once adequate anesthesia has been established, a thorough examination under anesthesia is performed on the affected knee with comparison to the unaffected knee. Examination includes inspection, range of motion, and stability testing to confirm the ligament instability as suspected preoperatively.

Technique

With the patient in the supine position, a tourniquet is placed on the upper thigh, and the lower extremity is prepped and draped free. The tourniquet is not generally inflated for the procedure, but is applied for the occasional case requiring assistance for hemostasis. Operative knee arthroscopy is performed initially with any intra-articular pathology addressed including chondral lesions, meniscal tears, or cruciate ligament injury. The tunnels are generally drilled for the ACL or PCL reconstruction before the posterolateral corner reconstruction is performed. In the acute setting, the lateral structures may be exposed initially to allow full egress of arthroscopic pump fluid from the lateral side of the knee and prevent overdistension of the soft tissues along the lateral knee and proximal anterior tibial muscular compartments. Once the intra-articular work is completed, the posterolateral cruciate and femoral collateral ligament reconstructions are performed.

A lateral curvilinear incision is made with the incision passing midway between Gerdy's tubercle and the fibular head on the lateral surface of the knee (Fig. 21-2). The subcutaneous tissues are pulled posteriorly using a dry lap sponge to expose the iliotibial (IT) band and the biceps femoris tendon. The peroneal nerve should be identified just posterior to the biceps tendon (Fig. 21-3). The surgeon should be aware of its position at all times during the reconstruction. The IT band is then incised in line with its fibers beginning at the point where it crosses the lateral femoral epicondyle and proceeding distally. This exposes the insertion point on the lateral femoral condyle of both the fibular collateral ligament as well as the popliteus tendon. The peroneal nerve is explored and freed as it dives beneath the fascia in the anterolateral compartment of the lower leg. In approximately 20% of cases, there is a very thick fascial band just deep to the anterolateral muscle compartment that may lead to common peroneal nerve palsy caused by postoperative swelling. The nerve is freed by incising this fascia for a distance of 2 to 3 cm into the anterolateral compartment to ensure the fascia will not entrap the nerve after completion of the procedure. A blunt retractor is then used to retract the biceps inferiorly and the lateral head of the gastrocnemius posteriorly to expose the popliteus muscle belly and posterolateral capsule (Fig. 21-4).

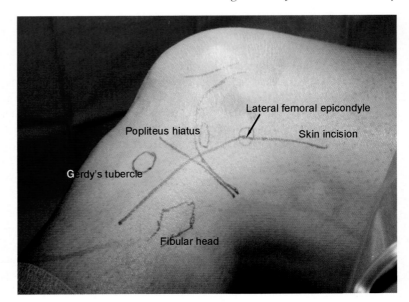

FIGURE 21-2

Photograph of the typical skin and bony landmarks with the intended incision from the lateral femoral epicondyle to a point between the fibular head and Gerdy's tubercle.

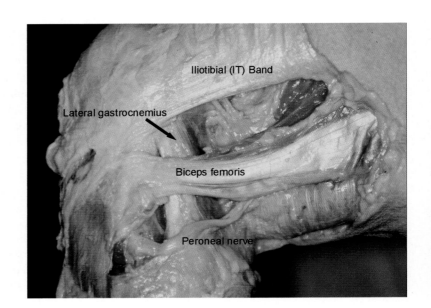

FIGURE 21-3

The initial layer of dissection for the PLCR including the peroneal nerve below the biceps femoris tendon, the iliotibial band, and lateral gastrocnemius tendon.

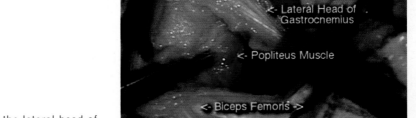

FIGURE 21-4

A blunt retractor retracts the biceps inferiorly and the lateral head of the gastrocnemius posteriorly to expose the popliteus muscle belly and posterolateral capsule.

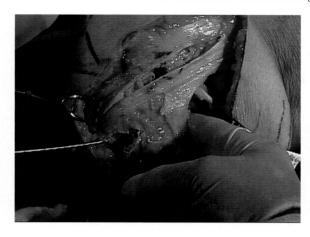

FIGURE 21-5

Tibial tunnel placement. A guidewire is placed through the tibia from just below Gerdy's tubercle to the musculotendinous junction of the popliteus muscle. A drill guide may be used, but we typically use direct visualization with a freehand technique for wire and tunnel preparation.

A portion of the anterior compartment musculature is dissected using sharp dissection off Gerdy's tubercle in the anterior proximal tibia. A guidewire is placed freehand from just below Gerdy's tubercle toward the posterolateral tibia with an attempt to exit the wire at the muscle tendon junction of the popliteus muscle belly (Figs. 21-5 to 21-7). This exit point should be 1 to 2 cm distal and 1 to 2 cm medial to the tibial articular surface and the proximal tibiofibular joint. Fluoroscopy may by used as a guide for placement of the guidewire; however, we have not generally felt that this is necessary. A tunnel is then drilled with a 10-mm cannulated reamer over the previously placed guidewire under careful visualization to prevent the guide pin from proceeding further posteriorly. A No. 5 doubled suture is passed from anterior to posterior through the tunnel using a Hewson suture passing device for later graft passage.

The femoral insertion of the popliteus tendon on the lateral aspect of the lateral femoral condyle is palpated. In most patients, the popliteus fovea is a palpable small groove running obliquely along the articular surface just posterior to the midline of the femoral condyle articular surface and is easily felt percutaneously. An incision previously made in the IT band at the lateral femoral epicondyle allows exposure of the popliteus tendon insertion in the area just distal to the peak of the lateral femoral epicondyle. A K-wire is placed at the anterior/superior insertion of the popliteus tendon for proximal placement of the bone block portion of the allograft. Work done in our laboratory previously has shown that a physiometric insertion site is located at the most anterior superior aspect of the popliteus tendon insertion into the fovea of the lateral femoral condyle just distal to the lateral epicondyle. For confirmation of the physiometric point, a suture can be fixed at this point and then passed under the fibular collateral ligament deep to the biceps tendon and IT band through the tibial tunnel, and the knee can be ranged to check for isometry. After many years of measuring this phys-

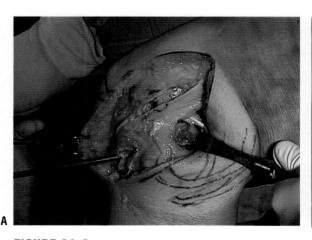
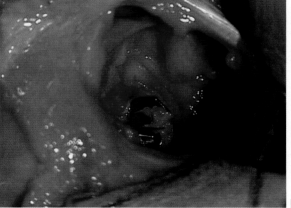

A   B

FIGURE 21-6

A: A 10-mm reamer is passed over the guidewire to exit at the popliteus muscle tendon junction. B: Close-up view of the reamer head exiting at the popliteus muscle tendon junction.

Posterior

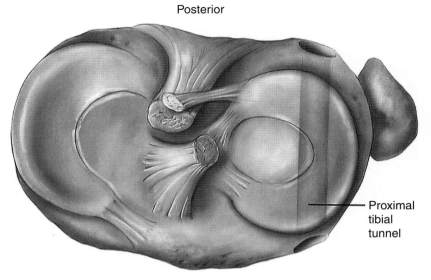

Proximal
tibial
tunnel

Anterior

FIGURE 21-7

Diagrammatic representation of the proximal
tibia, showing proper orientation of the
tibial tunnel.

iometric point, we no longer perform this step. A 10-mm wide × 20-mm depth tunnel is created using a 10-mm cannulated reamer (Fig. 21-8). Care is taken to ream perpendicular to the lateral aspect
of the femur to avoid entering the articular surface or damaging previously placed tunnels for ACL
reconstruction. An Achilles tendon allograft is prepared on the back table in the operating room with
the graft split in half, one half to be used for the posterolateral cruciate and the other half be used for
fibular collateral reconstruction, if necessary (Fig. 21-9). For the posterolateral cruciate, the bone is
fashioned to pass easily through a 10-mm cannula with a 20-mm bone block. A No. 5 running nonabsorbable suture is then placed through the tendon free edge. The graft is tubularized to aid in the
graft passage and fixation. If a double staple technique is to be used for tibial fixation, sutures are
placed in the free end of the tendon and the remaining tendon is resected at the conclusion of the procedure. If the graft is to be tied over a post, measurements must be made during the surgical procedure to determine appropriate length of the Achilles tendon allograft that is needed for graft fixation.
The graft is cut at that appropriate length and is tubularized and fixed with a No. 5 nonabsorbable
suture for later graft fixation to a post and washer. In general, a graft length of approximately 120
mm is appropriate for post fixation, whereas 150 mm of graft is required to use Dale Daniel's double staple technique for tibial fixation.

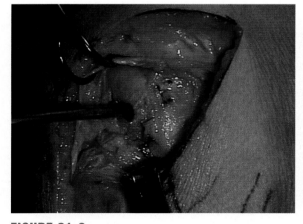

FIGURE 21-8

Femoral tunnel placement. A 10-mm wide × 20-mm
deep tunnel is created using a 10-mm cannulated
reamer at the anterior superior edge of the popliteus
fovea.

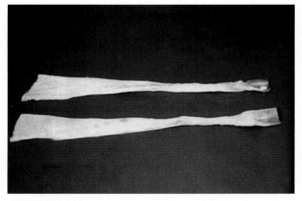

FIGURE 21-9

Achilles allograft preparation with graft divided into
two separate grafts with 9- × 20-mm bone plugs.

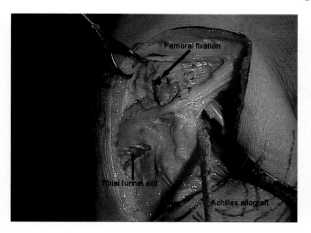

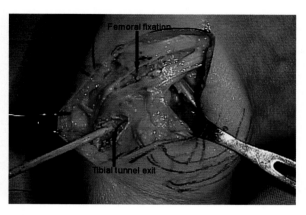

FIGURE 21-10

The graft is fixed in the femoral tunnel with a 9- × 20-mm interference screw, and the tendon is passed deep to the iliotibial band and fibular collateral ligament as well as the biceps tendon following the anatomic route of the popliteus tendon along the posterolateral tibia.

FIGURE 21-11

Graft passed through tibial tunnel from posterior to anterior and held tight while the knee is cycled through range of motion.

The bone block is placed in the femoral tunnel and fixed with a 9 × 20 mm interference screw. The interference screw is placed on the side of the bone block opposite the articular surface so that the tendon itself is more anterior and distal. The tendon is then passed deep to the iliotibial band and fibular collateral ligament as well as the biceps tendon following the anatomic route of the popliteus tendon along the posterolateral tibia (Fig. 21-10). The graft is passed into a plastic graft passing tube, which may aid in graft passage through the popliteus muscle belly and through the tibial tunnel. A No. 5 passing suture is used to deliver the graft from posterior to anterior through the tibial tunnel. The graft is then held taunt as the knee is taken through range of motion to assess isometric positioning and to cycle the graft (Fig. 21-11).

Fixation then depends on other ligaments to be reconstructed. If ACL or PCL reconstruction is performed at the same time, these grafts are fixed on the femoral side before fixation of the posterolateral corner graft. After femoral graft fixation for the cruciate reconstruction, the knee is held in approximately 30 degrees of knee flexion with internal tibial rotation and valgus stress applied. The fixation may be performed using Daniel's two staple belt buckle technique or by tying the sutures from the tendon end of the graft over a post and washer on the proximal lateral tibia (Figs. 21-12 and 21-13). Our current preference for tibial fixation includes intraoperative measurements using free suture as a ruler to ensure that the graft length ends within the tibial tunnel. The graft is prepared with a No. 5 nonabsorbable suture whip stitch and tied over a 30-mm cancellous screw and washer. The post and washer is placed along the anterolateral tibial crest under the anterior compartment muscles, which helps prevent symptoms from prominent hardware. Using this fixation technique, we have not needed to remove the tibial hardware.

The PLCR will restore rotational laxity but will not control excessive varus laxity. If varus laxity persists due to insufficiency of the FCL, the FCL may be reconstructed using the other half of the Achilles tendon allograft. Again, the remaining half of the allograft is prepared and easily passed through a 10-mm cannula with a bone block measuring 20 mm in length. A K-wire is then placed directly perpendicular into the lateral epicondyle through the epicondylar prominence. The origin of the fibular collateral ligament is just below the lateral femoral epicondyle and slightly posterior and proximal to the popliteus attachment. A 10-mm reamer is then used to create a tunnel 20 mm in depth. The bone block is affixed with a 9- × 20-mm interference screw so that the fibers of the graft are at the posterior edge of the tunnel, which will coincide with a normal insertion. The peroneal nerve has previously been identified and protected. The nerve should enter the anterior tibial musculature approximately 3 to 4 cm down the fibular neck. The nerve is visualized and protected throughout preparation of the fibular tunnel. A 7-mm tunnel is then drilled transversely from anterior and posterior through the widest portion of the fibular head. The tunnel is enlarged with progressively larger curets until it is large enough, typically 8 to 9 mm, to pass the soft tissue portion of

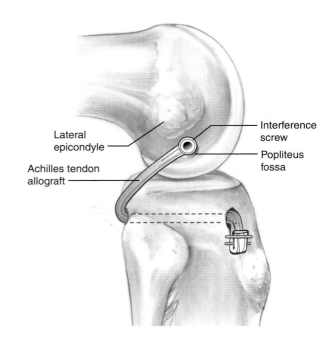

FIGURE 21-12
Schematic representation of completed posterolateral cruciate reconstruction with double staple tibial fixation.

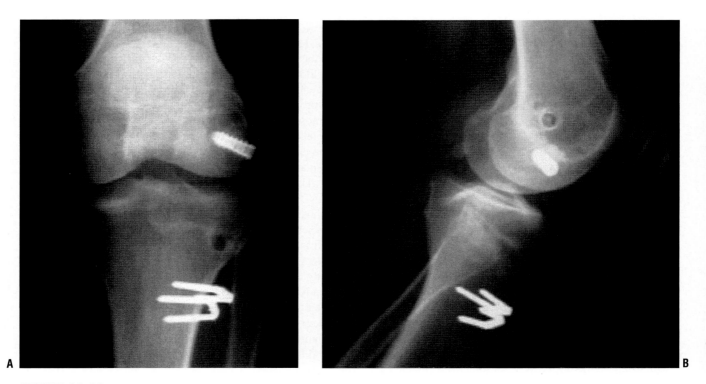

FIGURE 21-13
Anteroposterior (A) and lateral (B) radiographs following completion of the posterolateral cruciate reconstruction.

the Achilles tendon allograft. A suture passer is then used to pass the allograft from posterior to anterior, and the free end of the graft is then brought proximally onto itself. The graft is then tightened in slight valgus stress with 90 degrees of knee flexion. The graft is fixed to a suture anchor and then sewn to itself, or it can be fixed by using a double staple technique on the femoral surface. The anterior and posterior limbs of the graft are then sutured to themselves using nonabsorbable suture to produce a fibular collateral ligament reconstruction that proceeds directly from the lateral femoral epicondyle to the fibular head attachment (Fig. 21-14). After completion of PLCR and FCL reconstructions, tibial insertions of the cruciate ligaments are fixed, and the knee is cycled through range of motion and assessed for stability.

The wound is closed beginning with approximation of the IT band and biceps femoris using absorbable suture. The peroneal nerve is inspected to ensure that it is free of any restrictions or pressure throughout its course. Drains are placed deep within the lateral wound and brought out through separate stab incisions. The subcutaneous tissues are closed with 2-0 absorbable suture, and the wound is generally closed with skin staples. The patient is placed in a hinged knee brace locked in full extension and begins physiotherapy on postoperative day 1. If a PCL reconstruction is also performed, we prefer the knee to be placed in a spring-loaded dynasplint to counteract the posterior tibial forces that may tension the PCL graft.

Rationale for Using the PLCR Technique

This surgical technique creates a popliteal ligament to replace the popliteus muscle tendon complex with a much greater lever arm than the popliteofibular ligament. In addition, we believe that fibular-based techniques using a graft to create only a FCL will not adequately control PLRI over the long haul, resulting in late rotatory instability. Remember, many patients with symptomatic PLRI have no varus laxity or instability.

Pearls and Pitfalls

Proper tunnel placement is crucial as with other ligament reconstructions (ACL or PCL). The anterior-superior portion of the popliteus tendon attachment is the best physiometric position for the PLCR femoral tunnel, whereas the most prominent portion of the lateral femoral epicondyle is the best placement of the tunnel for the FCL femoral graft so the graft will lie at the inferior portion of the tunnel closest to the insertion point of the native FCL. Graft passage through the popliteus mus-

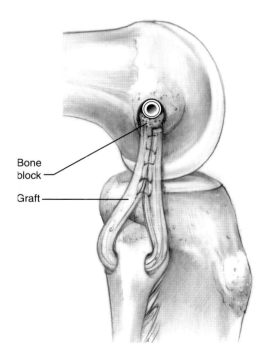

Bone
block

Graft

FIGURE 21-14

Schematic of fibular collateral ligament reconstruction with Achilles allograft. Note the suture connecting the anterior and posterior limbs.

cle belly is typically the toughest portion of the procedure, and may be helped by use of a plastic graft passage device (DePuy Mitek, Raynham, MA) to allow the Achilles tendon to slide through the muscle belly. Peroneal nerve exploration and particularly careful release of the fascial band of tissue at the entrance of the anterior compartment musculature will prevent the likelihood of postoperative peroneal neuropraxia.

POSTOPERATIVE MANAGEMENT

Initially, the patient is allowed to bear full weight in a brace locked in full extension with crutch ambulation. The patient performs range-of-motion exercises from 0 to 90 degrees of flexion three times a day for the first 2 weeks postoperatively, and usually goes to supervised physical therapy 2 to 3 days a week during this period. At 4 weeks, we allow full range of motion as tolerated and expect full range of motion about 6 weeks postoperatively. Active hamstring contractions are discouraged for the first 6 weeks to prevent excessive tibial translation or rotation and to prevent tension on the posterior cruciate or posterolateral corner grafts. The hinged knee brace is allowed to be unlocked during weightbearing at the 6-week mark based on ability of the patient to control his or her body weight with quadriceps contraction. The patient generally wears the hinged knee brace for 8 to 10 weeks postoperatively to protect the lateral and posterolateral structures. Quadriceps exercises are begun as soon as possible postoperatively. Running and plyometrics are generally started 16 weeks after surgery, with return to play anticipated approximately 6 to 8 months postoperatively. We do not routinely use functional postoperative braces for posterolateral corner reconstructions, although with certain contact sports, we use braces to protect the collateral ligaments.

COMPLICATIONS

Common Peroneal Nerve Palsy

Common peroneal nerve palsy is the most worrisome potential complication of posterolateral corner acute repair or reconstruction because of the proximity of the nerve during surgical exposure. In many cases of posterolateral and fibular collateral ligament injury, the peroneal nerve has been injured or has some damage at the time of initial traumatic event. During the surgical procedure, we generally explore the nerve proximally and distally to make certain that it is released from any restrictions within the anterior compartment of the tibia or along the posterior biceps tendon proximal to the area of injury. Since we began releasing the fibro-osseous tunnel at the anterior compartment of the tibia, we have not had any actual cases of peroneal nerve injury as an intraoperative complication.

If peroneal nerve palsy occurs postoperatively, this most likely is secondary to postoperative hematoma or surgical traction injury. In the case of large hematomeformation, re-exploration and evacuation of hematoma should be reconsidered if no improvement is seen by simple release of the bandages and dressings.

From 1977 to 1979, we were unaware of the potential presence of a fibrotic band distal to the entrance of the peroneal nerve into the anterolateral musculature. We have not had any cases of neuropraxia since we began exploring the anterior compartment entrance and releasing this band when present. In the cases of peroneal nerve palsy during the first 2 years of our case series, peroneal nerve weakness did not usually begin until postoperative day 3 and was completely resolved by 6 to 9 months. Sensation usually returns first, followed by anterior compartment muscle control. In our experience, the long toe extensor tendon function takes 2 to 3 months to recover, and the extensor halluces longus recovers at 6 to 9 months as the last muscle to improve. As a general rule, if no return of function has occurred by 6 weeks post injury, electrodiagnostic studies are done to determine the injury to the nerve as well as its regeneration potential. In addition, an ankle-foot orthosis (AFO) may be required for the involved foot for ambulation until there is adequate return of active dorsiflexion of the ankle.

Reconstruction Failure

In our previous technique for posterolateral corner reconstruction using biceps tenodesis procedure, biceps tendon rupture and failure were possible due to excess tension and tendon fixation using a spiked washer on the lateral femoral condyle (Fig. 21-15). With the current technique of posterolateral cruciate reconstruction, failure, if it occurs, is generally due to allograft reinjection or failure to

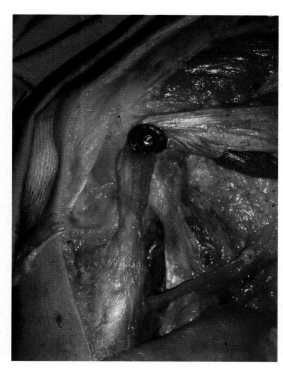

FIGURE 21-15

Intraoperative photograph of biceps tenodesis fixed to the lateral epicondyle with a spiked soft tissue washer.

incorporate. In the case of allograft rejection, the operative leg may remain swollen and painful and erythematous with no other clinical or laboratory evidence of infection. In the potential case of allograft rejection, the graft may have to be removed surgically followed by delayed alternative surgical procedures to restore mechanical stability. This has not occurred in our series.

Fixation Failure

With regard to graft fixation using a post and washer technique, appropriate length must be determined and the allograft must be prepared appropriately to allow fixation of sutures over a post and washer construct. If the double staple technique is used, adequate graft length must be present to allow a distal staple to be applied prior to the graft being folded onto itself and the proximal stable applied. We have had a case of graft failure due most likely to improper, insufficient tibial fixation of the graft which allowed slippage of the graft and loss of tension along the posterolateral corner. In cases where the graft is not long enough, we have placed several No. 5 Krackow-type nonabsorbable sutures tied to post and screw fixation with an additional back-up staple fixation or interference screw fixation. We have not used interference screw fixation as our primary mode of fixation on the tibial surface for the posterolateral cruciate reconstruction or fibular collateral ligament reconstruction.

Stiffness

Loss of motion is a rare complication with our current rehabilitation protocol, which allows 0 to 90 degrees of flexion immediately after PLCR. During the biceps tendon tenodesis procedure, stiffness was an issue because most patients were kept with limited range of motion for up to 6 weeks post surgery. Range of motion is encouraged with the PLCR rehabilitation protocol compared to the immobilization required for many of the other methods of posterolateral corner reconstruction. Although the multiple ligament injured knee can be a rehabilitation challenge, the occurrence of arthrofibrosis and need for manipulation or further surgery is rare with current techniques.

Infection

As with most open knee procedures, the risk of infection should be less than 1%. Prophylactic antibiotics are used as well as postoperative drainage to avoid hematoma formation. Copious irrigation and hemostasis are employed prior to wound closure.

CONCLUSIONS

Posterolateral corner instability is an often unrecognized, but extremely disabling injury that is usually misdiagnosed in the acute setting. Early repair of injured structures, including the FCL, biceps femoris, posterolateral capsule, popliteus, arcuate complex, and popliteofibular ligament generally results in return of knee stability. However, in cases of severe acute injury, or chronic posterolateral and/or varus instability, posterolateral cruciate ligament reconstruction and fibular collateral reconstruction with Achilles tendon allograft have proven to allow return of normal knee function and stability. Appropriate recognition and diagnosis are the keys to successful treatment.

RECOMMENDED READING

Clancy WG. Repair and reconstruction of the posterior cruciate ligament. In: Chapman MW, ed. *Operative Orthopaedics.* 2nd ed, vol 3. Philadelphia: JB Lippincott;1993:2093.

Clancy WG, Shelbourne KD, Zoellner GB, et al. Treatment of knee joint instability secondary to rupture of the posterior cruciate ligament: report of a new procedure. *J Bone Joint Surg.* 1983;65A:310–322.

Cooper DE. Tests for posterolateral instability of the knee in normal subjects. *J Bone Joint Surg.* 1991;73A:30–36.

Daniel DM, Stone ML, Barnett P, et al. Use of the quadriceps active test to diagnose posterior cruciate ligament disruption and measure posterior laxity of the knee. *J Bone Joint Surg.* 1988;70A:386–391.

Girgis FG, Marshall JL, Al Monajem ARS. The cruciate ligaments of the knee joint: anatomical, functional, and experimental analysis. *Clin Orthop.* 1975;106:216–231.

Gollehon DL, Torzilli PA, Warren RF. The role of the posterolateral and cruciate ligaments in the stability of the human knee: a biomechanical study. *J Bone Joint Surg.* 1987;69A:233–242.

Grood ES, Stowers SF, Noyes FR. Limits of movement in the human knee: the effects of sectioning the PCL and posterolateral structures. *J Bone Joint Surg.* 1988;70A:88–97.

Harner CD, Janaushek MA, Kanamori A, et al. Biomechanical analysis of a double-bundle posterior cruciate ligament reconstruction. *Am J Sports Med.* 2000;28:144–151.

Hughston JC, Andrews JR, Cross MJ. Classification of knee ligament instabilities, II: the lateral compartment. *J Bone Joint Surg.* 1976;58A:173.

Hughston JC, Jacobsen KE. Chronic posterolateral rotatory instability of the knee. *J Bone Joint Surg.* 1985;67A:351.

Jakob RP, Hassler H, Staeubli HU. Observations on rotatory instability of the lateral compartment of the knee. *Acta Orthop Scand.* 1981;191(suppl):1–32.

Noyes FR, Stowers SF, Grood ES. Posterior subluxations of the medial and lateral tibiofemoral compartments: an in vitro ligament sectioning study in cadaveric knees. *Am J Sports Med.* 1993; 21:407–414.

Veltri DM, Deng XH, Torzilli PA, et al. The role of the cruciate and posterolateral ligaments in stability of the knee: a biomechanical study. *Am J Sports Med.* 1995;23:436–443.

22 Medial Collateral Ligament Reconstruction

Christopher D. Harner, Anthony M. Buoncristiani, and Fotios P. Tjoumakaris

INDICATIONS/CONTRAINDICATIONS

Of the four major ligaments in the knee, the medial collateral ligament (MCL) has the greatest chance to heal after injury. This is in large part due to its anatomic and biologic properties. Because the MCL heals, there are few cases in which surgical intervention is required. In fact, it has been shown that surgery may even be detrimental in certain situations, since the risk of postoperative stiffness is significant.

Clinical classification of MCL injuries can be organized by timing, severity, and associated injuries. All these factors must be taken into account when formulating a treatment plan. Timing, although somewhat artificial, can be divided into acute (<3 weeks), subacute, and chronic (>4 to 6 weeks). This is based on the natural progression of the healing process, with the majority of MCL injuries healing to some extent within 3 to 4 weeks. Severity of the MCL injury is assessed by valgus stress testing at 0 and 30 degrees of knee flexion on physical examination. It is classified as per the guidelines established by the American Medical Association and discussed further later.

Finally, it is important to determine what other injuries are associated with an MCL tear. There are essentially three main scenarios: (a) no associated injuries (i.e., isolated); (b) associated with either anterior cruciate ligament (ACL) or posterior cruciate ligament (PCL) disruption alone; and (c) multiligementous injury. The anatomic location of the injury (i.e., femoral insertion, tibial insertion, or mid-substance tear) may be helpful in predicting the potential for healing. Femoral avulsions seem to heal better than tibial avulsions, although the risk of loss of motion is greater. The overall alignment of the limb also is an important factor, as an underlying genu varum alignment will protect the ligament more than genu valgum. Of course, patient activity level and expectations may also play a role in treatment.

Acute Cases

Isolated MCL Injuries   Isolated grade I and II MCL injuries are treated nonoperatively (Fig. 22-1). A guided program of early, protected (i.e., braced) motion, weight-bearing, and controlled exercises is instituted. The ACL acts as a secondary restraint to resist valgus load, and it is important to confirm its integrity before embarking on a course of nonoperative treatment.

Grade III, or "complete," tears may also be treated nonoperatively, but only after careful exclusion of any associated injuries that may necessitate surgical intervention. These would include cruciate ligament injury, meniscal tear requiring repair, and entrapment of the MCL (Figs. 22-2 and 22-3).

With ACL Disruption   The indications for ACL reconstruction remain the same despite the presence of an MCL injury. In cases of grade I or II MCL tears, if the ACL is to be reconstructed, it is delayed 4 to 6 weeks, giving the MCL a chance to heal and allowing the knee to recover from the initial

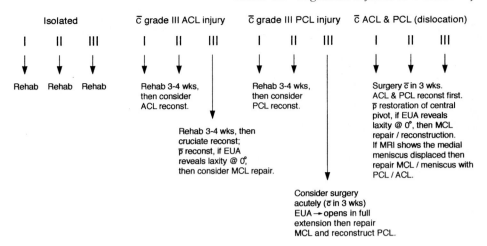

FIGURE 22-1

An algorithm for evaluating and treating injuries to the medial side of the knee.

trauma. Grade III MCL tears with ACL disruption pose more of a controversial scenario. There have been studies supporting acute surgery on both the MCL and the ACL as well as those supporting delayed reconstruction of the ACL along with nonoperative management of the MCL injury.

It has been our experience that most grade III MCL injuries heal if protected. The major risk with early surgery is the development of arthrofibrosis. However, in a certain subset of patients with this

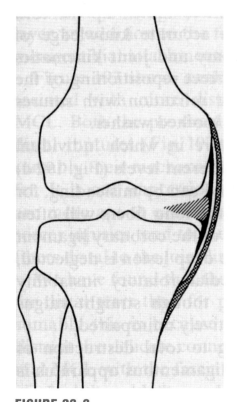

FIGURE 22-2

The normal anatomy of the MCL complex.

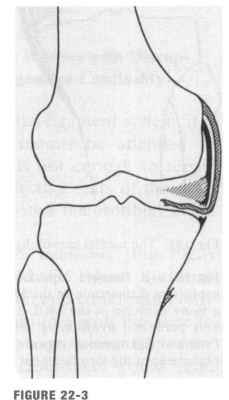

FIGURE 22-3

Entrapment of the superficial portion of the MCL.

combination of injury (grade III MCL/ACL), the MCL does not heal and there is residual valgus and rotatory laxity that is very difficult to correct later. We try to detect this group initially by physical examination and magnetic resonance imaging (MRI). If the patient has gross opening in full extension, he or she is considered a candidate for MCL repair. The MRI can be helpful in this setting, as it will reveal if the injury is an avulsion off of the tibia or the femur. We believe that the tibial avulsion is more problematic, as the synovial fluid has access to the ligament/bone interface, which may prevent healing. In this scenario, we do a surgical repair of the MCL through a limited approach to the tibial insertion combined with an ACL reconstruction. We prefer allograft tissue for the ACL to minimize iatrogenic trauma. Furthermore, if significant laxity is noted with an anterior drawer (>10 mm), we elect to repair the posterior oblique ligament (POL) at the site of injury to decrease anteromedial rotatory instability that may complicate the ACL reconstruction in this scenario. We also repair meniscal pathology at the same time. When we do elect to repair an MCL/ACL injury, we delay the surgery at least 10 to 14 days and brace the knee in the interim. This allows for the acute effects of the trauma to subside.

With PCL Disruption   Although a rare injury, this pattern can result in a very unstable knee. Because both the PCL and the MCL attach to the medial femoral condyle, complete disruption of both results in gross laxity of the medial side of the knee. In the setting of grade III injury to both of these structures, we recommend surgical treatment.

With ACL and PCL Disruption   In the setting of an ACL/PCL/MCL injury, we almost always repair or reconstruct all three injured ligaments. Delaying the intervention more than 3 weeks in this case often results in significant residual MCL laxity that is very difficult to correct. The only exception is if the MCL injury is only partial (i.e., grades I or II), in which case we postpone the surgery until final healing of the MCL occurs.

Chronic Cases

Chronic instability results following a grade III MCL injury that does not heal. There is usually more than single-plane (i.e., valgus) instability present with rotational and translational (i.e., cruciate ligaments) components. The overall alignment of the limb plays a critical part in the treatment. Knees with underlying genu valgum are more likely to have residual instability. In this setting both soft-tissue reconstruction and bony alignment may have to be addressed. The usual indication for reconstruction in chronic cases is persistent instability that affects activities of daily living.

PREOPERATIVE PLANNING

History

The MCL can be injured with valgus contact to the knee or through a twisting, noncontact mechanism. In the acute setting, depending on the severity and associated injuries, the patient will present with varying degrees of swelling, pain, and loss of motion. In combined ligament injuries, the patient is very uncomfortable and has significant loss of motion. The patient often presents with a large effusion and more pain than would be expected with an isolated ACL tear. If a combined ligament injury is suspected, the neurovasculature must be assessed, as a knee dislocation may have occurred. In the chronic setting, patients will present with instability, which usually affects activities of daily living and results in an inability to participate in athletic activities.

Examination

The goal of the examiner is to determine the degree of injury to the MCL as well as the presence of any associated injuries. In this regard, the examination of the MCL must be done in the setting of a comprehensive knee examination that includes assessment of the neurovascular status of the extremity. In the acute setting, the patient will have obvious discomfort, making the examination limited. The key to an informative examination is getting the patient to relax as much as possible. A pillow under the affected knee and gentle examination go a long way toward not only allowing the patient to guard less but also gaining his or her confidence.

The knee may or may not be grossly swollen, and the absence of a large effusion should not lead the examiner to a false sense of security. Tenderness to palpation over the MCL should be elicited.

Midsubstance tears may be associated with joint-line tenderness, creating potential difficulty in distinguishing meniscal from collateral injury. Concomitant injury to both structures, however, is possible.

Valgus stress testing of the affected knee in comparison to the contralateral knee is the cornerstone of the diagnosis. This is done at both 30 degrees of flexion and full extension, if possible. Flexing the knee to 30 degrees isolates the MCL. Putting the leg over the side of the examining table helps stabilize the femur, and placing a finger on the medial joint line helps in assessing the amount of opening. The amount of medial compartment opening is graded according to the American Medical Association (AMA) guidelines. A grade I injury allows 0 to 5 mm of opening with a firm end point; a grade II injury allows 5 to 10 mm with a firm end point; a grade III injury, or a "complete" tear of the superficial and the deep portions of the ligament, allows greater than 10 mm of opening and the end point is usually soft. These numbers are all with reference to the uninvolved side. The following figures demonstrate sequentially the Lachman (Fig. 22-4), posterior drawer (Fig. 22-5), positioning the knee at 30 degrees (Fig. 22-6) and then applying a valgus load (Fig. 22-7); then positioning the knee at 0 degrees (Fig. 22-8) and applying a valgus load (Fig. 22-9).

Any opening of the medial joint line to valgus stress with the knee at 0 degrees is a much more ominous sign and is seen only with grade III injuries. It implies a large magnitude of force to the knee and mandates careful scrutiny of cruciate ligaments, the menisci, and the patella for stability. The posteromedial capsule and the vastus medialis obliquus must also be suspected of involvement.

Another provocative test to determine the degree of injury is the external rotation anterior drawer test. This maneuver assesses the amount of anterior translation of the tibia under the femur at roughly 80 degrees of knee flexion and the foot in maximal external rotation. It is not always possible to perform this test on the acutely injured knee due to patient discomfort. It is positive if the amount of translation is significantly increased compared with the contralateral knee. The sine qua non for this test to be positive is disruption of the meniscotibial ligaments, allowing the meniscus to move freely. If the meniscotibial ligaments are intact, the meniscus remains firmly seated on the tibia, providing a buttress against the posterior femoral condyle and thus resisting anterior translation of the tibia.

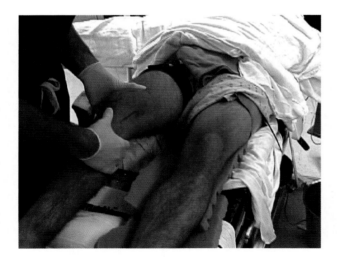

FIGURE 22-4

The Lachman test. With the knee at 30 degrees of flexion, an anterior stress is placed on the tibia. Note the position of the examiner's right thumb on the anteromedial joint line, allowing an accurate assessment of the degree of anterior translation of the tibia as well as the quality of the endpoint.

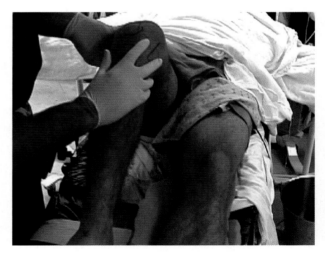

FIGURE 22-5

The posterior drawer test. With the knee at 90 degrees of flexion, a posteriorly directed force is placed on the tibia. Again, note the position of the examiner's right index finger on the anteromedial joint line, allowing an accurate assessment of tibial translation and the quality of the endpoint.

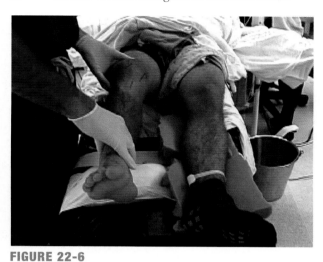

FIGURE 22-6

The knee is positioned at 30 degrees of flexion.

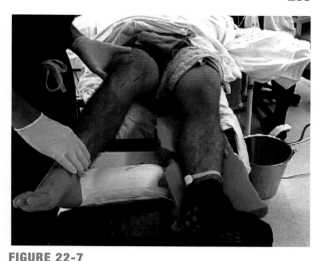

FIGURE 22-7

A valgus stress is placed on the knee at 30 degrees of flexion. The amount of medial joint space opening is assessed.

Imaging

A standard radiographic knee series is indicated in all cases of suspected MCL injury. This should include a 45-degree flexion weight-bearing view and lateral and sunrise views. If weight bearing is not possible, a simple anteroposterior view should be substituted. Avulsions or osteochondral fragments seen on radiograph could significantly affect the treatment plan. Any patient with increased laxity to valgus stress and open physes should have stress views to localize the source of the laxity. In chronic cases with instability, long-standing cassette radiographs of both lower extremities should be obtained to assess alignment.

Magnetic resonance imaging offers an abundance of information that may alter the treatment plan. The presence of meniscal tears, the location of the MCL tear, and any concomitant injuries, ligamentous or otherwise, can be discovered. This study is particularly useful when the physical examination is compromised but can also reveal pivotal information, such as the presence of an entrapped MCL lesion (Figs. 22-10 and 22-11), even in apparently straightforward cases.

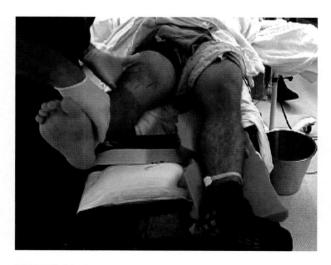

FIGURE 22-8

The knee is positioned at full extension.

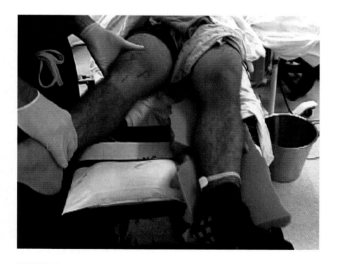

FIGURE 22-9

A valgus stress is placed on the knee at full extension. The amount of medial joint space is assessed.

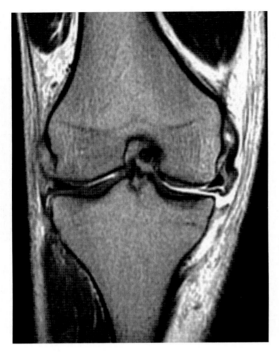

FIGURE 22-10

Magnetic resonance image demonstrating
entrapment of the superficial MCL in the joint
with displacement of the meniscus out of the
joint. Although a rare finding, this mandates
operative intervention to reduce and fix the MCL.

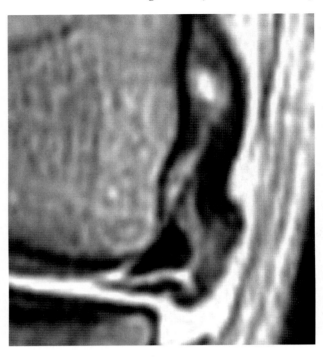

FIGURE 22-11

A magnified view of the area of interest in Figure 22-10.

In cases of disruption of the ACL, PCL, and MCL, careful consideration must be given to evaluating the vasculature by angiogram, as the incidence of vascular injury in the setting of knee dislocation is dangerously high. It is routine at our institution to obtain an angiogram in this setting.

SURGERY

Positioning and Draping

Position the patient supine on the operating room table (Fig. 22-12). We do not routinely use a tourniquet for this procedure, even in combined surgery. Examination under anesthesia is performed at this time. The anticipated surgical incisions are drawn on the skin along with appropriate anatomic landmarks (Fig. 22-13). The surgical sites are prepared with alcohol and betadine and then injected with lidocaine with epinephrine (1:100,000). The joint is injected as well. Allowing the epinephrine to sit for the few minutes while the remainder of the setup, preparation, and drape are completed achieves an excellent hemostatic effect. With this routine, the need for inflating a tourniquet is obviated. A 5-lb sand bag is taped to the table so that the foot can rest on it with the knee in 90 degrees of flexion. A side post is affixed to the table adjacent to the tourniquet to prevent the limb from abducting at the hip while the knee is flexed. The limb is prepared with Betadine and draped in standard fashion. After sterile draping has been completed, a bolster of soft goods is placed between the thigh and the side post so that the limb can be maintained at 90 degrees of flexion and vertically oriented throughout the case without assistance. Preoperative antibiotics are routinely administered.

In multiligament cases, the dorsalis pedis and posterior tibialis pulses are palpated and marked on the skin. If any difficulty is encountered with palpation, a sterile Doppler device is brought to the field and pulses are established before any surgical intervention. They are checked intermittently throughout the case. This setup allows for unencumbered physical examination of the limb at any time.

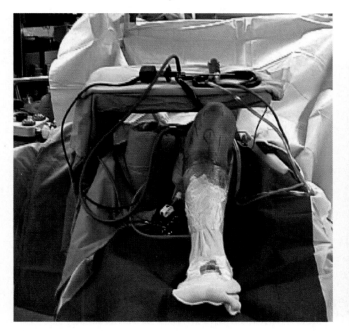

FIGURE 22-12

The limb is draped free for easy intraoperative access and examination. Range of motion is unencumbered. Note the window in the stockinette over the dorsalis pedis pulse for intermittent monitoring in multiligament cases.

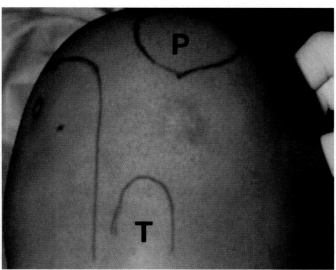

FIGURE 22-13

Anatomic landmarks of the knee for a medial approach.

Operative Technique

Acute Repairs   Acute repairs (<3 weeks) are performed in conjunction with cruciate ligament surgery. It is important to restore the central pivot (ACL and PCL) to optimize repair of the MCL. To restore normal knee stability, one must address all primary and secondary restraints that are injured. We begin by reconstructing the cruciates (ACL, PCL, or both). Our preferred graft for the ACL and PCL is tibialis anterior allograft. In most cases, the cruciate surgery is done arthroscopically. However, especially in the acute setting, fluid extravasation can be a problem. If there is any palpable increase in calf pressure during the case, then arthroscopy is abandoned and the case is performed in an open fashion. In performing these cases it is critical that the operating surgeon be skilled with both open and arthroscopic techniques.

Based on the examination under anesthesia, MRI, and arthroscopy, selective approaches with varying incisions are made. In most cases we use a medial hockey stick incision. In certain cases we can identify on the MRI either a femoral- or tibial-sided avulsion, and limited incisions directly over the injured area can be made (Figs. 22-10, 22-11, and 22-14 through 22-16).

In all cases of medial-sided repair, knowledge of the anatomy of the medial side of the knee is requisite to a successful operation. We endorse a layered approach to the medial side of the knee (Fig. 22-17). We use a variety of fixation devices to repair the MCL, but our most common material is sutures and/or suture attached to bone anchors. Our primary goal is to achieve an anatomic repair and to "seal off" the MCL from synovial fluid from the joint. The leakage of synovial fluid onto the injured MCL will cause delay and often complete cessation of the healing response.

The landmarks for the medial hockey stick incision include the adductor tubercle, the medial epicondyle, the medial joint line, and the patella. Often the knee is too swollen to palpate some of these superficial landmarks, and one must rely on an estimated path of the MCL from femur to tibia. This incision balances well and preserves the skin bridge between incisions (Fig. 22-18). We do not advocate a midline incision over the patella. Make the incision through the skin and subcutaneous fat to the level of the fascia of layer 1 (sartorial fascia). Gently sweep the fat layer off the fascia with a

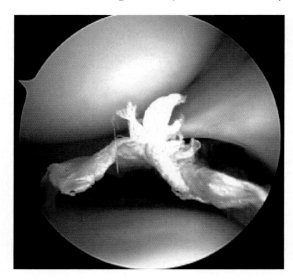

FIGURE 22-14

Intraoperative view of the entrapped MCL under the medial meniscus.

lap sponge to create skin flaps (Fig. 22-19). The infrapatellar branch of the saphenous nerve is always identified and preserved (Fig. 22-20). It emerges from under the anterior border of the sartorius and travels on the fascia. It can usually be found about 1 cm above the joint line. Tag the nerve with a vessel loop. The saphenous nerve and vein are rarely in the field and are easily avoided.

The fascia of layer 1 is incised in line with the skin incision. A convenient landmark proximally is between the adductor tubercle and the medial epicondyle. This incision extends from the epicondyle proximally to the gracilis distally. The sartorius muscle is retracted posteriorly along with the hamstring tendons, whereas the vastus medialis and the medial patellar retinaculum are taken medially. The pes bursa is teased away and this exposes layer 2, comprised of the superficial MCL, the POL, and the joint capsule anterior to the superficial MCL. Immediately deep to the superficial MCL is the deep MCL, which is considered part of layer 3 (see Fig. 22-17). Further access to the joint is established by performing an arthrotomy in the interval between the posterior border of the superficial MCL and the anterior border of the POL. Exercise caution when near the joint line to avoid transecting the meniscus. With the medial side of the knee exposed, the surgeon should carefully inspect all structures including the medial meniscus, the deep MCL, the superficial MCL, the POL, as well as the arms of the semimembranosus.

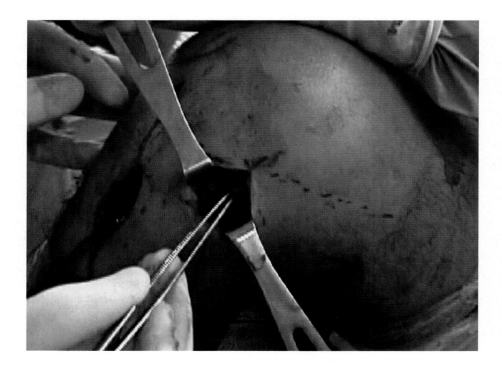

FIGURE 22-15

Limited approach to the tibial insertion of the MCL.

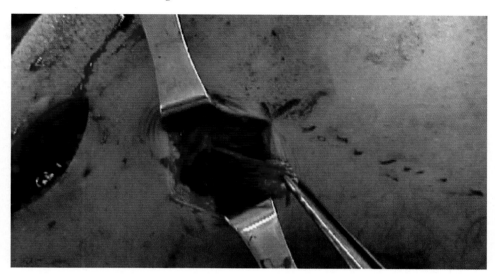

FIGURE 22-16

The avulsed tibial insertion of the superficial MCL. This was repaired with suture anchors anatomically.

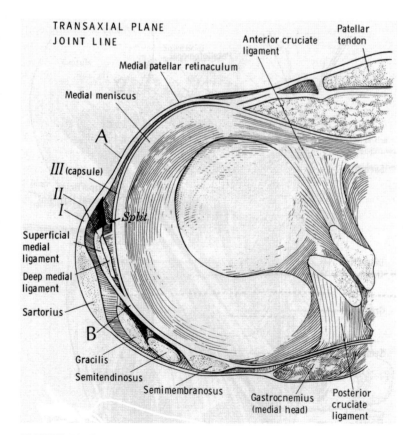

FIGURE 22-17

The anatomy of the medial side of the knee, organized by layers as described by Warren et al.

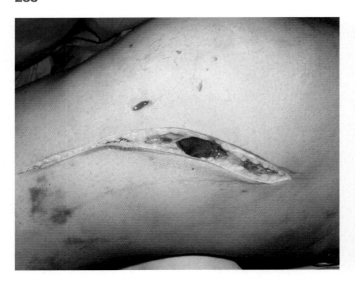

FIGURE 22-18

The skin incision.

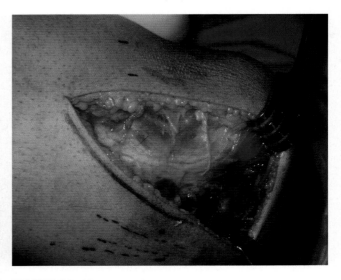

FIGURE 22-19

Sharp dissection is continued to layer 1. Fairly generous skin flaps are raised.

The joint may be inspected arthroscopically either before or after the approach to the medial side. Performing the exposure before the arthroscopy allows for easier identification of tissue planes, as there is no distortion of the tissue by extravasated fluid. However, the inconvenience of arthroscopy after opening the medial aspect of the joint must be weighed. The sequence of repair should follow an orderly progression from deep to superficial. First, repair meniscal tears that are accessible. This includes peripheral tears that must be repaired back to the overlying ligament or capsule using non-absorbable suture. The capsule or ligament to which the meniscus is being sewn must, of course, be reduced in an anatomic position as the sutures pass through the tissue to ensure proper placement. Position the knee in extension for this part of the case to avoid overconstraining the knee and restricting motion. Tag these sutures and tie them only after the medial side has been reconstructed.

Next, the MCL itself is repaired. At the time of the MCL repair, we place "soft goods" under the knee so that it remains reduced and is in 30 to 40 degrees of flexion. We take great care while repairing the MCL to not overconstrain the knee and cause a flexion contracture. If the MCL has been avulsed from its femoral insertion, repair both the superficial and the deep portion back to the epicondyle. A 0 or No. 1 nonabsorbable suture is used and the anatomy restored, sewing to the periosteum if available or using bone anchors (Fig. 22-21). If it has been torn midsubstance, then it is repaired anatomically. If the tibial insertion of the deep MCL is avulsed, this should be sutured back to the periosteum of the tibia under the superficial portion of the ligament. Fixing the deep MCL cre-

FIGURE 22-20

The infrapatellar branch of the saphenous nerve is identified and preserved.

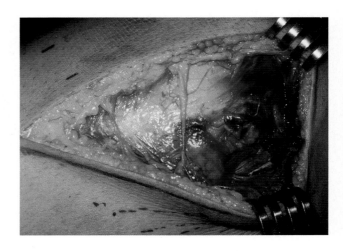

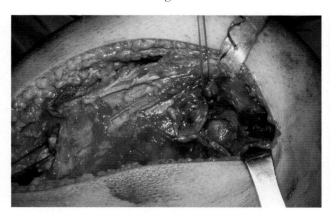

FIGURE 22-21
Suture anchors at the medial epicondyle.

ates a stable post on the medial side of the knee from which to continue the medial-sided repair. In the event that the tibial insertion of the superficial MCL has been avulsed as well, this should be repaired either with suture to the periosteum at its insertion or with suture anchors similarly placed. If the capsule has been avulsed, repair it with suture anchors placed just below and parallel to the joint line. Next, the POL is assessed.

If a POL repair is planned in isolation (as in anteromedial rotary instability [AMRI]), a limited incision can be employed (Fig. 22-22). The medial joint line is marked and an incision is carried down along the posterior one third of the medial femoral condyle. This incision is approximately 4 cm in length, with two thirds of the incision being placed below the joint line. A similar approach as used with the MCL repair is used through layer 1. Layer 2 is then identified and the junction of the superficial MCL and POL is located. This can be facilitated with an intraoperative valgus stress to the knee with palpation of the medial joint line. With this maneuver, the MCL becomes taught, and the POL remains lax allowing its identification. The junction between MCL and POL is then divided and the underlying capsule is exposed (Fig. 22-23). The capsule is incised superior to the medial meniscus, and the meniscus is tagged with nonabsorbable suture for later repair into the MCL (Fig. 22-24). The POL and MCL are separated off of the capsule with the use of an elevator. We use three to four braided, No. 2 nonabsorbable sutures through the POL in a horizontal mattress fashion and advance the POL to the MCL to recreate the posteromedial tension (Fig. 22-25). The repair is zone specific to the POL, advancing only the portion of the ligament that has been traumatized. The suture depth in the superficial MCL can be adjusted depending on the severity and location of the in-

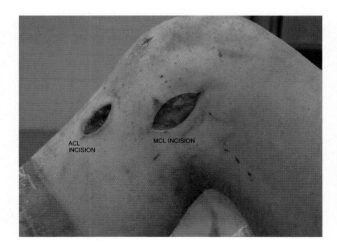

FIGURE 22-22
A limited medial incision can be employed when only repairing or imbricating the POL.

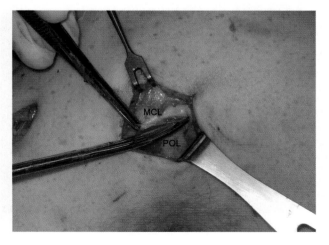

FIGURE 22-23
The demarcation between the POL and MCL is identified and split for the imbrication.

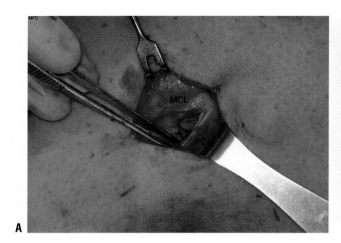
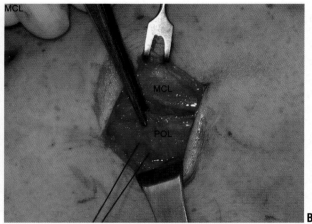

FIGURE 22-24

A: The capsule is incised superior to medial meniscus and the joint is exposed (MFC, medial femoral condyle; MM, medial meniscus). **B:** The medial meniscus is tagged (*black suture*) and this suture is incorporated into the final repair.

jury to vary the degree of imbrication that is achieved (Fig. 22-26). The sutures are then tied down over the MCL in slight flexion (15 degrees), and the repair is completed after repair of the sartorius fascia (layer 1) with absorbable suture (Fig. 22-27).

At this point, the knee is carefully taken through a full range of motion to ensure that the repair has not "captured" the knee. The tension can be adjusted if a full range of motion is not achieved. The surgeon must manually maintain anteroposterior reduction during this maneuver because the cruciate(s) has not been attached on the tibial side (in the setting of combined injury). Next, the knee is taken to 90 degrees extension and the PCL is tensioned and secured. Finally, the knee is brought out to full extension and the ACL graft is tied over a post. Closure is performed with the knee flexed to 90 degrees, and a postoperative drop-lock brace is applied with the knee in full extension.

Chronic Cases   In chronic cases, if surgery is indicated, every effort is made to repair the medial side primarily, and this is often possible. It is important to remember that the tissues in cases of chronic instability are not easily identified and are often severely attenuated. The surgeon must have several different techniques in his repertoire for managing chronic MCL laxity. The goal is to

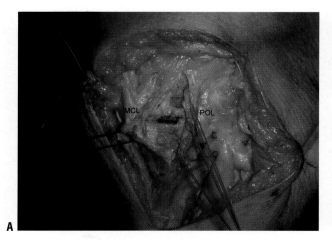
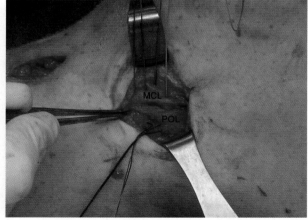

FIGURE 22-25

A: The mattress sutures have been placed in the POL and are ready for advancement through the MCL. The depth is varied depending on the degree of imbrication desired. The joint line is indicated by the blue marker (cadaver knee) **B:** The sutures have been passed and the repair is shown (live surgery).

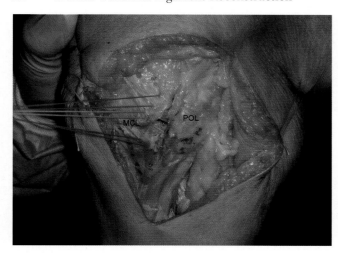

FIGURE 22-26

The sutures are passed and the depth is determined by the degree of instability present on examination (cadaver knee).

achieve an anatomic repair or reconstruction. This may necessitate the use of both primary repair and reconstructive techniques. Preoperatively, the MRI is helpful in identifying the location of the injury to the MCL. This can usually be seen on the coronal images and correlated with the arthroscopic view of the compartment under a valgus stress. Depending on where the pathology is (i.e., femoral, midsubstance, or tibial) the focus of the repair should be to this area.

On occasion the medial structures are attenuated to the point where repair is not possible, although in most cases we have been able to use existing tissue to repair the MCL. The underlying principle is to build off of the superficial and deep MCL and advance the POL on this complex if laxity persists. The choice of graft can be either allograft or autograft. We have used a number of different grafts, including Achilles tendon and tibialis anterior allograft, as well as semitendinosus autograft (Fig. 22-28). The principle of reconstruction remains the same regardless of graft choice.

The semitendinosus is easily harvested through the medial incision. Isolate it just inferior to gracilis and release it from its tibial insertion, preserving as much length as possible. Place a whipstitch of 0 suture in the free end. Carefully dissect the tendon free of all investing soft tissue with a combination of blunt and scissor dissection. In chronic cases, the tendon may be relatively adherent to surrounding scar, and patience is required, as careful preparation is crucial to successful harvesting. A closed-ended tendon stripper is used to harvest the tendon. Pay close attention to the direction of the tendon, cognizant that it inserts on the ischial tuberosity, and recreate that trajectory with the stripper. Once harvested, take the graft to the back table, divest it of all soft tissue, preserve all us-

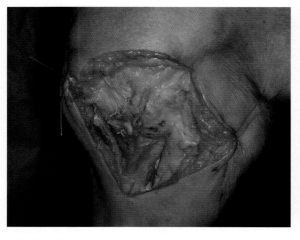

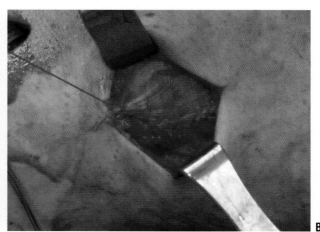

A   **B**

FIGURE 22-27

A: The sutures are tied over the MCL and the repair is completed (cadaver knee). **B:** The final repair after closure of the sartorial fascia (live surgery).

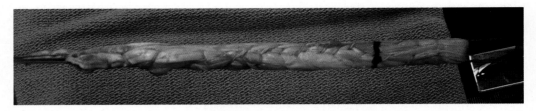

FIGURE 22-28

A prepared hamstring autograft.

able length, and place a whipstitch in the other end of the tendon. Fold the graft onto itself, doubling it over a piece of No. 5 suture, and then sew it into one bundle with 0 absorbable suture. It is obviously expedient if the graft preparation can be undertaken by a second assistant, so as not to interrupt the flow of the reconstruction.

Using the exposure as described previously, the medial epicondyle and the site of the tibial insertion of the superficial MCL should be clearly identified. The graft should recreate the path of the superficial MCL. The graft should also recreate the isometry of the native MCL. Toward this end, drill a hole at the tibial insertion site and place a screw with a soft-tissue washer through the graft into the pilot hole and tighten it. Next, palpate the medial epicondyle and hold the femoral side of the graft at the anticipated insertion. Take the knee through flexion and extension to assess whether the graft is placed isometrically. Adjust the femoral insertion point until the isometric point is found. Then drill a pilot hole at this site. Position the knee in full extension and apply gentle tension on the graft in an anatomically correct position. Thread a screw with a soft-tissue washer through the graft and secure it in the pilot hole. Trim the excess graft appropriately. Having established a stable post, the remainder of the medial-sided repair proceeds in an orderly sequence as described previously. It is our experience that the POL must be advanced more often in chronic cases than in acute cases. We assess it carefully and advance it onto the reconstructed MCL as necessary. Both the superior and inferior ends of the POL should be anatomically restored as shown in Figure 22-29. Take great care not to overtighten the POL, as this will result in a flexion contracture. Pass these sutures in a horizontal mattress-type stitch through the superficial MCL and into the underlying periosteum to increase the security of the repair. This portion of the procedure should be done with the knee at 20 to 30 degrees of flexion. The cruciate ligaments are tensioned and fixed in the same fashion as in the acute setting.

FIGURE 22-29

The POL is advanced according to the zone of injury. With femoral lesions, advancement is carried out along 1,2, and possibly 3 depending on the injury severity. With tibial lesions, 3,4, and 5 are more routinely advanced.

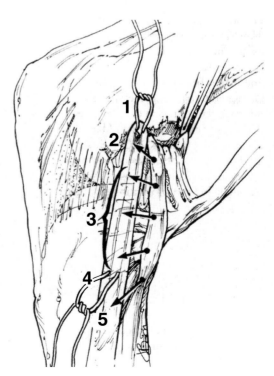

Pearls and Pitfalls

- Always be sure to maintain the knee at approximately 15 degress of flexion (near full extension) while the POL is advanced so as to not capture the knee and compromise postoperative motion.
- Identifying the POL from the MCL can be facilitated by a valgus stress at 30 degrees of knee flexion. With this maneuver, the POL remains lax while the MCL is placed under tension.
- In chronic cases, there is typically a substantial amount of AMRI contributing to the instability pattern, which can usually be addressed with POL advancement as described.
- Use the preoperative MRI to define where the MCL injury is and focus POL advancement at this point. For example, if it is on the femoral side, you would focus the advancement in this area.
- For reconstruction (using a graft), placing a K-wire in the medial epicondyle and looping a suture can help to locate the isometric point of the ligament prior to pilot hole placement.

POSTOPERATIVE MANAGEMENT

Cruciate ligament reconstruction takes precedence over the MCL with respect to the postoperative management. In general, the rehabilitation follows the regimen that is used for isolated ACL or PCL reconstructions, with careful attention to any decrease in range of motion. Achieving full extension is emphasized. If medial repair or reconstruction is the only procedure, the knee is braced in extension for 2 to 4 weeks to allow for healing. A slight varus bend can be applied to the brace to protect the repair. During this time, continuous passive motion is used two or three times a day. The brace is then unlocked, and range-of-movement exercises begun. Strengthening begins at 6 weeks. Bicycling and low-impact closed-chain exercises are an integral part of the strengthening phase. The brace is typically removed at 6 to 8 weeks. Small flexion contractures are tolerated through 8 to 12 weeks of rehabilitation, as it is thought to be protective of the repair and allows for maturation of scar tissue. A small flexion contracture is also postulated to allow the dynamic stabilization of the semimembranosus to strengthen the repair. If full extension is achieved in the operating room, it is possible to regain it through aggressive therapy at the appropriate time. Weight bearing is initially touch down and progresses to full gradually after 2 weeks. Crutches are discontinued only when ambulation is without a limp.

Complications

Complications regarding surgery of the medial collateral ligament itself are few. Certain risks are associated with anesthesia, surgery in general, and the procedures that may be performed concomitant with MCL repair. Specific to the medial-side reconstruction itself, the main complication is loss of motion. This is a problem that may occur with any knee surgery and, specifically, any knee ligament surgery. However, it has been recognized that MCL surgery is a particular risk factor for loss of motion after ligament reconstruction. Of course, technical aspects of the surgery come into play, as the repair of the medial side must not be so aggressive as to restrict motion. Tensioning the repaired or advanced tissue with the knee in full extension helps to prevent this complication. The timing of knee ligament reconstruction was also found to be important, as surgery less than 1 month after the injury was a risk factor, unless the knee was grossly unstable. In general, decreased postoperative range of motion can be avoided by operating on knees that have full range of motion preoperatively. In addition, an intraoperative confirmation of full knee excursion should be performed after the reconstruction is complete but before closure.

RESULTS

Not surprisingly, the less severe the injury, the better the prognosis. In cases of isolated MCL injury, rehabilitation is fairly aggressive, tempered by the severity of the injury to the knee. Return to sports is allowed when pain, tenderness, and instability are gone, range of motion is full, and strength and agility are nearly normal. This typically takes from 2 to 6 weeks for partial tears.

The prognosis for cases of acute, isolated grade III MCL tears is a bit less optimistic. The rehabilitative protocol is similar in nature to that for partial tears, but the progression is typically dramatically slower. The initial phase of pain and inflammation control may last up to 6 weeks in and of itself. The maintenance of range of motion is more difficult than it is for partial tears. Tears from the femoral insertion have been shown to heal quicker and more reliably than tears of the meniscotibial ligament with their associated capsular tears. The key to successful nonoperative management of isolated MCL injuries is ensuring that it is truly an isolated injury. Even so, return to sports may take more than 12 weeks.

For combined injuries, the prognosis is worse. MCL tears in the setting of a knee dislocation are potentially sport-ending injuries. Medial collateral ligament tears associated with only ACL tears are surmountable obstacles, but the risk of persistent residual laxity is not insignificant. The criteria for return to sport are the same as those described previously, but the time frame is longer. Return of full strength and proprioception may take up to a year.

RECOMMENDED READING

American Medical Association, Committee on the Medical Aspects of Sports. *Standard nomenclature of athletic injuries.* Chicago: The Association; 1966.

Baker CL, Liu SH. Collateral injuries of the knee: operative and nonoperative approaches. In: Fu FH, Harner CD, Vince KG, eds. *Knee surgery.* Baltimore: Williams & Wilkins; 1994:794–795.

Clayton ML, Weir GJ, Jr. Experimental investigation of ligamentous healing. *Am J Surg.* 1959;98:373–378.

Fetto JF, Marshall JL. Medial collateral ligament injuries of the knee: a rationale for treatment. *Clin Orthop.* 1978;132:206–218.

Frank C, Woo SL-Y, Amiel D, et al. Medial collateral ligament healing: a multidisciplinary assessment in rabbits. *Am J Sports Med.* 1983;11:379–389.

Harner CD, Irrgang JJ, Paul J, et al. Loss of motion after anterior cruciate ligament reconstruction. *Am J Sports Med.* 1992;20:499–506.

Hart DP, Dahners LE. Healing of the medial collateral ligament in rats: the effects of repair, motion, and secondary stabilizing ligaments. *J Bone Joint Surg Am.* 1987;69A:1194–1199.

Hughston JC, Andrews JR, Cross M J, et al. Classification of knee ligament instabilities. I. The medial compartment and cruciate ligaments. *J Bone Joint Surg Am.* 1976;58A:159–172.

Hughston JC, Barrett GR. Acute anteromedial rotatory instability: long-term results of surgical repair. *J Bone Joint Surg Am.* 1983;65A:145–153.

Hunter SC, Marascalco R, Hughston JC. Disruption of the vastus medialis obliquus with medial knee ligament injuries. *Am J Sports Med.* 1983;11:427–431.

Indelicato PA. Nonoperative management of complete tears of the medial collateral ligament. *Orthop Rev.* 1989;18:947–952.

Kannus P. Long-term results of conservatively treated medial collateral ligament injuries of the knee joint. *Clin Orthop.* 1988;226:103–112.

Mok DW, Good C. Nonoperative management of acute grade III medial collateral ligament of the knee: a prospective study. *Injury.* 1989;20:277–280.

Muller W. *The knee: form, function, and ligament reconstruction.* Berlin: Springer-Verlag; 1982.

Sandberg R, Balkfors B, Nilsson B, et al. Operative versus nonoperative treatment of recent injuries to the ligaments of the knee: a prospective randomized study. *J Bone Joint Surg Am.* 1987;69A:1120–1126.

Shelbourne KD, Patel DV. Management of combined injuries of the anterior cruciate and medial collateral ligaments. *Instr Course Lect.* 1996;45:275–280.

Shelbourne KD, Porter DA. Anterior cruciate ligament-medial collateral ligament injury: nonoperative management of medial collateral ligament tears with anterior cruciate ligament reconstruction—a preliminary report. *Am J Sports Med.* 1992;20:283–286.

Thornton GM, Johnson JC, Maser RV, et al. Strength of medial structures of the knee joint are decreased by isolated injury to the medial collateral ligament and subsequent joint immobilization. *J Orthop Res.* 2005;23:1191–1198.

Tipton CM, James SL, Mergner KW, et al. Influence of exercise on strength of medial collateral ligaments of dogs. *Am J Physiol.* 1970;218:894–902.

Warren LF, Marshall JL. The supporting structures and layers on the medial side of the knee. *J Bone Joint Surg Am.* 1979;61A:56–62.

Wilson TC, Satterfield WH, Johnson DL. Medial collateral ligament tibial injuries: indication for acute repair. *Orthopedics.* 2004;27:389–393.

Woo SL-Y, Inoue M, McGurk-Burleson E, et al. Treatment of the medial collateral ligament injury. II. Structure and function of canine knees in response to different treatment regimens. *Am J Sports Med.* 1987;15:22–29.

Woo SL-Y, Young EP, Ohland KJ, et al. The effects of transection of the anterior cruciate ligament on healing of the medial collateral ligament: a biomechanical study of the knee in dogs. *J Bone Joint Surg Am.* 1990;72A:382–392.

23 Surgical Technique for Knee Dislocations

Bryan T. Kelly, Struan H. Coleman, and Russell F. Warren

INDICATIONS/CONTRAINDICATIONS

Knee dislocations occur whenever the articular surfaces of the distal femur and proximal tibia displace completely from one another (Fig. 23-1). Dislocations are most usefully described according to the associated degree of local soft-tissue injury (e.g., closed or open grade I, II, III), and the primary direction of displacement. The direction of a particular knee dislocation is designated according to the direction of displacement of the tibia with respect to the femur (6,7). Anterior, posterior, medial, lateral, and rotatory dislocations have been described. Straight anterior or posterior dislocations are the most commonly reported. Other forms of dislocation (medial, lateral, or rotary) are far less common and are often combined with anterior or posterior dislocation (6,7,9,13–15).

The majority of reported dislocations of the knee occur in association with motor-vehicle accidents. The high velocity and ultra-high-force nature of this type of trauma often leads to associated head and thoraco/abdominal injuries of higher priority and, not uncommonly, to rapid mortality. Of primary importance in the multiple trauma victim is the immediate treatment of life-threatening conditions. Once these issues have been properly addressed, attention should be given to a dislocated knee.

We believe it is appropriate to attempt immediate closed reduction and immobilization of all knee dislocations if possible. The massive displacement of the bony architecture that occurs during dislocation causes extensive disruption of the joint capsule and ligaments. Usually, at least three major ligaments and the posterior joint capsule are damaged. Therefore, the degree of instability is usually so severe that gentle manipulation will easily achieve reduction. Once reduced, a thorough evaluation of the neurologic and vascular status of the injured extremity is critical. Adequate determination of pedal pulses, in addition to ankle-brachial indexes bilaterally, should be performed routinely in this setting. Failure of early diagnosis of vascular injuries has resulted in extremely high amputation rates, up to 90% in some series (2,4).

In some medial dislocations, it may be impossible to reduce the knee by closed manipulation, since the medial femoral condyle may have "button-holed" through the medial joint capsule and retinaculum. These cases require open reduction. Furthermore, the joint is often rendered so unstable in medial and lateral dislocations that closed reduction, once achieved, is very difficult to maintain. Under these circumstances, after a careful vascular and neurologic examination, the knee should be immediately immobilized in a brace, cast, or splint and a radiographic evaluation made of the reduction, with adjustment if required. In some cases placement of an external fixator is required to maintain the reduction. Immobilization in a significant degree of flexion (45 degrees or more) may be needed to achieve and maintain an adequate reduction. In contrast, reduction is often relatively easy to maintain after manual reduction of straight anterior or posterior dislocations in which the medial and lateral soft tissues have simply been "peeled off" anteriorly or posteriorly in a longitudinally intact sleeve of tissue. When these tissues are reduced to their original positions, they tend to provide enough stability to maintain adequate reduction with relatively minimal external support.

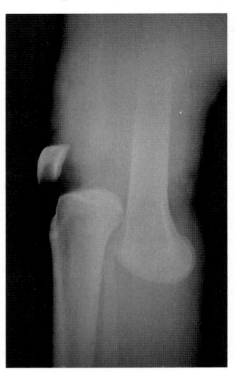

FIGURE 23-1

Lateral radiograph of an acute anterior knee dislocation.

NONOPERATIVE TREATMENT

In closed dislocations, without intra-articular fracture, and where a good reduction can be easily maintained in a cast or brace, nonoperative treatment with early range of motion (ROM) therapy may achieve an acceptable functional outcome. However, if this course is chosen, frequent radiographic assessment of the adequacy of the reduction must be performed during the first several weeks. This is because posterior subluxation will often lead to a poor outcome, and later attempts at surgical correction of this problem will have a low success rate once the soft tissues have "matured," creating a fixed, posteriorly subluxed position. A hinged external fixator may be used to prevent posterior subluxation but allow for progressive ROM in cases where the reduction is difficult to maintain.

Delayed Arthroplasty or Arthrodesis

In older patients with massively comminuted intra-articular fractures, the most prudent course of action may be to simply immobilize the knee in a position of acceptable alignment for a period of time, during the initial phase of bone and soft tissue recovery and healing, before performing a primary knee arthroplasty or arthrodesis as the definitive surgical treatment. Immobilization may take the form of a cast, brace, or external fixator device.

PREOPERATIVE PLANNING

It is of the utmost importance to assess the condition of the local skin and soft tissues (Fig. 23-2), neurologic status, and, particularly, the vascular status of the involved extremity, both initially and at frequent intervals after initial evaluation. Accurate monitoring of the pedal pulses is critical. Determination of the status of the knee ligaments, although of interest, is an issue of lower priority early after a knee dislocation. The evaluation and early management of a dislocation should be done in a manner that does not jeopardize or hinder the evaluation of the vascular status of the limb.

After the initial reduction, the factors that we consider most important in making surgical decisions about dislocations of the knee include:

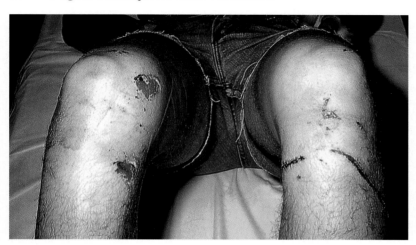

FIGURE 23-2
Typical skin trauma after closed knee dislocation.

1. *The adequacy of the reduction.* If closed reduction is impossible because of interposed soft tissue, open reduction should be performed at the earliest opportunity (within several hours after dislocation). If an adequate closed (or open) reduction can be achieved but cannot be maintained, the surgical repair of damaged ligaments should be performed as soon as the patient's general condition and the condition of the local soft tissues permit (from several hours or days to 2 weeks after dislocation). If the interval between injury and definitive fixation is anticipated to be a prolonged period, the use of an external fixator may be employed.

2. *The condition of the soft tissues.* In open injuries, surgical irrigation and debridement should be performed at the earliest opportunity (within several hours after injury). In most of these cases, and in closed dislocation with severe blunt injury to the local skin and soft tissues, attention to surgical stabilization of the knee should be delayed until the condition of these tissues improves to a level appropriate to the performance of extensive open-knee ligament surgery (within several days to 2 weeks after injury).

3. *The status of arterial blood flow to the distal extremity.* The impairment of popliteal arterial blood flow is the most common and severe complication of knee dislocations, with a reported incidence ranging from 5% with low energy trauma to 40% with high energy, anterior or posterior dislocations (2,5,15). Our plans for surgery are guided by the following criteria. The absence of pulses at the ankle and foot is an absolute indication for immediate surgical exploration and repair of the popliteal artery. Arterial blood flow must be re-established within 6 hours after the initial injury; otherwise, severe ischemic effects leading to amputation are inevitable in a great majority of cases. The absence or diminution of pulses obviates the need for preoperative angiography in favor of immediate exploration and repair of the popliteal artery, with intraoperative angiography, in this setting, reserved for identifying the site of injury. Patients with normal pulses may be monitored by careful vascular examination. In a study by Treiman et al (16), of 115 unilateral knee dislocations, the incidence of popliteal artery injury was 23%. However, there was a 79% incidence of popliteal injury associated with abnormal pedal pulses. In the remaining 86 patients with normal pulses, the arteriogram was normal in 77, showed spasm in 5 patients, and revealed an intimal flap in 4 patients. None of the patients with normal pedal pulses required arterial repair. Hollis et al (4) also concluded that routine arteriography is unnecessary in patients with a normal physical examination after reduction of the knee dislocation. The role of magnetic resonance angiography in making the diagnosis of a vascular injury in this setting remains to be determined, but appears to be particularly useful for evaluating those patients with extensive soft tissue injury and normal pulses when surgery is being planned (10,11).

In approaching soft-tissue reconstruction in a dislocated knee, the surgeon should consider and prepare options for repairing and grafting any or all of the main stabilizers of the knee, including the anterior cruciate ligament (ACL), posterior cruciate ligament (PCL), medial collateral ligament

(MCL), lateral collateral ligament (LCL), popliteus tendon and popliteofibular ligament, patellar tendon, patella, and quadriceps tendon. These may include autografts from the injured or contralateral knee, allografts and, very occasionally, ligament augmentation devices (LADs). The surgeon should assess the availability of these resources and obtain appropriate informed consent for their use before taking the patient to the operating room.

If vascular reconstruction has been performed, the use of a tourniquet may be contraindicated. Intraoperative fluoroscopy is often helpful in the placement of bone tunnels, which may be required for reconstruction of the PCL. Intraoperative plain radiographs should also be available to assess the correction of posterior subluxation before the conclusion of surgery.

Inspection of the menisci and articular surfaces, and preparation of the intercondylar notch for ligament reconstruction, is most easily and thoroughly accomplished arthroscopically. However, capsular disruption may preclude routine arthroscopy because of excessive extravasation of fluid into the soft tissues. Under these circumstances, we usually favor a brief arthroscopic inspection, with low-pressure flow and systemic wrapping of the calf, before proceeding to an open approach. We have also found "dry" or "semi-wet" arthroscopy, with intermittent fluid flushes, to be a viable option in inspection, debridement, and reconstruction in the intercondylar notch. The surgeon should be prepared, however, to perform the entire procedure in an open fashion, if necessary, and if arthroscopy is used, an awareness of fluid extravasation is paramount. Significant fluid extravasation may make open procedures (e.g., MCL and LCL reconstruction) more difficult, and can lead to a lower-leg compartment syndrome.

SURGERY

Technique

The patient is placed supine on an operating table that is adjustable to allow variable amounts of flexion at the hip and knee. We position the patient longitudinally on the table in such a way that the patient's knee-flexion crease is just distal to the distal flexion joint of the table, so that the foot of the table may be dropped to allow up to 90 degrees of knee flexion during the surgical procedure. If available, an operating table that has these features and is also designed for use with an image intensifier is optimal. Our preferred method of anesthesia is continuous lumbar epidural blockade. In our experience, this has provided excellent, adjustable, and long-lasting muscle relaxation and pain relief.

The first event after reaching an appropriate level of anesthesia should be a thorough examination of the knee. This should be done before prepping and draping the patient to allow easy manipulation of the knee and comparison with the opposite knee. A thorough assessment should be made of the status of the ACL, PCL, MCL, LCL, and posterolateral corner (Figs. 23-3 to 23-6).

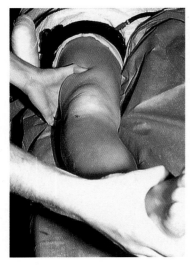

FIGURE 23-3
Assessment of lateral collateral ligament injury.

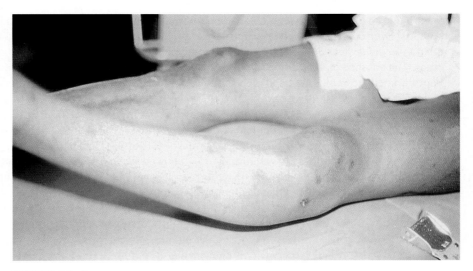

FIGURE 23-4
Severe posterior and lateral injury.

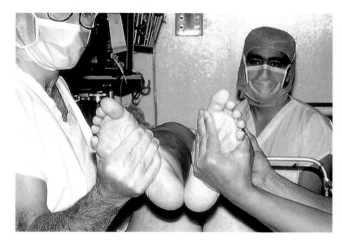

FIGURE 23-5

Assessment of external rotatory stability of the knee.

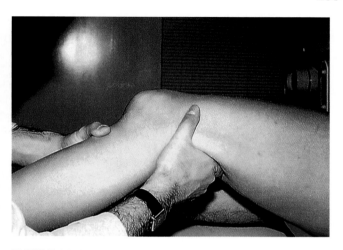

FIGURE 23-6

Assessment of posterior stability of the knee.

If possible, a tourniquet is then placed around the upper thigh at as high a level as possible, over a layer of protective cast-padding material. We then seal off the tourniquet area with adhesive plastic drapes to avoid the skin irritation occasionally seen when Betadine (povidone/iodine) solution seeps under the tourniquet and remains there during periods of tourniquet inflation. The entire extremity is then prepped by first scrubbing with Betadine scrub solution and then painting with concentrated-Betadine swabs. We seal off the lower leg and foot with an adhesive plastic dressing. Further standard draping is done with sterile paper drapes. If the use of contralateral autografts is anticipated, the opposite leg is also prepped and draped in the same manner.

A separate sterile table is set up away from the primary surgical field, at which an assistant is provided with the appropriate instruments for preparing graft material. If allografts are to be used, an assistant may begin graft preparation simultaneously with the start of the surgical procedure on the knee.

If arthroscopy is to be performed as part of the procedure, it is often done first. We occasionally harvest an autograft from the middle third of the patellar tendon, before the arthroscopic examination, to allow the assistant to prepare the graft while the rest of the procedure continues. We avoid using the tourniquet during arthroscopy by adding 1 mg of epinephrine to each 3,000-mL bag of arthroscopic irrigation solution, and have been quite satisfied with the level of hemostasis and clarity of visualization this affords. Arthroscopy begins with a routine visual inspection of the entire knee in a predetermined sequence as follows: suprapatellar pouch, patella, lateral gutter, popliteus recess, femoral trochlea, medial gutter, medial compartment, intercondylar notch and ligaments, and lateral compartment. Once the visual inspection is complete, we proceed to the required repairs (Fig. 23-7).

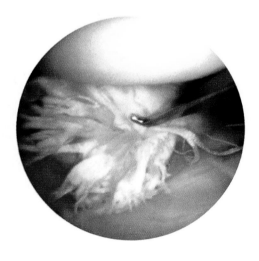

FIGURE 23-7

Arthroscopic view of midsubstance rupture of the PCL.

At this point, we may discontinue arthroscopy to harvest patellar tendon, semitendinosus, and gracilis grafts, as necessary. After the graft harvest is completed, we resume arthroscopy to perform any required meniscal work, as well as a debridement and preparation of the intercondylar notch. If fluid extravasation precludes further arthroscopy, we proceed to an open approach.

All remnants of ruptured ligaments, if unusable in the reconstruction, are removed. Enough bone is also removed from the roof and sides of the intercondylar notch to allow unencumbered movement of the knee so as to prevent impingement of the intended grafts.

At this stage, we prepare the tibial attachment site of the PCL arthroscopically using a posteromedial portal for visualization while debridement is performed through an anterior portal and the intercondylar notch (Fig. 23-8).

As previously mentioned, extensive capsular injury may compromise or even contraindicate arthroscopy in a fluid medium. If fluid loss is marked, the repair medially may be performed before addressing the ACL or PCL to allow better arthroscopic evaluation and ligament reconstruction. For open reconstruction of the knee ligaments, we have been satisfied with the utility of a long, oblique skin incision that courses over the front of the knee in a proximal-lateral to distal-medial direction (Figs. 23-9 and 23-10). With appropriate extension of the incision and the elevation of skin flaps, this type of incision allows access to all aspects of the knee.

Ligament Reconstruction

Our approach to multiple ligament reconstruction in the acute setting is guided by the following principles:

1. The sequence of reconstruction to which we adhere is PCL, ACL, MCL, posterolateral corner, LCL, and others (e.g., extensor mechanism, iliotibial band).

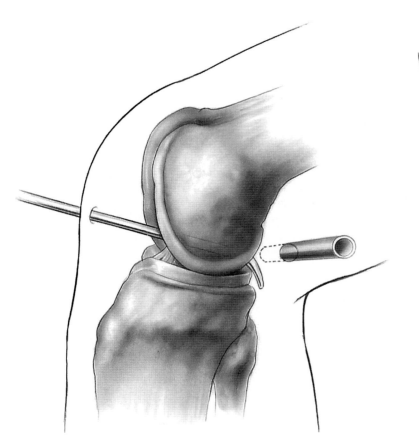

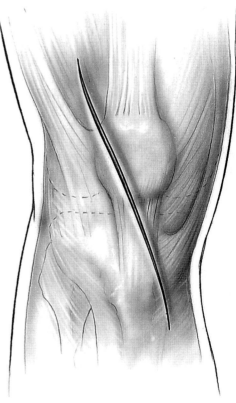

FIGURE 23-8

Preparation of the posterior tibial ledge may be accomplished arthroscopically by viewing through a posteromedial portal.

FIGURE 23-9

A long oblique skin incision for open multiple ligament reconstruction.

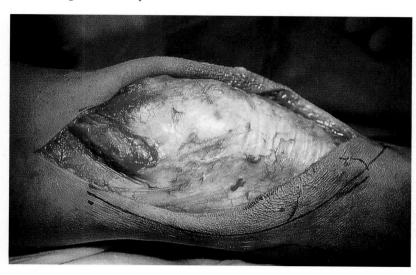

FIGURE 23-10
Initial exposure after long oblique skin incision.

2. Ligaments that have been avulsed from a bony attachment with little or no apparent intrasubstance injury are treated with primary repair and with augmentation if necessary (Figs. 23-11 and 23-12).
3. Allografts for PCL and ACL will greatly facilitate the reconstruction process. We prefer an Achilles allograft for the PCL reconstruction and a bone-tendon-bone (BTB) patella tendon allograft for ACL reconstruction.
4. Intrasubstance ruptures of the PCL and ACL are reconstructed with a BTB patella tendon, semitendinosus, or gracilis autograft. However, these autografts may be needed for the medial or lateral side reconstructions.
5. For combined ACL and PCL reconstructions, we make all of the required bone tunnels before passing any grafts, to avoid injury to the grafts.
6. Intrasubstance ruptures of other ligaments are treated with primary repair and augmentation.
7. If ipsilateral autografts are the only available biologic grafts, and both the ACL and PCL are ruptured, we give priority to a BTB autograft from the middle third of the patella in the PCL reconstruction. In these cases, we reconstruct the ACL with a semitendinosus-gracilis autograft.
8. Injuries to the MCL are treated with primary repair, advancement of posterior tissues (if appropriate), and/or augmentation with a hamstring tendon (Bosworth technique) or LAD.
9. Injuries to the popliteus tendon and popliteofibular ligament are usually treated with primary repair with augmentation, using a strip of iliotibial band. If the muscle-tendon junction has been disrupted, we perform a tenodesis of the tendon to the posterolateral tibia or posterior fibular head after ensuring the competence of the tendon's femoral attachment.
10. Injuries to the LCL are treated with primary repair and/or augmentation with a strip of biceps tendon graft. Reconstruction with an achilles tendon allograft has been used more recently.

Reconstruction of the Posterior and Anterior Cruciate Ligaments   We recommend using image intensification for making the tibial bone tunnel used for reconstruction of the PCL, especially if the procedure is to be done arthroscopically. In our experience, even a small portable system, used in conjunction with any standard drill guide, aids accurate and safe placement of a guidewire into the appropriate site on the posterior tibia. The anterior entry site for the tibial tunnel for the PCL is well distal to the usual ACL tunnel site. Alternatively, the tibial tunnel can be started lateral to the tibial tubercle to improve the tibial angle and thus decrease the angle posteriorly. The exit site of the tunnel, at the back of the tibia, is critical. Ideally, the guidewire should exit in the middle of the posterior facet of the natural PCL origin. This ensures that the reconstructed ligament will

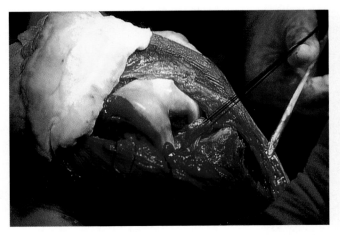

FIGURE 23-11

Open view of knee showing femoral avulsion of the ACL controlled with sutures before primary repair.

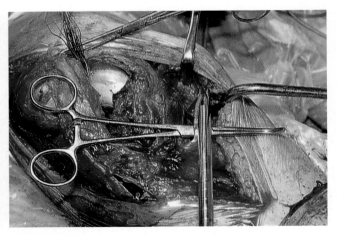

FIGURE 23-12

The semitendinosus tendon is being harvested for use as an augment for the ACL repair.

be anchored far enough posteriorly to function properly. A common error is to accept guidewire placement that is too close to the level of the joint line. The more proximally the wire is placed, the closer the top of the eventual tunnel will be to the articular cartilage of the joint. As the top of the tunnel is elevated superiorly, it also advances anteriorly owing to the geometry of the ledge, which has a gentle anterior slope. Furthermore, a tunnel exiting too close to the joint line has an area of weakness (a thin bone bridge) near its exit site, which will often break off during ligament tensioning, causing further anterior movement of the graft-attachment site on the tibia. A properly placed guidewire, when seen radiographically on a lateral view, parallels the angle made by the joint of the proximal tibia with the fibula and runs just superior and parallel to the posterior curve of the proximal tibial cortex, just underneath the posterior ledge (Fig. 23-13). Tips for this procedure are outlined in Table 23-1.

If the surgeon wants to create the tibial tunnel for the PCL reconstruction arthroscopically, we find that a posteromedial arthroscopic portal is helpful. With a posteromedial portal the surgeon can view with a 30- or 70-degree arthroscope either from the posteromedial position or through the notch, and obtain an excellent view of the posterior tibial ledge. Preparation of the area can then be easily accomplished by working through either an anterior portal or the posteromedial portal. We locate the position for the posteromedial portal by pushing the arthroscope to the posteromedial corner of the medial compartment, behind the MCL if it is present, or simply to the junction of the A and B zones of the medial meniscus. If the scope is pushed up against the capsule at this point, a correctly positioned portal can be placed by cutting in the area of skin transilluminated by the scope. Table 23-2 lists a few extremely helpful guides to PCL graft preparation (Fig. 23-14).

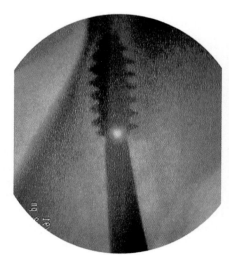

FIGURE 23-13

Fluoroscopic view of proper interference-screw placement for fixation of the PCL graft in the tibial tunnel. Note that the orientation of the screw is nearly parallel to the posterior tibial cortex and at the same level.

TABLE 23-1.   Pearls of Tibial Tunnel Creation

1. Set the initial length of the guidewire, from tip to drill chuck, such that when the guidewire has been advanced to the point at which the drill chuck hits the drill guide, the guidewire has just reached the inner table for the posterior tibial cortex.
2. Advance the guidewire under radiographic control from the beginning of the procedure. Stop advancement of the wire under power when the posterior cortex is reached.
3. Penetrate the posterior cortex slowly, viewing it directly from the posterior medial portal and radiographically.
4. Grasp the guidewire with an arthroscopic grasper or a clamp to ensure that it is not inadvertently driven further posteriorly during reaming over the wire.
5. Set the length of the reamer, from tip to drill chuck, to prevent inadvertent overpenetration of the reamer past the posterior tibial cortex. Drill over the guidewire while viewing the advancing reamer with frequent fluoroscopic radiographic spot pictures.
6. Chamfer the edges of the tunnel with a rasp.

TABLE 23-2.   Pearls of Posterior Cruciate Ligament Graft Preparation

1. In using a bone-tendon-bone graft, we have found that the lead bone plug on the graft should not exceed 20 mm in length or it will have a great degree of difficulty turning the corner at the tibial exit site to head up into the femoral tunnel.
2. We have also found it helpful to allow the trailing bone plug to be 30 to 40 mm long or longer. This makes fixation in the tibial tunnel, with an interference screw placed from anteriorly, much easier.
3. If an autograft from the middle third of the patellar tendon is being used, we fashion the short bone plug from the patella and the long one from the tibial tubercle, since the tibial tubercle can easily take such a long plug.
4. In passing the graft from the tibial tunnel to the femoral tunnel, it is helpful to manipulate the graft with an instrument that has a wide rolled edge that acts as a sort of "pulley" from anteriorly, so that as traction is applied to the draw-sutures, the pulley causes the part of the graft that has not emerged from the back of the tunnel to be drawn posteriorly. As this happens, the part of the graft that has already emerged from the tunnel curls around the instrument, following the actual traction vector, which is directed anteriorly toward the femoral bone tunnel (see Fig. 23-14).
5. Alternatively, an Achilles tendon allograft may be used for reconstruction of the PCL. In this case, we pass the free end first and impact the trailing bone plug into the tibial tunnel. The graft is fixed on the femoral side with an AO screw and washer.

The site for the femoral bone tunnel in PCL reconstruction is chosen at a point anterior and superior on the medial wall of the intercondylar notch. We have been satisfied with the results obtained by selecting a point for guidewire placement that corresponds to the anterolateral component of the PCL insertion (Fig. 23-15). When the notch is viewed with the knee flexed at 70 to 90 degrees, and is at the axilla (junction) of the medial wall and the roof of the notch (the notch usually lies approximately 1 cm proximal to the edge of the articular surface), the point of guidewire placement is optimal. The guidewire is placed from the anteromedial cortex of the distal femur into the chosen position in the intercondylar notch, using any standard drill guide, and the tunnel is made by reaming over the guidewire with the appropriate-sized reamer.

Whenever possible, we now prefer a double-bundle PCL reconstruction which recent reports have demonstrated to be biomechanically superior to a single bundle. The two femoral tunnels attempt to recreate the positions of the posteromedial bundle, which is tight in extension, and the anterolateral bundle, which tightens in flexion. An Achilles tendon graft is split to create the two components for the femoral attachment sites.

The following is a guide for the double-bundle PCL reconstruction technique:

1. The Achilles allograft bone plug is cut to 12 mm thick. The tendinous portion is then split into equal 8-mm halves (or into a 6-mm limb and a 10-mm limb to recreate the anterolateral and posteromedial bundles, respectively). The graft ends are tubularized and sized to fit into the 8-mm tunnel (Fig. 23-16).
2. The femoral footprint of the native PCL is identified arthroscopically, and a resection of the PCL stump is performed. A notchplasty is also performed if needed. A posteromedial arthroscopy portal is often used for the notchplasty.

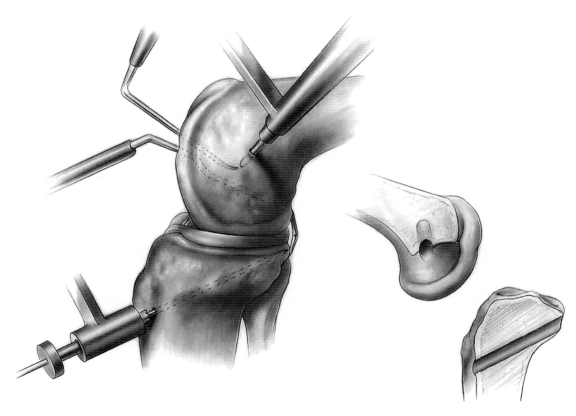

FIGURE 23-14
Lateral diagrams of proper tibial and femoral tunnel placement for PCL reconstruction.

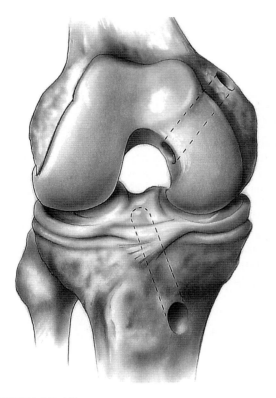

FIGURE 23-15
Anteroposterior diagram of proper tibial and femoral tunnel placement for PCL reconstruction.

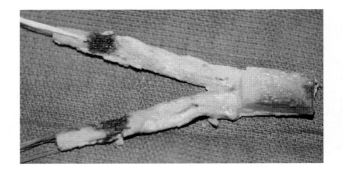

FIGURE 23-16
Split Achilles allograft used for a double-bundle PCL reconstruction before insertion.

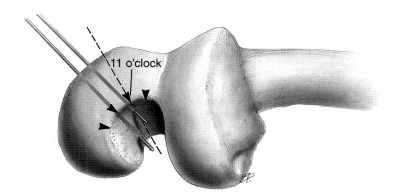

FIGURE 23-17

A diagram of guide pin placement for a double femoral tunnel PCL reconstruction.

3. A longitudinal incision is then made on the femur midway between the medial femoral epicondyle and the anteromedial articular margin. Two guide pins are then drilled from this region into the notch in an outside-in technique (Fig. 23-17). The two guide pins are placed a minimum of 12 mm apart such that the two 8-mm tunnels will be separated by at least a 4-mm bone bridge (Fig. 23-18). The anterolateral pin is placed first. The femoral drill guide targeting tip is positioned at the planned center of the tunnel in the notch (the "wall"-"roof" junction). The anterolateral guide pin is then placed. A pin guide is then placed over the first pin on the femoral cortex such that the drill hole for the second pin is 12 mm away. The second pin is then directed proximal and posterior to the first pin. Following pin placement, the tunnels are reamed to 8 mm (or to 6 mm and 10 mm). The tunnels are then smoothed with a shaver to aid the passage of the graft (Fig. 23-19).

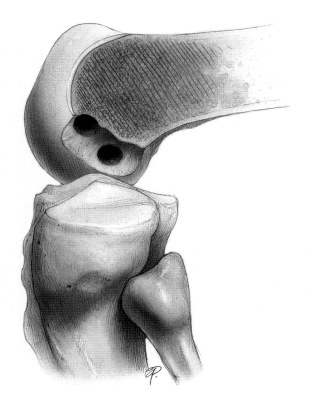

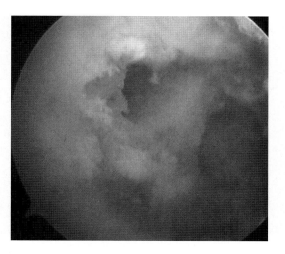

FIGURE 23-18

A diagram of two femoral tunnels.

FIGURE 23-19

An arthroscopic image of a double femoral tunnel before passage of the graft.

4. Mersilene tape is passed through the two tunnels in an outside-in technique and placed on the tibial plateau to approximate the required length of the graft. Bunnell stitches are then placed on the tendinous ends of the graft with No. 5 Ethibond (Ethicon, Inc., Somerville, NJ).

5. Immediately after the PCL tunnels are finished, we attend to the bonework required for ACL reconstruction. If the ACL is avulsed, we perform primary repair and augmentation with a hamstring tendon. If the ACL has suffered intraligamentous rupture, and the middle third of the patellar tendon has been used for the PCL, we reconstruct the ACL with a semitendinosus-gracilis graft or allograft.

The tibial tunnel for the ACL is made in typical fashion, using a standard drill guide and reamer system. A femoral tunnel for the ACL is also made in standard endoscopic fashion on the wall of the lateral femoral condyle.

When all required tunnels have been constructed, we prepare to pass the PCL and ACL grafts. The PCL graft is positioned first, followed by the ACL graft. Likewise, when both grafts are in place, the PCL graft is tensioned and fixed in place first, followed by tensioning and fixation of the ACL graft.

To facilitate passage of the PCL graft, we use a 22-gauge wire with a loop to lead the graft-draw sutures into the tunnels. We start by inserting the wire in an anterior-to-posterior direction through the tibial bone tunnel for the PCL. The leading end is grasped and brought into the area of the intercondylar notch, where a second grasper, reaching into the notch from the femoral tunnel for the PCL, can draw the wire up through the femoral tunnel. It is important during these maneuvers to control the trailing end of each wire with a clamp. Next, a second wire is looped through the looped end of the first wire and the first wire is used to draw the second wire back down through the knee. The second wire is then retracted to pull the PCL draw sutures, and the graft itself, into the tibial tunnel and intercondylar notch and out the femoral tunnel (Figs. 23-20 and 23-21).

To draw the ACL graft into position, we use a beath pin that is driven up through both the tibial and femoral tunnels and finally through the soft tissues of the distal, lateral thigh. The sutures that have been passed through the femoral bone plug of the graft are threaded through the end of the beath needle, and then the needle and sutures are advanced through the knee under direct visualization. A controlled tension is maintained on both sets of sutures as the femoral bone plug is guided into the femoral tunnel to the desired depth.

After both the PCL and ACL grafts have been positioned, the PCL graft is tensioned and fixed in place with interference screws. The knee must be properly reduced during fixation of the PCL graft to recreate the normal step-off. Proper tensioning of the PCL is best achieved with the knee at approximately 70 degrees of flexion. If the fixation of either interference screw is deemed tenuous, we provide additional fixation by fastening the draw sutures with either a ligament button or staples. If a double bundle technique is used for the PCL reconstruction, the anterolateral component is tensioned and fixed at 90 degrees of flexion, and the posteromedial component is tightened and fixed with the knee in extension.

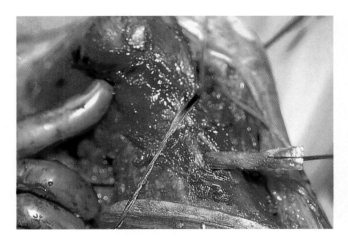

FIGURE 23-20
PCL graft being drawn into the tibial tunnel.

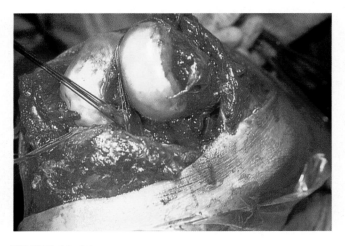

FIGURE 23-21
The ACL is controlled with several sutures in preparation for primary repair; the PCL graft is drawn forward in the notch in preparation for pulling it up into the femoral tunnel.

After the PCL graft has been fixed in place, the ACL graft is tensioned and fixed with interference screws with the knee in full extension and properly reduced. Again, if either screw appears tenuous, the fixation is reinforced by tying the sutures over an EndoButton (Smith & Nephew, Andover, MA) on either the femur or the tibia.

Reconstruction of the Medial Collateral Ligament   Reconstruction of the medial or lateral collateral ligaments requires a functional "central pivot" for accurate determination of isometricity. For this reason, we recommend performing the PCL reconstruction first, followed by the ACL reconstruction, and then the MCL and/or LCL-posterolateral reconstruction. Other repairs, such as to the iliotibial band or extensor mechanism, are left for last.

The first thing to do in approaching the MCL is to assess the type and amount of damage to the entire medial side. In cases in which the tibial attachment of the MCL has been relatively cleanly avulsed, a simple reattachment with a staple or a bone screw and ligament washer may be all that is necessary to effect a satisfactory repair. More often, the MCL injury is on the femoral side, leaving a frayed end that is much more difficult to control and repair. If the posterior MCL and capsular tissues appear to be intact and of good quality in such cases, we have often been satisfied with the results of suturing the remnants of the MCL back to bone with suture anchors, and anteriorly advancing or "reefing" the posterior tissues to establish medial stability. In knee dislocations, however, these tissues are often completely destroyed, and we find it necessary to augment the medial side with an ipsilateral semitendinosis tendon graft, as described by Bosworth, or use Achilles tendon allograft. The hamstring tendon graft is left attached at its tibial insertion and dissected proximally. The tendon is advanced to the center of rotation of the MCL on the femur, where it is fixed in place with an AO screw and washer or with a staple. If the tibial attachment site of the original MCL is still present, the graft should first be secured to the tibia directly over this site at a point that is approximately at the same level as the tibial insertion of the semitendinosus tendon. If the tibial attachment of the original MCL is no longer apparent, a site approximately 3 cm distal to the tibial joint line, at the level of the insertion of the semitendinosus tendon, will be effective. We prefer to use a cortical-bone screw with a ligament washer for fixation.

The next task is to determine the proper isometric femoral attachment site for the graft. We do this by first selecting a likely site on the medial cortex of the medial femoral condyle, approximately 25 mm proximal to the medial joint line. A guidewire is inserted into the femur at this site. Next, the graft is drawn taut over this wire at approximately 30 degrees of knee flexion. The knee is then taken through a range of motion from 0 to 100 degrees while the graft excursion over the wire is observed. For this observation, it is helpful to mark the graft where it lies directly over the wire when the knee is at 30 degrees of flexion. The proposed attachment site is then adjusted, according to whether the graft lengthens significantly in flexion or extension. If the graft lengthens in flexion, the attachment site is too far anterior. If the graft lengthens in extension, the site is too far posterior (Fig. 23-22). The guidewire is adjusted accordingly until minimal excursion (1 to 2 mm) is obtained. The graft should be attached to this site with a bone screw and ligament washer while the medial side of the knee is held closed at 30 degrees of knee flexion. The remaining remnants of MCL are then reefed over the "new" anterior band of MCL thus formed, and the posterior medial corner is repaired while keeping the tibia internally rotated and applying a varus stress.

Lateral Collateral Ligament and Posterolateral Corner   In approaching the posterolateral corner of the knee, our attention is first directed to the peroneal nerve. We routinely identify and expose the nerve to protect it from inadvertent injury during ligament reconstruction (Fig. 23-23). During exposure the nerve is inspected for signs of injury. If a nerve palsy was noted preoperatively, or an intraneural hematoma is seen, the epineurium is opened to allow blood to evacuate. It is particularly important to avoid traction on the peroneal nerve when dissecting the peroneal nerve from the neck of the fibula.

In cases of knee dislocation, the LCL, popliteus tendon, and popliteofibular ligament are often avulsed from their bony attachments, and may be reconnected directly to bone (Fig. 23-24). Recently, our basic science research has enabled us to appreciate a previously poorly recognized attachment of the popliteofibular ligament to the fibular head. Our anatomic dissections and biomechanical testing have shown us that the popliteofibular ligament is an important restraint to external rotation and posterior translation of the tibia (i.e., the "static" function of the popliteus tendon).

On the lateral side we restore the function of the popliteus tendon first. We perform a primary reattachment of the tendon to bone if the tendon is avulsed from its femoral attachment. More commonly

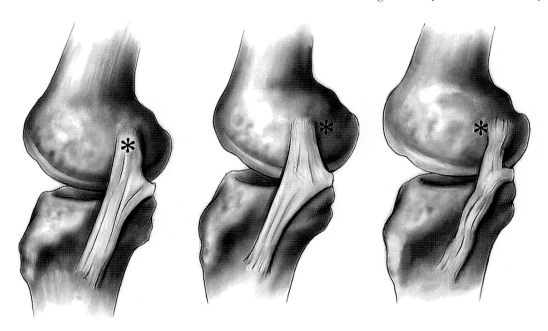

FIGURE 23-22

Reattachments of the MCL to the femur must be adjusted to obtain proper isometricity and function.

we find that the popliteofibular ligament and/or the popliteus muscle-tendon junction are severely damaged or destroyed, and we therefore tenodese the tendon to the posterolateral corner of the tibia or, preferably, the posterior part of the fibular head at the usual insertion of the popliteofibular ligament (Fig. 23-25). This attachment site is on the gently sloping surface of the posterior fibular head, approximately 8 to 10 mm posterior and 3 to 5 mm medial to the insertion of the LCL and biceps tendon. The attachment can be reconstructed by detaching part or all of the popliteus tendon from its muscular junction, controlling it with sutures, and fixing it to bone on the posterior fibula. The tension of the reconstruction should be set with the knee flexed at approximately 70 degrees and the lateral tibia drawn forward to its neutral position. It should be noted that after tightening the reconstruction in this position, it will become slightly slack when the knee is extended, owing to the cam effect of the femoral attachment site, since the latter is anterior to the center of rotation on the femur. The reconstruction will, however, continue to become taut and resist significant external rotation at

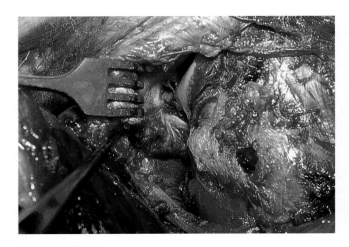

FIGURE 23-23

The peroneal nerve is exposed during the posterolateral repair.

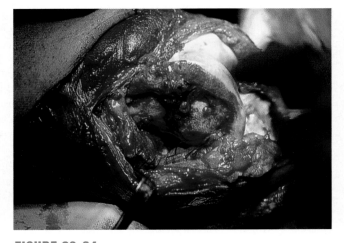

FIGURE 23-24

Open view of lateral side of knee showing where the popliteus and LCL have been avulsed from the bone.

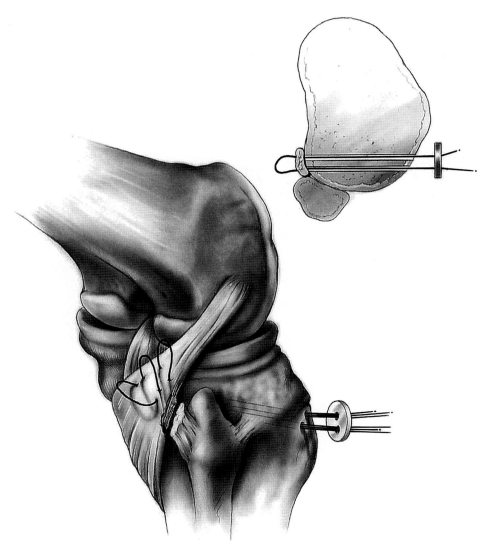

FIGURE 23-25
Popliteus tendon injury at the popliteofibular ligament or popliteus muscle-tendon junction may be treated with tenodesis of the popliteus tendon to the posterior lateral corner of the tibia.

all angles of knee flexion. If there is attenuation of the popliteus tendon, it may be repaired and augmented with a thin strip of iliotibial band left attached to Gerdy's tubercle. This is placed through a drill hole made from the anterior to the posterior of the tibia and then routed along the popliteus tendon (Fig. 23-26).

If the LCL is avulsed from its femoral insertion, it is reattached to the bone. If the proper site for reattachment is not obvious, it is determined in a manner that is completely analogous to the way in which the femoral attachment site is selected for reconstruction of the MCL. To do this, we use a guide pin at a level approximately 25 mm proximal to the joint line, with the knee at 30 degrees of flexion, to judge ligament excursion, and adjust the selected site accordingly. Next, we drill a shallow bone tunnel (about 5 to 10 mm deep) at the intended site of attachment with a one-quarter-inch (6 to 7 mm) bit, and then drive a Steinmann pin with holes in its trailing end (beath pin) through the bone tunnel, across the distal femur, and out the medial femoral cortex. We use the holes in the trailing end of the beath pin to draw the ligament sutures across the femur and advance the ligament into the bone tunnel. The sutures are then securely tied down over a ligament button.

In cases in which the LCL is avulsed from its fibular attachment, it may likewise be recessed into a shallow bone tunnel in the fibular head by using draw sutures taken through two drill holes brought

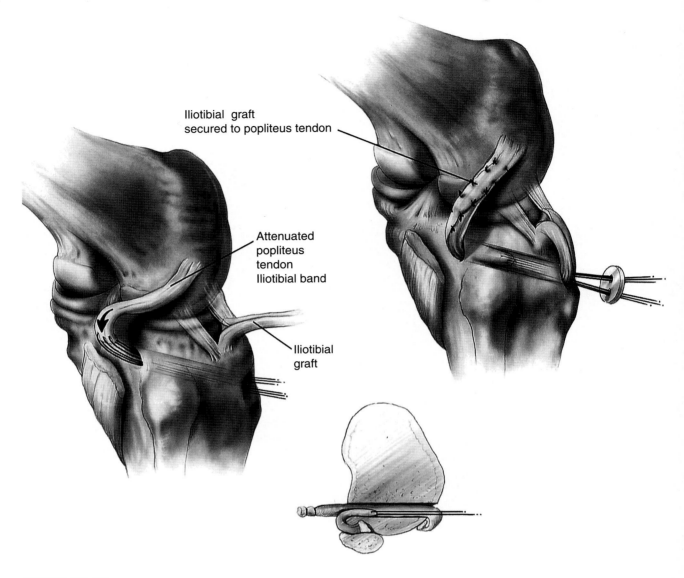

Iliotibial graft
secured to popliteus tendon

Attenuated
popliteus
tendon
Iliotibial band

Iliotibial
graft

FIGURE 23-26

Technique for popliteus tendon augmentation using an iliotibial band graft.

out distally on the fibula. Fixation is achieved by tying the sutures down over a bone bridge or ligament button (Fig. 23-27).

If direct repair of the LCL is impossible, the primary graft source for reconstructing the ligament is the biceps tendon, since the fibular insertion of this tendon actually envelops the fibular insertion of the LCL. To use the biceps tendon for LCL reconstruction, we first proceed by leaving the fibular insertion of the tendon undisturbed. We then elevate from the underlying muscle a segment of biceps tendon just proximal to the fibular insertion and approximately 20 mm wide and 8 to 10 cm long. Next, we "tubularize" this sheet of aponeurotic material by rolling one half to the midline and then rolling the other half around the first half. We secure the resulting tube with several simple sutures spaced a few millimeters apart along the length of the graft. The end of the graft is controlled by placing several loop sutures. Finally, the graft is attached to the femur (Fig. 23-28). It is our standard practice to perform anterior and lateral compartment releases at the completion of the reconstruction to decrease the chances of compartment pressure elevation.

Other graft materials that may be used for LCL reconstruction include hamstring tendon, tubularized iliotibial band, and a patellar allograft or the Achilles tendon. All of these graft sources are easily adapted to the techniques described previously, with the appropriate shaping of bone plugs when

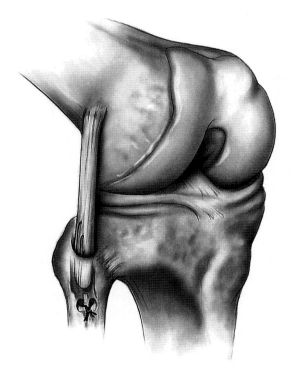

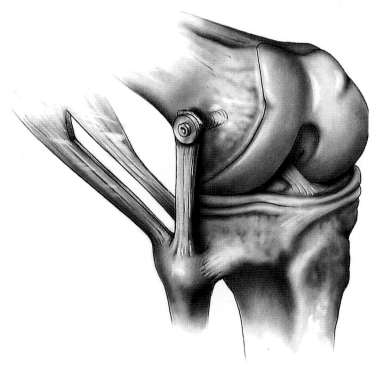

FIGURE 23-27
Repair of a fibular avulsion of the LCL.

FIGURE 23-28
Technique for LCL reconstruction using a biceps tendon graft.

used and the judicious use of draw sutures. When bone plugs are used as part of the graft construct, interference screws may be used to augment graft fixation.

Surgical dressings are loosely applied to avoid neurovascular compromise, and the leg may be braced and slightly elevated. Surgical drains should be left in place for as long as significant drainage (>50 mL/4 hr) persists. The wound should be observed and the dressing changed at least once daily. We maintain intravenous antibiotics for 48 hours postoperatively.

POSTOPERATIVE MANAGEMENT

Management of the hospitalized patient after surgical reconstruction of a dislocated knee focuses on the neurovascular status of the extremity and the condition of the wounds and local soft tissues. Frequent (every 4 hr) assessment of the pedal pulses, microcirculatory appearance of the foot, and distal sensorimotor function is top priority during the first several postoperative days. If difficulties arise, neurosurgical and vascular surgical consultations are promptly obtained. Repeat angiography and exploration of the popliteal artery should be performed rapidly if questionable symptoms arise.

After surgical reconstruction of a knee dislocation, we place the knee in a long-leg hinged brace before leaving the operating room, and we instruct that it is to be worn at all times. The brace is kept locked in full extension except during ROM exercises.

If possible, we begin continuous passive motion (CPM) immediately after surgical reconstruction. The arc of motion is started at 0 to 30 or 40 degrees and increased slowly until a 0- to 70- or 80-degree arc is established and comfortably maintained. Adjunctive cold therapy applied directly to the knee during passive motion has been effective in decreasing pain and edema, and allowing more rapid mobilization of the joint, especially in the early postoperative period.

In the absence of any wound or neurovascular complaints or severe associated traumatic injuries, most patients are ready to leave the hospital by 5 to 7 days after surgery. Ambulation is allowed on crutches, with no weight bearing on the affected side until 3 weeks after surgery. At 3 weeks, progression to partial weight bearing is allowed with the brace locked in full extension. At 6 weeks, the brace is unlocked to allow a 0- to 30-degree arc of motion and supervised gait training while the crutches are gradually discarded. Over 1 to 2 weeks, a long brace ceases to protect the posterolateral corner reconstruction.

After 6 weeks, aggressive therapy is begun to restore full ROM of the knee. Active isolated quadriceps and hamstring exercises (open kinetic-chain exercises) are avoided since they may create joint-shear forces and displacement. Closed kinetic-chain exercises are started, including leg presses, half squats, and stair exercises. Stationary bicycling is also an important part of the therapy program. Over the course of several months, exercises involving increasing resistance and various proprioceptive and agility drills are added to the therapeutic regimen.

Bracing and early motion are the hallmarks of our postoperative rehabilitation protocol. In this regard, we treat patients who have had a multiple ligament reconstruction more slowly and progressively than those who have had a routine ACL reconstruction, especially if there is lateral or posterolateral injury.

COMPLICATIONS

By far, the most common complication of dislocation of the knee is variable loss of knee motion. It is our impression that early surgical intervention and subsequent early motion therapy will lead to improved motion and stability that are reliably superior to what can be achieved with a program of cast immobilization as the definitive treatment for knee dislocations. The exception to this would apply in a straight anteroposterior dislocation in which there is sufficient stability to allow a nonsurgical approach and early motion. In older patients, a "wait and see" approach may also be advisable if there is sufficient stability after the knee is reduced.

Continuous passive motion is instituted early after surgery with the goal of achieving a 0- to 90-degree arc of knee flexion by 6 weeks postoperatively. If this goal is not achieved, we perform manipulation under anesthesia (MUA) to gently lyse adhesions. In general, our guidelines for MUA are to manipulate the knee at about 8 to 10 weeks postoperatively if the ROM is less than 70 to 80 degrees, and to manipulate at about 12 weeks if the ROM is less than 110 degrees. After MUA, we reinstitute CPM and resume the rest of the rehabilitation process.

A reasonable goal for ROM of the knee is an arc of 120 degrees. It is important to identify patients who might not be progressing toward this goal and to manipulate them at an early stage after surgery, since tissue maturation makes manipulation impossible and/or ineffective beyond 4 to 5 months postoperatively.

RESULTS

Knee dislocations often result in severe soft tissue injuries that make return of normal knee function challenging. Although surgical techniques have improved, a complete return to normal function remains difficult. In three recent studies (3,8,17) patients reported their postoperative function as nearly normal 39% of the time, abnormal in 40% of cases, and severely abnormal in 21% of the cases. In general, ROM and functional outcomes scores are better in patients treated with ligamentous reconstructions as outlined previously (1,12). However, residual impairment of function is the rule rather than the exception. The most common complications after surgical repair include postoperative stiffness, failure of some portion of the ligamentous reconstruction, and posttraumatic osteoarthritis (12).

CONCLUSION

Knee dislocations are challenging injuries that result in severe soft tissue injury around the knee joint. Surgical intervention appears to provide the most predictable return to improved function; however, despite newer surgical techniques, return to normal function is difficult. Close attention to complete presurgical evaluation is important to rule out associated neurovascular injury. Detailed surgical planning is critical for optimal outcomes. With appropriate preoperative planning and meticulous surgical technique return to near normal function can be anticipated.

REFERENCES

1. Dedmond BT, Almekinders LC. Operative versus nonoperative treatment of knee dislocations: a meta-analysis. *Am J Knee Surg.* 2001;14(1):33–38.
2. Green NE, Allen BL. Vascular injuries associated with dislocation of the knee. *J Bone Joint Surg Am.* 1977;59(2):236–239.
3. Harner CD, Waltrip RL, Bennett CH, et al. Surgical management of knee dislocations. *J Bone Joint Surg Am.* 2004;86-A(2):262–273.
4. Hollis JD, Daley BJ. 10-year review of knee dislocations: is arteriography always necessary? *J Trauma.* 2005;59(3):672–676.
5. Hoover NW. Injuries of the popliteal artery associated with fractures and dislocations. *Surg Clin North Am.* 1961;41:1099–1112.
6. Johner R, Ballmer PM, Rogge D, et al. Dislocation of the knee. In: Jacob RP, Stubli HU, eds. *The knee and the cruciate ligaments. Anatomy biomechanics. Clinical aspects reconstruction complications rehabilitation.* Berlin: Springer Verlag; 1990.
7. Kennedy JC. Complete dislocation of the knee joint. *J Bone Joint Surg Am.* 1963;45:889–904.
8. Liow RY, McNicholas MJ, Keating JF, et al. Ligament repair and reconstruction in traumatic dislocation of the knee. *J Bone Joint Surg Br.* 2003;85(6):845–851.
9. Meyers MH, Moore TM, Harvey JP, Jr. Traumatic dislocation of the knee joint. *J Bone Joint Surg Am.* 1975;57(3):430–433.
10. Potter HG. Imaging of the multiple-ligament-injured knee. *Clin Sports Med.* 2000;19(3):425–441.
11. Potter HG, Weinstein M, Allen AA, et al. Magnetic resonance imaging of the multiple-ligament injured knee. *J Orthop Trauma.* 2002;16(5):330–339.
12. Robertson A, Nutton RW, Keating JF. Dislocation of the knee. *J Bone Joint Surg Br.* 2006;88(6):706–11.
13. Shields L, Mital M, Cave EF. Complete dislocation of the knee: experience at the Massachusetts General Hospital. *J Trauma.* 1969;9(3):192–215.
14. Sisto DJ, Warren RF. Complete knee dislocation. A follow-up study of operative treatment. *Clin Orthop Relat Res.* Sep 1985(198):94–101.
15. Thomsen PB, Rud B, Jensen UH. Stability and motion after traumatic dislocation of the knee. *Acta Orthop Scand.* 1984;55(3):278–283.
16. Treiman GS, Yellin AE, Weaver FA, et al. Examination of the patient with a knee dislocation. The case for selective arteriography. *Arch Surg.* 1992;127(9):1053–1062.
17. Wascher DC, Dvirnak PC, DeCoster TA. Knee dislocation: initial assessment and implications for treatment. *J Orthop Trauma.* 1997;11(7):525–529.

24 High Tibial Osteotomy in Knees with Associated Chronic Ligament Deficiencies

Frank R. Noyes and Sue D. Barber-Westin

INDICATIONS/CONTRAINDICATIONS

Proximal tibial osteotomy has gained wide acceptance as a treatment option for patients with medial tibiofemoral osteoarthrosis and varus deformity of the lower extremity. Generally, high tibial osteotomy (HTO) provides beneficial results when performed early in the course of the arthrosis process in younger individuals (15,62). There are questions, however, about the level of physical activity that should be pursued after an HTO, as progression of the underlying knee arthrosis can be expected. The presence of varus angulation alone is not sufficient to justify a HTO. Rather, the symptoms, medial tibiofemoral arthrosis, and functional limitations are the primary indicators for the procedure. An added complexity in the varus angulated knee with medial compartment arthrosis is the presence of anterior cruciate ligament (ACL) deficiency. Patients who have these combined abnormalities often experience pain, swelling, giving-way, and functional limitations that sometimes result in a truly disabling condition. There may also be an associated deficiency of the lateral and posterolateral ligamentous structures that adds to the varus angulation and clinical symptoms.

The terms *primary, double,* and *triple* varus knee simplify the clinician's task in logically assessing the abnormal alignment and ligamentous deficiencies in a knee with varus alignment (Fig. 24-1). In short, primary varus refers to the overall tibiofemoral varus osseous alignment, including increased varus alignment due to loss of the medial meniscus and medial tibiofemoral articular cartilage.

As the tibiofemoral weight-bearing line (WBL) at the knee joint shifts onto the medial tibiofemoral compartment, a tendency is created for greater loads to be placed on the medial compartment, and less loads placed on the lateral compartment. The medial shift of the axis may result in excessive medial compressive loads, which may promote arthrosis in that compartment (5,68). Eventually, excessive tensile forces develop in the lateral ligaments, iliotibial tract, and other lateral soft tissues; and separa-

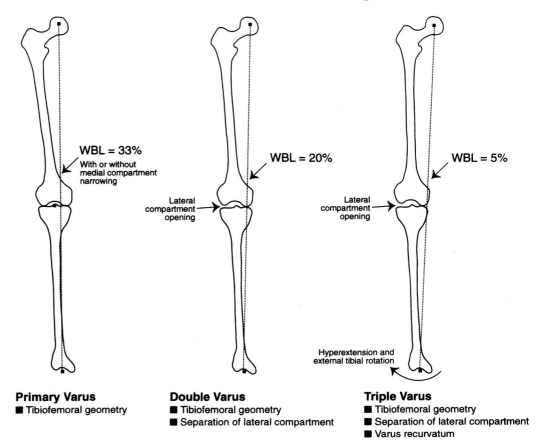

WBL = 33%
With or without
medial compartment
narrowing

WBL = 20%

WBL = 5%

Lateral
compartment
opening

Lateral
compartment
opening

Hyperextension and
external tibial rotation

Primary Varus
■ Tibiofemoral geometry

Double Varus
■ Tibiofemoral geometry
■ Separation of lateral compartment

Triple Varus
■ Tibiofemoral geometry
■ Separation of lateral compartment
■ Varus recurvatum

FIGURE 24-1

Schematic illustration of primary, double, and triple varus knee angulation (see text). WBL, weight-bearing line. (Reprinted with permission from Noyes FR, Simon R. The role of high tibial osteotomy in the anterior cruciate ligament-deficient knee with varus alignment. In: DeLee JC, Drez D, eds. *Orthopaedic Sports Medicine, Principles and Practice*, Philadelphia: WB Saunders, 1993.)

tion of the lateral tibiofemoral compartment will occur during standing and walking activities (lateral condylar lift-off) (30,68). This condition is termed the double-varus knee because the lower limb varus alignment results from two factors: the tibiofemoral osseous and geometric alignment and separation of the lateral tibiofemoral compartment due to lateral ligamentous damage.

There is a hierarchy of soft tissues on the lateral side that resists lateral tibiofemoral joint separation (9,36). The biceps femoris, quadriceps, and gastrocnemius muscles act in a dynamic manner to resist adduction moments on the knee during gait, maintaining lateral tibiofemoral contact (36). If the muscle forces do not provide a functional restraint due to excessive lateral tensile forces, separation of the lateral tibiofemoral joint occurs. While the fibular collateral ligament (FCL) will normally allow a few millimeters of lateral joint opening due to physiologic slackness, studies have found that the lateral ligamentous structures may stretch out in chronic varus angulated knees (5,22).

With injury to the posterolateral structures (FCL, popliteus muscle tendon-ligament unit, posterolateral capsule), a varus recurvatum position of the limb may occur (16). The triple varus knee refers specifically to varus alignment due to three causes: (a) tibiofemoral osseous alignment, (b) increased lateral tibiofemoral compartment separation due to deficiency of the FCL and popliteal muscle tendon-ligament complex, and (c) added varus recurvatum in extension due to the abnormal increase in external tibial rotation and knee hyperextension with involvement of the entire posterolateral ligament complex. An abnormal increase in hyperextension may also indicate damage to other ligamentous structures (ACL or posterior cruciate ligament [PCL], posterior capsule) (10). However, in some knees with physiologic slackness of the cruciate ligaments, there may be a significant varus recurvatum due to damage to the posterolateral ligamentous structures alone. The selection of an appropriate treatment must take into account the associated ligamentous injuries in addition to the varus malalignment.

Subjective symptoms of pain, swelling, and recurrent loss of stability related to activity are well-known effects of chronic ACL deficiency (56). What is unique to the varus-angulated ACL-deficient knee is that there may be two or three different knee subluxations that produce the symptoms of instability. Symptoms of instability may be due to subluxation of the anterior tibia, separation of the lateral tibiofemoral joint on walking (varus thrust), posterior subluxation of the lateral tibial plateau (with knee flexion and external tibial rotation), excessive hyperextension or varus recurvatum, or a combination of these subluxations. It is incumbent on the clinician to take a careful history to determine which of the symptomatic subluxations is present. A varus thrust on walking and a varus tibiofemoral osseous alignment are indications for a valgus-producing osteotomy. An ACL reconstruction in such knees would not address the instability and would be expected to fail due to the abnormal lateral joint opening. A varus recurvatum or "backknee" instability indicates a triple varus knee requiring reconstruction of the posterolateral ligamentous structures in addition to the ACL. The complaint of medial joint line pain may or may not correlate with the degree of medial compartment arthrosis (13,19). In the early stages, the patient usually complains of medial pain with sports activities but rarely with daily activities. When pain does occur with daily activity, the probability exists for extensive articular cartilage damage and exposed subchondral bone. Loss of the medial meniscus is the major risk factor for the progression of arthrosis of the medial compartment.

The timing of the HTO and ligament reconstructive procedures in knees with deficient knee ligaments is based on several factors (Table 24-1) (49). In double-varus knees, the gap test is used at arthroscopy to determine whether it is safe to proceed with ACL reconstruction concomitantly with the osteotomy, or whether it should be staged to allow adaptive shortening of posterolateral tissues. In knees that do not demonstrate abnormal lateral joint opening or external tibial rotation, the HTO and ACL reconstruction may be performed at the same setting. The tibial fixation of the ACL graft is performed by placing interference screws proximal to the osteotomy site and by adding sutures that are tied to a suture post for additional fixation. An ACL reconstruction should not be performed if there is excessive abnormal lateral tibiofemoral compartment opening because this would place the graft under undue forces. In triple-varus knees, we stage the ligament reconstructive procedures after the osteotomy. Performing all procedures (HTO, ACL reconstruction, and posterolateral ligament reconstruction) simultaneously results in a lengthy operation with increased risk of complications, prolonged rehabilitation, and knee motion problems (4,26,74). We perform the HTO and then, after adequate healing of the osteotomy, an arthroscopically assisted ACL reconstruction and open posterolateral ligament reconstruction. The ACL and posterolateral ligament reconstructive procedures must be performed together to allow both structures to function together to resist abnormal lateral tibiofemoral joint opening and varus recurvatum.

When a primary ACL reconstruction is performed with the HTO, our first graft choice remains a bone-patellar tendon-bone. In knees undergoing ACL revision reconstruction and osteotomy, we prefer to use a contralateral bone-patellar tendon-bone graft (44), followed by an ipsilateral quadriceps tendon-bone graft (43) (Fig. 24-2), or a four-strand semitendinosus-gracilis tendon autograft. We avoid allografts for ACL reconstructions in revision knees whenever possible due to the higher failure rates of these grafts compared to autografts (40,41,50). If an allograft is required and the knee demonstrates marked anterior displacement indicating involvement of the secondary ligament restraints, consideration may be given to also perform an iliotibial band extra-articular Losee-type procedure (41).

The recommendation for HTO is derived from careful consideration of subjective symptoms, findings on physical examination, radiographic findings of alignment and arthrosis, and gait analysis data when available. In our clinical setting the predominant indication for HTO is to obtain limb alignment in younger patients experiencing medial tibiofemoral joint pain and who wish to continue an active lifestyle. Unfortunately, a previous medial meniscectomy in a varus aligned knee is a major factor in the progression of the deterioration. Every attempt should be made to preserve and repair both simple and complex meniscal tears. We have described elsewhere techniques that allow for repair of meniscus tears that extend into the avascular region (34,67). After HTO, there is the necessity for modification of athletic activities and common sense guidelines as to what activities will be pursued. The goal of HTO is to allow a more active lifestyle, with recreational pursuits that impose a lower demand on the knee, avoiding strenuous and high-impact sports activities.

The second major indication for HTO is in a varus-aligned knee with combined cruciate injury and posterolateral ligament injury. It is necessary to achieve a normal axial alignment prior to the liga-

TABLE 24-1. Indications for and Timing of Ligament Reconstructive Procedures

Ligament Deficiency	Surgical Procedure	Timing Related to HTO	Indications/Comments
Anterior cruciate ligament	Autograft options: Central third bone-patellar tendon-bone Quadriceps tendon-patellar bone Semitendinosus-gracilis	At or preferably after HTO	Any patient who had instability before HTO should not risk a further trial of function and possible reinjury. Consider when secondary ligament restraints are lost (pivot shift 3 + impingement, >10 mm increased anterior displacement involved knee) and associated medial or lateral ligament deficiency is present. Consider when meniscus repair is performed. Athletically active patient desiring best knee possible for return to sports activities.
Lateral collateral ligament (posterolateral complex intact, no increased external rotation or varus recurvatum)	Usually not required		Expect adaptive shortening LCL in the majority of patients after valgus-producing osteotomy. At HTO, avoid disrupting proximal tibiofibular joint, which would allow proximal migration and laxity of posterolateral ligament structures.
Posterolateral complex, including lateral collateral ligament	Posterolateral complex proximal advancement LCL, posterolateral complex reconstruction with autograft or allograft (see text)*	Staged procedure: HTO first ACL, lateral/posterolateral reconstruction	Patients usually have increased lateral joint opening of 8 mm at the intercondylar notch (12 mm or more at periphery), increased external rotation of 10 to 15 degrees, and require posterolateral reconstruction at time of ACL reconstruction. Combined posterolateral reconstruction and ACL reconstruction always performed together to limit hyperextension and varus rotations.

*A biceps tendon transposition is contraindicated in these knees. The biceps muscle function is required to maintain compressive forces across the lateral tibiofemoral compartment and to allow active external tibial rotation. Both of these functions may be lost if the biceps tendon is transposed and fixated to the lateral femoral condyle.
Reprinted with permission from Noyes FR, Barber-Westin SD, Hewett TE. High tibial osteotomy and ligament reconstruction for varus angulated anterior cruciate ligament-deficient knees. *Am J Sports Med.* 2000;28:282–296.

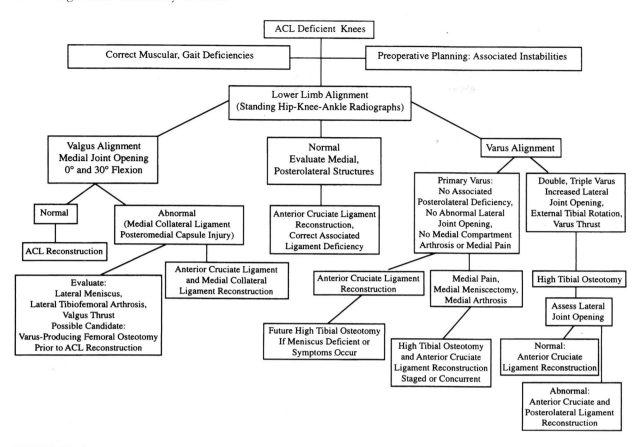

FIGURE 24-2

Algorithm for the treatment of ACL-deficient knees with varus or valgus malalignment requiring surgery.

ment reconstructive procedures. If there is no medial arthrosis, it is not necessary to produce a valgus overcorrection. Rather, a normal 50% weight-bearing line is achieved by corrective osteotomy.

Relative contraindications for HTO include:

- Medial tibiofemoral compartment bone exposure over an area >15 × 15 mm on both surfaces
- Prior lateral meniscectomy, or lateral tibiofemoral cartilage damage
- Extension deficit >10 degrees
- Significant lateral tibial subluxation
- Moderate to marked symptomatic patellofemoral arthrosis
- Depression and concavity of the medial tibiofemoral joint, due to advanced arthrosis which prevents loading the lateral compartment (teeter-totter knee)
- Poor motivation or unrealistic expectations of HTO by the patient. In this situation, the patient may do better with a joint replacement when the arthrosis advances, rather than with an HTO to buy time until a future total knee arthroplasty.

PREOPERATIVE PLANNING

The methodology for our preoperative evaluation and surgical planning is shown in Figure 24-3. The comprehensive physical examination includes particular attention to:

- Patellofemoral abnormalities, including extensor mechanism malalignment and arthrosis
- Detection of tibiofemoral crepitus on varus and valgus loading as an indicator of early articular cartilage damage prior to radiographic changes
- Palpation to detect inflammation, or neuroma of the soft tissues
- Detection of gait hyperextension abnormalities that require gait retraining preoperatively (46,57)
- Examination for abnormal motion limits and joint subluxations of the affected knee compared to the opposite knee

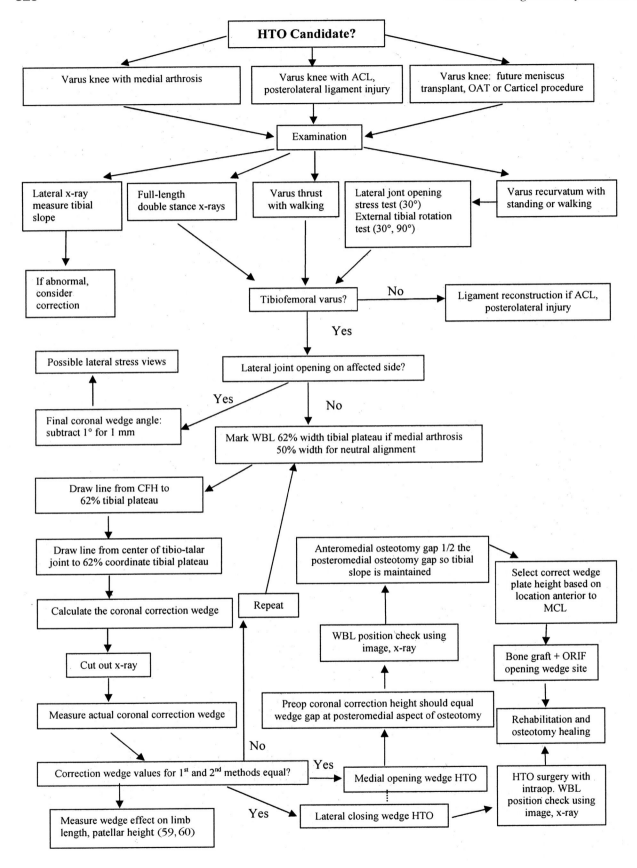

The clinician must determine three factors (54):

1. The abnormal motion limits (e.g., increases in tibial rotation and knee extension)
2. The subluxations that occur in the medial and lateral tibiofemoral joint in the physical examination, and the knee positions in which they occur
3. The anatomic ligament deficiencies that explain the abnormal motion limits and subluxations

The clinical test for FCL insufficiency is based on the varus stress test performed at 0 and 30 degrees of knee flexion. The examiner must estimate the amount (in millimeters) of joint opening from the initial closed contact position of each tibiofemoral compartment to the maximal opened position. The tibiofemoral rotation test, which we previously described (Fig. 24-4A,B), is performed at 30 and 90 degrees of knee flexion to diagnose posterior tibial subluxations in a qualitative manner after ligament injury (52). It is important at arthroscopy to perform a lateral and medial joint opening gap test to measure the amount of joint opening with a calibrated nerve hook (Fig. 24-5A,B). Knees that have insufficient posterolateral structures will demonstrate 8 mm of joint opening at the intercondylar notch, and 12 mm or more of joint opening at the periphery of the lateral tibiofemoral compartment.

Radiographic assessment of lower-limb alignment is based on an examination of radiographs of the full length of the extremity with the patient in the standing position. Separation of the lateral tibiofemoral compartment may occur, preventing a correct assessment of true tibiofemoral osseous alignment. We recommend double-stance, full-length anteroposterior radiographs showing both lower extremities from the femoral heads to the ankle joints (6). The knee is flexed 3 to 5 degrees to avoid a hyperextension position. If separation of the lateral tibiofemoral joint is observed, it is necessary to make appropriate calculations to subtract the lateral compartment opening so that the true tibiofemoral osseous alignment is determined (6). We also look for the "teeter-totter" effect in which simultaneous contact of the medial and lateral tibiofemoral compartments is not possible due to advanced changes of tibial obliquity and bone loss in the medial tibiofemoral joint. This finding indicates that overall limb alignment will probably remain in a varus position after HTO, since lateral tibiofemoral contact cannot be re-established. The required radiographic measurements include the tibiofemoral mechanical axis and tibiofemoral WBL (Fig. 24-6). It is possible for a patient to have a varus thrust on walking due to complete disruption of the posterolateral ligaments and still have a valgus tibiofemoral osseous alignment.

The results of our study (6) indicate that determination of the WBL at the knee joint represents the most precise method of preoperative planning. A WBL crossing the knee lateral to the 75% coordinate has the potential for a "lift-off" of the medial femoral condyle (23). Unicondylar weight-bearing resulting from distraction of the medial compartment is undesirable and could result in rapid lateral compartment deterioration, gradual medial collateral ligament (MCL) failure, and a possible progressive valgus deformity (21). The weight-bearing line-tibial intersection depends on two separate variables, the final mechanical axis angle and the femoral and tibial lengths of the patient.

We use two methods to determine the correction wedge on preoperative radiographs. First, the centers of the femoral head and tibiotalar joint are marked on the full-length radiograph (Fig. 24-7). The selected WBL coordinate of the tibial plateau is identified and marked. This is usually placed at 62% of the tibial width, which allows the WBL to pass through the lateral tibiofemoral compartment, providing a 3-degree angular overcorrection. The 62% WBL coordinate is used if there is medial tibiofemoral articular cartilage damage and the desire exists to transfer loads to the lateral compartment. A 50% WBL coordinate is chosen if there is no medial tibiofemoral joint damage and the surgeon wishes to correct to a normal axial alignment. One line is drawn from the center of the femoral head to the selected percent WBL intersection at the tibia, and a second line is drawn from the center of the tibiotalar joint to

---

FIGURE 24-3

Algorithm for preoperative planning in knees with angular malalignment and associated ligament injury. Tibial width 62% for valgus overcorrection if medial arthrosis, and 50% for neutral alignment. WBL, weight-bearing line. (Reprinted with permission from Noyes FR, Goebel SX, West J. Opening wedge tibial osteotomy. The 3-triangle method to correct axial alignment and tibial slope. *Am J Sports Med.* 2005;33:378–387.)

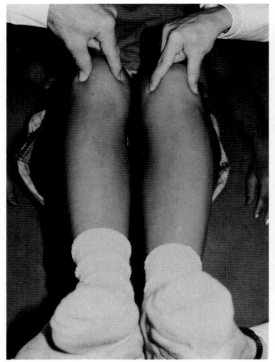
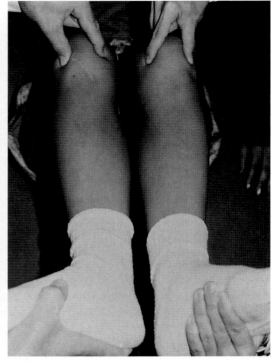

FIGURE 24-4

The tibiofemoral rotation test, shown at 90 degrees of knee flexion, during **(A)** neutral rotation and **(B)** external tibial rotation. The position of the medial and lateral tibial plateaus is palpated and compared with the normal knee to assess whether a subluxation (anterior or posterior) of the medial or lateral tibial plateau is present. The test is performed at 30 and 90 degrees of knee flexion. The position of the medial and lateral tibial plateau is assessed at the starting position (neutral tibial rotation) and at the final test position (external or internal tibial rotation). The axis of tibial rotation is also observed in the involved knee and compared with the normal knee to detect a shift to the medial or lateral tibiofemoral compartment during tibial rotation. (Modified with permission from Noyes FR, Simon R. The role of high tibial osteotomy in the anterior cruciate ligament-deficient knee with varus alignment. In: DeLee JC, Drez D, eds. *Orthopaedic sports medicine, principles and practice*. Philadelphia: WB Saunders; 1993.)

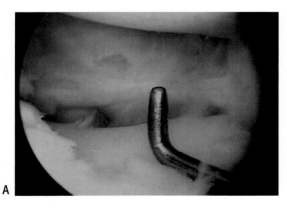

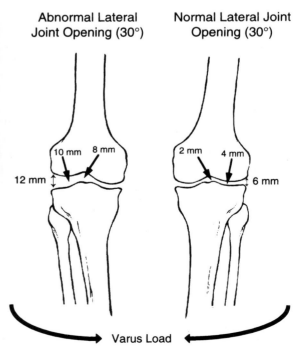

FIGURE 24-5

Arthroscopic gap test for determining the amount of lateral joint opening. A calibrated nerve hook is used to measure the millimeters of joint space. (Reprinted with permission from Noyes FR, Barber-Westin SD, Hewett TE. High tibial osteotomy and ligament reconstruction for varus angulated anterior cruciate ligament deficient knees. *Am J Sports Med.* 2000;28:282–296.)

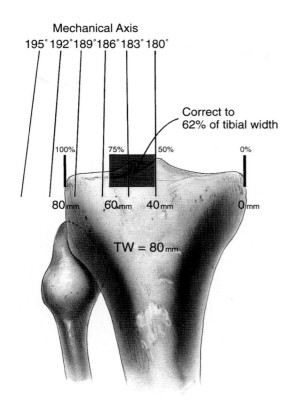

Mechanical Axis
195° 192° 189° 186° 183° 180°

Correct to 62% of tibial width

100%   75%   50%   0%

80 mm   60 mm   40 mm   0 mm

TW = 80 mm

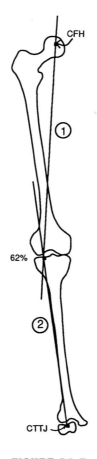

CFH

①

62%

②

CTTJ

STEPS:

① Draw line from CFH to 62% coordinate

② Draw line from CTTJ to 62% coordinate

Angle formed by the two lines equals the angle of correction required to result in weight-bearing line through the 62% coordinate

FIGURE 24-6

The weight-bearing line positions are shown for different degrees of the mechanical axis. In this example, a correction beyond 186 degrees results in a weight-bearing line lateral to the desired target area. TW, tibial width. (Reprinted with permission from Dugdale TW, Noyes FR, Styer D. Preoperative planning for high tibial osteotomy: effect of lateral tibiofemoral separation and tibiofemoral length. *Clin Orthop.* 1991;271:105–121.)

FIGURE 24-7

Graphic depiction of the method used to calculate the correction angle of an HTO using a full-length, non–weight-bearing anteroposterior roentgenograph of the lower extremity. (Reprinted with permission from Dugdale TW, Noyes FR, Styer D. Preoperative planning for high tibial osteotomy: effect of lateral tibiofemoral separation and tibiofemoral length. *Clin Orthop.* 1991;271:105–121.)

the same tibial coordinate position. The angle formed by the two lines intersecting at the tibia represents the angular correction required to realign the WBL through this coordinate.

The second method of determining the correction wedge involves cutting the full-standing radiograph horizontally through the line of the superior osteotomy cut (Fig. 24-8). A vertical cut of the lower tibial segment is then made to converge with the first cut at the level of the medial cortex. The distal portion of the radiograph is aligned until the center of the femoral head, the selected weight-bearing line coordinate point on the tibial plateau, and the center of the tibiotalar joint are all colinear. With the radiograph taped in this position, the angle of the wedge formed by the overlap of the two radiographic segments is measured and compared with the value obtained using the first method. The mechanical axis is measured to determine the angular correction. If there is a discrepancy between the two correction wedge angles, the procedures should be repeated.

Lateral radiographs are examined for abnormal tibial slope, such as an excessive posterior sloping of the tibial surface greater than 8 degrees. Abnormal posterior sloping of the tibia in the sagittal plane is usually seen after tibial fractures or growth abnormalities, and may increase forces on an ACL reconstruction, resulting in failure. It is important not to induce during the tibial osteotomy an abnormal tibial slope.

A high adduction moment may be anticipated in varus angulated knees; however, it is also known that the moments and loads on the knee joint cannot be reliably predicted from the static alignment of the lower limb measured on radiographs. We reported on the results of gait analyses in 32 patients

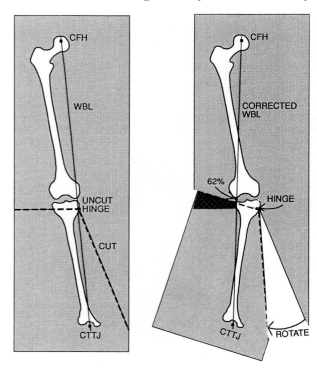

FIGURE 24-8

Graphic depiction of alternate method used to calculate the correction angle of a HTO using a full-length, non–weight-bearing radiograph of the lower extremity. (Reprinted with permission from Dugdale TW, Noyes FR, Styer D. Preoperative planning for high tibial osteotomy: effect of lateral tibiofemoral separation and tibiofemoral length. *Clin Orthop.* 1991;271:105–121.)

with ACL deficiency and varus angulation (57). The majority of patients (20 of 32) had an abnormally high adduction moment. The adduction moment showed a statistically significant ($p < .05$) correlation to predicted high medial tibiofemoral compartment loads and high lateral ligament tensile forces ($p < .01$). The data indicated the likelihood, in knees with high lateral ligament tensile forces, for separation of the lateral tibiofemoral joint to occur with "condylar lift-off" during periods of the stance phase. We also found that approximately one third of the patients had normal or low adduction moments and corresponding normal to low medial tibiofemoral compartment loads. These patients had gait characteristics or adaptations that tended to lower medial tibiofemoral loads despite the varus angulation of the knee joint. Gait analysis allowed identification of patients with very high medial joint loads suggesting a poorer prognosis for progression of the arthrosis. Alternatively, patients with a low adduction moment have a potentially better overall prognosis, and an HTO would result in a substantial lowering of these loads.

Opening Wedge HTO: Methodology for Correction of Axial Alignment and Tibial Slope

On cross-section, the proximal anteromedial tibial cortex has an oblique or triangular shape, whereas the lateral tibial cortex is nearly perpendicular to the posterior margin of the tibia. Because of this relationship, a medial opening wedge osteotomy that has an anterior tibial tubercle gap (width) equal to the gap (width) at the posteromedial margin would increase tibial slope, decrease knee extension, and potentially increase ACL tensile loads (13). A lateral closing wedge osteotomy that has an equal anterior-to-posterior gap along the lateral tibial cortex would have a small effect on tibial slope. Although authors have recognized that a change in tibial slope may occur when performing a medial opening wedge osteotomy, operative techniques or calculations have not been precisely defined to address this problem (8,14,24).

We conducted a study to mathematically calculate through three-dimensional analysis of the proximal tibia (using fine cut axial CT imaging) how the angle of the opening wedge along the anteromedial tibial cortex influences the tibial slope (sagittal plane) and valgus correction (coronal plane) when performing a medial opening wedge osteotomy (53). The obliquity of the anteromedial cortex of the proximal tibia relative to the posterior tibial cortex (Fig. 24-9) was measured on 35 magnetic resonance imaging (MRI) films in healthy young individuals (mean age, 32.7). Serial CT images of a cadaveric tibia were made in 1.25 mm slices and digitized using a computer-aided de-

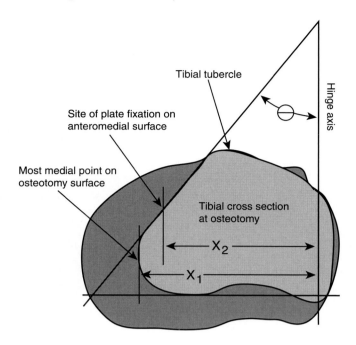

FIGURE 24-9

An axial cut of the proximal tibia at the diaphyseal-metaphyseal junction. The angle formed by the intersection of the medial-lateral axis along the posterior tibia and the axis along the anteromedial tibial cortex is called the anteromedial cortex oblique angle. This angle measures approximately 45 degrees to the coronal plane. (Reprinted with permission from Noyes FR, Goebel SX, West J. Opening wedge tibial osteotomy. The 3-triangle method to correct axial alignment and tibial slope. *Am J Sports Med.* 2005;33:378–387.)

sign package to create a solid model of the proximal tibia. A medial opening wedge osteotomy was created along the anterior-posterior axis to include a hinge axis on the lateral margin of the tibia. The open wedge osteotomy was just proximal to the tibial tubercle, ending 20 mm below the cortical margin of the lateral tibial plateau.

The distal portion of the tibia was rotated on the virtual model about the hinge axis (Fig. 24-10) through the lateral point of the osteotomy maintaining the anatomic tibial slope (sagittal plane). Measurements of the wedge angle and gap angle along the anteromedial tibial cortex were made from the resulting computerized model. Standard algebraic calculations were made using the law of triangles to determine the effect of different degrees of opening wedge osteotomy on coronal (valgus) and sagittal (tibial slope) alignment.

The MRI measurement of the anteromedial tibial cortex oblique angle at the site of the opening wedge osteotomy was 4 ± 6 degrees (range, 34 to 56 degrees) in the 35 patients.

The opening wedge angle, along the anteromedial tibial cortex to maintain the tibial slope, was found to be dependent on the angle of coronal valgus correction (HTO coronal angle) and the angle of obliquity of the anteromedial tibial cortex. In Figure 24-11, the results are shown for the calculation of the opening wedge angle (along the anteromedial tibial cortex) for five different osteotomy corrections in the coronal valgus plane (2.5 to 12.5 degrees). As an example, a 10-degree coronal valgus correction (assuming a 45-degree obliquity of the anteromedial tibial cortex with respect to the hinge axis) would result in a 7-degree opening wedge angle along the anteromedial tibial cortex. A larger wedge angle would decrease the tibial slope, and a smaller wedge angle would increase the tibial slope.

The gap angle is perpendicular to the anteromedial oblique surface of the tibia with a vertex on the hinge axis posterior to the tibia. This is shown in Figure 24-12, where the gap angle in degrees is shown for five different osteotomy corrections as a function of the obliquity of the anteromedial tibial cortex. As an example, a 10-degree coronal valgus correction (assuming a normal 45-degree obliquity of the anteromedial tibial cortex) would result in a 7-degree gap angle at the osteotomy site.

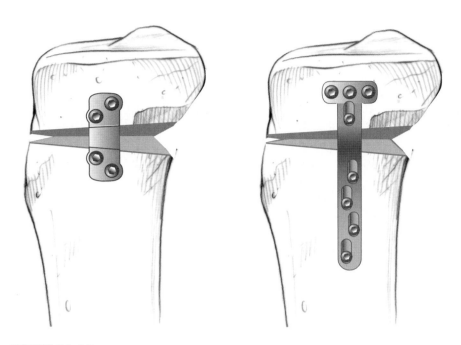

FIGURE 24-10

The distal portion of the tibia was rotated about an AP axis, which ran through the hinge point of the osteotomy to maintain the posterior tibial slope. A solid model of a high tibial osteotomy plate was placed at a series of positions around the medial aspect of the tibia, just anterior to the medial collateral ligament. (Reprinted with permission from Noyes FR, Goebel SX, West J. Opening wedge tibial osteotomy. The 3-triangle method to correct axial alignment and tibial slope. *Am J Sports Med.* 2005;33:378–387.)

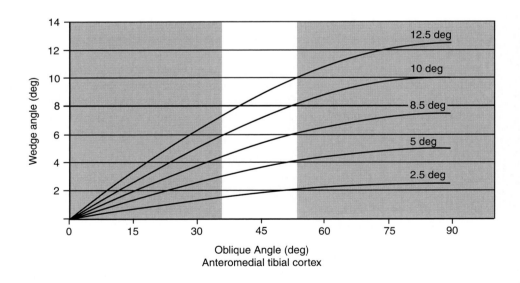

FIGURE 24-11

The anteromedial cortex opening wedge angle depends on the oblique angle of the tibial cortex with respect to the hinge axis. Each line represents the desired calculated degrees of correction for the opening wedge osteotomy in the true coronal (90-degree) plane. (Reprinted with permission from Noyes FR, Goebel SX, West J. Opening wedge tibial osteotomy. The 3-triangle method to correct axial alignment and tibial slope. *Am J Sports Med.* 2005;33:378–387.)

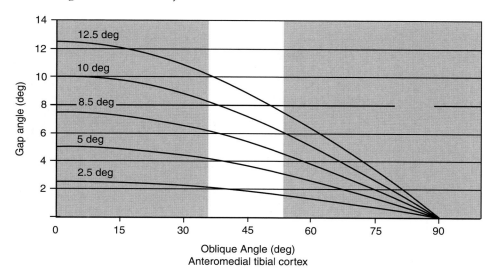

FIGURE 24-12

The magnitude of the gap angle changes with the obliquity of the anteromedial tibial cortex angle. Each line represents the calculated degrees of correction for the opening wedge osteotomy in the coronal plane. (Reprinted with permission from Noyes FR, Goebel SX, West J. Opening wedge tibial osteotomy. The 3-triangle method to correct axial alignment and tibial slope. *Am J Sports Med.* 2005;33:378–387.)

An error in the anteromedial tibial cortex opening wedge angle would result in an error in the tibial slope (Table 24-2). For example, an error of 5 mm in the Y_2 gap (Fig. 24-13) at the tibial tubercle, assuming the length of the anteromedial cortex (L) is 40 mm, would result in an unexpected change in the tibial slope of 10 degrees. As a general rule in this example, every millimeter of alteration in the gap height induces a change of 2 degrees in the tibial slope.

The opening wedge angle can be set at surgery by measuring and altering the vertical gap at two points along the osteotomy site, Y_1 and Y_2 (see Fig. 24-13). This has importance in determining that the correct wedge angle is obtained prior to internal fixation at the osteotomy site. The site at which the vertical gap measurement is taken depends on the coronal distance from the hinge axis, obliquity of the anteromedial tibial cortex, and the distance along the osteotomy site on the anteromedial surface (Tables 24-3 and 24-4). In Table 24-3, the millimeters of opening at the osteotomy site are based

TABLE 24-2.   Errors in the Tibial Slope Caused by Errors in Vertical Gap Height (Y_2)*

Error at Y_2 (mm)	Length of Anteromedial Cortex, mm							
	20	25	30	35	40	45	50	55
1	4.0	3.2	2.7	2.3	2.0	1.8	1.6	1.5
2	8.1	6.5	5.4	4.6	4.0	3.6	3.2	2.9
3	12.0	9.6	8.1	6.9	6.1	5.4	4.9	4.4
4	15.8	12.8	10.7	9.2	8.1	7.2	6.5	5.9
5	19.5	15.8	13.3	11.4	10.0	8.9	8.1	7.3
6	23.0	18.8	15.8	13.6	12.0	10.7	9.6	8.8
7	26.3	21.6	18.3	15.8	13.9	12.4	11.2	10.2
8	29.5	24.4	20.7	17.9	15.8	14.4	12.8	11.6
9	32.5	27.0	23.0	20.0	17.7	15.8	14.3	13.0
10	35.3	29.5	25.2	22.0	19.5	17.4	15.8	14.4

*Results are given in degrees.
Reprinted with permission from Noyes FR, Goebel SX, West J. Opening wedge tibial osteotomy. The 3-triangle method to correct axial alignment and tibial slope. *Am J Sports Med.* 2005;33:378–387.

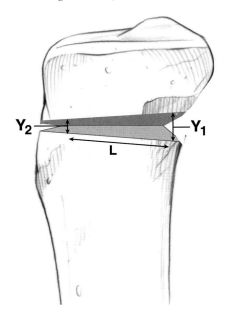

FIGURE 24-13

The opening wedge angle along the anteromedial tibial cortex can be calculated using the three linear measurements along the osteotomy opening wedge. Y_2, posterior gap; Y_1, gap anterior to Y_2; L, length between Y_1 and Y_2. (Reprinted with permission from Noyes FR, Goebel SX, West J. Opening wedge tibial osteotomy. The 3-triangle method to correct axial alignment and tibial slope. *Am J Sports Med.* 2005;33:378–387.)

on the width of the tibia and the angle of correction. In Table 24-4, an average 45-degree oblique angle of the anteromedial cortex and a tibial width of 60 mm are assumed. This allows the surgeon to calculate at the time of surgery making simple measurements, the desired gap height at two points along the osteotomy to maintain the tibial slope. For example, the measurement of the posterior tibial width is made at the osteotomy site (X_1). The opening height at the most posteromedial point (Y_1) and the distance between the two measurement points (Y_1 to Y_2) is used in Table 24-4 to determine the second opening height at a defined distance (L) along the osteotomy site to maintain tibial slope.

If a buttress wedge plate is used, the appropriate size plate may be selected for the opening wedge depending on the site where the plate is placed. An example is given if the surgeon selects to place the buttress plate just anterior to the superficial MCL on the anteromedial tibial cortex approximately 20 mm anterior to the most posteromedial point of the osteotomy. In Table 24-4, with a 10-

TABLE 24-3. Millimeters of Opening at the Osteotomy Site Based on the Width of the Tibia and the Angle of Correction

	Degrees of Angular Correction								
TW*	5	6	7	8	9	10	11	12	13
50	4.37	5.25	6.15	7.00	8.00	8.80	9.70	10.85	11.55
55	4.81	5.78	6.77	7.70	8.80	9.68	10.67	11.94	12.71
60	5.25	6.30	7.38	8.40	9.60	10.56	11.64	13.02	13.86
65	5.69	6.83	8.00	9.10	10.40	11.44	12.61	14.11	15.02
70	6.12	7.35	8.61	9.80	11.20	12.32	13.58	15.19	16.17
75	6.56	7.88	9.23	10.50	12.00	13.20	14.55	16.28	17.33
80	7.00	8.40	9.84	11.20	12.80	14.08	15.52	17.36	18.48
85	7.44	8.93	10.46	11.90	13.60	14.96	16.49	18.45	19.64
90	7.87	9.45	11.07	12.60	14.40	15.84	17.46	19.53	20.79
95	8.31	9.98	11.69	13.30	15.20	16.72	18.43	20.62	21.95
100	8.75	10.50	12.30	14.00	16.00	17.60	19.40	21.70	23.10

*TW, coronal tibial width at osteotomy site.
Reprinted with permission from Noyes FR, Goebel SX, West J. Opening wedge tibial osteotomy. The 3-triangle method to correct axial alignment and tibial slope. *Am J Sports Med.* 2005;33:378–387.

TABLE 24-4. Opening Wedge Height Measurements*						
		Tibial Width at Osteotomy (X$_1$), mm				
Opening at Osteotomy (Y$_1$), mm	**L, mm**	**50**	**55**	**60**	**65**	**70**
8	0	8.0	8.0	8.0	8.0	8.0
	20	5.7	5.9	6.1	6.3	6.4
	25	5.2	5.4	5.6	5.8	6.0
	30	4.6	4.9	5.2	5.4	5.6
	35	4.0	4.4	4.7	5.0	5.2
	40	3.5	3.9	4.2	4.5	4.8
	45	2.9	3.4	3.8	4.1	4.4
10	0	10.0	10.0	10.0	10.0	10.0
	20	7.2	7.4	7.6	7.8	8.0
	25	6.5	6.8	7.1	7.3	7.5
	30	5.8	6.1	6.5	6.7	7.0
	35	5.1	5.5	5.9	6.2	6.5
	40	4.3	4.9	5.3	5.6	6.0
	45	3.6	4.2	4.7	5.1	5.5
12	0	12.0	12.0	12.0	12.0	12.0
	20	8.6	8.9	9.2	9.4	9.6
	25	7.8	8.1	8.5	8.7	9.0
	30	6.9	7.4	7.8	8.1	8.4
	35	6.1	6.6	7.1	7.4	7.8
	40	5.2	5.8	6.3	6.8	7.2
	45	4.4	5.1	5.6	6.1	6.5

*By measuring the width of the tibia, the opening wedge height at the most medial point (Y$_1$), and the distance between vertical measurement points (L), the vertical height at the second measurement point (Y$_2$) can be found on the table. Calculations based on 45-degree angle of the anteromedial tibial cortex at osteotomy site.
Reprinted with permission from Noyes FR, Goebel SX, West J. Opening wedge tibial osteotomy. The 3-triangle method to correct axial alignment and tibial slope. *Am J Sports Med.* 2005;33:378–387.

mm posteromedial opening (Y$_1$), the correct width of the buttress plate would be 7.6 mm (tibial width 60 mm). For a 12-mm posteromedial opening, the correct width of the buttress plate would be 9.2 mm. A wider buttress plate gap would result in excessive valgus alignment and altered tibial slope. The overall method to follow to correct lower limb alignment is summarized in Table 24-5.

The change in the oblique angle of the anteromedial cortex, within the standard deviations reported, would have only a small and negligible effect on the width measurements of the opening wedge (see Table 24-4). For example, assuming a 10-mm width to achieve the desired valgus correction, the computed width for the buttress plate (20 mm anteriorly) and width at the tibial tubercle (45 mm anteriorly) would be 7.6 mm and 4.7 mm, respectively. For a 40-degree oblique angle, the width would be 7.4 mm and 4.3 mm, respectively. For a 50-degree oblique angle, the width would be 7.9 mm and 5.2 mm, respectively, at the two sites.

In general, the rules to maintain tibial slope are:

- The most anterior gap of the osteotomy wedge at the tibial tubercle should be one half of the posteromedial gap to maintain the tibial slope.
- Every millimeter of gap error at the tibial tubercle results in approximately 2 degrees of change in the tibial slope.
- Preoperative radiographic measurement of the tibial slope is recommended.
- The buttress plate height at Y$_2$ (placed anterior to the MCL; see Fig. 24-13) will be 2 to 3 mm less than the posteromedial height at Y$_1$ (gap) to maintain tibial slope during the coronal valgus correction.
- Since small millimeters of change at the osteotomy site affect slope and coronal angulations, radiographic confirmation of final alignment at surgery and postoperatively is required.

TABLE 24-5. Proposed Method to Follow for Opening Wedge Osteotomy to Correct Coronal and Sagittal Malalignment

1. Determine the coronal valgus angular correction in degrees based on preoperative full-standing radiographs for the desired placement of the weight-bearing line at the tibial plateau and measure the tibial slope based on a lateral radiograph.
2. Determine the millimeters of opening at the posteromedial osteotomy site at surgery (Y_1 gap) using the width of the tibia (X_1 distance) for the coronal valgus correction based on the law of triangles (first triangle; Table 24-3).
3. Determine the proper gap width of the osteotomy opening wedge along the anteromedial cortex to maintain tibial slope and the proper width of the tibial buttress plate based on its location along the anteromedial cortex (Table 24-4). If the tibial slope is to be increased or decreased, the effect on the degrees of tibial slope is shown in Table 24-2.
4. Confirm final angular correction based on intraoperative radiographs and later, postoperative full-standing and lateral radiographs.

Reprinted with permission from Noyes FR, Goebel SX, West J. Opening wedge tibial osteotomy. The 3-triangle method to correct axial alignment and tibial slope. *Am J Sports Med.* 2005;33:378–387.

SURGICAL TECHNIQUE

Selection of Opening Wedge or Closing Wedge Osteotomy

Currently, the two most frequently used techniques for correcting varus deformity are the opening and closing tibial wedge osteotomies. We recommend opening wedge osteotomy under the following circumstances:

- When a small angular correction is indicated, the lateral dissection and fibular osteotomy are avoided
- When a large angular correction greater than 12 to 15 degrees is required to avoid excessive tibial shortening
- When distal advancement or reconstruction of the MCL is also required
- When an extensive FCL and posterolateral reconstruction is required, avoiding proximal fibular osteotomy since ligament grafts are anchored to the proximal fibula
- When patella alta or leg length shortening is positively affected by the millimeters of opening wedge osteotomy

There are disadvantages of the opening wedge osteotomy in that appropriate autograft or allograft bone is required at the opening wedge site to restore the anteromedial and posteromedial cortex to add fixation strength and promote osseous union. We prefer autogenous bone grafting of the open defect, which aids in achieving stability at the osteotomy site. There are no published clinical trials we are aware of on the outcome of opening wedge osteotomy where bone allografts were used to fill the osteotomy site. Numerous authors have reported on the outcome of opening wedge osteotomy where autogenous bone was used to fill the gap site (31,63,65,79). We believe the potential problem of early varus collapse of an opening wedge osteotomy due to delayed union may be lessened by autogenous iliac crest bone grafting. In addition, a T- or L-shaped tibial buttress plate with locking screws may be required to achieve more rigid fixation (71).

There is a greater chance of increasing the posterior tibial slope if the opening wedge buttress plate is placed in a more anterior position. However, with attention to this problem at surgery, the normal tibial slope in the sagittal plane can be preserved. Another disadvantage of an opening wedge osteotomy is that transection of the superficial MCL's distal attachment is usually required. In an opening wedge osteotomy of 5 to 7.5 mm, the MCL fibers may be incompletely transected at several different levels (pie-crust approach) to maintain the distal attachment, effectively lengthening the ligament.

The closing wedge osteotomy has the advantage of faster healing and earlier resumption of weight bearing, since contact of two large cancellous surfaces of the proximal tibia is achieved. The initial internal fixation of the osteotomy is more secure than an opening wedge procedure, and there is less chance for a change in osteotomy position and loss of correction. The closing wedge osteotomy does involve more dissection and a meticulous approach and osteotomy of the proximal fibular neck region avoiding the peroneal nerve. It is also somewhat more tedious to resect more bone and alter the lower limb correction at surgery, should it be necessary.

In the preoperative planning, the surgeon should measure the height of the patella on lateral radiographs to determine if an abnormal patella infera or alta position exists which may contraindicate an opening or closing wedge osteotomy, respectively, as these procedures would further decrease or elevate the patella position. The use of an external fixator has been advocated with tibial osteotomy (80); it has the advantage of allowing minor adjustments to be made in lower limb alignment, which is postoperatively helpful in difficult or biplanar corrections. A disadvantage of an external fixator is the risk of pin tract infections and the 10- to 12-week period of time that the fixator is used.

Authors' Preferred Technique for Closing Wedge Tibial Osteotomy

In preparing for the HTO, the entire lower extremity is prepped and draped free. Arthroscopy is performed at the time of the HTO to evaluate articular surfaces of the medial and lateral tibiofemoral compartments and patellofemoral joint. Anterior cruciate ligament–deficient knees frequently have associated meniscus tears that require repair (67) or partial removal. Appropriate debridement of tissues, inflamed synovium, and notch osteophytes limiting knee extension is performed. A sterile tourniquet is inflated before the skin incision. An oblique incision is made from the head of the fibula to the anterior crest of the tibia, 2 cm distal to the tibial tubercle (Fig. 24-14A). The subcutaneous tissues are incised down to the fascia of the anterolateral tibial musculature. A fascial incision is made from the lateral aspect of the tibial tubercle sloping up proximally to the distal aspect of Gerdy's tubercle, and is then extended posteriorly and laterally to the anterior bare area of the fibula (Fig. 24-14B). The anterior bare area of the fibula is an important and safe anatomic landmark. The FCL and peroneal nerve are safely avoided when one identifies this bare area to initiate the limited subperiosteal exposure of the fibular neck for the fibular osteotomy.

Subperiosteal dissection on the tibia is initiated just distal to Gerdy's tubercle, using a scalpel followed by a Cobb elevator. The dissection is continued just lateral to the patellar tendon, and should

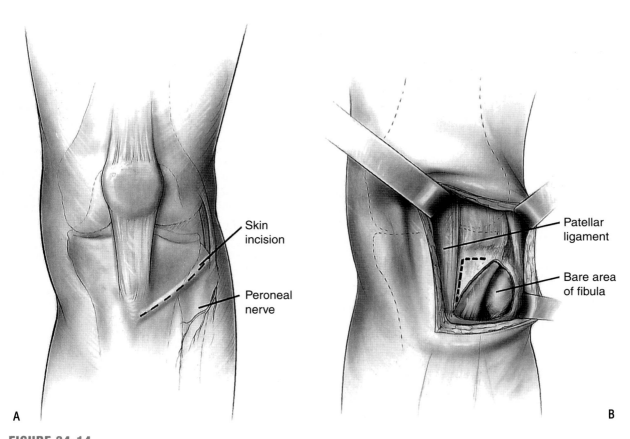

A   B

FIGURE 24-14

A: Oblique skin incision. **B:** Dome-shaped fascial incision.

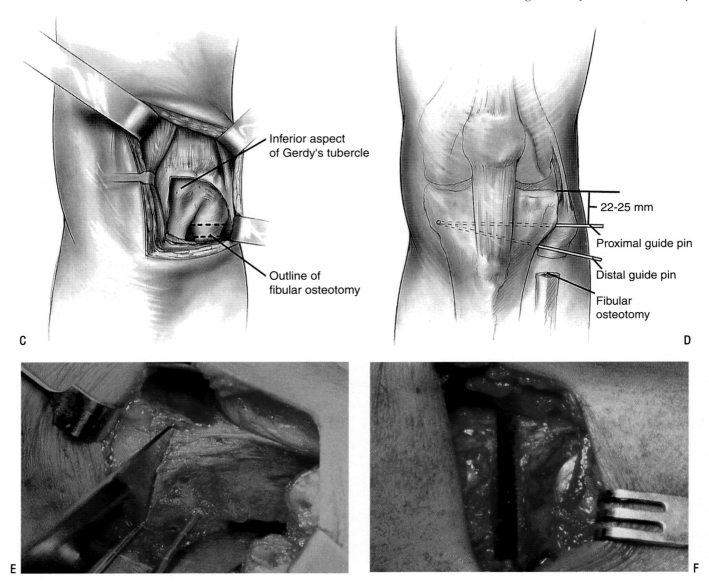

FIGURE 24-14

(Continued) **C:** The proximal fibula is subperiosteally dissected and the peroneal nerve is identified and protected in preparation for the proximal fibular osteotomy. **D:** The proximal guide pin is placed parallel to the joint and 2.5 cm from it. The width of the proximal tibial is determined by measuring the length of this pin. The preoperative planning notes are consulted to determine the starting point for the distal guide pin with reference to the proximal pin, which has been computed for the desired angle of correction. The distance between the two guide pins is essentially the width of the base of the osteotomy wedge. **E:** The proximal tibial osteotomy is made by using the two guide pins as an external jig system to guide the osteotome. **F:** The outer half of the tibial width of the wedge of bone is removed as a single piece.

be done cleanly, with a relatively bloodless field and without damage to muscle tissue. The retinaculum adjacent to the patellar tendon is incised and the retropatellar space entered. The patellar tendon is retracted anteriorly. The dissection is continued posteriorly on the tibia. It is important to remain in a subperiosteal plane because of the proximity of neurovascular structures. Posteriorly, the dissection is completed across the width of the tibia in one location, and is then carefully extended proximally and distally in this safe subperiosteal plane.

There are three basic options for the fibula when performing a HTO: proximal slide, proximal fibular osteotomy, and distal fibular osteotomy. A proximal slide (disruption of tibiofibular joint) is strongly contraindicated in ACL-deficient knees as this shortens the lateral and posterolateral ligaments and may lead to a posterolateral instability in an already unstable knee. Our procedure of choice is a proximal fibular osteotomy through the fibular neck region (Fig. 24-14C,D). Meticulous surgical technique, and protection and palpation of the peroneal nerve, are essential. To protect the peroneal nerve, the lateral and posterior periosteal sleeve is carefully preserved and not retracted under tension. If there is any question as to potential peroneal nerve damage, exposure of the nerve is indicated with direct visualization and protection. The fibular bone wedge that is removed is 2 to 3 mm less than the computed tibial wedge to allow compaction of the fibula osteotomy. Excellent bony apposition is achieved when the osteotomy is closed, and it is not necessary to add internal fixation.

An alternative choice for a fibular osteotomy is at the junction of the middle and distal thirds of the fibula through a 3-cm posterolateral incision. The peroneal tendons are retracted anteriorly and two bunion retractors can be used for exposure after subperiosteal exposure. A portion of the medial cortex of the proximal fibula is preserved to maintain bone contact and promote union. A bone graft from the tibial site is added.

The proximal tibial closing wedge osteotomy may be performed using a commercially available calibrated osteotomy guide system (3) (NexGen Osteotomy System, Zimmer, Warsaw, IN). As an alternative, bone cuts can be determined using a freehand method (Fig. 24-14E,F). A smooth guide pin is placed transversely just through but not beyond the medial cortex, 25 mm distal to the joint line with the use of an image intensifier to ensure proper placement. It is critical to leave at least 25 mm of proximal tibia to avoid a tibial plateau fracture. The transverse length of the guide pin determines proximal tibia width. The method described by Slocum (70) involving a series of congruent right triangles is used to determine the entry point of the second guidewire, again confirming proper positioning of the guidewires with fluoroscopy. These guide pins determine the osteotomy triangular bone wedge that is removed to achieve the desired correction.

We prefer to make our initial osteotomy cuts using a micro-oscillating saw to only cut the outer cortex and then complete the osteotomy with thin osteotomes. An oscillating saw in the cancellous bone may wander and potentially change the correction angle. A malleable retractor is placed in the subperiosteal tissues posteriorly to protect the neurovascular structures, and the knee is flexed 15 degrees. The lateral one half of the wedge is removed as a single piece. This wedge of bone may occasionally need to be replaced if an inadvertent overcorrection is obtained at surgery. The remaining wedge of bone is removed under direct visualization. The surgeon is seated, using a headlamp to view the depth of the osteotomy. The osteotomy plane is maintained in a perpendicular manner, noting that at the midpoint of the tibia, the tibial width is one half of that at the lateral cortex.

The medial 7 to 10 mm of the wedge adjacent to the medial cortex is not disturbed. The medial cortex is preserved to provide stability and prevent tibial medial or lateral translation or varus recurrence. The posterior tibial cortex of the wedge is removed under direct visualization, with a retractor placed subperiosteally at all times to protect the neurovascular structures. The patellar tendon is carefully protected.

Two to three perforations of the medial cortex with a guidewire are often required before the osteotomy gap can be closed with a gentle valgus force which is applied over a few minutes to gradually deform the remaining medial cortex. Apposition of the bony surfaces of the tibia and fibula should be visualized and inspected.

It is important as already stressed that HTO does not increase or decrease the normal posterior tibial slope. An increase in the posterior tibial slope would result in a loss of knee extension and place higher forces on an ACL reconstruction. A decrease or reverse in the tibial slope (anterior tibia slopes distally) would produce knee hyperextension and place high forces on a PCL reconstruction. The sagittal plane of the osteotomy should be perpendicular to the long axis of the tibia with an equal width of cortex removed both anteriorly and posteriorly to preserve the normal posterior tibial slope. In rare cases, usually after a tibial shaft fracture that healed in an abnormal anterior or posterior position, a biplanar osteotomy for correction of an abnormal tibial slope may be required.

Using fluoroscopy, an alignment guide rod (rigid 3 to 4 mm rod, 1 m in length) is positioned over the center of the femoral head and the center of the tibiotalar joint to determine the newly corrected WBL intersection at the tibial plateau. A large single staple may be placed across the lateral tibial osteotomy site for provisional fixation. During this procedure the lower limb is axially loaded at the foot to maintain closure of both the medial and lateral tibiofemoral compartments. The knee is held at 5 degrees of flexion to avoid hyperextension. The alignment guide rod represents a new WBL which should agree with preoperative calculations. If necessary, further bone may be removed from the osteotomy to adjust the WBL as required. Internal fixation of the osteotomy is achieved using an L-shaped plate. Two 6.5-mm cancellous screws are placed in the proximal tibia, and two to three cortical screws are placed distal to the osteotomy (Fig. 24-15A,B). Rarely, a 6.5-mm cancellous screw is placed in a lag fashion across the osteotomy site into the medial aspect of the proximal tibial bone for additional fixation. The final WBL is determined after fixation.

The tourniquet is released and hemostasis obtained. The fascia of the anterior compartment musculature is loosely reattached to the anterolateral aspect of the tibial border. A Hemovac drain is used for 24 hours. A soft Jones-type dressing is applied. The patient is admitted overnight for ice, elevation, pain control, and monitoring of the neurovascular status.

Authors' Preferred Technique for Opening Wedge Tibial Osteotomy

The same preoperative calculations are made as described for the closing wedge technique, except the correction is achieved by performing an oblique opening wedge just proximal to the tibial tubercle. The lower limb is positioned and arthroscopy performed as already described. The ipsilateral anterior iliac crest is also prepped.

A 4-cm incision is made over the anterior iliac crest and deepened to the periosteum (Fig. 24-16A, B), which is sharply incised and reflected medially only to the pelvic brim. Laterally, meticulous subperiosteal dissection is carried along the outer table of the pelvis. The graft size is defined on the bone using electrocautery. In most patients, the graft dimension is 40 mm in length, 10 mm in width, and 30 mm in depth. However, in smaller patients, the graft may be smaller in width, approximately 8 mm in depth. Patients undergoing large osteotomies may require a longer graft in length of ap-

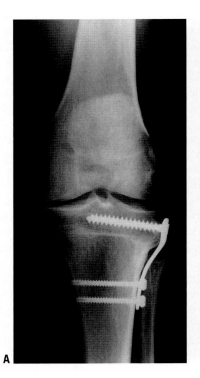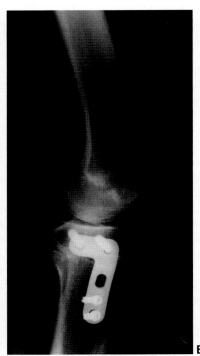

FIGURE 24-15

Anteroposterior **(A)** and lateral **(B)** radiographs show the postoperative appearance after proximal tibial osteotomy, fibular osteotomy, and internal fixation. (Reprinted with permission from Noyes FR, Barber-Westin SD, Hewett TE. High tibial osteotomy and ligament reconstruction for varus angulated anterior cruciate ligament-deficient knees. *Am J Sports Med.* 2000;28:282–296.)

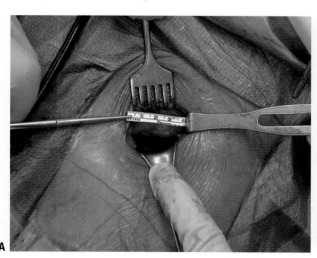
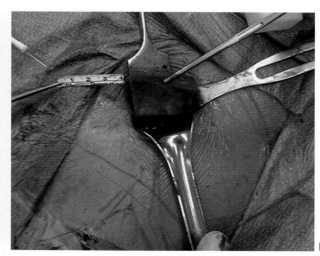

FIGURE 24-16

A: A 4-cm incision over the anterior iliac crest is made to harvest the iliac crest bone graft. The graft is comprised of the anterior crest and outer iliac cortex; the inner table is not removed. **B:** The usual iliac crest bone graft dimensions are 40 mm in length, 10 to 12 mm in width, and 30 mm in depth. (Reprinted with permission from Noyes FR, Mayfield W, Barber-Westin SD, et. al. Opening wedge high tibial osteotomy. An operative technique and rehabilitation program to decrease complications and promote early union and function. *Am J Sports Med.* 2006;34:1262–1273.)

proximately 45 mm. The inner iliac cortex is not dissected, the muscle attachments are not disturbed, and a spacer of the outer table defect is not required. Additional cancellous bone is removed from the inner pelvic cortex. The graft is later fashioned into three triangles. One triangle is placed posterior to the plate to close the gap at the posterior tibial cortex; one triangle is placed in the midportion of the osteotomy deep to the plate; and the smaller triangle is placed in the gap in the anterior tibial cortex. A drain is not required at the iliac crest harvest site.

A 5-cm vertical skin incision is made medially midway between the tibial tubercle and posteromedial tibial cortex, starting 1 cm inferior to the joint line (Fig. 24-17). The sartorius fascia is incised in line with its fibers, proximal to the gracilis tendon. The sartorius and pes anserinus are retracted posteriorly, exposing the superficial medial collateral ligament (SMCL) and posterior border of the tibia. The SMCL is transected at its most distal tibial attachment. Anteriorly, the retropatellar bursa is entered by incising the medial patellar retinaculum, allowing the patellar tendon to be lifted to expose the anterior tibia. A small portion of the patellar tendon fibers attaching medially may be incised at the tibial tubercle to achieve an oblique osteotomy line.

A sharp periosteal incision is made at the posteromedial tibial border, just posterior to the SMCL, to allow meticulous posterior tibial subperiosteal dissection by a Cobb elevator. Care is taken to protect the inferior medial geniculate artery which lies just beneath the distal fibers of the SMCL. A malleable retractor is placed in the subperiosteal posterior tibial space. Only sufficient posterior tibial subperiosteal dissection is used to protect the neurovascular structures, and wide dissection is not necessary (Fig. 24-18).

Management of Superficial Medial Collateral Ligament   There are three surgical approaches for management of the SMCL. In a small opening wedge osteotomy of 5 to 7.5 mm, a "pie-crusting" procedure using multiple transverse incisions at different places may effectively lengthen the SMCL. In larger opening wedge osteotomies, it is necessary to transect the distal attachment, usually 6 cm from the joint, and perform a distal elevation of the attachment in a subperiosteal plane. This allows for the SMCL to be reattached distally after the opening wedge osteotomy with the posteromedial portion of the SMCL bridging the osteotomy site. Transecting the SMCL at the most distal attachment site preserves its length, allows excellent exposure and bone grafting, and allows the tibial fixation plate to be placed in a correct midline position. The tibial slope is not altered, and function of the SMCL is retained.

A third approach is used when distal advancement of the SMCL is required as a reconstructive procedure due to SMCL insufficiency and abnormal medial joint opening. The SMCL is dissected

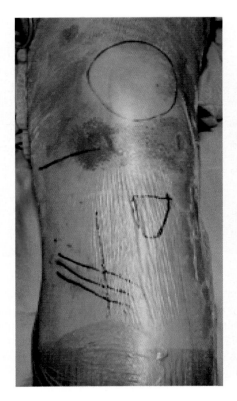

FIGURE 24-17

Skin incision over opening wedge
osteotomy midway between the tibial
tubercle and posterior tibia along the
anterior border of the superficial
medial collateral ligament. The gracilis
and semitendinosus tendon insertions
are marked.

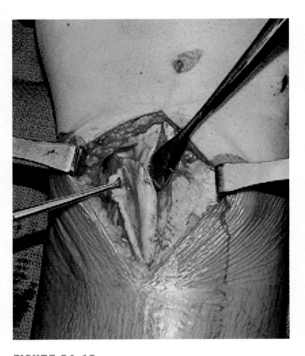

FIGURE 24-18

Subperiosteal dissection of the superficial medial
collateral ligament which is later transected at its
distal attachment in cases where a large opening
wedge osteotomy is necessary.

to the medial joint which is entered anterior and posterior to the SMCL fibers. The posterior incision
is at the junction of the SMCL and posteromedial capsule (short oblique fibers). The anterior incision preserves the attachment of the medial patellofemoral ligament. The medial meniscus position
is carefully examined when a distal advancement of the SMCL is performed. It may be necessary to
incise the medial meniscus capsular attachments and then resuture the attachment to preserve the
correct anatomic location of the meniscus when the SMCL is advanced. The SMCL should appear
relatively normal without scar replacement, as advancement of only scar tissue would be expected
to fail and not provide medial stability. In select cases, a semitendinosus tendon augmentation of the
SMCL may be necessary. The tendon is detached proximally, passed through a small drill hole at
the femoral attachment just anterior and posterior to the SMCL femoral attachment, and then both
anterior and posterior tendon arms are sutured to the SMCL after the osteotomy is completed. The
distal attachment of the semitendinosus is not disturbed. In some instances, both the gracilis and
semitendinosus tendons may be used. The need to surgically reconstruct the SMCL is infrequent;
however, the details as presented should allow for restoration of function when required. At the conclusion of the SMCL reconstruction, plication of the posteromedial capsule anteriorly to the SMCL
is performed to remove any abnormal redundancy with the knee at full extension. Overtightening of
the SMCL and posteromedial capsules is avoided; the repair allows for full knee extension, and a
normal range of flexion.

Placement of Tibial Guide Pins   The patellar tendon and retropatellar bursa are exposed medially. The superior attachment of the tendon is recessed 5 mm using a scalpel to provide adequate exposure for the osteotomy. Retractors are placed anteriorly and posteriorly to complete the exposure. A Keith needle is placed in the anterior medial joint just above the tibia, and the distance is marked on the desired point of the osteotomy along the anteromedial cortex. A second Keith needle is placed at the posteromedial tibial joint space, and the same millimeters are marked to provide a measurement of the tibial slope (Fig. 24-19).

A commercial guide system (Arthrex Opening Wedge Osteotomy System, Arthrex Inc., Naples, FL) is used to facilitate guidewire placement (Fig. 24-20A–D). A 2-mm guide pin is placed at the posteromedial cortex at the marked line and advanced across the tibia at an oblique angle. This pin is usually placed at approximately 15 degrees of obliquity to the tibial shaft and is verified by intraoperative fluoroscopy. To prevent fracture of the lateral tibial plateau, it is important to retain as much lateral tibial width as possible. The error is to have too much obliquity to the guide pin compromising postoperative tibial internal fixation. A second pin is placed anterior and parallel to the first pin. At this point, it is imperative to ensure that the medial osteotomy line (from anterior to posterior) is perpendicular to the joint line. A measurement of the perpendicular cut is accomplished to confirm the distance of each guide pin from the articular surface of the tibia. The distances should be equal in order to maintain the original posterior tibial slope. The length of the posterior pin is measured and used following the law of triangles (53) to determine the millimeters of osteotomy opening to obtain the desired angular correction.

The osteotomy is performed using an oscillating saw for the outer medial and anterior cortices, followed by a 3/4-inch osteotome, placed over the guide pin and verified by fluoroscopy (Fig. 24-21A,B). A 1/2-inch osteotome is used for the posterior cortex, with the edge palpated posterior to the tibia as the osteotome is advanced. The osteotomy is carried to within 10 mm of the lateral cortex. Calibrated opening wedges are then gently inserted into the osteotomy site to achieve the de-

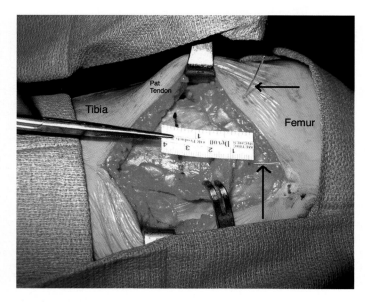

FIGURE 24-19

The intraoperative photograph shows the placement of two Keith needles (*arrows*) at the joint line, which assists the surgeon in obtaining an osteotomy that is perpendicular to the normal tibial slope. In the photograph, the Army-Navy retractor is beneath the patellar tendon. The osteotomy site starts at the anteromedial cortex, 35 mm from the joint line in an oblique manner just proximal to the tibiofemoral joint. This maintains sufficient width of the proximal tibia and limits the risk of a tibial plateau fracture. (Reprinted with permission from Noyes FR, Mayfield W, Barber-Westin SD, et al. Opening wedge high tibial osteotomy. An operative technique and rehabilitation program to decrease complications and promote early union and function. *Am J Sports Med.* 2006;34:1262–1273.)

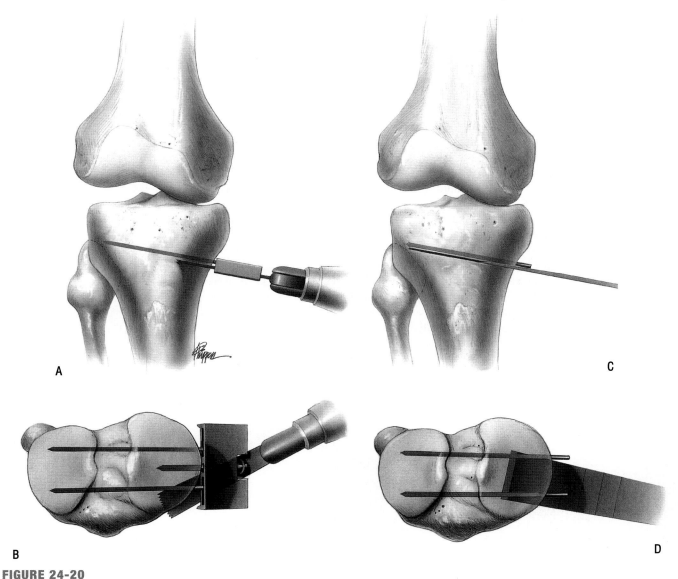

A

B

C

D

FIGURE 24-20

Correct placement for guide pin and subsequent osteotomy with a thin osteotome. The lateral cortex is preserved.

sired angular correction, hinging on the intact posterolateral cortex. This step requires several minutes to prevent fracture of the lateral tibial pillar. Intraoperative fluoroscopy verifies the correct hip-knee-ankle weight-bearing line at the tibia. In addition, the surgeon should determine that there is closure of the medial and lateral tibiofemoral compartments using axial weight bearing against the foot with the knee at 5 to 10 degrees of flexion. The alignment is verified and adjusted if required to achieve the desired angular correction. The anterior gap of the osteotomy site should be one half of the posterior gap, following rules previously described to maintain the tibial slope (53). The width of the tibial buttress plate along the anteromedial cortex is measured and is always less than the millimeters at the posterior medial gap due to the angular inclination of the anteromedial tibial cortex. In select cases, the slope may be purposefully increased in PCL-deficient knees or decreased in ACL-deficient knees.

The three cancellous bone graft triangular segments are impacted tightly into the osteotomy site to obliterate the space and provide added stability, particularly in the sagittal plane (Fig. 24-22A,B). An appropriately sized plate with trapezoidal block is selected and secured with 6.5-mm cancellous screws proximally and 4.0-mm cortical screws distally (Fig. 24-23A–C). We avoid the use of plates with a square buttress block, since this geometry increases the posterior tibial slope. For osteotomies 15 mm or greater, a low-profile T- or L-shaped locking plate is used.

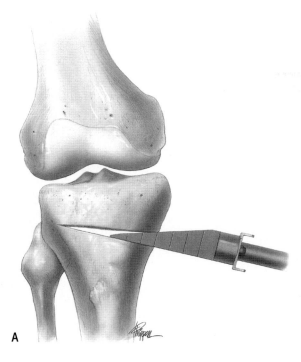

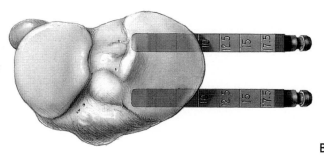

FIGURE 24-21

The use of a commercial (Arthrex Opening Wedge Osteotomy System, Arthrex Inc., Naples, FL) osteotomy wedge to gradually open the osteotomy site.

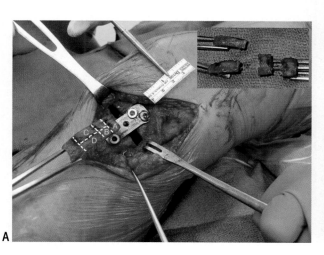

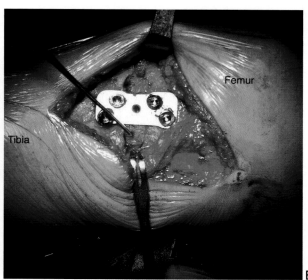

FIGURE 24-22

A: The opening wedge triangular osteotomy opening is shown, along with the harvested and prepared (see inset) iliac crest bone grafts. The bone segments are oversized by 1 to 2 mm to achieve impaction into the osteotomy site. One graft is placed along the posterior tibial cortex at the osteotomy site **(A)**, one is wedged beneath the buttress plate **(B)**, one graft is placed anteriorly at the tibial tubercle (which is one-half the width of the posterior segment to maintain tibial slope) **(C)**, and the remaining bone graft is packed deep into the osteotomy site to promote healing. **B:** The final appearance at the osteotomy site. The iliac crest bone grafts have been placed to restore the entire medial cortex from posterior to anterior to provide a buttress at the osteotomy site. The senior author now prefers a locking path design for more secure fixation. (Reprinted with permission from Noyes FR, Mayfield W, Barber-Westin SD, et al. Opening wedge high tibial osteotomy: an operative technique and rehabilitation program to decrease complications and promote early union and function. *Am J Sports Med.* 2006;34:1262–1273.)

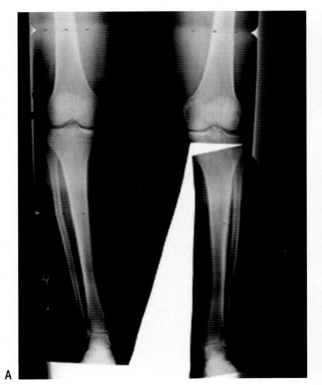

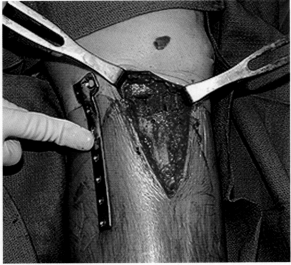

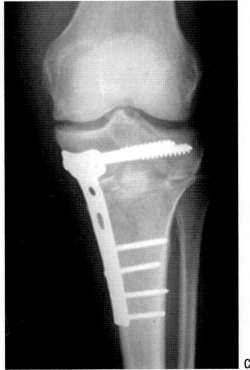

FIGURE 24-23

Demonstration of a 15-mm opening wedge osteotomy, with incorporation of a large tibial plate. **A:** Standing bilateral preoperative radiograph shows the desired opening wedge (gap) to be obtained at the proximal tibia. **B:** An AO tibial side plate is shown, with cortical iliac crest autograft implanted. **C:** Immediate postoperative anteroposterior radiograph. **D:** Tibial locking screw plate designs are available for superior fixation as shown. (Reprinted with permission from Noyes FR, Mayfield W, Barber-Westin SD, Albright JC, Heckmann TP. Opening wedge high tibial osteotomy. An operative technique and rehabilitation program to decrease complications and promote early union and function. *Am J Sports Med.* 2006;34:1262–1273.)

The SMCL fibers are sutured distally and secured to either the plate screws or to suture anchors to maintain tension. The pes anserine tendons and sartorius fascia are reapproximated.

Pearls and Pitfalls

To avoid complications and inadequate correction following opening wedge osteotomy, the following technical pearls are suggested:

- Avoid too proximal placement of guide pin and osteotomy, as this can lead to lateral tibial plateau fracture.
- Verify the osteotomy starting point at the medial cortex and use anterior and posterior Keith needles to verify tibial slope.
- Perform subperiosteal dissection to protect the superficial medial collateral ligament.
- Ensure a secure fixation of the medial collateral ligament repair to avoid valgus instability.

- Use iliac crest bone graft, especially for larger opening wedges.
- Use newer screw locking plate designs for secure fixation.
- Measurement pitfalls: anterior tibial gap should be one half of the posteromedial gap. Downsize plate from the posteromedial coronal gap measurement.
- Begin immediate knee motion and patellar mobilization to avoid arthrofibrosis.
- Avoid too oblique of an osteotomy by maintaining a 15-degree pin angulation to the tibial axis.

Careful preoperative planning is required to avoid inadequate correction. During surgery, confirmation of adequate correction should be accomplished under fluoroscopy. The knee will be placed in an overall excessive valgus position if excessive tibiofemoral joint opening is not evaluated on preoperative standing radiographs. Even though an ideal position is verified at surgery, there may be a change when postoperative full-standing radiographs are taken under the patients' partial or full weight postoperatively. These radiographs should be obtained by 6 to 8 weeks postoperatively (or sooner if there is a concern) to document the surgical correction under weight-bearing conditions. If necessary, it is relatively easy to correct the coronal and sagittal angles at the osteotomy by reoperation early, before bone healing.

The incidence of delayed or nonunion after osteotomy may be reduced by attention to technical details. We do not perform the osteotomy distal to the tibial tubercle. The cancellous surfaces should be cut in a manner that will maximize the amount of surface area that will be in opposition. Adequate internal fixation is believed important with toe-touch weight-bearing in the initial 4-week postoperative period to protect the osteotomy site. Any loss in the overall alignment is an indication for a reoperation. From an empirical standpoint, we insist that no nicotine be consumed for at least 16 weeks before surgery with total abstinence until healing of the osteotomy is evident.

Most if not all of the complications reported in the literature regarding iliac crest bone graft harvest may be avoided by the surgical technique described in this report. For example, we limit the dissection to include only 10 mm of the superior iliac crest. A meticulous subperiosteal exposure of the outer iliac crest is performed without violating the muscle plane. The inner iliac cortex is never dissected, and the muscle attachments are kept intact. We acknowledge that the iliac crest harvest procedure can be painful with trunk flexion activities for up to 4 weeks postoperatively, and patients are advised accordingly. The advantage of the autogenous bone graft is prompt healing, less time on crutches, less overall disuse, and lowered incidence of delayed or nonunion (55).

Peroneal nerve palsy most commonly results from pressure from a tight bandage or lying with the lower limb in external rotation postoperatively. The nerve may also be directly injured during surgery. Osteotomy of the fibula is performed at different sites by different authors depending on the operative technique. There is a risk of injuring the peroneal nerve if the osteotomy is performed in the proximal third of the fibula (77). Fibular osteotomy in the middle portion of the fibula may injure the peroneal nerve innervation to the extensor hallicus longus.

A patella infera condition may develop postoperatively due to quadriceps weakness and concomitant contracture of peripatellar and fat pad tissues. If not recognized and treated promptly, developmental patella infera can rapidly progress to a permanent patella infera and disabling patellofemoral arthrosis (59,60). A diagnosis is established by measuring a decrease in the vertical height ratio of the patella, either from preoperative measurements or from the opposite knee, of 11% to 15%, depending on the method used (60).

We use immediate knee motion and patellar mobilization exercises, and a rehabilitation protocol of straight-leg raises, multiangle isometrics, and electrical muscle stimulation to decrease the incidence of quadriceps weakness and knee motion limitation following HTO. In addition, a phased rehabilitation treatment program for limitations of motion is implemented early postoperatively when restriction of either extension or flexion is noted (51). We had no cases of patella infera in our prospective HTO studies following this program. Any suspect case where there is a postoperative limitation of knee motion and patellar mobility requires lateral radiographs to determine the patellar vertical height (ratio).

Fracture of the tibial plateau can be avoided by meticulously following the previously described operative techniques. The proximal osteotomy should remain parallel to the joint surface and maintain a minimum of 25 mm of tibial width proximally. The medial cortex may be penetrated by a few drill holes, avoiding forceful closure of the wedge. If plateau fracture does occur during a closing wedge osteotomy, anatomic reduction and internal fixation of the plateau fragments may be performed and the osteotomy completed. In an opening wedge osteotomy, the osteotomy is not completed, but delayed until adequate healing of the tibial plateau fracture is demonstrated.

Recognition of the anatomic relationship of the vessels to the surgical dissection is imperative. The anterior tibial artery is at risk because it pierces the proximal interosseous membrane. Injury to this artery may result in an anterior compartment syndrome, which must be recognized and dealt with promptly. The popliteal artery is at risk during posterior dissection and osteotomy of the posterior tibial cortex. By flexing the knee and gently retracting the popliteal structures, the risk of injury to these structures will be significantly reduced.

POSTOPERATIVE REHABILITATION

The protocol for rehabilitation following HTO is shown in Table 24-6. The program includes immediate range of motion (0 to 90 degrees), quadriceps muscle isometric exercises, straight-leg raises, patellar mobilization, and electrical muscle stimulation (49). For 1 week after surgery, ice or a commercial cooling system, mild compression, and maximal elevation are used to prevent edema and swelling. Patients are ambulatory for short periods of time, but are instructed to elevate their limb, remain home, and not resume usual activities. Prophylaxis for deep venous thrombosis includes intermittent compression foot boots in both extremities, immediate knee motion exercises, antiembolism stockings, ankle pumps performed hourly, and aspirin (600 mg daily for 10 days). Doppler ultrasound is routinely performed at 5 days postoperative and at any time the patient demonstrates abnormal calf tenderness, a positive Homan's sign, or increased edema.

A long-leg postoperative brace is worn for the first 8 weeks postoperatively. Initially, patients are only allowed toe-touch weight bearing. At 4 weeks, 25% weight bearing is allowed and gradually increased to full by week 8 if radiographs demonstrate adequate healing and maintenance of the osteotomy position. If allograft bone is used in an opening wedge osteotomy, a delay in full weight bearing is advocated until radiographic evidence of healing is demonstrated. This may take 12 to 16 weeks for osteotomies greater than 10 mm. The protocol emphasizes strengthening of the quadriceps, hamstring, hip, and gastrocsoleus musculature. Closed-chain exercises and stationary bicycling are begun at week 4 postoperatively, and weight machine exercises are begun at week 7 to 8 postoperatively. Excessive use of bicycling and weight machines is not allowed in patients with articular cartilage damage. By week 9 to 12 postoperatively, other aerobic conditioning exercises are begun as appropriate including swimming, ski machines, and walking.

Patients who express the desire to return to sports activities are advised of the risk of further cartilage deterioration if damage was present at the index procedure. Muscle strength tests should demonstrate quadriceps and hamstring strength values of at least 70% that of the contralateral limb. We advise that there should be no pain or swelling with activities. The majority of patients who undergo HTO usually return to only light recreational activities.

COMPLICATIONS

Inadequate or Loss of Correction of Lower Limb Alignment

Inadequate or overcorrection of lower limb alignment has been reported by many authors (13,18,19,61). Hernigou et al reported persistent varus occurred in 10 of 93 knees immediately following closing-wedge osteotomy (13). At 10 to 13 years postoperatively, 71 of 76 knees showed some degree of recurrent varus deformity. Magyar et al reported a loss of correction after closing-wedge osteotomy (28). Although normal alignment was demonstrated immediately postoperatively, 9 of 16 knees in this series had collapsed into valgus by 1 year postoperatively.

Loss of the axial alignment obtained at surgery may be attributed to several factors, including lack of internal fixation, inadequate internal fixation, or collapse of the distal fragments settling into the cancellous bone of the plateau. Bauer et al reported that 15 of 65 knees (23%) experienced shifting of the distal fragments medially after HTO; no internal fixation was used (2). Hernigou et al reported that 21 of 93 patients (23%) lost correction within the first postoperative year; displacement of the osteotomy prior to healing occurred in 11 knees, and the osteotomy failed to correct the varus deformity in 10 knees (13). Stuart et al evaluated standing tibiofemoral angles, which decreased from a mean of 9.3 degrees of varus to 7.8 degrees of valgus at final follow-up (73). Using the Kaplan-Meier survival analysis method, the authors predicted that varus alignment was likely to occur in 18% of knees; lateral compartment arthrosis was likely to progress in 60%; and medial and lateral compartment arthrosis was likely to progress in 83% by 9 years after surgery. Recent survival rates

TABLE 24-6.   Cincinnati Sportsmedicine and Orthopaedic Center Rehabilitation Protocol Summary for High Tibial Osteotomy

	Postop Weeks					Postop Months		
	1–2	3–4	5–6	7–8	9–12	4	5	6
Brace: Long-leg postoperative	X	X	X	X				
Range of motion minimum goals:								
0–110 degrees	X							
0–135 degrees		X						
Weight bearing:								
None to toe touch	X							
1/4 body weight		X						
1/2 to 3/4 body weight			X					
Full				X				
Patella mobilization	X	X	X	X				
Modalities:								
Electrical muscle stimulation	X	X	X					
Pain/edema management (cryotherapy)	X	X	X	X	X	X	X	X
Stretching:								
Hamstring, gastrocsoleus, iliotibial band, quadriceps	X	X	X	X	X	X	X	X
Strengthening:								
Quad isometrics, straight-leg raises, active knee extension	X	X	X	X	X			
Closed-chain: gait retraining, toe raises, wall sits, minisquats		X	X	X	X	X		
Knee flexion hamstring curls (90 degrees)					X	X	X	X	X
Knee extension quads (90–30 degrees)					X	X	X	X	X
Hip abduction-adduction, multi-hip					X	X	X	X	X
Leg press (70–10 degrees)			X	X	X	X	X	X
Balance/proprioceptive training:								
Weight-shifting, minitrampoline, BAPS, KAT, plyometrics					X	X	X	X
Conditioning:								
UBE		X	X	X				
Bike (stationary)			X	X	X	X	X	X
Aquatic program			X	X	X	X	X	X
Swimming (kicking)					X	X	X	X
Walking					X	X	X	X
Stair climbing machine					X	X	X	X
Ski machine					X	X	X	X
Running: straight								X
Cutting: lateral carioca, figure 8								X
Full sports								X

BAPS, Biomechanical Ankle Platform System (BAPS, Camp, Jackson, MI); KAT, Kinesthetic Awareness Trainer (Breg, Inc., Vista, CA); UBE, upper body ergometer.
Reprinted with permission from Noyes FR, Mayfield W, Barber-Westin SD, et al. Opening wedge high tibial osteotomy. An operative technique and rehabilitation program to decrease complications and promote early union and function. *Am J Sports Med.* 2006;34:1262–1273.

reported by authors following closing and opening wedge osteotomy are shown in Tables 24-7 and 24-8.

Delayed Union and Nonunion

Jackson and Waugh reported 19 of 226 (8%) patients had a delayed union following closing wedge HTO; 14 were immobilized for more than 12 weeks before union was achieved, and the remaining five required bone grafting (20). Naudie et al reported 15 of 106 (14%) patients had a delayed union or nonunion after HTO (38).

Warden et al reported low incidence rates of delayed union and nonunion (6.6% and 1.8%, respectively) in 188 opening wedge osteotomies where an iliac crest bone autograft was used in the

TABLE 24-7.	Survival Rates Following Closing Wedge High Tibial Osteotomy					
			Survival Rates			
Study	Number of Patients, Age at HTO	End Points for Survival Analysis	5 Years Postoperative	10 Years Postoperative	15 Years Postoperative	Factors Correlated with Survival Rate
Koshino 2004	N = 75 59 y (46–73 y)	1. TKA or unicompartmental arthroplasty 2. Moderate pain at final f.u. >15 y p.o.	97.8%	96.2%	93.2%	None
Aglietti 2003	N = 91 58 y (36–69 y)	1. TK A 2. HSS score <70 points	96%	78%	57%	Alignment at healing, muscle strength, male gender
Sprenger 2003	N = 76 69 y (47–81 y)	1. TKA 2. HSS score <70 points 3. Patient dissatisfaction	86%	74%	56%	Alignment at 1 y p.o.
Billings 2000	N = 64 49 y (23–69 y)	1. TKA	85%	53%	NA	None
Naudie 1999	N = 106 55 y (16–76 y)	1. TKA	73%	51%	39%	Body weight, delayed or nonunion, age, preop flex
Coventry 1993	N = 87 63 y (41–79 y)	1. TKA 2. Moderate or severe pain in patients who declined TKA	87%	66%	NA	Body weight, alignment at 1 y p.o.
Stuart 1990*	N = 75 58 y (33–75 y)	1. Recurrence varus deformity >5 degrees from femorotibial angle achieved at HTO 2. Medial compartment radiographic arthritic progression 3. Lateral compartment radiograpic arthritic progression	96% 62% 81%	82% 17% 40%	NA NA NA	None

HTO, high tibial osteotomy; TKA, total knee arthroplasty; y, years; f.u., follow-up; HSS, Hospital for Special Surgery; p.o., postoperative.
*Follow-up for survival rates calculated at 9 years postoperative.

TABLE 24-8.	Survival Rates Following Opening Wedge High Tibial Osteotomy					
			Survival Rates			
Study	Number of Patients, Age at HTO	End Points for Survival Analysis	5 Years Postoperative	10 Years Postoperative	15 Years Postoperative	Factors Correlated with Survival Rate
Sterett 2004	N = 38 51 y (34–79 y)	1. TKA 2. Revision HTO	84%	NA	NA	None
Weale 2001	N = 76 54 y (36–70 y)	1. TK A 2. Waiting for TKA 3. Postoperative sepsis precluded revision	88.8%	63%	NA	None
Hernigou 2001	N = 215 61 y (48–72 y)	1. TKA	94%	85%	68%	None

HTO, high tibial osteotomy; TKA, total knee arthroplasty; y, years.

majority of knees (79). There was a trend toward an increased incidence of delayed union or nonunion when a coral wedge was used either alone or in conjunction with the autogenous graft (15%, 5 of 33 knees) compared to when an iliac crest graft was used alone (6%, 8 of 128 knees). No problems with union were reported by Marti et al (32), Pace and Hofmann (63), or Patond and Lokhande (65) following opening wedge osteotomy and iliac crest bone autograft procedures.

The effectiveness of allograft or other bone substitute materials for opening wedge osteotomy has not been adequately determined, even though the introduction of commercially available triangular-shaped cortical-cancellous allografts (along with rigid plate designs) has led to their increased usage. The clinical presumption that large osteotomy gaps would proceed to union with the use of allograft or other bone substitute materials without loss of correction cannot be currently answered. A porous hydroxylapatite wedge was used in conjunction with a fibular autograft in 21 knees in one series, with no problems reported with union (24). The patient population in that study averaged 66.6 years of age, and the osteotomies were small in magnitude (maximum, 10 mm). A high 55% rate of complications was reported by one investigation in which tricalcium phosphate was used to fill the wedge defect in 20 knees during opening wedge osteotomy (66). Nonunions occurred in 35%; loss of correction in 15%; infections in 10%; and material failure in 30%. Hernigou and Ma described the implementation of a block of acrylic bone cement which was placed into the posteromedial portion of the osteotomy, in combination with an anteromedial plate, in 203 knees (12). Only two patients had a delayed union with loss of correction, and one patient had nonunion of the osteotomy. To our knowledge, no report published to date has provided results using allograft bone to fill the defect during opening wedge osteotomy.

Staubli et al reported on 92 opening wedge osteotomy cases in which no bone or bone substitutes was used to fill the gap; a medial tibial plate with locking screws provided fixation and support to the osteotomy site (71). There was a small (2%) incidence of delayed union and a 2% incidence of loss of correction; however, 40% required removal of the implant. Many investigators have demonstrated that external fixators can accomplish adequate union and correction, such as the series reported by Sterett et al., in which only 1 of 33 patients had a loss of correction early postoperatively (72). However, pin tract infections were reported in 45% by these authors, which were similar to the pin tract infection rate reported by Weale et al of 38% (28 of 73 knees) (80) and Magyar et al of 51% (157 of 308 cases) (29).

Peroneal Nerve Injury or Palsy

In 1974, Jackson and Waugh reported 27 of 226 (12%) cases of partial or complete injury to the peroneal nerve during osteotomy (20). There was a higher incidence of injury during curved osteotomies located below the tibial tuberosity, and the authors concluded that osteotomy in this location was too dangerous. A 7% incidence of peroneal nerve injury was reported by Sundaram et al (75), and a 6% incidence was described by Harris and Kostuik (11). The rate of injury is extremely high (25%) after dome osteotomy below the tibial tubercle (20). In three reports by Noyes et al (42,49,55) of 137 osteotomies (including both opening and closing wedge), no peronal nerve injuries were reported.

Arthrofibrosis and Patella Infera

Arthrofibrosis and developmental patella infera after knee surgery require prompt recognition and treatment (59,60,69). Many early HTO studies cited unacceptably high rates of arthrofibrosis and patella infera following postoperative immobilization. Windsor et al reported that 80% of 45 knees had patella infera following closing wedge HTO and postulated that postoperative plaster immobilization allowed the quadriceps muscle to relax and the patellar ligament to shorten (82). Westrich and colleagues reported that 16 of 34 knees (47%) treated with cast immobilization developed patella infera, compared with only 3 of 35 (8%) that received immediate postoperative motion (81).

A decrease in the patellar height Blackburn-Peel ratio may be expected following opening wedge osteotomy. Wright et al reported that all 28 patients in their series of medial opening wedge osteotomies had a decrease in patellar height; however, no significant change in patellar ligament length was detected using the Insall-Salvati ratio (17,83). The authors reasoned that because the osteotomy increased the distance between the tibial tubercle and tibial articular surface, the patella migrated distally. Other authors have reported similar findings in decreased patellar height following opening wedge osteotomy (12,37,39,76). Patella infera has been noted to correlate with the magnitude of angular correction after HTO (76,83).

Tibial Plateau Fracture

The incidence of tibial plateau fracture following osteotomy has been reported from 1% to 20% (13,33). Matthews et al reported that 8 of 40 patients (20%) sustained a tibial plateau fracture intraoperatively, which became the obvious cause for recurrence of the varus deformity in five of these patients (33). Bauer et al (2) reported that six fractures occurred in 61 patients (10%), and a similar incidence was published by Hernigou et al (13) (10 of 93 knees, 11%).

Tibial plateau fracture appears to be a rare problem following opening wedge osteotomy, although Amendola et al reported 7 of 37 patients (19%) in their initial series of opening wedge osteotomies had intra-articular fractures that extended into the lateral compartment (1). The fractures were believed to be caused by a combination of a vertical osteotomy site (closer to the lateral tibial plateau joint line than the lateral cortex) and use of thick osteotomes. After adjusting the obliquity of the osteotomy and switching to thin, flexible osteotomes, the authors did not experience any further cases of fracture.

Vascular Injury

Vascular complications are exceedingly rare following osteotomy (2,7,13,32). Flierl et al reported the incidence of neurologic complications after two opening wedge osteotomy techniques, one which used a conventional oscillating saw and another that created multiple drill holes and osteoclasis (7). In the conventional sawing method group, acute transient peroneal nerve palsy developed in 15.7% of 89 patients, with persistent deficits found in 12.4% 6 months postoperatively. In the osteoclasis group, 14% had acute transient events, and 4.7% reported permanent weakness. Other than the report by Flierl et al, nerve injury after opening wedge HTO appears to be extremely rare (13,32).

Deep-Vein Thrombosis

The incidence of deep-vein thrombosis (DVT) has not been adequately studied following HTO. Turner et al reported a 41% rate of DVT using venography after HTO in 84 patients; only 15% of these had been diagnosed clinically (78). Only calf clots were diagnosed clinically; three proximal and 12 mixed clots were diagnosed with a venogram. Leclerc et al performed a randomized, prospective trial comparing low-molecular-weight heparin (LMWH) to placebo after 129 osteotomies (27). The incidence of DVT was 17% in the LMWH group compared to 58% in the placebo group. While 19% of the placebo group had femoral vein clots, none were detected in the treatment group.

RESULTS

We completed three prospective studies assessing treatment results for closing wedge (42,49) and opening wedge (55) osteotomies. The first study reported the results of 41 patients (100% follow-up) who were followed for an average of 58 months after closing wedge osteotomy (range, 23 to 86 months) (42). These patients also had ACL-deficiency, of which 30 were treated with a reconstructive procedure. Significant improvements were found at follow-up for pain, swelling, and giving-way ($p < .001$) and 24 patients (59%) had returned to mostly light sports with no symptoms. Thirty-six patients (88%) stated they would undergo the HTO again and 32 (78%) felt that their knee condition was improved compared to its preoperative status. The radiographic evaluation showed that 37 (90%) patients were surgically corrected with a WBL between 50% and 80%. Patients who had advanced arthrosis with bone exposure in the medial tibiofemoral compartment avoided ACL reconstruction by returning only to activities of daily living.

The second study determined the results of patients with double or triple varus knees who had varus malalignment treated by closing wedge osteotomy, ACL-deficiency treated by bone-patellar tendon-bone graft reconstruction, and lateral ligament deficiency treated in certain cases with a posterolateral ligament reconstruction (49). Forty-one patients remained in follow-up a mean of 4.5 years (range, 2 to 12 years) after the HTO. At follow-up, significant improvements were found for pain, swelling, and giving-way ($p < 0.001$) (Fig. 24-24A–C). Twenty-nine patients (71%) had improvements in their pain score, and 27 patients (66%) had returned to mostly light athletics without symptoms. The preoperative mean adduction moment of the study group was 35% higher ($p <$

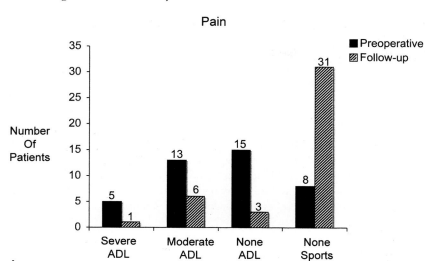

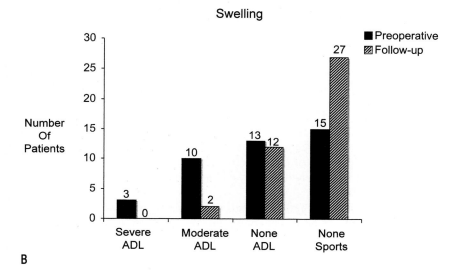

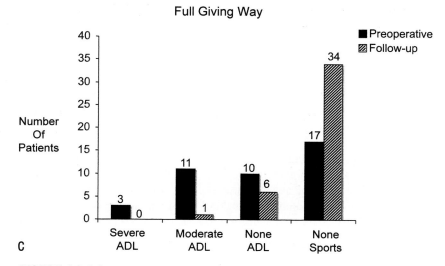

FIGURE 24-24

Statistically significant improvements were found for pain **(A)**, swelling **(B)**, and giving-way **(C)** from preoperative to follow-up ($p < 0.01$). ADL, activities of daily living. (Reprinted with permission from Noyes FR, Barber-Westin SD, Hewett TE. High tibial osteotomy and ligament reconstruction for varus angulated anterior cruciate ligament–deficient knees. *Am J Sports Med.* 2000;28:282–296.)

0.001) than the control group value; 10 of the 17 patients (59%) had values that were greater than 1 standard deviation above control values. Postoperatively, the adduction moment decreased to significantly lower than control values. At surgery, all knees were corrected to a WBL of 62%. At the most recent follow-up, 33 knees (80%) remained in an acceptable position. We noted, as reported by other authors (13,18,19,61), a gradual return to a varus alignment in certain knees due to continued wear and collapse of the medial tibiofemoral compartment despite achieving an initial valgus correction.

Our third study followed 55 consecutive patients who underwent opening wedge osteotomy to determine the rate of complications including nonunion, delayed union, alteration in tibial slope, patellar infera, and arthrofibrosis (55). The patients were observed a mean of 20 months (range, 6 to 60 months) postoperatively. All underwent the technique described in this report, followed by the rehabilitation program detailed in Table 24-6. The osteotomy opening size ranged from 5 to 17.5 mm; 35 knees (64%) had openings of 10 mm or less, and 20 knees (36%) had openings greater than 11 mm. The osteotomy united in all patients. Three knees had a delay in union, which resolved by 6 to 8 months postoperatively. The iliac crest bone graft healed without complications. There were no infections, loss of knee motion, nerve or arterial injuries, alterations in tibial slope, or cases of patellar infera. Full weight bearing was achieved a mean of 8 weeks (range, 4 to 11 weeks) postoperatively. A loss of fixation occurred in one patient who admitted to resuming full weight bearing immediately after surgery, and the osteotomy was successfully revised.

Reconstruction of the Posterolateral Knee Structures

Indications for reconstruction of the posterolateral structures include abnormal lateral joint opening, increased external tibial rotation, and a varus recurvatum position with hyperextension of the knee. The primary functioning posterolateral structures are the FCL and popliteus muscle-tendon-ligament unit (PMTL), including the popliteofibular ligament (PFL) and posterolateral capsule. These structures function together to resist lateral joint opening, posterior subluxation of the lateral tibial plateau with tibial rotation, knee hyperextension, and varus recurvatum (10,58,64). We previously described in detail the surgical options for correcting deficiency or ruptures to the posterolateral structures (45–47). These options are based on the quality and integrity of these tissues determined at the time of surgery (Fig. 24-25A,B).

In cases of acute ligamentous disruptions, primary repair of the FCL is only indicated for bony avulsions that are amendable to internal fixation. Otherwise, graft reconstruction of the FCL is recommended, especially if an immediate knee motion program is to be used postoperatively, as will be detailed following. We prefer to perform acute posterolateral reconstruction procedures within the first 10 days of injury. Since posterolateral ruptures are usually accompanied by injuries to one or both cruciates and may represent a knee dislocation, we observe these patients for 1 week to evaluate the neurovascular structures and skin condition. This short delay also allows appropriate planning of the surgical procedure and most importantly, the institution of rehabilitation to initiate supervised range of motion and muscle exercises before surgery.

Our preferred reconstruction for either acute posterolateral injuries not amendable to primary repair, or chronic ruptures with abnormal lateral joint opening, external tibial rotation, and varus recurvatum is an anatomic FCL reconstruction with a bone-patellar tendon-bone graft. The posterolateral reconstruction is performed using a straight lateral incision, approximately 12 to 15 cm in length centered over the lateral joint line (Fig. 24-26A–C). The incision is extended distally to allow exposure of the fibular head and proximally to allow exposure of the femoral attachment of the FCL. The skin flaps are mobilized beneath the subcutaneous tissue and fascia to protect the vascular and neural supply. An incision is made along the posterior border of the iliotibial band and continued proximally, overlying the vastus lateralis. The attachment of the iliotibial band to the lateral intramuscular septum is preserved. The posterolateral structures are identified both proximally at their femoral attachment (25) and distally. The interval anterior to the lateral gastrocnemius tendon and muscle and posterior to the posterolateral capsule is entered. The approach is similar to that described for meniscus repairs (34,35). This allows exposure of the PMTL junction, posterolateral capsule, and PFL. The peroneal nerve is protected throughout the procedure and usually is not dissected from its anatomic position.

The lateral joint capsule is incised vertically 10 mm anterior to the popliteal tendon's femoral attachment site. An incision is made in the posterolateral capsule posterior to the FCL femoral attach-

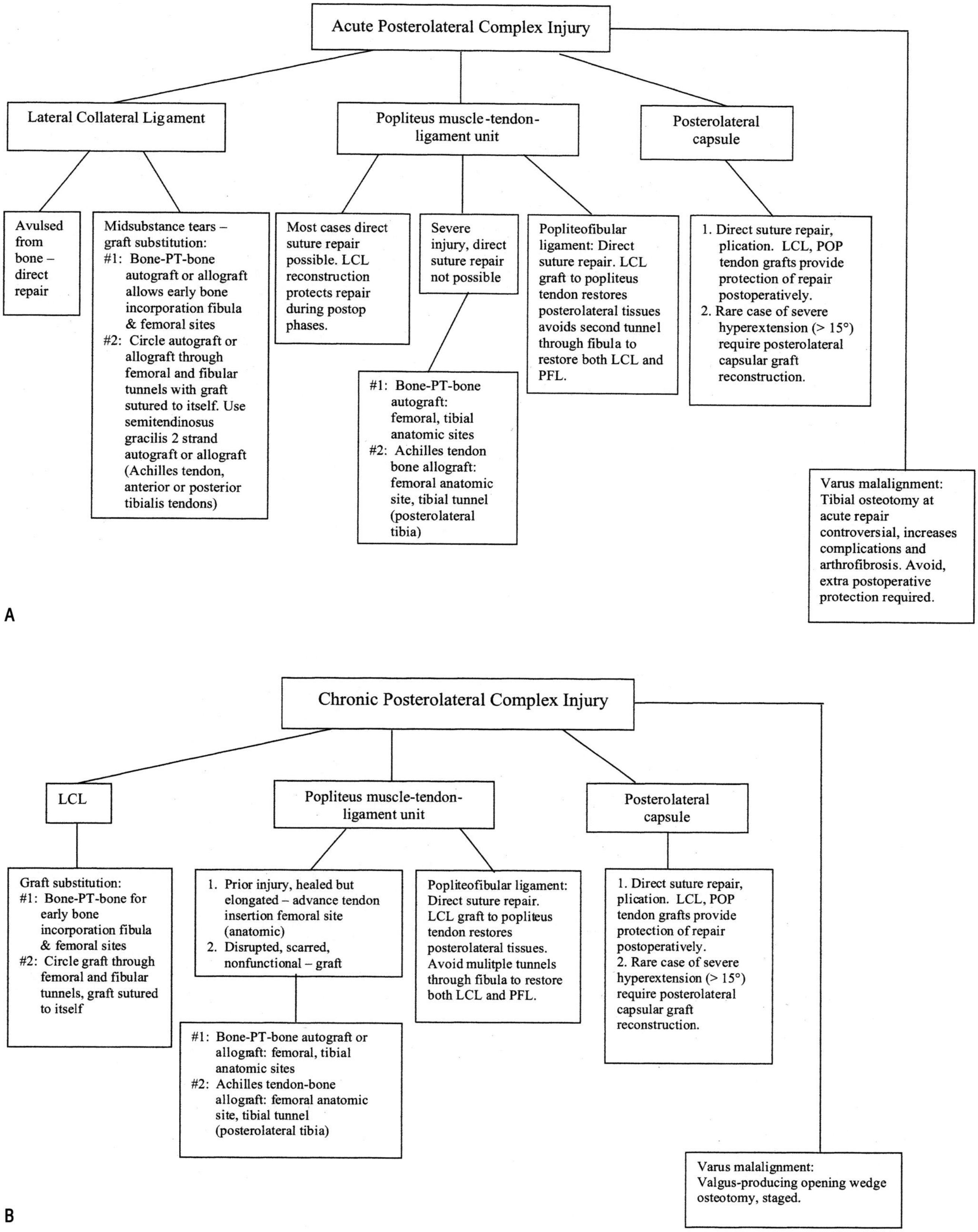

FIGURE 24-25

Algorithm for the treatment of acute **(A)** and chronic **(B)** posterolateral injuries. (Reprinted with permission from Noyes FR, Barber-Westin SD, Albright JC: An analysis of the causes of failure in 57 consecutive posterolateral operative procedures. *Am J Sports Med.* 2006;34:1419–1430.)

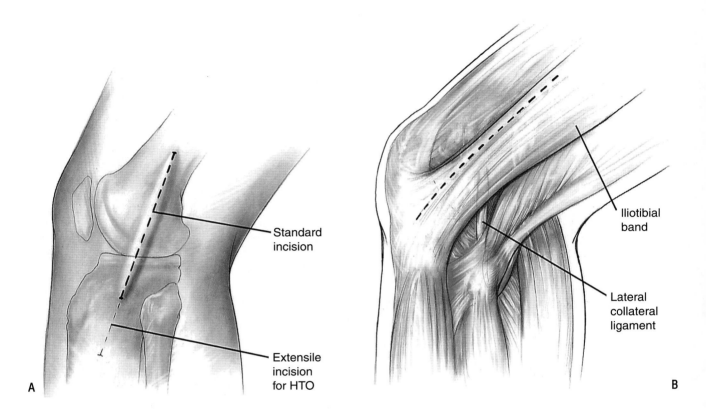

Standard incision

Extensile incision for HTO

Iliotibial band

Lateral collateral ligament

B

Lateral intramuscular septum

Lateral collateral ligament

Tendon of lateral gastrocnemius

Popliteus tendon

C

FIGURE 24-26

A: Straight lateral incision over the epicondyle, extended distally for an HTO. **B:** Exposure of the posterolateral structures through an iliotibial band-splitting approach. **C:** The posterolateral structures are identified and their quality and size determined.

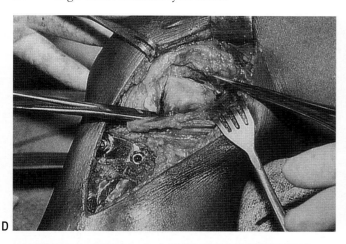

D

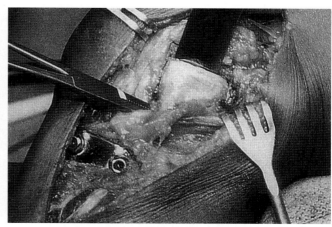

E

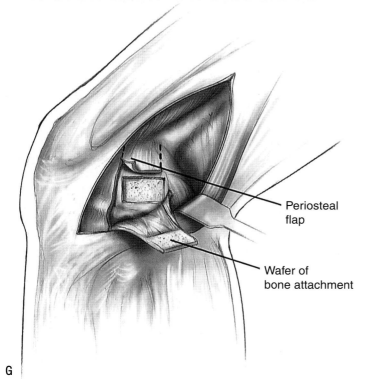

F

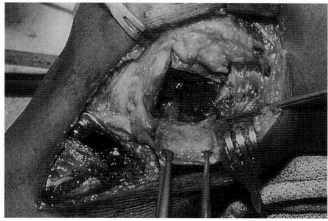

Periosteal
flap

Wafer of
bone attachment

G

FIGURE 24-26

(Continued) **D:** Incision just proximal and superior to the attachment of the LCL to the epicondyle. **E:** Elevation of a 6- to 7-mm wedge of bone. **F:** Alice clamps placed on the wafer of bone. **G:** Release of the posterolateral capsule.

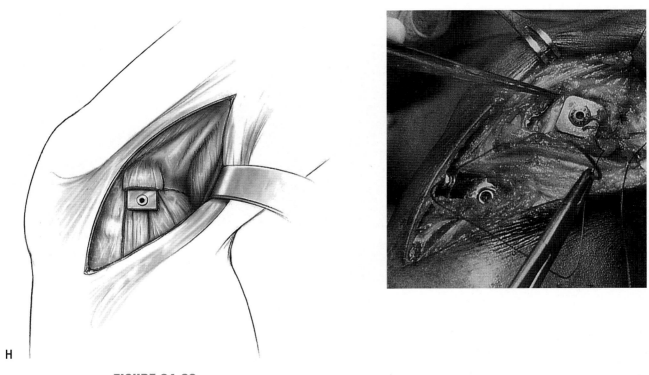

FIGURE 24-26

(Continued) H, I: Reattachment of the bone with a four-pronged staple.

ment, avoiding the popliteus tendon, to expose the lateral meniscus attachments and popliteal tendon recess.

A 9 to 10 mm bone-patellar tendon-bone autograft or allograft may be used to replace the FCL. The collagenous portion of the graft is usually 50 mm in length. The approximate length required for the FCL bone-patellar tendon-bone graft is determined before surgery by measuring the distance from the anatomic femoral insertion site to the anatomic fibular insertion site on a lateral radiograph (using appropriate magnification markers). The length is also verified intraoperatively. In some patients, the autogenous patellar tendon is insufficient in size and, therefore, an allograft of the desired size is required for the procedure.

A tunnel at the proximal fibular attachment site is made over a guide pin that matches the same depth and diameter of the bone portion of the graft. Only the anterior and proximal portion of the fibula is exposed. The bone portion of the graft is gently tapped into the fibular tunnel and attached with two 3.5-mm cortical screws. A guide pin is placed 5 mm proximal and eccentric to the FCL femoral attachment to allow the collagenous portion of the graft to be anatomically placed at the femoral attachment site. The femoral tunnel is drilled with a beath pin, and a suture is attached to the bone to tension the graft. The FCL graft is tensioned at 30 degrees of knee flexion with the lateral joint closed by placing approximately 9 newtons on the graft to avoid overconstraining the lateral tibiofemoral compartment. An interference screw is placed at the femoral anatomic insertion site of the FCL (Fig. 24-27A,B).

In some patients, the autogenous patellar tendon is insufficient in size and therefore, an allograft of the desired size is required for the FCL anatomic replacement procedure. We ensure that sufficient allograft tissue is available during surgery if required. There are two methods available for femoral fixation of the graft. While we normally use tunnel fixation with an interference screw as described in this study, an inlay technique may be used with a four-prong staple for grafts in which secure tunnel fixation may not be accomplished. The FCL graft reconstruction forms the cornerstone and, along with repair or substitution of the posterolateral structures, provides sufficient tensile strength for an immediate protected knee motion program.

The use of a bone-patellar tendon-bone graft provides the advantages of bony incorporation at the femoral and fibular insertion sites, avoiding the potential prolonged incorporation that may occur with soft tissue grafts. Even so, asymmetrical loading at the bone-patellar tendon-bone interface could be expected to occur with knee flexion-extension cycles. We believe that this graft remodels at the insertion sites in a manner similar to that seen in bone-patellar tendon-bone ACL reconstruction due to these sagittal plane motions. This is our current graft of choice for FCL replacement.

In our experience, there are two procedures for restoration of the PMTL. The first, indicated in chronic cases in which the distal attachments of the PMTL are elongated but intact, is a proximal advancement of the popliteus tendon at its femoral attachment. The popliteus tendon is transected at its femoral attachment site and recessed into a 7-mm tunnel using a beath needle with one suture at the tendon end. Internal fixation is done with a reabsorbable interference screw. In severe cases of acute ruptures of the posterolateral tissues or in chronic cases in which the distal attachments of the PMTL are disrupted or deficient with scar tissue, it is necessary to perform a graft substitution of the PMTL. We prefer to use an Achilles tendon-bone allograft and place the bone portion of the graft at the anatomic femoral insertion site. An alternative graft to consider is a bone-patellar tendon-bone allograft or a semitendinosus and gracilis two-strand autograft. The graft is brought out through an 8-mm tunnel placed at the most lateral tibia margin, 15 mm distal to the joint line, adjacent to the popliteus muscle. Fixation is accomplished with a soft-tissue interference screw and suture post at the tibia (Fig. 24-28A–E). This represents a reconstruction of the static portion of the popliteal-tibial attachments. The graft is passed through an appropriately sized drill hole at the femoral anatomic attachment of the popliteus tendon (25) and fixated by a soft tissue interference screw and suture post if required. The graft is tensioned at 30 degrees of knee flexion in neutral tibial rotation under approximately 9 newtons of force to avoid overconstraining the normal amount of external tibial ro-

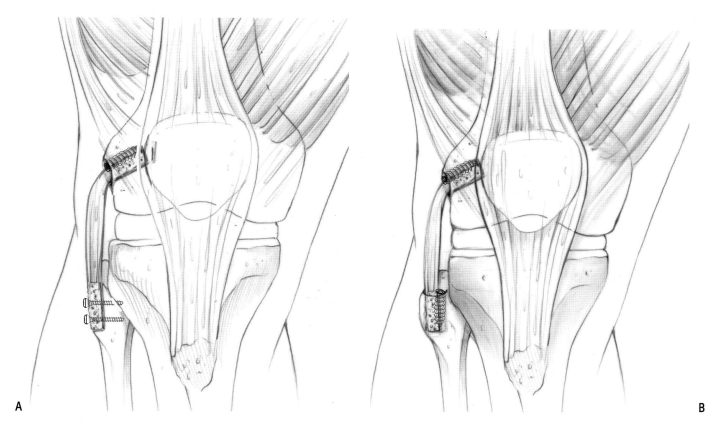

A   B

FIGURE 24-27

Internal fixation of the LCL bone-patellar tendon-bone graft is accomplished on the femur by an interference screw and on the fibula by two small cortical screws **(A)**. Ideally, the graft is placed at the femoral site in a tunnel which is angulated 30 degrees to decrease stress concentration effects. Alternatively, the fibula fixation may be accomplished with an interference screw (with or without additional suture fixation) **(B)** in certain cases such as revision knees where osteopenia may weaken graft fixation strength. (Redrawn with permission from Noyes FR and Barber-Westin SD: Treatment of complex injuries involving the posterior cruciate and posterolateral ligaments of the knee. *Am J Knee Surg.* 1996;9:200–214.)

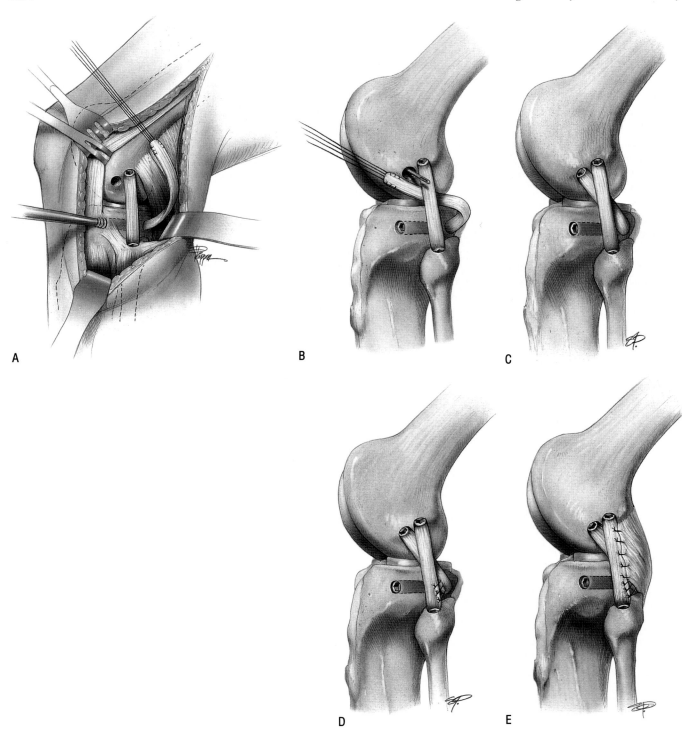

FIGURE 24-28

Popliteus tendon-ligament reconstruction with two-strand semitendinosus autograft and lateral collateral ligament reconstruction with bone-patellar tendon-bone autograft. **A:** A soft tissue interference screw is used for tibial fixation of the popliteus semitendinosus autograft. **B:** Passage of popliteus semitendinosus graft beneath lateral collateral ligament bone-patellar tendon-bone autograft. The posterior exit tunnel is at the posterolateral corner of the tibia. **C:** Final fixation of the popliteus and lateral collateral ligament graft reconstructions. **D:** Suture of popliteus two-strand semitendinosus graft to posterior margin of lateral collateral ligament autograft at the fibular attachment site to restore the popliteal fibular ligament. **E:** Suture plication of posterolateral capsule to posterior margin of lateral collateral ligament bone-patellar tendon-bone autograft.

tation. We do not recommend drilling a second tunnel for the PMTL reconstruction at the fibula, as this may compromise the fixation strength of the FCL graft at the fibular attachment site. Two nonabsorbable sutures placed between the PMTL graft and FCL graft secure the static arm of the popliteus tendon to the fibula (PFL). We prefer to place the popliteus tendon graft on the posterolateral aspect of the tibia at the popliteus muscle attachment.

In our experience, most knees require a combined reconstruction of the posterolateral structures and cruciate ligaments (Fig. 24-29A,B). The order of the reconstruction of multiple ligament procedures is as follows. First, the cruciate ligaments are reconstructed; however, the tibial or femoral attachment site for the ACL or PCL, respectively, is not fixated. Second, the posterolateral dissection is performed and the graft tunnels are drilled. Third, the knee is reduced in the anteroposterior plane and the cruciate grafts secured (48). Finally, the FCL and PMTL grafts are passed and the final fixation of the posterolateral structures is performed.

A second operative option we described for chronic posterolateral instability is a nonanatomic femoral-fibular graft reconstruction. This procedure is indicated when the FCL is intact but deficient and the PMTL does not require graft substitution. In addition, the procedure is advantageous when operative time needs to be considered in dislocated knees and a relatively easy stabilizing procedure can be performed (45). An Achilles tendon allograft is passed from anterior to posterior through the anatomic FCL fibular attachment site and 3 to 4 mm anterior and posterior to the FCL femoral attachment site. The circular graft provides the first arm of the reconstruction and replaces important tensile bearing tissues laterally. The plication or advancement of the posterolateral structures produces a dense collagenous plate of tissues extending from the FCL and posterolateral corner of the knee joint. We described the results of this operation in a consecutive group of patients (45). Twenty of 21 patients (95%) were followed a mean of 42 months postoperatively (range, 24 to 73 months). The success rate of the operative procedure was 76% as determined by stress radiographs and knee stability examinations. The postoperative program of immediate knee motion restored 0 to 135 degrees of motion in all knees and was not deleterious to the reconstructions. Significant improvements were noted for functional limitations in sports activities ($p < 0.05$), symptoms ($p < 0.01$), and in the overall rating score ($p < 0.0001$).

A third operative approach may be considered in knees in which chronic insufficiency of the posterolateral structures results from either a minor injury (without a traumatic disruption) or from varus osseous malalignment and a varus recurvatum thrust on walking (46). The posterolateral insufficiency is due to interstitial tearing, as a definitive FCL of normal width and integrity (although lax) can be identified and the PMTL appears functionally intact even though elongated. A graft reconstruction is not indicated in these knees. Instead, the posterolateral tissues are proximally advanced in a more simplified manner that avoids the added operative complexity and morbidity that may occur with major graft reconstructive procedures. Note that the FCL must be at least 5 to 7 mm in width, and the posterolateral structures must be at least 3 to 4 mm thick, to be functional when the residual slackness is removed by the advancement procedure. This procedure will not be effective if the posterolateral structures consist of scar tissue or if the distal attachment site has been disrupted. One advantage of the proximal advancement technique is that the ligamentous tissues are tightened in a more simplified manner without the added operative complexity and morbidity that occurs with major graft reconstructive procedures. We described the outcome of this procedure in a consecutive series of knees (46). Twenty-one of 23 patients (91%) were followed a mean of 42 months (range, 23 to 94 months) postoperatively. The posterolateral advancement was found to be fully functional in 64%, partially functional in 27%, and nonfunctional in 9%. Overall, 71% of the patients showed improvement in the pain score ($p = 0.02$), and all but one showed improvement in the overall rating score ($p = 0.0001$).

Rehabilitation

The postoperative rehabilitation protocol following posterolateral reconstruction allows immediate knee motion the first postoperative day, but includes protection against excessive joint loads to prevent graft stretching and failure. Patients are warned to avoid hyperextension and activities that would incur varus loading, external tibial rotation, or lateral joint opening. Patients are placed initially in a bivalved cylinder cast for 4 weeks, which is removed for careful active-assisted range of

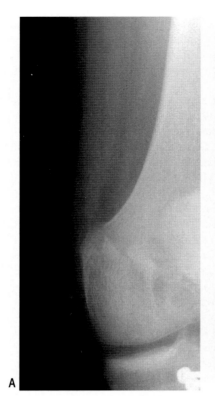
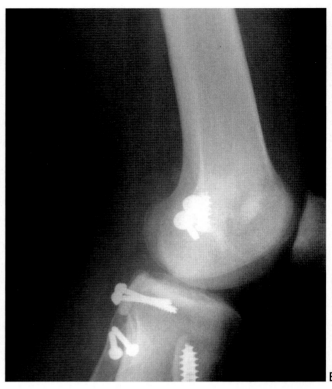

FIGURE 24-29

Postoperative anteroposterior **(A)** and lateral **(B)** radiographs of a 22-year-old male who underwent a PCL tibial inlay two-strand reconstruction, an ACL reconstruction, and a posterolateral reconstruction. The LCL bone-patellar tendon-bone graft fixation is shown. The method of fixation at the femur was a bone inlay at the anatomical LCL fixation site and at the fibula by two small fragment screws. An advancement of the popliteus tendon at the femur and repair of the PFL were also performed. (Reprinted with permission from Noyes FR, Barber-Westin SD. Posterolateral knee reconstruction with an anatomical bone-patellar tendon-bone reconstruction of the fibular collateral ligament. *Am J Sports Med.* 2007;35:259–273.)

motion exercises in a range of 0 to 90 degrees 4 times a day. The cast is used in this time period instead of a soft-hinged postoperative brace, as we think a brace will not provide sufficient protection against excessive lateral joint opening that could occur with ambulation. At 4 weeks postoperatively, a lower extremity, hinged, double-upright brace is applied locked at 10 degrees of extension. The brace is removed 4 times daily for range of motion exercises. At 6 weeks, the brace is unlocked, motion from 0 to 110 degrees is encouraged, and partial weight bearing from 25% to 50% of the patient's body weight is allowed. At 7 to 8 weeks, a custom medial unloading brace is applied as weight bearing progresses to full and flexion is advanced to 120 degrees. The brace is also used as the patient returns to activity to provide some protection against knee hyperextension and excessive varus loads.

In select athletes, a running program is begun at approximately 9 months postoperatively, and plyometric and sports-specific training programs are initiated at 12 months postoperatively. However, the majority of patients who require multiple ligament reconstructive procedures do not want to return to high-impact sports and therefore, this advanced conditioning and training is usually not required. We advise patients who have articular cartilage damage to return to low-impact activities only to protect the knee joint.

REFERENCES

1. Amendola A, Fowler PJ, Litchfield R, et al. Opening wedge high tibial osteotomy using a novel technique: early results and complications. *J Knee Surg.* 2004;17:164–169.
2. Bauer GC, Insall J, Koshino T. Tibial osteotomy in gonarthrosis (osteoarthritis of the knee). *J Bone Joint Surg.* 1969;51A:1545–1563.
3. Billings A, Scott DF, Camargo MP, et al. High tibial osteotomy with a calibrated osteotomy guide, rigid internal fixation, and early motion. Long-term follow-up. *J Bone Joint Surg Am.* 2000;82:70–79.
4. Boss A, Stutz G, Oursin C, et al. Anterior cruciate ligament reconstruction combined with valgus tibial osteotomy (combined procedure). *Knee Surg Sports Traumatol Arthrosc.* 1995;3:187–191.
5. Chao EYS. Biomechanics of high tibial osteotomy. In: Evarts CM, ed. AAOS Symposium on Reconstructive Surgery of the Knee. St. Louis: Mosby; 1978;143–160.
6. Dugdale TW, Noyes FR, Styer D. Preoperative planning for high tibial osteotomy: the effect of lateral tibiofemoral separation and tibiofemoral length. *Clin Orthop Relat Res.* 1992;274:248–264.
7. Flierl S, Sabo D, Hornig K, et al. Open wedge high tibial osteotomy using fractioned drill osteotomy: a surgical modification that lowers the complication rate. *Knee Surg Sports Traumatol Arthrosc.* 1996;4:149–153.
8. Fowler PJ, Tam JL, Brown GA. Medial opening wedge high tibial osteotomy: how I do it. *Oper Tech Sports Med.* 2000;8:32–38.
9. Grood ES, Noyes FR, Butler DL, et al. Ligamentous and capsular restraints preventing straight medial and lateral laxity in intact human cadaver knees. *J Bone Joint Surg Am.* 1981;63:1257–1269
10. Grood ES, Stowers SF, Noyes FR. Limits of movement in the human knee. Effect of sectioning the posterior cruciate ligament and posterolateral structures. *J Bone Joint Surg Am.* 1988;70:88–97.
11. Harris WR, Kostuik JP. High tibial osteotomy for osteoarthritis of the knee. *J Bone Joint Surg.* 1970;52A:330–336.
12. Hernigou P, Ma W. Open wedge tibial osteotomy with acrylic bone cement as bone substitute. *Knee.* 2001;8:103–110.
13. Hernigou P, Medevielle D, Debeyre J, et al. Proximal tibial osteotomy for osteoarthritis with varus deformity. A ten- to thirteen-year follow-up study. *J Bone Joint Surg.* 1987;69A:332–354.
14. Hernigou P, Ovadia H, Goutallier D. Mathematical modelling of open-wedge tibial osteotomy and correction tables. *Rev Chir Orthop Reparatrice Appar Mot.* 1992;78:258–263.
15. Holden DL, James SL, Larson RL, et al. Proximal tibial osteotomy in patients who are fifty years old or less. A long-term follow-up study. *J Bone Joint Surg.* 1988;70A:977–982.
16. Hughston JC, Jacobson KE. Chronic posterolateral rotatory instability of the knee. *J Bone Joint Surg Am.* 1985;67:351–359.
17. Insall J, Salvati E. Patella position in the normal knee joint. *Radiology.* 1971;101:101–104.
18. Insall JN, Joseph DM, Msika C. High tibial osteotomy for varus gonarthrosis. A long-term follow-up study. *J Bone Joint Surg Am.* 1984;66:1040–1048.
19. Ivarsson I, Myrnerts R, Gillquist J. High tibial osteotomy for medial osteoarthritis of the knee. A 5- to 7- and 11- to 13-year follow-up. *J Bone Joint Surg.* 1990;72B:238–244.
20. Jackson JP, Waugh W. The technique and complications of upper tibial osteotomy. A review of 226 operations. *J Bone Joint Surg.* 1974;56B:236–245.
21. Johnson F, Leitl S, Waugh W. The distribution of load across the knee. A comparison of static and dynamic measurements. *J Bone Joint Surg.* 1980;62B:346–349.
22. Kettelkamp DB. Tibial osteotomy. In: Evarts CM, ed. *Surgery of the musculoskeletal system.* New York: Churchill Livingstone; 1990;3551–3567.
23. Kettelkamp DB, Jacobs AW. Tibiofemoral contact area—determination and implications. *J Bone Joint Surg Am.* 1972;54:349–356.
24. Koshino T, Murase T, Saito T. Medial opening-wedge high tibial osteotomy with use of porous hydroxyapatite to treat medial compartment osteoarthritis of the knee. *J Bone Joint Surg Am.* 2003;85-A:78–85.
25. LaPrade RF, Ly TV, Wentorf FA, et al. The posterolateral attachments of the knee: a qualitative and quantitative morphologic analysis of the fibular collateral ligament, popliteus tendon, popliteofibular ligament, and lateral gastrocnemius tendon. *Am J Sports Med.* 2003;31:854–860.
26. Lattermann C, Jakob RP. High tibial osteotomy alone or combined with ligament reconstruction in anterior cruciate ligament-deficient knees. *Knee Surg Sports Traumatol Arthrosc.* 1996;4:32–38.
27. Leclerc JR, Geerts WH, Desjardins L, et al. Prevention of deep vein thrombosis after major knee surgery—a randomized, double-blind trial comparing a low molecular weight heparin fragment (enoxaparin) to placebo. *Thromb Haemost.* 1992;67:417–423.
28. Magyar G, Toksvig-Larsen S, Lindstrand A. Changes in osseous correction after proximal tibial osteotomy: radiostereometry of closed- and open-wedge osteotomy in 33 patients. *Acta Orthop Scand.* 1999;70:473–477.
29. Magyar G, Toksvig-Larsen S, Lindstrand A. Hemicallotasis open-wedge osteotomy for osteoarthritis of the knee. Complications in 308 operations. *J Bone Joint Surg Br.* 1999;81:449–451.
30. Markolf KL, Bargar WL, Shoemaker SC, et al. The role of joint load in knee stability. *J Bone Joint Surg.* 1981;63A:570–585.
31. Marti CB, Gautier E, Wachtl SW, et al. Accuracy of frontal and sagittal plane correction in open-wedge high tibial osteotomy. *Arthroscopy.* 2004;20:366–372.
32. Marti RK, Verhagen RA, Kerkhoffs GM, et al. Proximal tibial varus osteotomy. Indications, technique, and five to twenty-one-year results. *J Bone Joint Surg Am.* 2001;83-A:164–170.
33. Matthews LS, Goldstein SA, Malvita TA, et al. Proximal tibial osteotomy. Factors that influence the duration of satisfactory function. *Clin Orthop Relat Res.* 1988;229:193–200.
34. McLaughlin JR, Noyes FR. Arthroscopic meniscus repair: recommended surgical techniques for complex meniscal tears. *Techniques in Orthopaedics.* 1993;8:129–136.
35. Medvecky MJ, Noyes FR. Surgical approaches to the posteromedial and posterolateral aspects of the knee. *J Am Acad Orthop Surg.* 2005;13:121–128.
36. Muller W. Kinematics of the cruciate ligaments. In: J.A. Feagin, ed. *The cruciate ligaments. Diagnosis and treatment of ligamentous injuries about the knee.* New York: Churchill Livingstone; 1988:217–233.
37. Nakamura E, Mizuta H, Kudo S, et al. Open-wedge osteotomy of the proximal tibia with hemicallotasis. *J Bone Joint Surg Br.* 2001;83:1111–1115.

38. Naudie D, Bourne RB, Rorabeck CH, et al. Survivorship of the high tibial valgus osteotomy. A 10- to 22-year followup study. *Clin Orthop Relat Res.* 1999;367:18–27.

39. Naudie DD, Amendola A, Fowler PJ. Opening wedge high tibial osteotomy for symptomatic hyperextension-varus thrust. *Am J Sports Med.* 2004;32:60–70.

40. Noyes FR, Barber SD. The effect of a ligament-augmentation device on allograft reconstructions for chronic ruptures of the anterior cruciate ligament. *J Bone Joint Surg Am.* 1992;74:960–973.

41. Noyes FR, Barber SD. The effect of an extra-articular procedure on allograft reconstructions for chronic ruptures of the anterior cruciate ligament. *J Bone Joint Surg Am.* 1991;73:882–892.

42. Noyes FR, Barber SD, Simon R. High tibial osteotomy and ligament reconstruction in varus angulated, anterior cruciate ligament-deficient knees. A two- to seven-year follow-up study. *Am J Sports Med.* 1993;21:2–12.

43. Noyes FR, Barber-Westin SD. Anterior cruciate ligament revision reconstruction. Results using a quadriceps tendon-patellar bone autograft. *Am J Sports Med.* 2006;34:553–564.

44. Noyes FR, Barber-Westin SD. Revision anterior cruciate surgery with use of bone-patellar tendon-bone autogenous grafts. *J Bone Joint Surg Am.* 2001;83-A:1131–1143.

45. Noyes FR, Barber-Westin SD. Surgical reconstruction of severe chronic posterolateral complex injuries of the knee using allograft tissues. *Am J Sports Med.* 1995;23:2–12.

46. Noyes FR, Barber-Westin SD. Surgical restoration to treat chronic deficiency of the posterolateral complex and cruciate ligaments of the knee joint. *Am J Sports Med.* 1996;24:415–426.

47. Noyes FR, Barber-Westin SD. Treatment of complex injuries involving the posterior cruciate and posterolateral ligaments of the knee. *Am J Knee Surg.* 1996;9:200–214.

48. Noyes FR, Barber-Westin SD, Grood ES. Newer concepts in the treatment of posterior cruciate ligament ruptures. In: Insall JN, Scott WN, eds. *Surgery of the knee.* Philadelphia: WB Saunders; 2001:841–877.

49. Noyes FR, Barber-Westin SD, Hewett TE. High tibial osteotomy and ligament reconstruction for varus angulated anterior cruciate ligament-deficient knees. *Am J Sports Med.* 2000;28:282–296.

50. Noyes FR, Barber-Westin SD, Roberts CS. Use of allografts after failed treatment of rupture of the anterior cruciate ligament. *J Bone Joint Surg Am.* 1994;76:1019–1031

51. Noyes FR, Berrios-Torres S, Barber-Westin SD, et al. Prevention of permanent arthrofibrosis after anterior cruciate ligament reconstruction alone or combined with associated procedures: a prospective study in 443 knees. *Knee Surg Sports Traumatol Arthrosc.* 2000;8:196–206.

52. Noyes FR, Cummings JF, Grood ES, et al. The diagnosis of knee motion limits, subluxations, and ligament injury. *Am J Sports Med.* 1991;19:163–171.

53. Noyes FR, Goebel SX, West J. Opening wedge tibial osteotomy: the 3-triangle method to correct axial alignment and tibial slope. *Am J Sports Med.* 2005;33:378–387.

54. Noyes FR, Grood ES, Torzilli PA. Current concepts review. The definitions of terms for motion and position of the knee and injuries of the ligaments. *J Bone Joint Surg Am.* 1989;71:465–472.

55. Noyes FR, Mayfield W, Barber-Westin SD, et al. Opening wedge high tibial osteotomy: an operative technique and rehabilitation program to decrease complications and promote early union and function. *Am J Sports Med.* 2006;34:1262–1273.

56. Noyes FR, Mooar PA, Matthews DS, et al. The symptomatic anterior cruciate-deficient knee. Part I: the long-term functional disability in athletically active individuals. *J Bone Joint Surg Am.* 1983;65:154–162

57. Noyes FR, Schipplein OD, Andriacchi TP, et al. The anterior cruciate ligament-deficient knee with varus alignment. An analysis of gait adaptations and dynamic joint loadings. *Am J Sports Med.* 1992;20:707–716

58. Noyes FR, Stowers SF, Grood ES, et al. Posterior subluxations of the medial and lateral tibiofemoral compartments. An in vitro ligament sectioning study in cadaveric knees. *Am J Sports Med.* 1993;21:407–414

59. Noyes FR, Wojtys EM. The early recognition, diagnosis and treatment of the patella infera syndrome. In: Tullos HS, ed. Instructional Course Lectures. Rosemont, IL: AAOS; 1991:233–247.

60. Noyes FR, Wojtys EM, Marshall MT. The early diagnosis and treatment of developmental patella infera syndrome. *Clin Orthop.*1991;265:241–252.

61. Odenbring S, Egund N, Knutson K, et al. Revision after osteotomy for gonarthrosis. A 10-19 year follow-up of 314 cases. *Acta Orthop Scand.* 1990;61:128–130.

62. Odenbring S, Tjornstrand B, Egund N, et al. Function after tibial osteotomy for medial gonarthrosis below aged 50 years. *Acta Orthop Scand.* 1989;60:527–531.

63. Pace TB, Hofmann AA, Kane KR. Medial-opening high-tibial osteotomy combined with Magnuson intraarticular debridement for traumatic gonarthrosis. *J Orthop Tech.* 1994;2:21–28.

64. Pasque C, Noyes FR, Gibbons M, et al. The role of the popliteofibular ligament and the tendon of popliteus in providing stability in the human knee. *J Bone Joint Surg Br.* 2003;85:292–298.

65. Patond KR, Lokhande AV. Medial open wedge high tibial osteotomy in medial compartment osteoarthrosis of the knee. *Nat Med J India.* 1993;6:105–108.

66. Patt TW, Kleinhout MY, Albers RG, et al. Paper #142. Early complications after high tibial osteotomy—A comparison of two techniques (open vs. closed wedge). *Arthroscopy.* 2003;19:74.

67. Rubman MH, Noyes FR, Barber-Westin SD. Arthroscopic repair of meniscal tears that extend into the avascular zone. A review of 198 single and complex tears. *Am J Sports Med.* 1998;26:87–95.

68. Schipplein OD, Andriacchi TP. Interaction between active and passive knee stabilizers during level walking. *J Orthop Res.* 1991;9:113–119.

69. Scuderi GR, Windsor RE, Insall JN. Observation on patellar height after proximal tibial osteotomy. *J Bone Joint Surg.* 1989;71A:245–248.

70. Slocum DB, Larson RL, James SL, et al. High tibial osteotomy. *Clin Orthop Relat Res.* 1974;104:239–243.

71. Staubli AE, De Simoni C, Babst R, et al. TomoFix: a new LCP-concept for open wedge osteotomy of the medial proximal tibia—early results in 92 cases. *Injury.* 2003;34(suppl 2):B55–62.

72. Sterett WI, Steadman JR. Chondral resurfacing and high tibial osteotomy in the varus knee. *Am J Sports Med.* 2004;32:1243–1249.

73. Stuart MJ, Grace JN, Ilstrup DM, et al. Late recurrence of varus deformity after proximal tibial osteotomy. *Clin Orthop Relat Res.* 1990;260:61–65.

74. Stutz G, Boss A, Gachter A. Comparison of augmented and non-augmented anterior cruciate ligament reconstruction combined with high tibial osteotomy. *Knee Surgery Sports Traumatology Arthroscopy.* 1996;4:143–148.

75. Sundaram NA, Hallett JP, Sullivan MF. Dome osteotomy of the tibia for osteoarthritis of the knee. *J Bone Joint Surg.* 1986;68B:782–786.
76. Tigani D, Ferrari D, Trentani P, et al. Patellar height after high tibial osteotomy. *Int Orthop.* 2001;24:331–334.
77. Tjornstrand BE, Egund N, Hagstedt BV. High tibial osteotomy: a seven-year clinical and radiographic follow-up. *Clin Orthop Relat Res.* 1981;160:124–135.
78. Turner RS, Griffiths H, Heatley FW. The incidence of deep-vein thrombosis after upper tibial osteotomy. A venographic study. *J Bone Joint Surg Br.* 1993;75:942–944.
79. Warden SJ, Morris HG, Crossley KM, et al. Delayed- and nonunion following opening wedge high tibial osteotomy: surgeons' results from 182 completed cases. *Knee Surg Sports Traumatol Arthrosc.* 2005;13:34–37.
80. Weale AE, Lee AS, MacEachern AG. High tibial osteotomy using a dynamic axial external fixator. *Clin Orthop Relat Res.* 2001;382:154–167.
81. Westrich GH, Peters LE, Haas SB, et al. Patella height after high tibial osteotomy with internal fixation and early motion. *Clin Orthop Relat Res.* 1998;354:169–174.
82. Windsor RE, Insall JN, Vince KG. Technical considerations of total knee arthroplasty after proximal tibial osteotomy. *J Bone Joint Surg.* 1988;70A:547–555.
83. Wright JM, Heavrin B, Begg M, et al. Observations on patellar height following opening wedge proximal tibial osteotomy. *Am J Knee Surg.* 2001;14:163–173.

25 Guidance System for ACL Reconstruction

Jason L. Koh

Anterior cruciate ligament (ACL) reconstruction is a commonly performed operation, with over 175,000 procedures performed in the United States with a cost of more than $1 billion. Precise graft placement has a significant effect on clinical outcomes, with poor tunnel location related to pain, loss of motion, impingement, graft failure, and arthritis. According to the American Orthopedic Society for Sports Medicine (AOSSM), there is a relatively high revision rate (10% to 20%), and these failures are usually associated with technical factors, specifically tunnel placement. Several studies have documented the difficulty in manually placing ACL tunnels, even in the hands of experienced surgeons.

Current computer-aided navigations systems primarily use optical tracking of markers attached to the femur, tibia, and instruments. Almost all systems will allow the use of any graft choice or type of fixation, and standard manual instruments can be used, and position verified with navigation. Navigation systems provide additional information about the location of tunnels, isometry, and impingement data. They also can document movement in multiple planes, such as rotational stability as well as pure anterior-posterior stability.

Computer-aided navigation systems improve the accuracy of ACL tunnel placement and can reliably document translational and rotational outcomes. Reasons for navigation include:

- Manual tunnel placement has been demonstrated to have errors.
- Navigation improves accuracy of ACL tunnel placement.
- Real time information about impingement is provided.
- Real time information about isometry is provided.
- Real time information about location from the over-the-top position is provided.
- Postoperative stability is improved with navigation.
- Navigation allows documentation of rotation and translation.

INDICATIONS/CONTRAINDICATIONS

Indications

Indications for computer-aided navigation are knee ligament reconstructions where accuracy and precision are desired. My preference is to use navigation in almost every case. Particular situations in which navigation is useful include:

- Revision ACL reconstruction, where the anatomy may be altered and navigation may provide additional information about alternative tunnel locations
- Single-bundle (anteromedial or posterolateral bundle) reconstruction of partial ACL tears
- Double-bundle ACL reconstruction
- Combined osteotomy/ligament reconstruction procedures

Contraindications

Relative contraindications for computer-aided navigation are situations where there is an inability to palpate and register intra-articular landmarks accurately, or when kinematic data are unable to be obtained. The result would be potential errors in parts of the navigation; however, some of the data will remain useful. Caution should be used when there is significant bony loss or inability to obtain consistent flexion-extension data. When used in cases of multiple ligament injury, it is critical to keep the tibia reduced on the femur during acquisition of data. If this cannot be accomplished in the grossly unstable knee, the projection of the intercondylar notch on the tibia (impingement screen) will be incorrect, and the isometry data will also be incorrect.

PREOPERATIVE PLANNING

Essentially no preoperative preparation is needed for the Orthopilot system. All measurements can be obtained intraoperatively. Optional preoperative radiographic data can be input into the machine, but I typically do not find this necessary.

SURGERY

In many ways the technique is identical to the standard ACL procedure, except that prior to the drilling of tunnels, points are registered in the computer and kinematic data are obtained. It is important to remember that navigation serves as a precise measuring tool; it does not dictate the course of surgery or tunnel position. Typically, to improve workflow, all intra-articular work such as stump removal and notch preparation is performed prior to marker placement.

Marker Placement

Reflective balls are attached to the tibial, femoral, and instrument trackers, and the trackers are then placed in a secure location on the back table. The surgeon's preferred graft type is harvested and prepared as usual. Data regarding the type of graft and size of graft are input into the computer. The computer is carefully positioned opposite the operative leg toward the foot of the bed with the camera facing the operative site (Fig. 25-1). Two stab incisions are made in the distal tibia, and two unicortical K-wires are placed into the tibia distally to avoid the tibial tunnel site (Fig. 25-2). Arthroscopy fluid can be used to irrigate and cool the K-wires as they are drilled in to the tibia. A pin clamp is attached to the K-wires and the tibial tracker is then attached to the clamp. Two K-wires are then drilled into the medial epicondyle, and the femoral tracker is attached to a clamp attached to the pins. I prefer to place the femoral tracker in an area with relatively less soft tissue motion to avoid stress on the pins.

Registration

Extra-articular landmarks including the tibial tubercle, anterior tibial spine, and medial and lateral tibial plateau are registered in the computer by using a pointer with attached markers. The tip of the pointer is placed on the structure and stabilized by the finger of the surgeon, and the right foot pedal is used to register the data. This is followed by acquisition of kinematic data. The tibia is reduced onto the femur and the knee is evaluated in full extension, at 90 degrees of flexion, and through an arc of motion. This is followed by acquisition of intra-articular landmarks. The anterior portion of the posterior cruciate ligament (PCL) is lightly touched with the tip of the probe and registered, followed by the medial tibial eminence and anterior horn of the lateral meniscus. It is important to make sure that the tibia is not anteriorly subluxated when the PCL is palpated, since this will falsely place the PCL more posterior than its normal anatomic position with respect to the ACL footprint. The anterior edge of the intercondylar notch is then sequentially palpated and registered. The instrument tracker is then attached to the hook probe, and the over-the-top position is palpated at 12 o'clock (Fig. 25-3) and 1:30/10:30 with the tip of the instrument at the junction of the bone and soft tissue fringe. This step is particularly useful in avoiding palpation of "resident's ridge" since instantaneous feedback on the length of Blumensaat's line is provided. (Standard length is approximately 30 to 32 mm; values of 25 to 26 mm suggest that there is too anterior palpation of the over-the-top position). The ACL origin points are then acquired. Preoperative kinematic data are then acquired by placing the reduced knee at the desired angle (typically 30 degrees) and applying an anterior and posterior

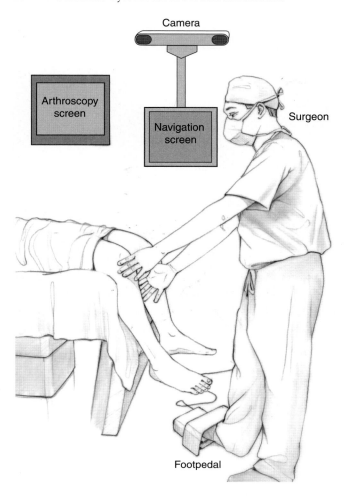

FIGURE 25-1

Operating room setup.

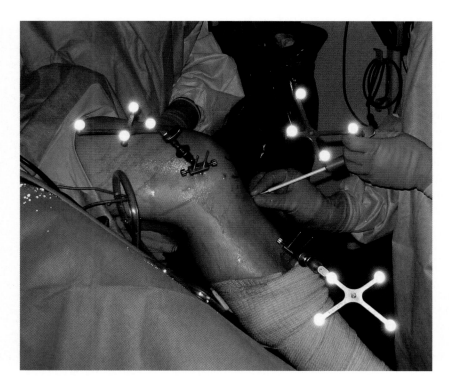

FIGURE 25-2

Tracker placement and palpation. Note that tibial tracker pins are placed relatively distal to the origin of the tibial tunnel and that the femoral pins are placed near the epicondyle.

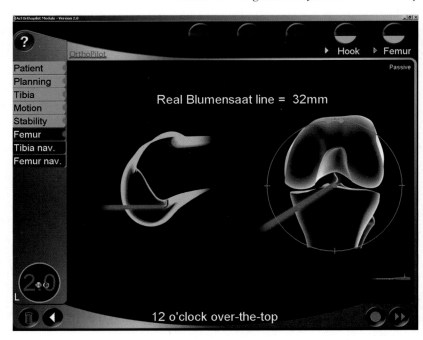

FIGURE 25-3

Palpation of the over the top position (Blumensaat's line). Average length is 30 to 32 mm; shorter distances suggest incorrect palpation.

force. The rotational laxity of the tibia with respect to the femur is also registered by internally and externally rotating the tibia.

Tibial Tunnel Mapping

The tibial drill guide is then placed intra-articularly, and an approximate position for the tibial tunnel is chosen. The instrument tracker is attached to the drill guide, and the relationship of the proposed tunnel to intra- and extra-articular landmarks is seen on the navigation screen (Fig. 25-4). Information provided includes the location of the intercondylar notch with the knee in full extension projected onto the tibial plateau; the distance from the PCL, and the location of the medial tibial eminence and the anterior horn of the lateral meniscus. The amount and location of any impingement are also shown. The percentage of the medial-lateral distance is calculated. The coronal and sagittal angle of the tibial tunnel with respect to the tibia is also shown, which aids in aiming the tunnel to the appropriate position on the femur. Taking the provided information into account, the surgeon chooses a tunnel location, and a guidewire is drilled into the elbow of the guide. The tunnel location is then registered using the foot pedal. The tibial tracker can be removed from the tibial pin clamp at this point prior to drilling the tunnel, and reattached at the end of the case for evaluation of knee stability.

Femoral Tunnel Mapping

Typically, a standard manual offset guide is used to identify an approximate position for the femoral tunnel, and a dimple is made by placing a guide pin through the guide. The offset guide can be placed transtibially or through a low anterior portal; alternatively, an outside-in technique can be used and a pin placed. The instrument tracker is then attached to the femoral probe, and the approximate starting point is palpated. The femoral navigation screen (Fig. 25-5) provides real-time information on the distance to the over-the-top position, graft isometry, location on the clock face, and the location and amount of any potential impingement. Using this information the surgeon can decide on and register an appropriate starting point. The guidewire is then drilled into this point and the reamer is used to create the femoral tunnel.

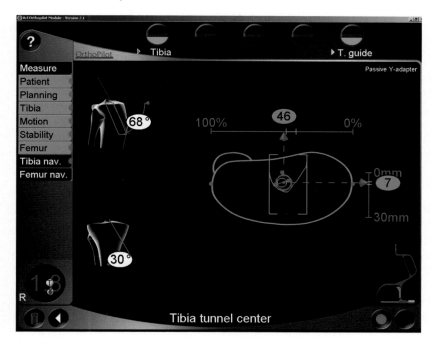

FIGURE 25-4

Tibial navigation screen demonstrating the projected notch, indicating areas of impingement, distance from the PCL, anterior horn of the lateral meniscus, and medial tibial eminence. The coronal and sagittal angle of the tunnel are also shown.

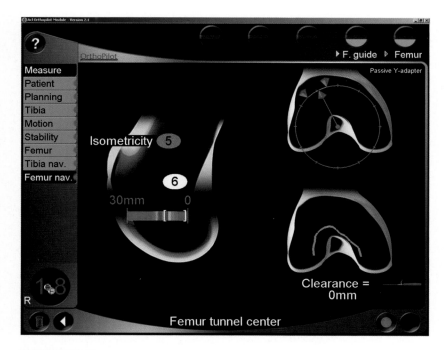

FIGURE 25-5

Femoral navigation screen demonstrating the areas of potential impingement, isometry, distance from the over-the-top position, and location on the clock face.

Final Evaluation

After tunnel creation, the graft is passed into the knee, tensioned and cycled, and secured with the surgeon's preferred fixation devices. The tibial tracker is reattached to the tibial pin clamp, and knee is placed in the appropriate degree of flexion to retest anterior-posterior and rotational stability. Similar forces are applied to the reconstructed knee to evaluate laxity, and the pre- and postoperative anteroposterior (AP) translation in millimeters and the degrees of rotation are displayed (Fig. 25-6). These measurements are then recorded, and then the markers and pins can be removed. A summary data sheet can be printed out. Typically, the AP stability improves from a mean of 15 to 5 mm, and the rotational arc improves from 28 to 18 degrees. Steristrips are placed over the pin sites.

Pearls and Pitfalls

- The markers should be positioned to avoid interfering with tunnel drilling and placement, and the pins should be securely fastened to bone. Slightly divergent pins improve the stability of the clamps. The markers can be attached to a larger screw if sufficient bony stability cannot be achieved. Placing the femoral pins in an area with relatively less soft tissue motion over bone will decrease the chance of pin loosening. If the pins become loose, they can be reinserted, but reregistration should be performed.
- The reflective markers need to be kept dry during the case. Placing gauze or a sponge on the shaft of instruments exiting the joint can help reduce spray of fluid onto the trackers. If the markers get wet, a dry sponge and a quarter turn of the reflective ball can improve the ability of the camera to track the marker.
- Intra-articular palpation must be done accurately. During palpation of the PCL, it is important to keep the tibia appropriately reduced, avoiding anterior translation of the tibia. The tip of the probe should be barely touching the anterior fibers of the PCL. The notch palpation can proceed in only one direction. If there are obvious discrepancies between the navigation screen and the arthroscopic appearance of the tibia or femur, it is recommended to reregister data points. In addition, anterior translation of the tibia on the femur during the kinematic registration will result in abnormal impingement and isometry data.
- At any point during the registration and measurement process, previous screens can be accessed and points can be removed using the left foot pedal. Pressing both the pedals will allow screenshots or the use of an intra-articular measuring tool.

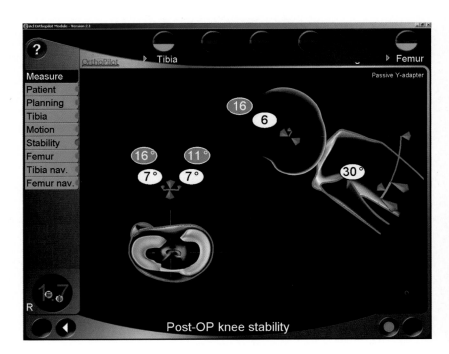

FIGURE 25-6

Postoperative knee stability screen showing both pre- and postoperative anterior translation and rotation values.

POSTOPERATIVE MANAGEMENT

The surgeon's standard postoperative protocol can be used.

COMPLICATIONS

The goal of navigation is to reduce the rate of improperly placed tunnels. Complications associated with computer-assisted navigation can be associated with equipment or software. The information displayed on computer navigation screens is only as accurate as the registration points input by the user. The surgeon should always correlate the information on the screen with the anatomy visualized arthroscopically. In its current format, the Orthopilot system is quite robust and rarely has a significant error or freezes. If at any point there is a discrepancy between the navigation screens and actual anatomy, re-registration should be performed. If there are persistent abnormalities, the surgeon always has the option to perform the standard manual instrumentation technique.

The only other complication noted has been some minimal discomfort associated with the unicortical tibial pin sites. One patient developed superficial erythema and some drainage associated with one site that resolved over a period of 2 weeks. Given the size of the K-wires used to attach the trackers, it is unlikely that fracture will occur through the pin sites.

RESULTS

Results using a variety of computer-aided navigation systems have consistently demonstrated improved tunnel position and clinical measurements. My experience (4,5) has demonstrated improved tunnel placement, with the tibial tunnel located slightly more anterior in the anatomic footprint and a substantial improvement in both anterior-posterior and rotational stability when compared to injured knees. Eichhorn has demonstrated improved tunnel position, with precision to within 1.6 mm on the tibia and 2 mm on the femur; and a more anatomic tibial and femoral tunnel placement at 1:30/10:30 clock face position. Picard and the Pittsburgh group (6) demonstrated on foam knees that the manual instrumentation had errors on the tibia of 4.9 mm and femur of 4.2 mm that decreased to 3.4 mm and 2.7 mm. Plaweski (7) showed radiographic impingement decreased from 75% to 0% with navigation, and that 96.7% have less than 2 mm translation postoperatively, compared to 83% with manual tools.

RECOMMENDED READING

Koh JL. Computer-assisted navigation and anterior cruciate ligament reconstruction: accuracy and outcomes. *Orthopaedics*. 2005; 28(10)(suppl):S1283–1287.

Koh JL, Koo SS, Leonard J, Kodali P. Anterior cruciate ligament (ACL) tunnel placement: a radiographic comparison between navigated versus manual ACL reconstruction. *Orthopaedics*. 2006;29(10)(suppl):S122–124.

Picard F, DiGioia AM, Moody J, et al. Accuracy in tunnel placement for ACL reconstruction. *Comp Aid Surg*. 2001;6(5):279–289.

Plaweski S, Cazal J, Rosell P, et al. Anterior cruciate ligament reconstruction using navigation. *Am J Sports Med*. 2006;34(4):542–552.

REFERENCES

1. Eichhorn H-J. Image-free navigation in ACL replacement with the OrthoPilot System. In: Stiehl JB, Konermann WH, Haaker RG, eds. *Navigation and robotics in total joint and spine surgery*. Berlin: Springer-Verlag; 387–396.
2. Eichhorn J. Three years of experience with computer-assisted navigation in anterior cruciate ligament replacement. http://www.aclstudygroup.com/Powerpoint-pdf02/Eichhorn.pdf.
3. Eichhorn J. Three years of experience with computer navigation–assisted positioning of drilling tunnels in anterior cruciate ligament replacement (SS-67). *Arthroscopy*. 2004;20(5)(suppl):31–32.

PART FOUR

ARTICULAR CARTILAGE AND SYNOVIUM

26 Arthroscopic Chondroplasty and/or Debridement

Douglas W. Jackson

INDICATIONS/CONTRAINDICATIONS

Chondroplasty is defined as the "surgical shaping of cartilage." This shaping includes contouring and removing devitalized or detached cartilage fragments. The debridement of loose or fragmented articular cartilage may relieve mechanical symptoms associated with the diseased articular surfaces.

Chondroplasty of the knee is usually always part of an overall debridement procedure, and at the same time is an associated joint lavage and irrigation. This washout removes small particulate debris and bioactive molecules that may include inflammatory mediators and enzymes. Although the natural history of the arthritic process in the knee joint is probably unaffected by arthroscopic chondroplasty, debridement, and lavage, in selected patients the procedure may reduce or eliminate certain mechanical symptoms.

A definition for arthroscopic debridement of the knee when used in the treatment of degenerative articular cartilage disease (degenerative arthritis) has not been defined in the literature. Therapeutic arthroscopic techniques for knee joint osteoarthritis include debridement and/or chondroplasty, partial meniscectomy, osteophyte excision, joint lavage, and loose-body removal. At the time of the arthroscopic assessment, in addition to a chondroplasty and debridement of the articular surfaces, the surgeon may also address exposed subchondral bone.

Several of these associated or concomitantly performed procedures are described in other chapters in this book, including the microfracture technique to stimulate localized repair over the exposed boney surface (Chapter 27), chondrocyte transplantation (Chapter 29), osteochondral autografts (Chapter 28), osteochondral allografts (Chapter 33) and associated osteotomy (Chapters 24, 30, and 31).

The indications for considering arthroscopic chondroplasty and debridement are primarily for mechanical symptoms in the knee that are felt to be secondary to articular cartilage fragmentation and loosening, loose bodies, meniscal fragments, and tears and impingements. These symptoms may include localized joint pain with specific rotation and/or flexion, catching or locking, and recurrent effusions associated with the shedding of articulate cartilage debris and fragments. These symptoms should be interfering with daily activities and adversely affecting the patient's quality of life. The symptoms have not been responsive or relieved by nonsurgical treatments, including activity modification, anti-inflammatory medication, and/or glucosamine sulfate, viscosupplementation, corticosteroid injection (with or without aspiration), physical therapy, stress off-loading with bracing or orthotics, and activity restriction.

The long-term management of degenerative articular disease involves patient education and weight loss (if appropriate). The photos (images) of patient's articular surfaces taken at the time of chondroplasty (debridement) can be used to reinforce the need to lose weight, build and maintain lower extremity strength, and proactively select nonaggravating activities and exercises.

While arthroscopic chondroplasty and debridement can provide palliative treatment to reduce symptoms from knee osteoarthritis in carefully selected individuals, it is often difficult to predict which patients will definitely benefit. The patient and surgeon should have realistic expectations regarding its possible outcome. The duration of symptomatic relief following chondroplasty is variable and is influenced by the natural history and predisposing factors of the individual's underlying articular cartilage disease. This is further impacted by the patient's future use of the knee and subsequent aggravating injuries. Symptomatic improvement is less likely in the presence of more advanced articular cartilage disease (articulating exposed bone particularly on opposing sides of the joint), altered subchondral bone, extremity malalignment, and obesity. Those patients with more advanced articular cartilage degeneration can on occasion experience worsening of their preoperative symptoms following this procedure.

PREOPERATIVE PLANNING

While imaging techniques for articular cartilage lesions are improving, arthroscopy remains the best method for assessing the grade, size, and location of degenerative articular cartilage changes in the knee joint. Most patients presenting for an orthopaedic surgeon's evaluation with symptomatic articular cartilage disease have mild to moderate osteoarthritis of the knee and are between 40 and 70 years of age. They usually are coming because of the sudden onset or significant change in their mechanical symptoms and/or effusion. Their assessment begins with a history and physical examination. The duration and severity of symptoms should be established. The onset of the pain related to symptomatic degenerative articular cartilage disease may be insidious; it may develop following an aggravating activity or be associated with a specific traumatic event. The patients who have a more sudden onset tend to respond better to arthroscopic chondroplasty and debridement. In addition to their pain, common symptoms include grinding, clicking, and catching. The mechanical symptoms may be related to loose fragments of cartilage and/or their interaction with degenerative meniscal tissue. Patients may describe a feeling of tightness and/or a sense of swelling related to intra-articular effusions after aggravating activities. The effusion often contributes to their difficulty when squatting or kneeling.

The patient's discomfort may be exacerbated by twisting motions of the knee, when squatting and turning over in bed at night. The pain is often increased with prolonged standing, walking, or running. The symptoms are usually relieved by rest and restrictions in motion of the knee. The severity of the associated pain may escalate with certain activities and motion and interfere with activities of daily living; night pain can interrupt sleep.

Physical examination includes documentation of the standing lower-extremity alignment in both coronal and sagittal planes. An associated genu varum malalignment is a more common deformity in symptomatic osteoarthritic knees than those with abnormal genu valgus. The presence of a fixed flexion deformity is not unusual in those patients with more advanced joint involvement.

An effusion may be palpable, and the affected joint may feel warmer in the presence of an underlying inflammatory process. The ranges of active and passive motion of the knee without effusion are usually within normal limits in the early stages of articular cartilage disease. Localized joint-line pain may be present on palpation, and the McMurray test may elicit some discomfort in the involved compartment. Associated degenerative meniscal tears and articular cartilage disease are commonly associated with older patients. The knee is usually stable to ligament evaluation in most patients, but excluding underlying ligamentous instability is an important part of the examination and future management.

Aspiration of the joint, with appropriate synovial fluid analysis, should be considered when an effusion is a persistent finding. The shedding of particulate debris from degenerative articular surface(s), and its subsequent digestion and removal, may evoke an inflammatory response within the joint. The synovial aspiration may show particulate debris on gross examination if the needle bore for aspiration is of adequate size. (I prefer an 18-gauge needle for aspirations of symptomatic synovial effusions). Crystal analysis (gout and pseudogout), cell count, and other synovial fluid studies should be performed when an aspirate is sent for laboratory evaluation.

In assessing the patient's complaints, it is helpful to establish clinically whether the medial, lateral, or anterior compartment(s) of the knee are involved. Is the problem related to predominantly one compartment, or is a tricompartment problem contributing to the patient's disability? Weight-bearing radiographs are useful adjuncts to supplement the clinical findings. They document leg alignment and the extent of articular cartilage interval narrowing, subchondral bone changes, and osteophyte formation.

Radiographic imaging of knees with chondral disease should include weight-bearing views. The joint space is best evaluated with a posteroanterior (PA) view, taken of the weight-bearing knees in 20 to 30 degrees of flexion. These PA flexion views may give narrowing changes on weight-bearing views that are not apparent on the same knee fully extended. They document the most frequent region of earlier joint space narrowing (i.e., the middle one third of the femoral condyle) (Fig. 26-1). Radiologic features such as sharpening of the tibial spines, squaring of the joint margins, subchondral sclerosis, and cyst formation may be associated with more advanced degeneration. Tibiofemoral alignment can be assessed on the weight-bearing views of the knee, but a full-length-extremity film may be required to assess the mechanical axis (if thought to be needed). The greater the varus or valgus deformity and the closer to bone on bone articulation, the less likely the arthroscopic chondroplasty will provide symptomatic relief. The reader is referred to the accompanying chapters on osteotomy, which discuss treatment options for these patients.

Magnetic resonance imaging (MRI) is a useful noninvasive means that may help demonstrate symptomatic articular cartilage lesions. There is often a high correlation with radiographs, but MRI may be particularly helpful when standard radiographs appear normal. A wide variety of MRI pulse sequences have been investigated with regard to their utility in assessment of cartilage image. Among the most useful are fat suppressed proton density (FSPD) and T2-weighted sequences (FST2). A number of gradient recalled sequences continue to be used although no clear consensus on the best pulse sequence has emerged. An example of a MRI grading system is shown in Table 26-1. Current techniques are more accurate in detecting partial or full-thickness cartilage loss (grades III or IV). Experience suggests that MRI and arthroscopic findings may not always correlate. A clinically practical and reproducible system of staging cartilage loss using MRI on a wide scale has yet to emerge.

Nevertheless, MRI is excellent for demonstrating the integrity of the meniscus in the degenerative compartment being evaluated. Magnetic resonance imaging is also capable of providing information on the condition of the underlying subchondral bone and adjacent marrow space (Fig. 26-2).

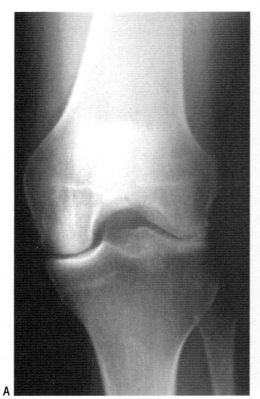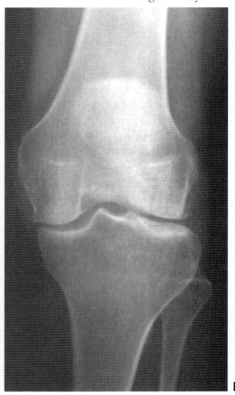

A   B

FIGURE 26-1

Radiographs of a single knee. Weight-bearing posteroanterior view with knee flexion **(A)** illustrates complete loss of joint space in the lateral compartment, whereas the weight-bearing view with the knee in extension **(B)** suggests the presence of a reasonable joint space.

A radionuclide bone scan may provide additional information in those patients whose pain is out of proportion to the objective findings. As an indicator of increased blood flow, radiotracer uptake may be localized to a single joint surface or compartment. A more generalized uptake may indicate more advanced changes, or even at times an alternate pathology. Recent advances in nuclear medicine techniques include the use of tomographic techniques (SPECT imaging) in conjunction with performing the bone scan. This technique offers increased sensitivity for lesion depiction compared with conventional planar nuclear imaging methods.

The MRI and/or bone scan can be very helpful in the diagnosis of avascular necrosis and its variants of localized bone involvement. Its presence should be explained preoperatively to the patient. Some of these patients may eventually need partial or total knee replacement regardless of what is done. The natural history as best it is known should be explained to the patient, giving the patient the option of additional watchful waiting with possible limited weight bearing.

TABLE 26-1.   Grading of Cartilage Lesions

Grade	MRI	Arthroscopy
I	Signal heterogeneity	Softening
II	Fissuring	Fraying or fissuring
III	Partial thickness loss	Partial thickness loss
IV	Complete loss of cartilage	Full thickness loss (exposed bone)

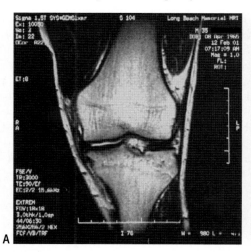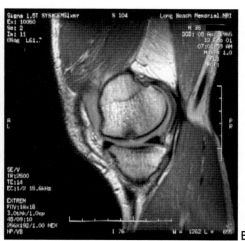

FIGURE 26-2

MRI images demonstrating chondropathy. Articular cartilage thinning over the middle third of the medial femoral condyle is shown on a coronal image **(A)**. The sagittal image **(B)** shows changes in the subchondral bone with articular cartilage breakdown.

Eighty-five percent of early symptomatic chondral lesions occur in the medial tibiofemoral compartment. Chondral lesions are most commonly encountered during arthroscopy on the femoral side of the joint, and less commonly cartilage changes are noted on the opposing tibial surface. When there is disruption of the chondral surface (grade IV) encountered during arthroscopy, an associated degenerate meniscal tear in the involved compartment is present at least 70% of the time.

Whenever arthroscopy of the knee is performed, particularly in middle-aged and older patients, the surgeon should be prepared to perform some type of arthroscopic chondroplasty and/or debridement. This includes the debridement and/or removal of loose, undermined, and partially detached articular cartilage, lavage out articular cartilage debris, and excise abnormally mobile and/or degenerative meniscus fragments leaving smoothly contoured and stable rims. The lavage provided at the time of arthroscopy is a method of irrigating and removing the smaller particulate intra-articular cartilaginous debris and degradative enzymes present in the joint.

The informed and written consent obtained before surgery should explain the possibility of this additional procedure(s), risks, rehabilitation, and prognosis. We try to give a clear understanding to each patient of the possibility of the debridement of a potentially symptomatic articular cartilage. This includes an explanation of degenerative cartilage disease and the objectives of a chondroplasty in trying to reduce certain specific symptoms. Patients are also informed that there is a small chance that their knee may be made more symptomatic following the procedure. In our patients we think this risk is less than 5%. The poor results that are seen following arthroscopic debridement are more often in those knees with advanced degenerative disease. This is common when there are articulating bone-on-bone surfaces, significant malalignment, obesity, and in those patients with secondary gain factors (legal or industrial injury) related to their symptoms.

Since there is a possibility of performing the microfracture technique in association with the chondroplasty, this should be discussed, particularly in relation to the postoperative course. See Chapter 27 on the indications and details of microfracture. Surgeons should be prepared to deal with fragmented and loose articular cartilage as well as exposed bone.

SURGERY

On the day of surgery, the "correct" limb is confirmed and marked. The patient's medical history should be reviewed for allergies to drugs that may be used during and after surgery. We seldom inflate a tourniquet during this procedure; but if is to be used, special attention should be made regarding patients with underlying vascular disease, vascular grafts, or previous deep vein thrombosis.

The patient is placed on the operating table in a supine position, and the correct limb is once again confirmed. General, regional, or local anesthesia can be used, depending on patient and surgeon preference. If local anesthesia is used, we prefer an anesthesiologist present to provide sedation if necessary and additional pain relief and muscle relaxation if needed. If the patient prefers to observe the procedure on the television monitor, sedation is minimized or eliminated.

An examination of the knee is routinely performed at the beginning of the case before anesthesia is complete to document the preoperative passive range of motion and ligamentous stability in the affected and contralateral knee. A tourniquet is applied proximally on the thigh but is only inflated during the case if intra-articular bleeding slows the progress of the surgical procedure. If this circumstance occurs during the case, we inflate the tourniquet to a pressure of 300 mm Hg after elevating the leg for 60 seconds. We prepare and drape the leg in the usual orthopaedic manner using iodine solution and impervious arthroscopy drapes. The foot and entire lower extremity are placed in a sterile impervious stocking. An adhesive elastic wrap is used to contour the stocking to the leg and seal the opening below the knee to prevent fluid accumulation within the sterile stocking.

The operating room and equipment are arranged to facilitate the surgical procedure. We prefer to stand beside the affected limb and view the TV monitor placed on the opposite side of the operating table. This allows a straight, unobstructed view of the arthroscopic image for the surgeon. The surgical assistant, if present, stands beside the patient's waist to assist with limb positioning. The presence of skilled and experienced operating room personnel is invaluable.

We prefer to use gravity-flow irrigation to maintain knee joint distension and fluid pressure throughout the procedure, and we do not use an automated (pump) inflow system. The circulating nurse has the role of obtaining additional instrumentation as needed, overseeing the fluid delivery and suction system, and facilitating the documentation procedure. The relevant arthroscopic findings are documented with photographic prints and hand drawn on a specific form at the conclusion of the case. Both of these are included as a part of the operative record in our office charts. The grading and description of articular cartilage lesions are helpful in the future management of the patient's symptoms. The improved technology in the integrated operating suites, digital imaging and computerized documentation, can be used to enhance patient education, medical and operative records, and report generation and billing (Fig. 26-3).

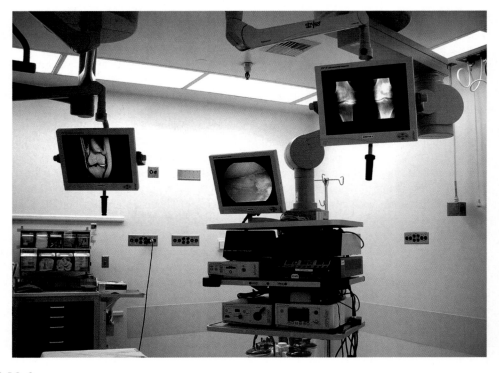

FIGURE 26-3

The new integrated operating rooms enable enhanced digital documentation for the medical records, operative report, patient education, coding, billing, transmission to an off-site office, and for use in education forums.

Technique

The same systematic approach is used for all our knee arthroscopies. After the lower extremity has been prepared and draped in the usual orthopaedic manner, the desired portals are infiltrated with a solution containing equal amounts of Xylocaine (1%) and Marcaine (0.25%), with epinephrine (1:200,000) to minimize portal site bleeding and reduce postoperative pain.

An anterolateral portal is created for the placement of the arthroscope. With the knee flexed in a 90-degree position, the portal site is identified as a "soft spot" located at the lateral border of the patella tendon, one fingerbreadth above the lateral tibial plateau. The skin is incised with a No. 11 scalpel blade. My preference is to make a puncture that is oriented vertically and directed centrally toward the intercondylar notch as it penetrates the joint capsule. A blunt trochar is then used to pass the arthroscopic cannula into the joint. Having penetrated the joint capsule, the trochar is carefully inserted into the suprapatellar pouch, while extending the knee. Gently inserting a blunt trochar with the knee in extension minimizes the risk of damaging the patellar, trochlear, and condylar articular surfaces. The camera and light source are attached to the arthroscope, and the camera image is "white balanced" before placing it into the sheath.

The 30-degree (4-mm) arthroscope is inserted through the high-flow cannula placed in the anterolateral portal. The inflow tubing is then attached to the cannula, and the joint is distended with saline. The caliber of the cannula is large enough to allow sufficient irrigation during the procedure. Intra-articular placement of the scope is confirmed visually on screen. An outflow tubing is attached to the cannula's second tap to allow suction drainage as required. Initial joint lavage may be required to disperse intra-articular bleeding so that a clear image is visible on the TV monitor. The amount of intra-articular cartilaginous debris present during initial washout is noted (Fig. 26-4). A more extensive lavage can be achieved by introducing a large bore in flow cannula or suction via an anteromedial or superior portal. We do not hesitate to create additional portals, including posterior medially, if necessary to facilitate adequate visualization, irrigation, and removal of loose bodies and/or fragments.

Inspection   Once the arthroscope position and image are satisfactory, a diagnostic arthroscopy is performed. This involves a complete inspection of the knee joint, made in a sequential and systematic fashion. Each compartment is evaluated, and the status of the articular cartilage on both sides of the joint compartment; the integrity of the meniscus, anterior cruciate ligament (ACL), and posterior cruciate ligament (PCL); the condition of the synovium; and the presence of osteophytes are documented.

We begin with inspection in the suprapatellar pouch, noting any synovial changes, plicae, intra-articular debris, or loose bodies. The articular surfaces of the patellofemoral joint are inspected with the knee in full extension. Each facet of the patella is viewed, and the contour of the femoral sulcus

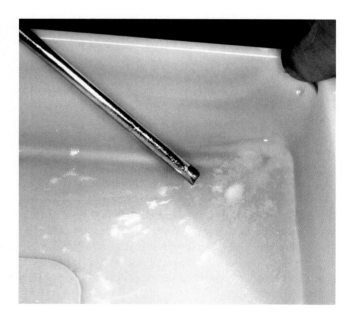

FIGURE 26-4

Initial drainage of knee joint effusion containing particulate debris.

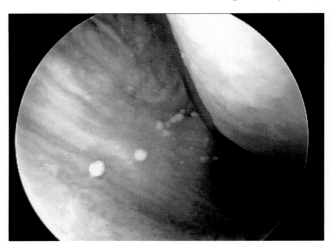

FIGURE 26-5

Particulate debris located in medial gutter.

is followed downward to the intercondylar notch. Special attention is directed to the trochlear groove and the tracking of the patella during 40 degrees of knee flexion and extension. The presence of enlarged or impinging synovial plica is evaluated before passing the arthroscope into the medial gutter, and the presence of osteophytes and articular debris is documented (Fig. 26-5).

The arthroscope is then passed into the medial compartment to assess the articular surfaces of the medial femoral condyle and tibial plateau. Inspection of the medial meniscus is also undertaken. To visualize the entire articulating surface of the femoral condyle, the knee is observed as it is moved from extension into flexion. Maximum knee flexion affords the best visualization of the posterior third of the condylar articular surface. A gentle valgus force, generated by controlled manual pressure, is usually required to view the posterior horn of the medial meniscus adequately. This opening of the medial joint space can be facilitated by a leg holder, lateral post, and/or knowledgeable assistant.

Inspection of the intercondylar notch is carried out with the knee in a flexed position. The ACL and PCL are observed, and the presence of notch osteophytes is noted. Once the structures of the intercondylar notch have been visualized, the scope is carefully passed into the posteromedial compartment of the knee to ensure there are no loose bodies. The integrity of the posterior attachment of the medial meniscus and status of the synovium are also assessed.

The arthroscope is then directed across the notch to inspect the lateral compartment and gutter. To improve visualization of the lateral compartment, the knee is moved into the figure-4 position. With the knee at 90 degrees or less, the ankle can be held or rested on the contralateral tibia. Under its own weight, the leg falls outward, externally rotating and abducting the femur, creating a varus force that opens up the lateral joint. In this position, the articular surfaces and lateral meniscus are inspected by rotating the arthroscope to take advantage of the 30-degree lens. Finally, the lateral joint margin and its gutter are inspected for osteophytes, debris, and loose bodies.

Intra-articular Probing and Palpation   The purpose of initial visual inspection is to identify areas of pathology within the joint. However, a diagnostic arthroscopy is not complete unless the intra-articular structures are palpated and probed. We prefer to use a blunt nerve hook as the probing instrument to assess articular cartilage defects and the mobility of meniscal fragments or tears.

The probe is usually inserted through the second portal, most frequently created anteromedially. With the knee in 90 degrees of flexion, the "soft spot" is palpated adjacent to the medial edge of the ligamentum patella. This location is confirmed by transillumination with the arthroscope tip positioned at the intra-articular site of the portal. Precise placement of the portal is enhanced by first using an 18-gauge spinal needle to determine the position and trajectory of subsequent instrumentation and its ability to access the target tissue (Fig. 26-6). Surgical instruments should be as parallel to the tibial plateau as possible. To be certain that the meniscus is not damaged when creating the portal, the lens of the arthroscope is rotated to view the position of the penetrating knife blade. A No. 11 blade is used to create a vertically oriented portal. By creating these surgical portals under direct arthroscopic visualization, injury to the menisci can be avoided, and the most advantageous angles of approach with the instrumentation can be achieved.

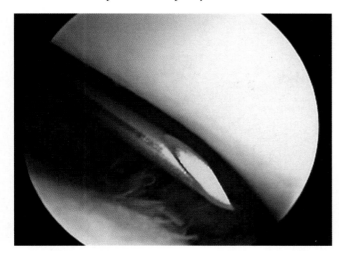

FIGURE 26-6
An 18-gauge spinal needle is used for selective portal placement. Operative portals are best created under direct arthroscopic vision.

With the nerve hook placed through the anteromedial portal, palpation of the articular surfaces and the menisci is performed. It is important to characterize and describe the chondral lesions. The extent of the segments of loose or undermined cartilage may only become apparent when probed (Fig. 26-7). This process is helpful to grade chondral pathology more accurately. Each compartment of the knee is palpated. At times, it may be advantageous to switch portals for the arthroscope and nerve hook to improve visualization and instrumentation.

Documentation   Depending on the surgeon's preference and available equipment, documentation can be in the form of written text, diagrams, arthroscopic photography, videotape, or digital image recording. Articular cartilage lesions are recorded in terms of grade/stage, size, and location. The size of the lesion is measured for length and width. Using the 5-mm tip of the nerve hook probe may be helpful as a sizing tool (Fig. 26-8). We grade chondral lesions according to the Outerbridge classification I to IV (Figs. 26-9 to 26-12), although numerous other grading systems exist. We prefer to record the data using a diagram and photography. To ensure documentation is complete, all intra-articular structures are recorded in a systematic fashion on our postoperative data sheet.

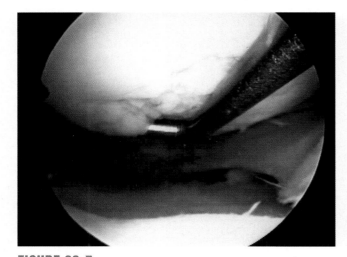

FIGURE 26-7
A blunt hook is used to palpate undermined cartilage.

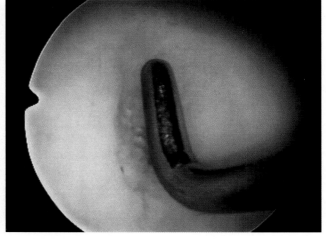

FIGURE 26-8
Probe may be used to size chondral lesions.

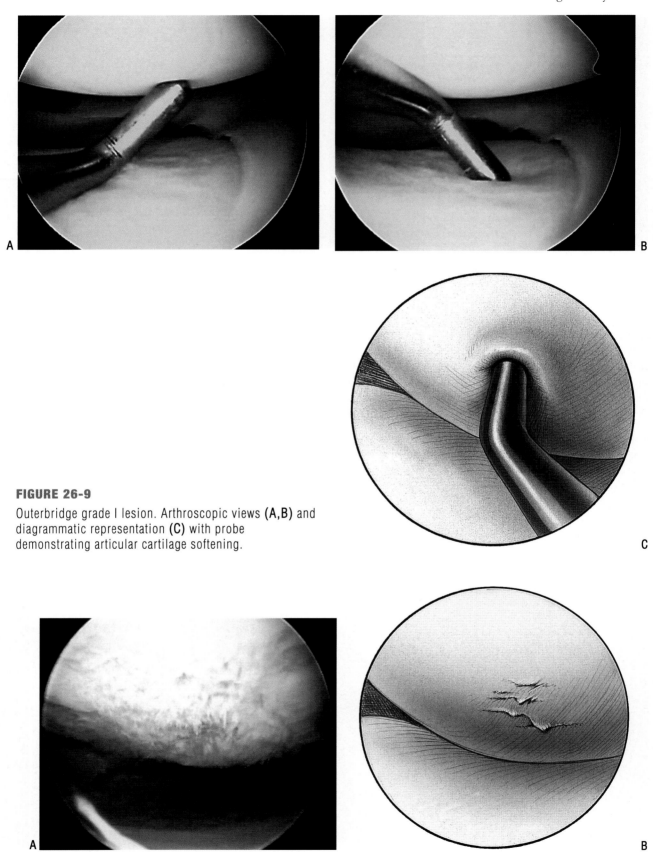

FIGURE 26-9
Outerbridge grade I lesion. Arthroscopic views **(A,B)** and diagrammatic representation **(C)** with probe demonstrating articular cartilage softening.

FIGURE 26-10
Outerbridge grade II lesion. Arthroscopic view **(A)** and schematic diagram **(B)** demonstrating cartilage fibrillation.

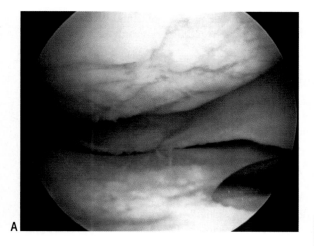

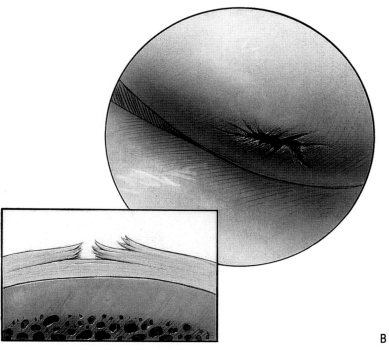

FIGURE 26-11

Outerbridge grade III lesion. Arthroscopic view **(A)** and diagram **(B)** showing partial-thickness cartilage loss.

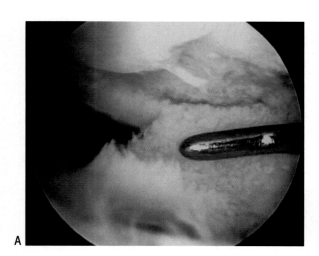

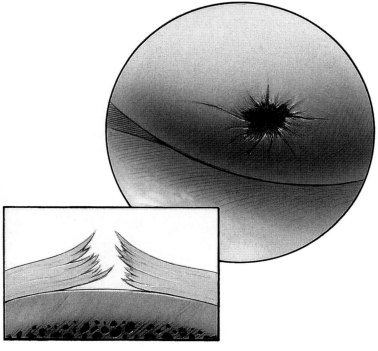

FIGURE 26-12

Outerbridge grade IV lesion. Arthroscopic view **(A)** and diagram **(B)** showing full-thickness loss of articular cartilage and exposed underlying bone.

Chondroplasty and Debridement   Using a combination of manual and powered arthroscopic tools, the surgical techniques that may be applicable to osteoarthrosis include the following:

- Lavage of intra-articular debris
- Loose body removal
- Partial meniscectomy
- Debridement of loose and fragmented articular cartilage
- Shaving and contouring of detaching cartilage surfaces
- Occasional selective excision of osteophyte(s)
- Limited synovectomy
- Microfracture of selected grade IV exposed bone (see Chapter 27)

Following the diagnostic palpation with the nerve hook, if indicated the debridement of chondral lesions is undertaken. The goal is to excise loose articular cartilage and remove that represent undermined lesions. Larger fragments may be detached using a hand-held punch, cutting forceps, or curette. Smaller partial-thickness lesions of the condyle are smoothed with a power shaver. A non-aggressive tip has less risk of causing unwanted damage to healthy cartilage. The tip is glided across the contoured surface of the condyle, with the cutting surface at right angles to the articular surface (Fig. 26-13). It should be kept under direct visualization. With suction applied to the power tool, the debrided cartilage will be sucked into the resector tip. Care is always taken to avoid damage to healthy, normal-appearing articular cartilage.

There is usually a gradual transition from normal to abnormal articular cartilage in degenerative knee joints. If, however, there is an abrupt transition between the diseased and normal areas, the ridge separating the two zones is tapered with the power shaver or curette. The treated area is re-probed to ensure there are no remaining undermined flaps of loose articular cartilage.

In regions where the underlying subchondral bone is exposed, the procedure is the same, and then the surgeon decides if in addition to debridement, marrow-stimulation techniques may be employed. The exposed bone of the grade IV lesion may be penetrated using microfracture. This technique penetrates the subchondral bone, inducing clot formation and the potential migration of marrow cells. If a healing response is initiated, the defect is repaired with fibrocartilage scar tissue, which has inferior structural and functional properties to hyaline cartilage. The reader is referred to Chapter 27, which covers the microfracture technique in detail.

Joint margin osteophytes can occasionally be the source of localized pain or popping as soft tissue rolls over them. Impinging osteophytes within the notch or on the tibial shelf can occasionally contribute to restricting knee extension. Removal of symptomatic or impinging osteophytes can be done arthroscopically and may include using a small intra-articular osteotome, curette, or a power tool fitted with an arthroscopic burr or other aggressive resector tip.

Radiofrequency (RF) energy has also been used to ablate diseased articular cartilage, in place of the usual mechanical shaving methods for debridement. A variety of monopolar and bipolar probes are available to deliver the thermal energy, and lower RF settings appear to inflict less thermal damage. We do not use it on articular cartilage. Studies on the effect of RF have shown the potential for deleterious

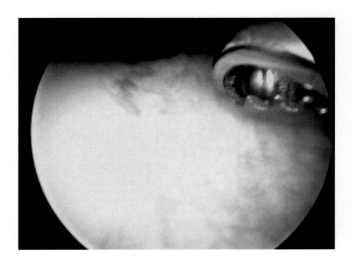

FIGURE 26-13

Arthroscopic power-shaver with nonaggressive resector tip glides over condylar surface, excising loose fibrillated cartilage drawn into its jaws with suction.

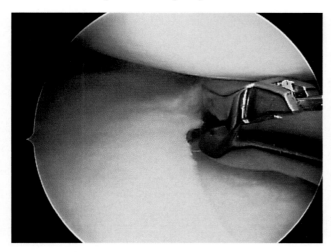

FIGURE 26-14

Arthroscopic view of a basket forceps making the initial cut across the anterior base of a flap tear of the meniscus.

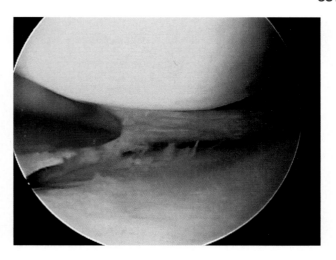

FIGURE 26-15

Powered meniscal resector contours stable meniscal rim.

alterations in adjacent chondrocytes, cartilaginous matrix, and even the subchondral bone. Caution is advised until definitive guidelines emerge for the application of RF electrodes in thermal-assisted chondroplasty. Currently, we prefer mechanical techniques for articular cartilage debridement.

Dealing with symptomatic degenerative meniscus pathology is an important part of the arthroscopic treatment of knee osteoarthritis. The meniscal tears found in association with chondral disease often have associated degenerative flap tears of the posterior and/or middle one third of the meniscus. Debridement of mobile meniscus fragments or flap-based resection is performed using basket forceps (Fig. 26-14) and/or power instruments with suction (Fig. 26-15). The remaining unstable rim is then trimmed and balanced with a basket forceps or power shaver (Fig. 26-16). A probe can be used at this point to test for stability of the remaining meniscal rim and to confirm there are no undersurface flaps or residual irregularities of the meniscus. While attending to meniscal pathology, care must be taken not to inflict damage to adjacent articular surfaces. Often degenerative meniscal and cartilage lesions are present in the same compartments.

The techniques of arthroscopic debridement may be used in all three compartments of the knee. During patellofemoral chondroplasty, instrumentation through the standard portals may not be satisfactory to gain access to the involved chondral surface. To facilitate surgical access in these cases, it may be necessary to create additional portals into the suprapatellar pouch (Fig. 26-17). Superior

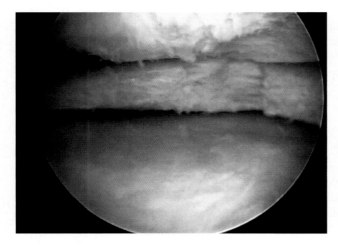

FIGURE 26-16

Completed partial meniscectomy and chondroplasty.

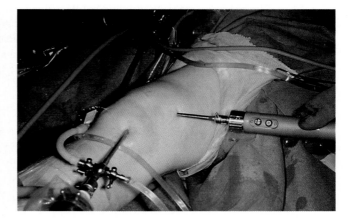

FIGURE 26-17

Suprapatellar portal for better access to involved articular cartilage in the patellofemoral joint.

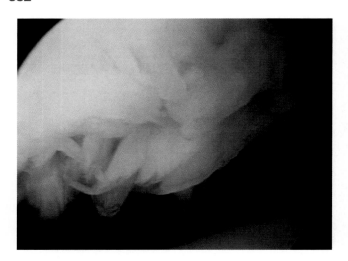

FIGURE 26-18

Arthroscopic view of frayed patellar articular cartilage.

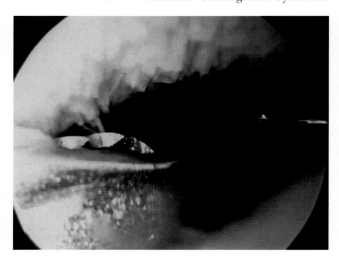

FIGURE 26-19

Patella chondroplasty.

portals can be placed medially or laterally, and the trajectory for instrumentation through a portal can be determined using an 18-gauge needle technique to confirm access to the desired surface. This additional portal facilitates the application of the techniques of arthroscopic chondroplasty to the femoral trochlea and undersurface of the patella (Figs. 26-18 and 26-19).

A final inspection of the knee joint is made to seek residual loose fragments of menisci, intra-articular debris, and loose pieces of articular cartilage. Particular attention is paid to joint recesses where debris may collect, namely, the suprapatellar pouch, medial and lateral gutters, the popliteus tendon sheath, and the posteromedial and posterolateral compartments. Larger loose bodies may require extraction using a grasping forceps, and the exit portal may require enlargement, depending on the fragment's size. If indicated, synovial biopsy or partial synovectomy may be performed.

Lavage   Joint lavage is a part of arthroscopic chondroplasty and debridement. The same irrigation fluid that distends the joint flushes out the smaller debris generated during the debridement process. Frequently, 3 to 4 L of irrigation fluid are used during a routine arthroscopic chondroplasty and debridement. In addition to the clearance of particulate intra-articular debris, irrigation can wash out inflammatory mediators and enzymes.

When arthroscopic instrumentation has been completed, the fluid inflow is turned off. The remaining intra-articular fluid is flushed out with any residual debris (Fig. 26-20). If desired, the fluid inflow is turned back on and the cannula is inserted into another compartment to repeat the final irrigation process. Before removing the cannula at the end of the procedure, we prefer that all the fluid is drained from the joint. To aid postoperative analgesia, we inject the knee with a 25-mL solution containing a long-acting local anesthetic (bupivacaine, 0.25%) and morphine (Duramorph, 5 mg). We close each portal with an interrupted suture. Band-Aids and gauze dressing are placed over the wounds. A long leg support hose secures the dressing in place and applies pressure to the knee (Fig. 26-21).

Pearls and Pitfalls

- My experience has been that up to 5% of patients who undergo chondral debridement describe increased knee symptoms following the procedure. It is important to discuss the possibility of increased symptoms postoperatively with the patient before surgery to avoid any patient surprise. This is particularly true in patients with malalignment who have areas of bone on bone articulation. Often these patients should have had a knee replacement; instead, the surgeon performed the debridement in hopes of prolonging the use of the knee before the need for replacement.
- One area to be cautious of in extensive debriding is the femoral sulcus that has a large area of loosening and degenerating articular cartilage. These lesions are often an incidental finding or have been mildly symptomatic. These patients may have a sudden increase in symptoms when their degenerating articular cartilage in the femoral sulcus is aggressively debrided. On occasion, follow-

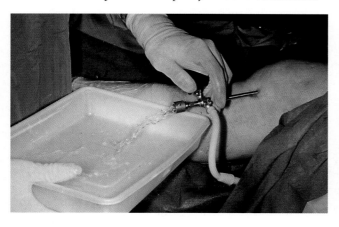

FIGURE 26-20
Lavage: pressurized distension fluid flushes out the debris through the cannula into a sterile basin.

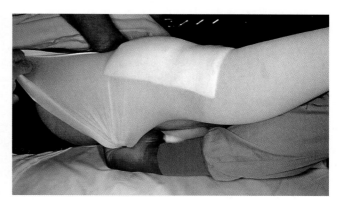

FIGURE 26-21
Long-leg support hose to maintain pressure and hold dressing in place.

ing extensive debridement of the femoral sulcus articular cartilage, the patella can start mechanically giving a catching or giving-way sensation to some of these patients.
- Be alert for those patients who have knee symptoms related to the early phases of osteonecrosis or avascular changes in the subchondral bone. These can usually be identified by a preoperative MRI. I see patients every year who have an MRI after an arthroscopic debridement and feel their MRI changes of osteonecrosis and increasing symptoms were caused by their arthroscopic debridement.

POSTOPERATIVE MANAGEMENT

Patients undergoing arthroscopic chondroplasty and debridement are treated on an outpatient basis. Elevation and cooling of the knee are provided in the recovery room, and the patient is instructed in the use of crutches with partial weight bearing on the affected limb. Nonnarcotic oral analgesia is all that is usually required following this procedure. At discharge, the patient is given an instruction sheet explaining the postoperative protocol, with specific mention of symptoms suggestive of postoperative complications.

Patients are advised to elevate and intermittently ice the knee during the first 48 hours postoperatively. They may change the Band-Aid dressings on the day after surgery, and showering of the extremity is permitted after 48 hours. At 1 week most patients are able to ambulate without crutches, and weight bearing is allowed as tolerated. We suggest crutches and partial weight bearing for those who have persistent effusions. The first postoperative office visit is scheduled 3 to 5 days following surgery. A wound check is performed and sutures are removed. We explain the surgical findings and treatment, and discuss the prognosis.

Rehabilitation

Our patients begin exercises at home without supervision following surgery. Printed instructions are provided outlining the techniques of isometric and limited-arc quadriceps- and hamstring-strengthening exercises. Range of motion is gradually increased, aiming to achieve full active extension and flexion within 1 to 2 weeks. At this stage, the patient is allowed to weight bear as tolerated on the operated limb. Should an effusion persist and prevent active range-of-motion exercises, aspiration of the joint may be performed. The patient is instructed to return to crutch walking for any distance outdoors, until the joint effusion abates.

Once the acute reaction to surgery subsides, patients are encouraged to begin bicycling, swimming, or water aerobics. For most patients, a home program of unsupervised rehabilitation is sufficient for recovery, provided that the surgeon monitors the patient's progress. Those patients lacking either the motivation or the facility to rehabilitate without supervision are referred to a rehabilitation therapist for a supervised program. Rehabilitation for this group of patients differs from the aggressive approach offered to the young athlete. It involves progressive resistance exercises and may need to be restricted to limited-arc exercises, rather than using full-arc strengthening programs. The importance of maintaining body weight within reason, general conditioning, and strength of the leg musculature on a regular basis has been stressed preoperatively and is stressed again before the patient is discharged from care. Patients are advised to avoid jogging as their form of endurance exercising and preferably substituting activities that reduce axial and impact loading of the knee joint.

COMPLICATIONS

The morbidity of arthroscopic surgery is low. Complications such as hemarthrosis (2%), deep venous thrombosis (0.5%), and septic arthritis (0.1%) require early detection and intervention. Cutaneous nerve injury can occur during portal skin incision, resulting in a small area of postoperative paresthesia. Sinus formation at the portal site is uncommon, and significant vascular injury during arthroscopic chondroplasty is unusual. Patients need to have realistic expectations and know that 30% to 40% of patients may have no improvement in their symptoms.

RESULTS

The literature is lacking prospective and/or randomized studies that apply defined techniques of arthroscopic chondroplasty and debridement with long-term follow-up. There are many retrospective articles that report patient benefits. When performed for the indications outlined, I tell our patients that arthroscopic debridement and lavage may provide symptomatic improvement 60% to 70% of the time. The postoperative result may take as long as 3 months to be apparent, and the relief of pain and stiffness can last 5 years or more. Approximately 30% to 40% of my patients have no change in preoperative symptoms and may require further surgery or choose to live with their disability until it becomes worse. A small percentage of patients (5%) report they are more symptomatic following a chondroplasty and debridement.

Several factors determine the prognosis after arthroscopic chondroplasty. Those patients who benefit the most present with mechanical symptoms of shorter duration and do not have pronounced angular deformity of their lower extremity, with only mild to moderate radiographic evidence of osteoarthritis.

Arthroscopic lavage and debridement can be a successful temporizing treatment for the symptomatic osteoarthritic knee. The natural history of the arthritic process is probably not altered, and it is important to counsel patients that the goal of surgery is to reduce symptoms in the knee joint during non-aggravating activities.

RECOMMENDED READING

Browne JE, Branch TP. Surgical alternatives for the treatment of articular cartilage lesions. *J Am Acad Othrop Surg.* 2000;8:180–189.

Ewing JW. Arthroscopic treatment of degenerative meniscal lesions and early degenerative arthritis of the knee. In: Ewing JW, ed. *Articular cartilage and knee joint function: basic science and the arthroscope.* New York: Raven Press; 1990:137–145.

Hanssen AD, Stuart MJ, Scott RD, et al. Surgical options for the middle-aged patient with osteoarthritis of the knee joint. *J Bone Joint Surg.* 2000;82-A:1768–1781.

Harwin SF. Arthroscopic debridement for osteoarthritis of the knee: predictors of patient satisfaction. *Arthroscopy.* 1999;15:142–146.

Jackson DW, Simon TM, Aberman HA. Symptomatic articular cartilage degeneration: the impact in the new millennium. *Clin Orthop Relat Res.* 2001;391S:S14–S25.

Jackson RW. Arthroscopic surgery and a new classification system. *Am J Knee Surg.* 1998;11:51–54.

Jackson RW, Dieterichs C. The results of arthroscopic lavage and debridement of osteoarthritic knees based on the severity of degeneration: a 4- to 6-year follow-up. *Arthroscopy.* 2003;19:13–20.

Lu Y, Edwards RB, Cole BJ, et al. Thermal chondroplasty with radiofrequency energy: an in vitro comparison of bipolar and monopolar radiofrequency devices. *Am J Sports Med.* 2001;29:42–49.

McCauley TR, Disler DG. Magnetic resonance imaging of articular cartilage of the knee. *J Am Acad Orthop Surg.* 2001;9:2–8.

Mosely JB, O'Malley K, Petersen NJ, et al. A controlled trial arthroscopic surgery for osteoarthritis of the knee. *N Engl J Med.* 2002;347:81–88.

Puddu G, Cipolla M, Cerulio G, et al. Arthroscopic treatment of flexed arthritic knee in active middle-aged patients. *Knee Surg Sports Traumatol Arthrosc.* 1994;2:73–75.

Simon TS, Jackson DW. Articular cartilage: injury pathways and treatment options. *Sports Med Arthrosc Rev.* June 2006.

27 Microfracture Technique: Treatment of Full-Thickness Chondral Lesions

J. Richard Steadman and William G. Rodkey

The "microfracture" technique was developed to enhance chondral resurfacing by providing a suitable environment for new tissue formation and to take advantage of the body's own healing potential. Specially designed awls are used to make multiple perforations, or "microfractures," into the subchondral bone plate. Microfracture is our preferred method to treat chondral defects. The senior author (JRS) first described this technique more than 20 years ago. He has treated more than 3,000 patients with the microfracture procedure.

INDICATIONS/CONTRAINDICATIONS

Indications

Microfracture was designed initially for patients with posttraumatic articular cartilage lesions of the knee that had progressed to full-thickness chondral defects. The microfracture technique still is most commonly indicated for full-thickness loss of articular cartilage in either a weight-bearing area between the femur and tibia or in an area of contact between the patella and trochlear groove. Unstable cartilage that overlies the subchondral bone is also an indication for microfracture. If a partial thickness lesion is probed and the cartilage simply scrapes off down to bone, we consider this to be a full-thickness lesion. Degenerative joint disease in a knee that has proper axial alignment is another common indication for microfracture. These lesions all involve loss of articular cartilage at the bone-cartilage interface.

Patients with acute chondral injuries are treated as soon as practical after the diagnosis is made, especially if the knee is being treated concurrently for meniscus or anterior cruciate ligament (ACL) pathology. Patients with chronic or degenerative chondral lesions often are treated nonoperatively (conservatively) for at least 12 weeks after a suspected chondral lesion is diagnosed clinically. This treatment regimen includes activity modification, physical therapy, nonsteroidal anti-inflammatory drugs, viscosupplement injections, and perhaps dietary supplements that may have cartilage-stimulating properties. If nonoperative treatment is not successful, then surgical treatment is considered.

No limitations are placed on how large an acute lesion can be and still be considered suitable for microfracture. We have observed that even very large acute lesions respond well to microfracture. We have noted empirically that traumatic lesions, acute or chronic, less than 400 mm^2 tend to respond better to microfracture than those lesions greater than 400 mm^2, but we have not observed this difference to be statistically significant. Treatment of chronic degenerative lesions is not specifically limited by size, but more emphasis is placed on proper axial alignment and the presence of global degenerative changes throughout the knee.

General considerations for use of the microfracture procedure include patient age, acceptable biomechanical alignment of the knee, the patient's activity level, and the patient's expectations. If all of these criteria define a patient who could benefit from chondral resurfacing, then microfracture is considered.

Contraindications

Specific contraindications for microfracture include axial malalignment (as described following), patients unwilling or unable to follow the required strict and rigorous rehabilitation protocol, partial thickness defects, and inability to use the opposite leg for weight bearing during the minimal or non-weight-bearing time. Other specific contraindications include any systemic immune-mediated disease, disease-induced arthritis, or cartilage disease. A relative contraindication is for patients older than 65 years because the authors have observed that some patients older than 65 years experience difficulty with crutch walking and the required rigorous rehabilitation. Other contraindications to microfracture include global degenerative osteoarthrosis or if the cartilage surrounding the lesion is too thin to establish a perpendicular rim to hold the marrow clot. In these advanced degenerative cases, axial malalignment is often a confounding factor (Table 27-1).

PREOPERATIVE PLANNING

Patients who present with knee pain undergo a thorough physical and orthopaedic examination. The cartilage lesions can be on the joint surfaces of the femur, tibia, and/or patella. At times the physical diagnosis can be difficult and elusive, especially if only an isolated chondral defect is present. Identification of point tenderness over a femoral condyle or tibial plateau is a useful finding, but in itself is not diagnostic. If compression of the patella elicits pain, this finding might be indicative of a patellar or trochlear lesion.

For diagnostic imaging, we use long-standing radiographs as described following to observe for angular deformity and for joint space narrowing that is often indicative of loss of articular cartilage. We also obtain standard anteroposterior (AP) and lateral radiographs of both knees as well weight-bearing views with the knees flexed to 30 to 45 degrees. Patellar views are also useful to evaluate the patellofemoral joint. Magnetic resonance imaging (MRI) that employs newer diagnostic sequences specific for articular cartilage has become a mainstay of our diagnostic workup of patients with suspected chondral lesions.

Two methods for radiographic measurement of the biomechanical alignment of the weight-bearing axis of the knee are used in our facility: (a) the angle made between the femur and tibia on AP views obtained with the patient standing, and (b) the weight-bearing mechanical axis drawn from the center of the femoral head to the center of the tibiotarsal joint on long standing (approx. 51 in/130 cm) radiographs. If the angle drawn between the tibia and femur is greater than 5 degrees of varus or valgus compared to the normal knee, this amount of axial malalignment would be a relative contraindication for microfracture. Preferably the mechanical axis weight-bearing line should be in the central quarter of the tibial plateau of either the medial or lateral compartment. If the mechanical axis weight-bearing line falls outside the central-most quarter of the plateaus, medial or lateral, this weight-bearing shift also would be a relative contraindication if left uncorrected (Fig. 27-1). In such cases, a realignment procedure should be included as a part of the overall treatment regimen.

TABLE 27-1. Indications and Contraindications for Microfracture

Indications	Contraindications
Full-thickness defect (grade IV), acute or chronic	Partial thickness defects
Unstable full-thickness lesion	Uncorrected axial malalignment
Degenerative joint disease lesion (requires proper knee alignment)	Unable to commit to rehabilitation protocol
Patient capable of rehabilitation protocol	Global degenerative osteoarthrosis

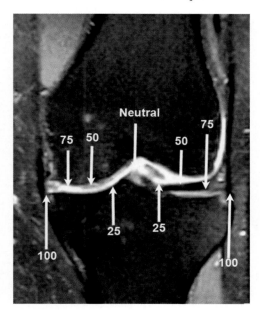

FIGURE 27-1

If the mechanical axis weight-bearing line falls outside the central-most quarter of the plateaus, medial or lateral, this weight-bearing shift also would be a relative contraindication if left uncorrected.

TECHNIQUE

The patient is placed supine, and routine skin preparation and draping are completed. Standard arthroscopic portals can be used for microfracture; however, we find that making the portals slightly higher and slightly further off the midline may provide additional visualization (Fig. 27-2). We make three portals: a superior and medially placed inflow portal and medial and lateral parapatellar portals (Fig. 27-3). Accessory portals may occasionally be made for lesions in difficult-to-reach locations. Typically we do not use a tourniquet during the microfracture procedure; instead, we adjust the arthroscopic fluid pump pressure to control bleeding. An initial thorough diagnostic examination of the knee should be done before beginning the actual microfracture. We carefully inspect all geographic areas of the knee including the suprapatellar pouch, the medial and lateral gutters, the patellofemoral joint, the intercondylar notch and its contents, and the medial and lateral compartments including the posterior horns of both menisci. We do all other intra-articular procedures before completing microfracture, with the exception of ACL reconstruction. This sequence helps prevent loss of visualization when the fat droplets and blood enter the knee from the marrow cavity via microfracture holes. This technique also decreases the amount of time that the microfractured bone is exposed to the elevated intra-articular pressures and fluid flow that possibly could decrease the formation of the surgically induced marrow clot ("super clot") that is critical to the success of the microfracture procedure. We pay particular attention to soft tissues such as plicae and the lateral retinaculum that potentially could produce increased compression between cartilage surfaces.

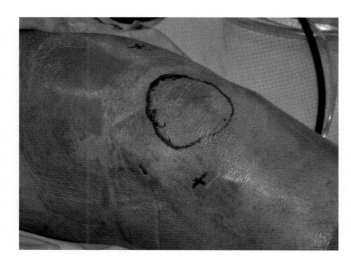

FIGURE 27-2

Standard arthroscopic portals can be used for microfracture; however, we find that making the portals slightly higher and slightly further off the midline may provide additional visualization.

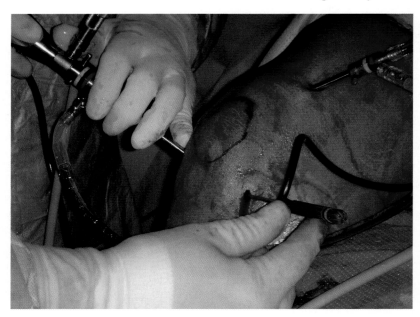

FIGURE 27-3

We make three portals: a superior and medially placed inflow portal and medial and lateral parapatellar portals.

After carefully assessing the full-thickness articular cartilage lesion, we debride the exposed bone of all remaining unstable cartilage using a hand-held curved curette and a full radius resector. It is critical to remove all loose or marginally attached cartilage from the surrounding rim of the lesion (Fig. 27-4). Establishment of a stable full-thickness border of cartilage surrounding a central lesion is optimal for microfracture to provide some degree of protection to the regenerating tissue that is forming in the treated lesion. The calcified cartilage layer that remains as a cap to many lesions must be removed, preferably by using a curette (see Fig. 27-4). Thorough and complete removal of the calcified cartilage layer is extremely important based on animal studies we have completed. Care should be taken to maintain the integrity of the subchondral plate by not curetting too deeply; otherwise, the joint shape and geometry might be negatively altered. This prepared lesion, with a stable perpendicular edge of healthy well-attached viable cartilage surrounding the defect, provides a pool that helps hold the "super clot." After preparation of the lesion, we use an arthroscopic awl to make multiple holes, or "microfractures," in the exposed subchondral bone plate. We use an awl with an angle that permits the tip to be approximately perpendicular to the bone as it is advanced, typically 30 or 45 degrees (Fig. 27-5). There also is a 90-degree awl that should be used only on the patella or

FIGURE 27-4

It is critical to remove all loose or marginally attached cartilage from the surrounding rim of the lesion. The calcified cartilage layer that remains as a cap to many lesions must be removed, preferably by using a curette.

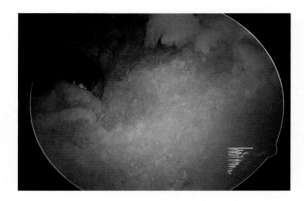

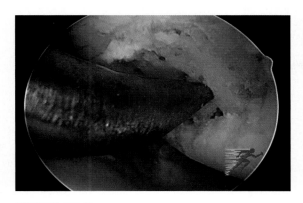

FIGURE 27-5

We use an awl with an angle that permits the tip to be approximately perpendicular to the bone as it is advanced, typically 30 or 45 degrees.

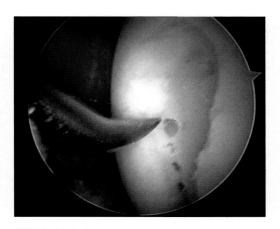

FIGURE 27-6

When fat droplets can be seen coming from the marrow cavity, the appropriate depth (approx. 2 to 4 mm) has been reached. We make microfracture holes around the periphery of the defect first, immediately adjacent to the healthy stable cartilage rim.

other soft bone. The 90-degree awl should be advanced only manually, not with a mallet. The holes are made as close together as possible, but not so close that one breaks into another, thus damaging the subchondral plate between them and potentially altering the joint shape. This technique usually results in microfracture holes that are approximately 3 to 4 mm apart. When fat droplets can be seen coming from the marrow cavity, the appropriate depth (approx. 2 to 4 mm) has been reached (Fig. 27-6). The arthroscopic awls likely produce no thermal necrosis of the bone compared with hand-driven or motorized drills. We make microfracture holes around the periphery of the defect first, immediately adjacent to the healthy stable cartilage rim (see Figs. 27-5 and 27-6). Then, we complete the process by making the microfracture holes toward the center of the defect (Fig. 27-7). We assess the treated lesion at the conclusion of the microfracture to ensure a sufficient number of holes have been made before reducing the arthroscopic irrigation fluid flow (Fig. 27-8).

After the arthroscopic irrigation fluid pump pressure is reduced, under direct visualization we are able to observe the flow of marrow fat droplets and blood from the microfracture holes into the prepared lesion (Fig. 27-9). The quantity of marrow contents flowing into the joint is judged to be adequate when we observe marrow elements flowing from all microfracture holes (Fig. 27-10). We

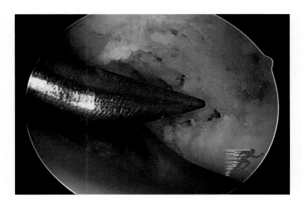

FIGURE 27-7

We complete the process by making the microfracture holes toward the center of the defect.

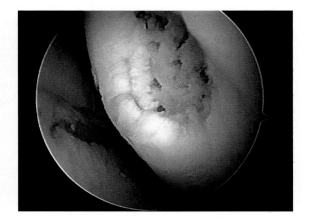

FIGURE 27-8

We assess the treated lesion at the conclusion of the microfracture to ensure a sufficient number of holes have been made before reducing the arthroscopic irrigation fluid flow.

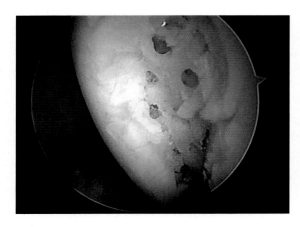

FIGURE 27-9

After the arthroscopic irrigation fluid pump pressure is reduced, under direct visualization we are able to observe the flow of marrow fat droplets and blood from the microfracture holes into the prepared lesion.

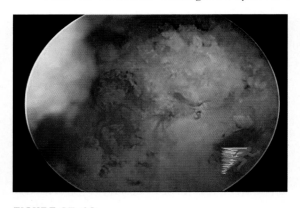

FIGURE 27-10

The quantity of marrow contents flowing into the joint is judged to be adequate when we observe marrow elements flowing from all microfracture holes.

then remove all instruments from the knee and evacuate the joint of fluid. Intra-articular drains should *not* be used because the goal is for the super clot rich in marrow elements to form and to stabilize while covering the lesion.

Chronic degenerative chondral lesions commonly have extensive eburnated bone and bony sclerosis with thickening of the subchondral plate, thus making it difficult to do an adequate microfracture procedure. In these instances and when the axial alignment and other indications for microfracture are met, we first make a few microfracture holes with the awls in various locations of the lesion to assess the thickness of the sclerotic or eburnated bone. We often use a motorized burr to remove the sclerotic bone until punctate bleeding is evident. After the bleeding appears uniformly over the surface of the lesion, a microfracture procedure can be performed as previously described. We have observed noticeably improved results for these patients with chronic chondral lesions since we began using this technique. However, if the surrounding cartilage is too thin to establish a perpendicular rim to hold and protect the super clot, then likely we would not do a microfracture procedure in patients with such advanced degenerative lesions.

The microfracture awl produces a rough surface in the subchondral bone to which the marrow clot can adhere more easily, yet the integrity of the subchondral plate is maintained for joint surface shape and geometry (see Fig. 27-8). The microfracture procedure virtually eliminates thermal necrosis and provides a roughened surface for blood clot adherence. The different angles of arthroscopic awls available provide easier access to difficult-to-reach areas of the knee. The awls not only provide perpendicular holes but also improved control of depth penetration compared to drilling. We believe that the key to the entire procedure is to establish the surgically induced marrow clot to provide the optimal environment for the body's own pluripotent marrow cells (mesenchymal stem cells or progenitor cells) to differentiate into stable tissue within the lesion.

Pearls and Pitfalls

- Complete a thorough arthroscopic diagnostic examination, inspecting all geographic areas of the knee. Perform all other intra-articular procedures before completing microfracture, with the exception of ACL reconstruction.
- Assess the chondral lesion. Remove all loose or marginally attached cartilage down to exposed bone.
- Thoroughly and completely remove the calcified cartilage layer with a hand held curette, but do not penetrate the subchondral bone.
- Use a microfracture awl to make microfracture holes in the subchondral bone, first working all the way around the periphery and then into the center of the lesion.

- Microfracture holes should be about 3 to 4 mm apart so that one does not break into another, and they should penetrate approximately 2 to 4 mm deep to access the marrow elements.
- Reduce the irrigation pump pressure (or tourniquet) and observe for marrow element flow from all holes.
- Remove all instruments and evacuate the joint. Do not use a drain in the joint.

POSTOPERATIVE MANAGEMENT

We have designed the postoperative management program to promote the ideal physical environment in which the newly recruited mesenchymal stem cells from the marrow can differentiate into the appropriate articular cartilage-like cell lines. These differentiation and maturation processes must occur slowly but consistently. Our animal studies have confirmed that both cellular and molecular changes are an essential part of the development of a durable repair tissue. Our experience and clinical research data indicate that improvement can be expected to occur slowly but steadily for at least 2 years. During this protracted period, the repair tissue matures, pain and swelling resolve, and the patient regains confidence and comfort in the knee during increased levels of activity.

The rehabilitation program after microfracture for treatment of chondral defects in the knee is crucial to optimize the results of the surgery. The surgically induced marrow clot provides the basis for the most ideal chemical environment to complement the physical environment. This newly proliferated repair cartilage then fills the original defect. The postoperative rehabilitation program after microfracture necessitates consideration of several factors. The specific protocol recommended depends on both the anatomic location and the size of the defect. These factors are critical to determine the ideal postoperative plan. For example, if other intra-articular procedures are done concurrently with microfracture, such as ACL reconstruction, we will alter the rehabilitation program as necessary. All of the possible variations of the rehabilitation program are not within the scope of this chapter, but here we describe two different protocols.

Rehabilitation Protocol for Patients with Lesions on the Femoral Condyle or Tibial Plateau

After microfracture of lesions on the weight-bearing surfaces of the femoral condyles or tibial plateaus, we initiate immediate motion with a continuous passive motion (CPM) machine in the recovery room. The initial range of motion (ROM) typically is 30 to 70 degrees, and then it is increased as tolerated by 10 to 20 degrees, until full passive ROM is achieved. The rate of the machine is usually 1 cycle per minute initially, but the rate can be varied based on patient preference and comfort. Many patients tolerate use of the CPM machine at night. For those who do not, we have observed that intermittent use during the day is as beneficial. Regardless of when the CPM machine is used, the goal is to have the patient in the CPM machine for 6 to 8 hours every 24 hours. If the patient is unable to use the CPM machine, then instructions are given for passive flexion and extension of the knee with 500 repetitions three times per day. We encourage patients to gain full passive ROM of the injured knee as soon as possible after surgery. We also prescribe cold therapy for all patients postoperatively. Our experience and observations indicate that the cold helps control pain and inflammation, and most patients state that the cold provides overall postoperative pain relief. Cold therapy is typically used for 1 to 7 days postoperatively. Crutch-assisted touchdown weight-bearing ambulation (10% of body weight initially) is prescribed for 6 to 8 weeks, depending on the size of the lesion. For most patients, 6 to 8 weeks is adequate time to limit weight bearing. However, for patients with small lesions (<1 cm diameter), weight bearing may be initiated earlier. Patients with lesions on the femoral condyles or tibial plateaus rarely use a brace during the initial postoperative period. However, we may prescribe an unloading type brace when the patient becomes more active and the postoperative swelling has resolved.

The patient begins therapy immediately after surgery with an emphasis on patellar mobility and range of motion. Patients are instructed to perform medial to lateral and superior to inferior movement of the patella as well as medial to lateral movement of the quadriceps and patellar tendons. This mobilization is essential to prevent patellar tendon adhesions and associated increases in patellofemoral joint reaction forces. Range-of-motion exercises (without range-of-motion limitations), quadriceps sets, straight-leg raises, hamstring stretching, and ankle pumps are also initiated the day of surgery.

Stationary biking without resistance and a deep water exercise program are initiated at 1 to 2 weeks postoperatively. The deep water exercises include use of a flotation vest for deep water running. It is imperative that the foot of the injured leg does not touch the bottom of the pool during this exercise to avoid placing excessive loads on the microfracture site.

After 8 weeks of touchdown weight bearing, the patient is progressed to weight bearing as tolerated, typically weaning off crutches within 1 week. Restoration of normal muscular function through the use of low-impact exercises is emphasized during weeks 9 through 16. Stationary biking with increasing resistance, treadmill walking on a 7% incline, and elliptical training are all initiated during this phase. Closed-chain double knee bends and elastic cord exercise are added to the regimen at about 12 weeks. Our observations indicate that the ability to achieve predetermined maximum levels for sets and repetitions of elastic resistance cord exercises is an excellent indicator for progressing to weight training.

We permit free or machine weights when the patient has achieved the early goals of the rehabilitation program, but not before 16 weeks after microfracture. We strongly emphasize the importance of proper technique when beginning a weight program. The patient is instructed to avoid pain during weight training and may be counseled to avoid ranges of motion that stress the microfracture site. A progressive run-walk program and initial agility drills start between 16 to 24 weeks postoperatively. Initial running is completed on a forgiving surface, using a ratio of 1 minute running followed by 4 minutes walking. Once the patient can perform 20 minutes at a 1:4 ratio, the ratio is gradually progressed to 4 minutes running and 1 minute walking before the patient is allowed to run continuously. Initial agility drills include single plane activities completed at 25% speed with increases in duration made before increases in intensity. Depending on the clinical examination, size of the patient, the sport, and the size of the lesion, we usually recommend that patients do not return to sports that involve pivoting, cutting, and jumping until at least 4 to 9 months after microfracture.

Rehabilitation Protocol for Patients with Patellofemoral Lesions

Without exception, all patients treated by microfracture for patellofemoral lesions must use a brace set at 0 to 20 degrees for the first 8 weeks postoperatively. This brace limits compression of the regenerating surfaces of the trochlea or patella, or both. We allow passive motion with the brace removed, but otherwise the brace must be worn at all times. Patients with patellofemoral lesions are placed into a continuous passive motion machine set at 0 to 50 degrees immediately postoperatively. Apart from the ROM setting, parameters for the CPM are the same as for tibiofemoral lesions. We also use cold therapy as described previously. With this regimen patients typically obtain a pain-free and full passive ROM soon after surgery.

For patients with patellofemoral joint lesions, we carefully observe joint angles at the time of arthroscopy to determine where the defect comes into contact with the patellar facet or the trochlear groove. We make certain to avoid these areas during strength training for approximately 4 months. This avoidance allows for training in the 0- to 20-degree range immediately postoperatively because there is minimal compression of these chondral surfaces with such limited motion. Patients are allowed to weight bear as tolerated in their brace 2 weeks after surgery. After 8 weeks, we open the knee brace gradually before it is discontinued. When the brace is discontinued, patients are allowed to advance their training progressively. Stationary biking without resistance is allowed 2 weeks postoperatively; resistance is added at 8 weeks after microfracture. Starting 12 weeks after microfracture, the exercise program is the same as used for femorotibial lesions.

COMPLICATIONS

Most patients progress through the postoperative period with little or no difficulty. However, some patients present with mild transient pain, most frequently after microfracture in the patellofemoral joint. Small changes in the articular surface of the patellofemoral joint may be detected by a grating or "gritty" sensation of the joint, especially when a patient discontinues use of the knee brace and begins normal weight bearing through a full ROM. Patients rarely complain of pain at this time, and this grating sensation usually resolves spontaneously in a few days or weeks. Similarly, if a steep perpendicular rim was made in the trochlear groove, patients may notice "catching" or "locking" as the apex of the patella rides over this lesion during joint motion. Some patients may even perceive these symptoms while in the CPM machine. These symptoms usually gradually dissipate within 3 months. If this perceived locking is painful, the patient is advised to limit weight bearing and avoid the symptomatic joint angle for an additional period.

Swelling and joint effusion typically resolve within 8 weeks after microfracture. Occasionally, a recurrent effusion develops between 6 and 8 weeks after microfracture, most commonly when a patient begins to bear weight on the injured leg after microfracture of a defect on the femoral condyle. While this effusion may mimic the preoperative or immediate postoperative effusion, usually it is painless. We treat this type of painless effusion conservatively. It usually resolves within several weeks after onset. Rarely has a second arthroscopy been required for recurring effusions.

RESULTS

We published the first long-term outcomes paper on the microfracture technique. This study followed 72 patients an average of 11 years following microfracture, with the longest follow-up being 17 years. This study included knees with no joint space narrowing, no degenerative arthritis, and no ligament or meniscus pathology which required treatment. All patients were under 45 years of age. The microfracture technique used on these patients did not include recent improvements to the technique as described in the technique section of this chapter. With a 95% follow-up rate, the results showed improvement in symptoms and function. Patient-reported pain and swelling decreased at postoperative year 1, continued to decrease at year 2, and the clinical improvements were maintained over the study period. The study identified age as the only independent predictor of functional (Lysholm) improvement. Patients over 35 years of age improved less than patients under 35; however, both groups showed improvement.

We also have documented the outcome of microfracture in patients who played professional football in the United States. Twenty-five active National Football League players were treated with microfracture between 1986 and 1997. The study found that 76% of players returned to play the next football season. Following return to play, those same players played an average of 4.6 additional seasons. All players showed decreased symptoms and improvement in function. Of those players who did not return to play, most had pre-existing degenerative changes of the knee.

Arthroscopic treatment of the degenerative knee is controversial. However, we documented outcomes at 2 years in patients with degenerative chondral lesions treated with microfracture. Our goals were to alleviate pain, maximize function, and prevent further degenerative changes. With strict patient selection, proper surgical technique, and compliance with a well-defined rehabilitation program, patients showed improvement in their function and had decreased symptoms. Pain and swelling significantly decreased with most patients reporting only mild symptoms, and patients were highly satisfied with their results. Factors that were associated with less functional improvement included bipolar lesions, lesions greater than 400 mm^2, and meniscus-deficient knees. Failures, as defined by revision microfracture or total knee replacement, were documented in 6% of the patients. These results confirm excellent short-term outcomes; however, further studies will be needed to determine how long the results last. A contraindication to microfracture in the degenerative knee is axial malalignment of the joint. Medial opening wedge high tibial osteotomy (HTO) has gained popularity as a means of correcting malalignment in patients with medial compartment arthrosis and varus malalignment who wish to stay active. We recently reported on 39 patients who underwent an opening wedge osteotomy on the medial side of the proximal tibia in conjunction with the microfracture procedure in their degenerative varus knee. Patients showed improvement in function and activity level, as well as decreased symptoms. Most patients had a greater than 20-point increase in their Lysholm score. This study also showed that patients with no prior surgeries had more improvement. Two patients went on to total knee replacement at 3 years and 5 years following the HTO. The study concluded that at a minimum of 2 years following surgery, patients with varus alignment and chondral surface lesions of the knee can be treated effectively with the high tibial osteotomy and microfracture. These patients returned to an active lifestyle as demonstrated by their significantly higher activity (Tegner) scores.

RECOMMENDED READING

Frisbie DD, Morisset S, Ho CP, et al. Effects of calcified cartilage on healing of chondral defects treated with microfracture in horses. *Am J Sports Med.* 2006;34:1824–1831.

Frisbie DD, Oxford JT, Southwood L, et al. Early events in cartilage repair after subchondralbone microfracture. *Clin Orthop.* 2003;407:215–227.

Frisbie DD, Trotter GW, Powers BE, et al. Arthroscopic subchondral bone plate microfracture technique augments healing of large osteochondral defects in the radial carpal bone and medial femoral condyle of horses. *J Vet Surg.* 1999;28:242–255.

Hagerman GR, Atkins JA, Dillman C. Rehabilitation of chondral injuries and chronic degenerative arthritis of the knee in the athlete. *Oper Tech Sports Med.* 1995;3:127–135.

Kocher MS, Steadman JR, Briggs KK, et al. Reliability, validity, and responsiveness of the Lysholm knee scale for various chondral disorders of the knee. *J Bone Joint Surg.* 2004;86A:1139–1145.

Miller BS, Steadman JR, Briggs KK, et al. Patient satisfaction and outcome after microfracture of the degenerative knee. *J Knee Surg.* 2004;17:13–17.

Steadman JR, Briggs KK, Rodrigo JJ, et al. Outcomes of microfracture for traumatic chondral defects of the knee: average 11-year follow-up. *Arthroscopy.* 2003;19:477–484.

Steadman JR, Miller BS, Karas SG, et al. The microfracture technique in the treatment of full-thickness chondral lesions of the knee in National Football League players. *J Knee Surg.* 2003;16:83–86.

Steadman JR, Rodkey WG, Briggs KK, et al. Debridement and microfracture for full-thickness articular cartilage defects. In: Scott WN, ed. *Insall & Scott surgery of the knee.* Philadelphia: Elsevier; 2006:359–366.

Steadman JR, Rodkey WG, Briggs KK. Microfracture chondroplasty: indications, techniques, and outcomes. *Sports Med Arthrosc Rev.* 2003;11:236–244.

Steadman JR, Rodkey WG, Briggs KK. Microfracture to treat full-thickness chondral defects. *J Knee Surg.* 2002; 15:170–176.

Steadman JR, Rodkey WG. Microfracture in the pediatric and adolescent knee. In: Micheli LJ, Kocher M, eds. *The pediatric & adolescent knee.* Philadelphia: Elsevier; 2006:308–311.

Steadman JR, Rodkey WG. Microfracture technique: treatment of full-thickness chondral lesions. In: Jackson DW, ed. *Reconstructive knee surgery.* 2nd ed. New York: Lippincott Williams & Wilkins; 2002:329–335.

Steadman JR, Rodkey WG, Rodrigo JJ. "Microfracture": surgical technique and rehabilitation to treat chondral defects. *Clin Orthop.* 2001;391S:S362–S369.

Sterett WI, Steadman JR. Chondral resurfacing and high tibial osteotomy in the varus knee. *Am J Sports Med.* 2004;32:1243–1249.

28 Osteochondral Plug Transplantation

László Hangody, Zsófia Duska, and Zoltán Kárpáti

INDICATIONS/CONTRAINDICATIONS

Efficacious treatment of full-thickness cartilage defects of the weight-bearing surfaces represents a multifaceted challenge for the orthopaedic surgeon. During the recent decade many efforts have been made to improve the quality of different cartilage repair techniques aiming to provide a hyaline-like surface in the resurfaced area. Autologous osteochondral transplantation represents one solution, enabled by promotion of a hyaline or hyaline-like repair of the affected area. Several series of dog and horse experiments and 14 years of clinical experience proved that autologous osteochondral mosaicplasty is a useful alternative in the treatment of full-thickness cartilage defects. Open and arthroscopic use of the mosaicplasty technique has already extended clinical experience, and recent data suggest both indications and contraindications. Besides femoral and tibial condylar and patellotrochlear applications, talar, femoral head, humeral head, and capitulum humeri implantations were carried out. Preclinical animal studies and subsequent clinical practice have confirmed the survival of the transplanted hyaline cartilage as well as fibrocartilage filling of the donor sites (located on the non–weight-bearing and less–weight-bearing surfaces of the knee joint). Clinical scores, several types of different imaging techniques, control arthroscopies, histologic examination of biopsy samples, and cartilage stiffness measurements have been used to evaluate the clinical outcome and quality of the transplanted cartilage, and have confirmed the clinical efficacy of the mosaicplasty technique. This chapter discusses the indications, contraindications, technical details, rehabilitation, and pitfalls and complications of the procedure.

If the preoperative differential diagnosis includes a small or medium-sized focal defect of the weight-bearing surfaces, the patient should be advised of the possibility of an autologous osteochondral mosaicplasty. In such cases, the patient should also be prepared for an open procedure. The site or the size of the lesion can require a miniarthrotomy or an open procedure; however, the main goal should be an arthroscopic approach for this type of cartilage transplantation. Open procedures can lead to an overnight stay and altered weight-bearing status for several weeks.

Transplantation of osteochondral autografts is not new, but its clinical application was restricted because of certain technical difficulties, such as congruency and donor site problems. Osteochondral autograft donor sites must be taken from relatively non–weight-bearing surfaces, which limits the procurement field. On the other hand, use of large grafts can cause certain incongruities at the recipient site, permanently altering the biomechanics of the joint. Instead of single-block transfer, the use of small multiple cylindrical grafts may permit more tissue to be transplanted while preserving donor site integrity, and their use in a mosaic-like implanting fashion would allow progressive contouring of the new surface. Autologous osteochondral mosaicplasty has been introduced in clinical practice in 1992 in Hungary. This type of resurfacing can be indicated for 1- to 4-cm^2 focal chondral or osteochondral defects of the weight-bearing area. The most common recipient sites are the femoral condyles, but clinical experience with the patellotrochlear, tibial, and talar applications is fairly extensive. As far as exceptional applications are concerned, a few implantations for certain osteochondral defects of the humeral and femoral head as well as the capitulum humeri were carried out.

As with other types of resurfacing, mosaicplasty requires the elimination of the underlying causes (if this is possible) in the same step. According to clinical experience, anterior cruciate ligament (ACL) reconstruction, meniscus surgery, and femorotibial realignment procedures are the most common concomitant procedures, but patellofemoral realignment techniques, lateral release, and so on, may also be required.

Any disadvantageous condition hindering the survival of the transplanted hyaline cartilage on the recipient site can be a contraindication, such as the following:

- Generalized arthritis, rheumatoid and/or degenerative type
- Lack of appropriate donor area
- Infectious or tumor defects
- Age greater than 50 years
- Osteochondral defects deeper than 10 mm

PREOPERATIVE PLANNING

Localized full-thickness cartilaginous lesions are usually defined at arthroscopy, but preoperative clinical investigation may also give some useful information. Anamnestic data and actual clinical findings (e.g., tenderness in the medial joint space, swelling, clicking) may support the presence of a cartilage defect, but there are no specific signs for determining the exact type and location of existing chondral damage. Osteochondral lesions usually show more expressed complaints. Despite that small- or medium-sized chondral and osteochondral damages do not give a characteristic picture, the clinical examination is necessary to eliminate the actual biomechanical problems. Stability of the affected knee, femorotibial alignment, and patellofemoral traction conditions should be cleared at the clinical examination.

Standard and standing radiographic examinations are basic elements of the preoperative diagnostics. Computed tomography (CT) may inform about the subchondral bony condition. Ultrasound investigation or special sequences of magnetic resonance imaging (MRI) can give useful information about the location and extension of the chondral defects, but severity cannot always be determined exactly. The last step is usually the arthroscopic examination, which should determine the exact location and stage of the damage, evaluate the quality of the donor area, and check all the other intra-articular conditions.

Preoperative preparations should include antibiotic prophylaxis. General or local anesthesia with tourniquet control is recommended.

SURGERY

The patient is positioned supine with the knee capable of 120 degrees of flexion. The contralateral extremity is placed in a stirrup. Standard arthroscopic instrumentation and MosaicPlasty Complete System (Smith & Nephew, Inc., Endoscopy Division, Andover, MA) are required. Beside these reusable instruments, disposable chisels, drillbits, and tamps are also available to provide ideal conditions for precise graft harvest and tunnel preparation (Dispoposplasty System, Smith & Nephew, Inc., Endoscopy Division, Andover, MA). A fluid management system may support the procedure.

Choosing a procedure (arthroscopic or miniarthrotomy) depends on the type, size, and exact location of the defect determined during arthroscopy. As placing the grafts perpendicular to the surface is paramount to the success of the operation, the first task is to determine whether an arthroscopic or open procedure is required. Although certain trochlear defects can be resurfaced arthroscopically, patellotrochlear and tibial lesions always require an open procedure. Most of the femoral condylar defects can be managed arthroscopically. As for most of these lesions, central anterior medial and central anterior lateral portals will allow correct perpendicular access.

An open procedure may be chosen in the learning curve or when an arthroscopic approach is not practical due to size or location of the lesion. Arthroscopic or open mosaicplasties have the same steps and technique.

Arthroscopic Mosaicplasty

Portal Selection   As has been emphasized previously, perpendicular access to the lesion is critical to proper insertion of the grafts. Take care in making the viewing and working portals. Use a

1.2-mm K-wire or 18-gauge spinal needle initially to locate the portal sites. It should be noted that these portals tend to be more central than the standard portals due to the inward curve of the condyles (Fig. 28-1). For osteochondritis dissecans on the medial femoral condyle, the approach should be from the lateral side. Standard lateral portal is sometimes too oblique. Therefore, use the central patellar tendon portal, which gives good access to the inner positions of both the medial femoral condyle and the lateral femoral condyle.

Defect Preparation   Use a full-radius resector or curette and a knife blade to bring the edges of the defect back to good hyaline cartilage at a right angle. Clean the base of the lesion with an arthroscopic burr (Abrader, Acromionizer) or half-round rasp to viable subchondral bone (Fig. 28-2). Abrasion arthroplasty of the defect site promotes fibrocartilage grouting from the bony base. Because tapping the cutting edge of the guide into the bony base and removal of it can mark the defect site, use the drill guide to determine the number and size of grafts needed (Fig. 28-3). Filling of the defect by same-sized contacting rings allows a filling rate of about 70% to 80%, but use of additional sizes to cover the dead spaces and cutting the grafts into each other can improve the coverage to 90% to 100% (Fig. 28-4). Finally, measure the depth of the defect with the laser marks of the dilator.

Graft Harvest   The medial femoral condyle periphery of the patellofemoral joint above the line of the notch is the preferred arthroscopic harvest site. The lateral femoral condyle above the sulcus terminalis and, in exceptional cases, the notch area can serve as additional donor areas (Fig. 28-5). Grafts harvested from the notch area are less favorable features, as they have concave cartilage caps and less elastic underlying bone. The medial patellofemoral periphery has easier access than the lateral one as fluid distension can promote lateral positioning of the patella and may provide easier perpendicular positioning for the harvesting chisel.

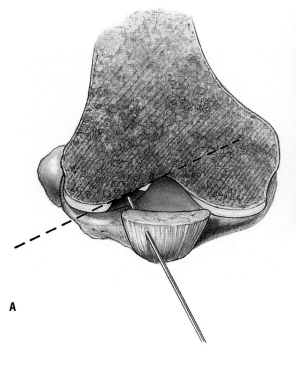

A

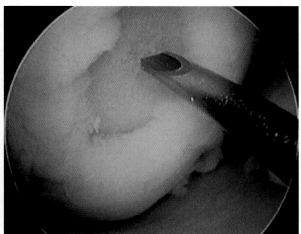

B

FIGURE 28-1

A: Use of a spinal needle to determine the perpendicular access to the defect. **B:** Arthroscopic picture of the same step.

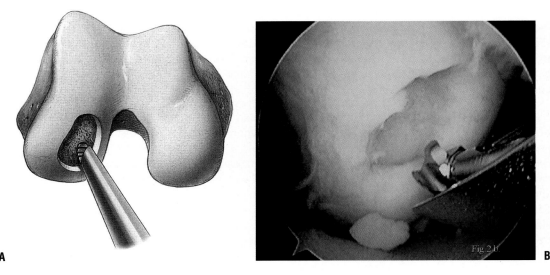

FIGURE 28-2

A: Abrasion arthroplasty of the bony base of the defect. **B:** Arthroscopic picture of the same step.

The best view for harvesting grafts is obtained by introducing the scope through the standard contralateral portal. Extend the knee and use the standard ipsilateral portal to check the perpendicular access to the donor site. Extended position should provide perpendicular access to the most superior donor hole. Step-by-step flexion allows the harvest of additional grafts from the lower portions of the patellofemoral periphery. If the standard portals do not allow a perpendicular approach, use a spinal needle or a K-wire to determine the location of additional harvesting portals.

Once the necessary portal has been determined, introduce the proper-sized tube chisel filled with the appropriate harvesting tamp. Once the site has been clearly identified, the chisel is located per-

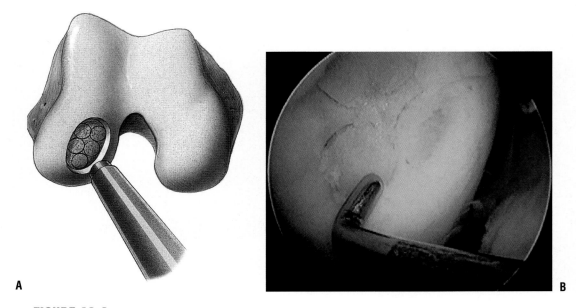

FIGURE 28-3

A: Abrasion arthroplasty of the bony base of the defect. **B:** Arthroscopic picture of the same step.

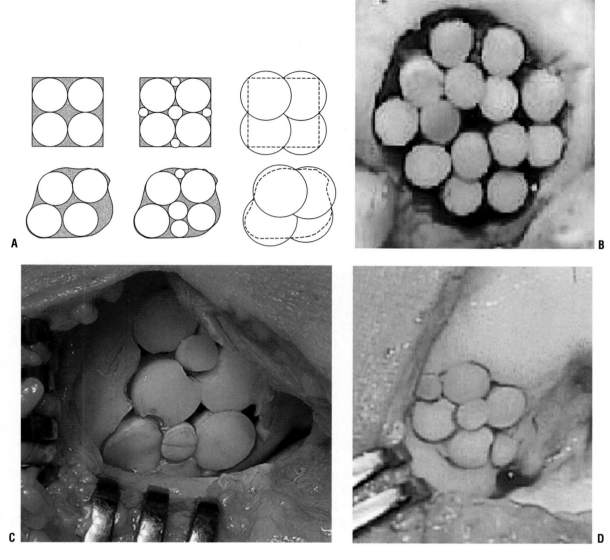

FIGURE 28-4

A: Eighty percent, 90%, and 100% filling of a defect. **B–D:** Intraoperative pictures of the same filling rates.

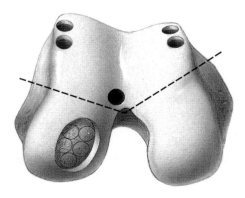

FIGURE 28-5

Location of the recommended donor sites.

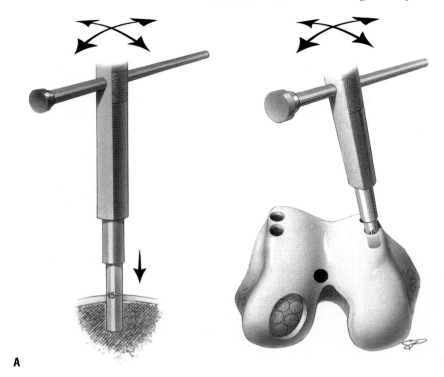

FIGURE 28-6

A,B: Graft harvest by toggling the harvesting chisel.

pendicular to the articular surface and driven by a hammer to the appropriate depth. The minimal length of the graft should be at least two times its diameter, but, as a rule, take l5-mm-long grafts to resurface chondral lesions and 25-mm-long plugs for osteochondral defects. It is important to hold the chisel firmly to avoid its shifting at the cartilage–bone interface, producing a crooked graft. By flexing the knee, lower sites can be obtained. The lower limit is the level of the top of the inter-condylar notch (sulcus terminalis). Insert the appropriate harvesting tamp into the cross-hole in the tubular chisel and use it as a lever. The chisel should be toggled, not rotated, causing the graft to break free at the chisel tip (Fig. 28-6). Eject the grafts from the chisel by sliding the appropriately sized chisel guard over the cutting end. Use the tamp to push out the graft onto gauze in a saline-wetted basin (Fig. 28-7). The donor site holes will eventually be filled up with initial repair tissue by bleeding mediated mesenchymal stem cell invasion in a few hours. Proper rehabilitation during the first postoperative weeks may support a transformation of the primary repair tissue into cancel-lous bone and fibrocartilage as final coverage.

During the learning curve, the grafts can also be obtained through a miniarthrotomy (1.5 to 2.0 cm).

Implantation of the Grafts: "Drill-Dilate-Deliver" (Three-Dimensional Grafting)

DRILL Flex the knee and establish good distension. Reintroduce the drill guide using the dilator as an obturator. Place these tools perpendicularly to the defected surface. By rotating the arthro-scope, the drill guide and the perpendicularity of the laser mark can be seen from different angles, ensuring proper orientation. Tap the cutting edge of the guide into the subchondral bone. Insert the appropriate size drill bit and drill to the desired depth (Fig. 28-8). Generally, a recipient hole a few millimeters deeper than the length of the graft is desirable to minimize high intraosseal pressure. Re-duce the inflow to minimize leakage. Finally, remove the drill bit.

DILATE Insert again the conical-shaped dilator into the drill guide. Tap it to the desired depth, de-pending on the actual features of the recipient bone. Stiff bone needs more dilation than normal or soft bone. Hold the drill guide firmly and remove the dilator from the hole (Fig. 28-9).

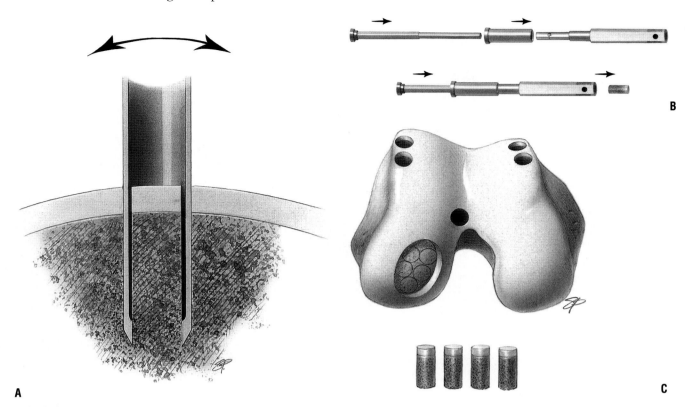

FIGURE 28-7

A–C: Graft removal from the harvesting chisel.

DELIVER Adjust the delivery tamp by turning the handle to initially allow the graft to sit slightly higher than the depth of the defect. This will minimize the likelihood of overpenetrating the graft. Stop the inflow; otherwise, fluid flow can push the graft out of the tube. Deliver the graft under direct visualization into the recipient hole through the drill guide with the delivery tamp (Fig. 28-10). Insert the graft deeper by turning the delivery tamp handle counterclockwise. The graft should be flush with the original articular surface. Remove the drill guide to inspect the graft. If the graft is proud, reinsert the drill guide and tap the graft down gently with the tamp of the appropriate size. Insert the subsequent grafts in a similar fashion by placing the drill guide immediately adjacent to the previously placed grafts. Such step-by-step graft implantation has several advantages. Dilation of the actual recipient hole allows an easy graft insertion (low insertion force on the hyaline cap), but dilation of the next hole affects the surrounding bone to the previously implanted grafts, which can result in a very safe press fit fixation (Fig. 28-11).

When all the holes are filled and the grafts are in place, put the knee through a range of motion, creating varus or valgus stress, depending on the site of the resurfacing (Fig. 28-12). Close the portals and introduce suction drainage into the joint through a superior portal. Use an elastic bandage to fix the appropriate dressing.

Complications

One of the most common problems is to neglect the main requirement of the operation. Perpendicular harvest and implantation of the grafts are crucial for successful transplantation. Oblique harvest and insertion may result in steps on the surface. Careful control by the arthroscope from different angles should help avoid such problems.

Another frequent mistake is to implant a graft deeper than the desired level. First of all, appropriate use of the delivery tamp can help to avoid deep insertion of the grafts. If the graft has been inserted too deep, the following steps are recommended: Insert the drill guide next to the previously implanted graft. Drill the appropriate recipient hole. Remove the guide and use the arthroscopic

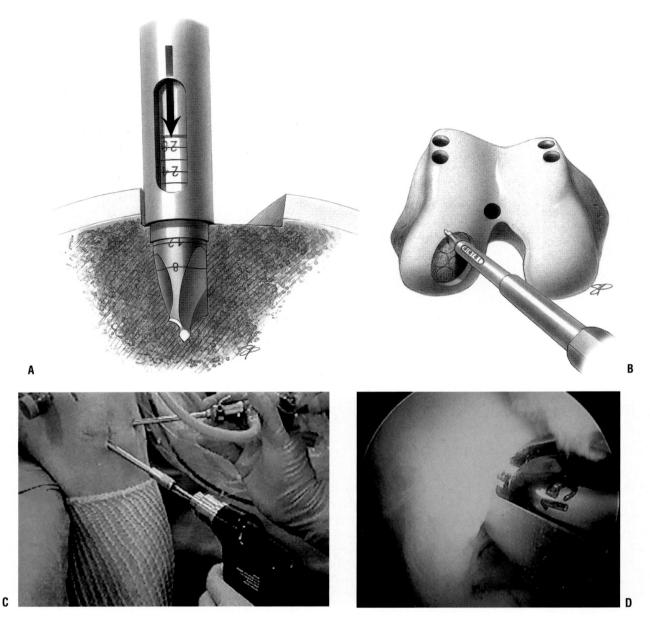

FIGURE 28-8
A–C: Drilling of the recipient tunnel. D: Arthroscopic picture of the same step.

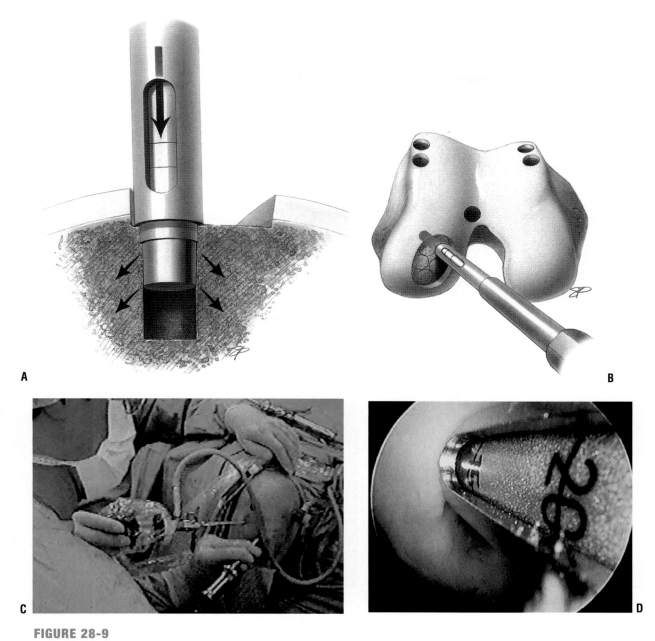

FIGURE 28-9

A–C: Dilating of the recipient tunnel. **D:** Arthroscopic picture of the same step.

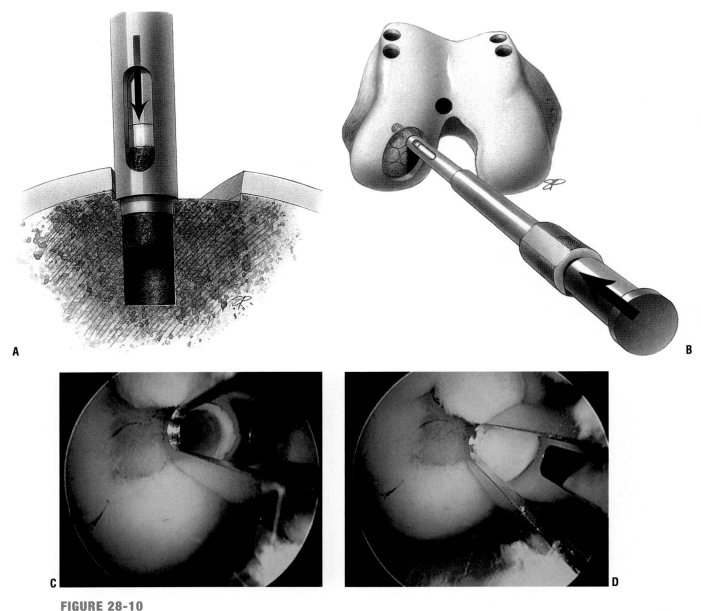

FIGURE 28-10

A,B: Insertion of the graft. **C,D:** Arthroscopic pictures of the same step.

probe to remove the previously implanted graft to the proper level (Fig. 28-13). The recipient hole adjacent to the implanted graft should allow such manipulation. As soon as the expected graft level has been achieved, continue the recommended sequence for the other insertions. Dilation of the adjacent tunnel will provide perfect press fit fixation of the previously implanted graft.

Open Mosaicplasty

If an arthroscopic approach is impractical, it may be necessary to create a medial or lateral anterior sagittal incision or an oblique incision to perform a miniarthrotomy mosaicplasty (Fig. 28-14). Patellotrochlear and tibial implantations may require an extended anteromedial approach. Further steps and technique of the implantation are identical to those for the open procedure.

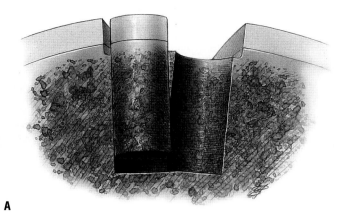

A

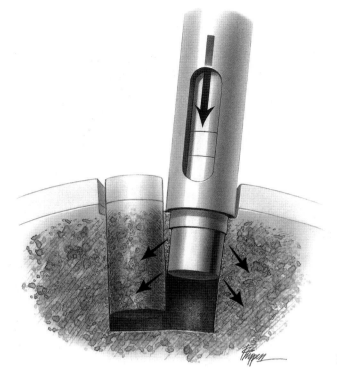

B

FIGURE 28-11
A,B: Step-by-step implantation supports a safe press fit fixation.

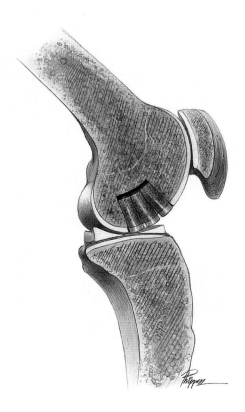

A

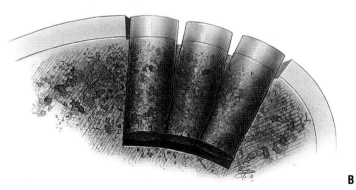

B

FIGURE 28-12
A,B: Functional test of the resurfaced area.

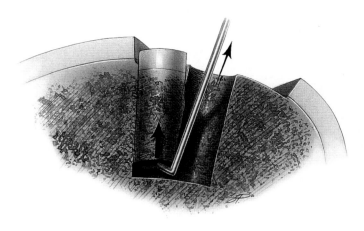

FIGURE 28-13

Elevation of a too deeply implanted graft.

POSTOPERATIVE MANAGEMENT

Postoperatively, the drain should be removed at 24 hours. Appropriate pain and cool therapy as well as nonsteroidal anti-inflammatory drugs can lessen patient discomfort. Postoperative thrombosis prophylaxis is recommended.

Rehabilitation

In the rehabilitation protocol following mosaicplasty at our institutions, *there is no immobilization.* The main point of the rehabilitation is to ensure the early motion of the treated joint to promote appropriate nutrition of transplanted cartilage. Cool therapy can be used during the first week to avoid postoperative bleeding and to decrease pain. In the case of a concomitant procedure requiring external fixation of the affected joint (e.g., meniscus reinsertion), limitation of range of motion for a short period by bracing can be allowed. Table 28-1 provides the details of our rehabilitation protocol.

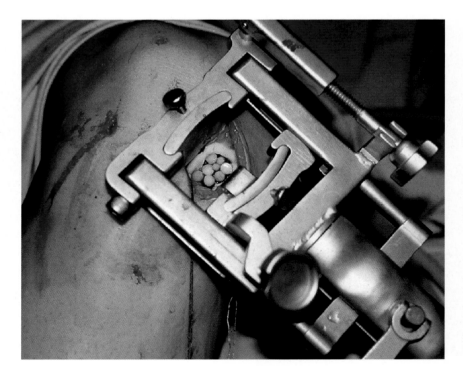

FIGURE 28-14

Intraoperative picture of a miniarthrotomy mosaicplasty.

TABLE 28-1.   Mosaicplasty Rehabilitation Protocol (Uzsoki Hospital and Sanitas Private Clinic, Budapest, Hungary)

Ambulation

Extent, type (chondral or osteochondral), and location of the defect may modify weight bearing.

Two-crutch ambulation, non–weight bearing	Immediately
Two-crutch ambulation, partial loading (30 to 40 kg/sec)	2 to 4 weeks
Discontinue crutches, full weight bearing	4 to 5 weeks

Functional Exercises

Form walking, gait evaluation	4 to 5 weeks
Step-up	4 to 5 weeks
Step-down	5 to 6 weeks

Range of Motion

Early range of motion is encouraged.

CPM for 2 to 4 cm^2 lesions (in painless range)	Immediately (first week)
Full extension, flexion as tolerated	Immediately
Stationary bicycle	3 weeks

Strength Return

Quadriceps

Open-chain exercises, leg raises	Immediately
Concentric contraction to full extension	1 week (or earlier if tolerated)
Concentric contraction against resistance	2 weeks
Isometric exercises at different angles	Immediately
Excentric exercises against resistance	3 to 4 weeks

Hamstrings

Isometric exercises in different angles	Immediately
Concentric and excentric strengthening	1 to 2 weeks
Against resistance	3 to 4 weeks

Closed-Chain Exercises

Partial loading promotes the transformation of connecting tissue (between transplanted plugs) into fibrocartilage, so these exercises are important, especially in the half–weight-bearing period. However, with some closed-chain exercises (e.g., cycling) it is possible to ensure cyclic loading that makes the fluid and nutrition transport much more efficient between synovial fluid and hyaline cartilage.

Pushing a soft rubber ball with foot	Immediately
Closed-chain exercises with half weight bearing	2 to 3 weeks
With full weight bearing	5 to 6 weeks
Stationary bicycle with resistance	2 to 4 weeks (if 90 degrees knee flexion achieved)
Stair Master	6 to 8 weeks

Proprioception Return

Balance exercises standing on both feet	5 to 6 weeks
Standing on one foot (hard ground)	6 to 8 weeks
Standing on one foot (trampoline or aerostep)	8 to 10 weeks

Return to Activity

Jogging	10 weeks
Straight-line running	3 months
Directional changes	4 to 5 months
Shear forces	5 months (approx. 4 to 5 months are needed to form a composite hyaline-like surface on a transplanted area that tolerates shear forces)
Sport-specific adaptations	5 months
Sport activity	5 to 6 months (depending on depth and extent of the defect; if strength, power, endurance, balance, and flexibility are not sufficient, sport activity is allowed later)

Special Viewpoints

(continued)

TABLE 28-1. *continued* Mosaicplasty Rehabilitation Protocol (Uzsoki Hospital and Sanitas Private Clinic, Budapest, Hungary)	
Weight Bearing at Different Defects of the Knee	
Femur or tibia condyle, chondral defect, d <15 mm	
Non–weight bearing	1 week
Partial weight bearing	1 to 3 weeks
Femur or tibia condyle, chondral defect, d ≥15 mm	
Non–weight bearing	2 weeks
Partial weight bearing	2 to 4 weeks
Femur or tibia condyle, osteochondral defect	
Non–weight bearing	3 weeks
Partial weight bearing	3 to 5 weeks
Patellar defect, d <15 mm	
Partial weight bearing	2 weeks
Patellar defect, d ≥15 mm	
Partial weight bearing	3 weeks
Quadriceps Strengthening and Patellar Mobilization—Differences at Patellar Defects	
Vastus medialis strengthening	
Isometric exercises in extension	Immediately
Patellar mobilization	Immediately
Isometric exercises in different angles	1 week
Open-chain exercises	2 weeks
Against resistance	3 to 4 weeks
Eccentric exercises against resistance	4 to 5 weeks
Closed-chain exercises	2 to 3 weeks
The treatment of underlying causes can also modify the rehabilitation program. The most frequent combinations at knee applications follow.	
Anterior Cruciate Ligament (ACL)—Reconstruction Combined with Mosaicplasty	
2 to 4 weeks non–weight bearing (up to the mosaicplasty)	
2 more weeks of partial weight bearing	
0 to 90 degrees ROM for 3 weeks	
Mainly closed-chain exercises for quadriceps strengthening	
Hamstring strengthening in open and closed chain	
Proprioceptive training	
Meniscus Reinsertion Combined with Mosaicplasty	
4 weeks of non–weight bearing	
2 more weeks of partial weight bearing	
5 to 45 degrees ROM for 4 weeks	
Retinaculum Patellae Reconstruction Combined with Mosaicplasty	
2 to 4 weeks of non–weight bearing (up to the mosaicplasty)	
2 more weeks of partial weight bearing	
0 to 45 degrees ROM for 4 weeks	
High Tibial Osteotomy (HTO) Combined with Mosaicplasty	
Weight bearing (for 4 weeks only with crutches and only in extension) is up to the mosaicplasty, pain, and degree of the correction of the varus (undercorrection—non–weight bearing, overcorrection—early weight bearing).	

COMPLICATIONS

Septic or thromboembolic complications may result in a negative influence on the clinical outcome. Correct aseptic conditions, one-shot antibiotics, and thrombosis prophylaxis can decrease the chance of these complications.

According to 14 years of follow-up, long-term donor site morbidity does not occur frequently. Patellofemoral complaints, such as pain or swelling after strenuous physical activity, follow the mosaicplasty procedure in fewer than 3% of cases. However, excessive postoperative bleeding occurred in 8%. Precise postoperative drainage, cool therapy, and elastic bandages can lessen the chance of this complication.

RESULTS

Between February 1992 and February 2002, 831 mosaicplasties were accomplished at our institutions. These implantations involved the femoral condyles in 597 procedures, the patellofemoral joint in 118, the talar dome in 76, the tibial condyles in 25, the capitulum humeri in 6, the femoral head in 9, and later, the humeral head in 3 cases as well. Two thirds of the patients underwent surgery because of a localized grade III or grade IV cartilage lesion, according to the Outerbridge classification system, whereas one-third underwent surgery because of osteochondral defects. In 85% of the patients, concomitant surgical interventions also were done, including ACL reconstructions, realignment osteotomies, and meniscal surgery. In most of the patellar or trochlear graftings, patellofemoral realignment or lateral release was also done. The results of the resurfacing procedures were evaluated at regular intervals with use of standardized clinical scores and radiography, and selected patients were also assessed with MRI, second-look arthroscopy, histological analysis of biopsy materials, and cartilage stiffness measurement. Femoral, tibial, and patellar implants were evaluated according to the modified Hospital for Special Surgery scoring system, the modified Cincinnati knee-rating scale, the Lysholm scale, and the International Cartilage Repair Society scoring system, and donor-site disturbances were evaluated according to the Bandi score system. According to our investigations, good-to-excellent results were achieved in more than 92% of the patients treated with femoral condylar implantations, 87% of those treated with tibial resurfacing, 79% of those treated with patellar and/or trochlear mosaicplasties, and 94% of those treated with talar procedures. Long-term donor-site discrepancies, assessed with use of the Bandi score, showed that patients had 3% morbidity after mosaicplasty.

Nineteen patients had a second-look arthroscopic examination performed between 2 months and 6 years postoperatively because of persistent or recurrent pain, swelling, or postoperative intra-articular bleeding; 23 had arthroscopy performed between 1 and 9 years postoperatively because of a second trauma; and 41 had arthroscopy performed between 2 and 4 months postoperatively to evaluate the quality of the resurfaced area and to determine the earliest date to return to a professional sports activity. Sixty-nine of the 83 patients who were followed arthroscopically showed congruent gliding surfaces, histologic evidence of the survival of the transplanted hyaline cartilage, and fibrocartilage filling of the donor sites. In a limited series involving 23 patients, cartilage stiffness measurements were performed with use of a computerized arthroscopic indentometric device, the Artscan 1000 (Artscan Oy, Helsinki, Finland), at a pressure of 10 N. Nineteen of them had similar values to the healthy hyaline cartilage.

RECOMMENDED READING

Bodó G, Hangody L, Módis L, et al. Autologous osteochondral grafting (mosaic arthroplasty) for the treatment of subchondral cystic lesions in the equine stifle and fetlock.*Vet Surg.* 2004;33:588–596.

Feczkó P, Hangody L, Varga J, et al. Experimental results of donor site filling for autologous osteochondral mosaicplasty. *Arthroscopy.* 2003;19(7):755–761.

Hangody L. Mosaicplasty. In: Insall J, Scott N, eds. *Surgery of the knee.* New York: Churchill Livingstone; 2000:357–361.

Hangody L. The mosaicplasty technique for osteochondral lesions of the talus. *Foot Ankle Clin North Am.* 2003;8:259–273.

Hangody L, Feczkó P, Kemény D, et al. Autologous osteochondral mosaicplasty for the treatment of full thickness cartilage defects of the knee and ankle. *Clin Orthop.* 2001;391(suppl):328–337.

Hangody L, Kish G. Surgical treatment of osteochondritis dissecans of the talus. In: Duparc, J, ed. *European textbook on surgical techniques in orthopaedics and traumatology. Editions Scientifiques et Medicales.* New York: Elsevier; 2000.

Hangody L, Kish G, Kárpáti Z, et al. Arthroscopic autogenous osteochondral mosaicplasty for the treatment of femoral condylar articular defects. *Knee Surg Sports Traumatol Arthros.* 1997;5: 262–267.

Hangody L, Kish G, Kárpáti Z, et al. Osteochondral plugs: autogenous osteochondral mosaicplasty for the treatment of focal chondral and osteochondral articular defects. *Oper Tech Orthop.* 1997;7:312–322.

Hangody L, Kish G, Kárpáti Z, et al. Treatment of osteochondritis dissecans of talus: the use of the mosaicplasty technique. *Foot Ankle Int.* 1997;18:628–634.

Hangody L, Ráthonyi G, Duska Zs, et al. Autologous osteochondral mosaicplasty—surgical technique. *J Bone Joint Surg.* 2004;86-A(suppl I):65–72.

Kish G, Módis L, Hangody L. Osteochondral mosaicplasty for the treatment of focal chondral and osteochondral lesions of the knee and talus in the athlete. *Clin Sports Med.* 1999;18:45–61.

Kordás G, Szabó J, Hangody L. Primary stability of osteochondral grafts used in mosaicplasty. *Arthroscopy.* 2006;22(4):414–422.

29 Chondrocyte Transplantation

Lars Peterson

INDICATIONS/CONTRAINDICATIONS

Lesions of the articular cartilage in the knee joint present great diversity in size, location, depth, and containment. These factors have to be evaluated to decide the right treatment. Autologous chondrocyte transplantation (ACT) is a treatment option for symptomatic full-thickness chondral or osteochondral lesions (OCD). The patients (15 to 55 years old) often present with pain and catching or locking on activity and pain and swelling after activity.

Chondral lesions possible for treatment with ACT should be between 1 to 2 and 16 cm^2 with grade III or IV Outerbridge classification (grade 3 or 4 ICRS classification). The opposing articular surface has to be undamaged or have only minor cartilage pathology (grade I or II Outerbridge classification, grade 1 or 2 ICRS classification).

Autologous chondrocyte transplantation is indicated for lesions on the femoral condyles, the femoral trochlea, and patella. Patients with tibial plateau defects treated with ACT are showing improved results over time; therefore, this locale can be considered for ACT. Long-term follow-up on kissing lesions (i.e., bipolar lesions in the femurotibial and patellotrochlear joints) show at 4 to 10 years postoperatively satisfactory results in 75% of the cases. Autologous chondrocyte transplantation can be tried in these cases in younger patients as a salvage procedure. Multiple lesions, two or more lesions in one joint excluding kissing lesions, have shown satisfactory results in 84% at 5 to 11 years postoperatively. Almost all of these patients needed concomitant procedures to create optimal environment for the transplanted chondrocytes. Stabilizing or unloading procedures will improve the short- and long-term survival of the repair tissue in the injured surfaces. Autologous chondrocyte transplantation is not a treatment for osteoarthritis (general joint disease), gout, and rheumatoid arthritis or other systemic joint diseases.

Autologous chondrocyte transplantation is indicated for osteochondritis dissecans (OCD) with unstable fragments, osteochondral flaps and empty defects, and a size between 1 to 2 and 16 cm^2. If the bony defect is between 6 and 8 mm deep, ACT alone can be used. If the bony defect is deeper, concomitant autologous bone grafting (sandwich technique) has to be used.

PREOPERATIVE PLANNING

The preoperative planning includes a careful history to find out the cause of the cartilage lesion: traumatic or microtraumatic. Clinical assessment of symptoms and signs, radiologic imaging including standing radiographs, and arthroscopic assessment are essential.

Examination and Evaluation

The preoperative assessment is important when deciding if ACT is an option for the patient and should include all pathology of the knee; but an arthroscopic evaluation must precede the final decision. Try to find out the cause of the cartilage defect, since this affects the treatment. Crepitations during extension and flexion against resistance may indicate cartilage pathology. Check for any ligament instability or malalignment that might need surgical correction. It is important to have a stable joint since instability greatly decreases the chances of a successful surgery.

Regarding lesions to the patella, it is very important to examine for possible patellar instability, malalignment, or maltracking, since this often is the cause of the cartilage damage.

Radiography, Magnetic Resonance Imaging, Arthrography

Radiologic imaging is useful to rule out patients with osteoarthritis. Standing radiographs in 45 degrees of knee flexion and extension and hip-knee-ankle radiographs show joint space reduction and varus or valgus malalignment that may need surgical correction. Computerized tomography with and without quadriceps contraction may reveal patellofemoral dysplasia or instability. Magnetic resonance imaging (MRI) with or without contrast medium (gadolinium) may be helpful to assess the articular cartilage and pathology of the underlying bone.

Arthroscopic Evaluation

If ACT so far is the choice of treatment, the next step is an arthroscopic examination performed by the surgeon. The examination proceeds as follows:

- Administer general or spinal anesthesia.
- Test the joint stability.
- Examine all the articular surfaces, the menisci, the synovial lining, and the cruciate ligaments using an arthroscopic probe.
- Remove loose bodies or debris in the joint, if present.
- Evaluate the location, size, containment, and depth of the cartilage lesion (Fig. 29-1).
- Make sure the lesion is accessible through an optimal arthrotomy.
- Harvest cartilage if the lesion is suitable for chondrocyte transplantation.
- Slice cartilage specimens from the unloaded proximal, medial edge of the trochlea using a ring curette or a gouge and (Fig. 29-2).
- When necessary use other locations for the cartilage biopsy, such as the proximal, lateral edge of the trochlea or the lateral intercondylar notch.
- Cut down through the subchondral bone to cause a bleeding, so the donor site area may heal with fibrocartilage.
- Let one end of the specimen still be attached, then use a grasper to take out the specimen.
- Harvest cartilage from a surface of approximately 5 by 10 mm is, resulting in the required 200 to 300 mg of cartilage.
- Place the specimens in a sterile tube containing a medium of DMEM with phenolred and gentamycin.
- Treat meniscal injuries after the harvesting of cartilage.

The harvested cartilage is enzymatically digested and the chondrocytes are isolated and cultured for 2 weeks, which results in an increase in cell number by 20 to 30 times (Fig. 29-3). The implantation of the chondrocytes can thus at the earliest take place 2 weeks after the harvesting. If the implantation is scheduled at a later date, the chondrocytes can be frozen after 1 week of culturing, and then thawed and cultured for another week before the implantation.

SURGERY

Chondral Lesions

Preparation and Approach
- Place the patient supine on the operating table.
- Use general or spinal anesthesia and a tourniquet-controlled bloodless field.
- Perform medial or lateral parapatellar miniarthrotomy to open the joint.
- Adjust the arthrotomy for good access to the defect.
- To expose multiple femoral or patellar lesions, the patella may have to be dislocated.
- Consider the approach for concomitant procedures, for example, high tibial osteotomy.

Debridement of Defect
- Excise all damaged and undermined cartilage.
- Get vertical edges to healthy cartilage.
- Cut down to the subchondral bone around the lesion using a knife with a No. 15 blade.
- Keep the lesion contained by cartilage, if possible.

ICRS Grade 0 - Normal

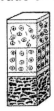

ICRS Grade 1 – Nearly Normal

Superficial lesions. Soft indentation (A) and/or superficial fissures and cracks (B)

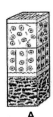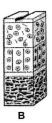

A   B

ICRS Grade 2 – Abnormal

Lesions extending down to <50% of cartilage depth

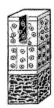

ICRS Grade 3 – Severely Abnormal

Cartilage defects extending down >50% of cartilage depth (A) as well as down to calcified layer (B) and down to but not through the subchondral bone (C). Blisters are included in this Grade (D)

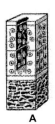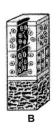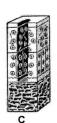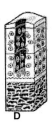

A   B   C   D

ICRS Grade 4 – Severely Abnormal

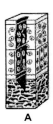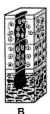

A   B

A

FIGURE 29-1

A–C: ICRS classification of the location and depth of a cartilage lesion. (With permission from International Cartilage Repair Society, ICRS Cartilage Injury Evaluation Page, 2000.)

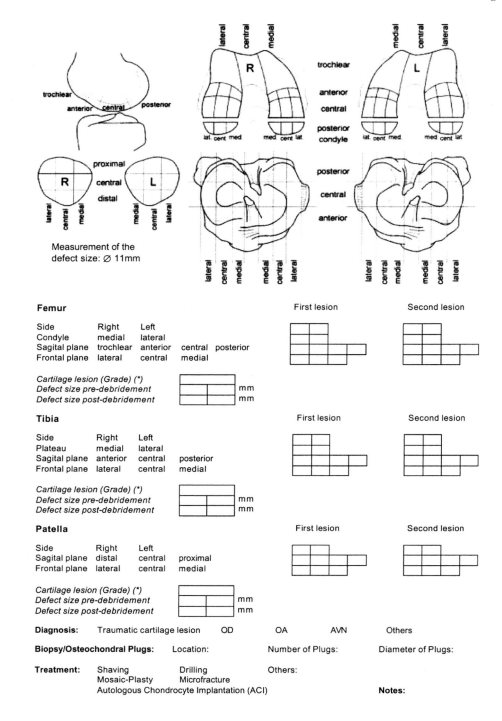

FIGURE 29-1
(Continued)

ICRS OCD I

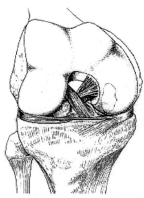

Stable, continuity: Softened area covered by intact cartilage.

ICRS OCD II

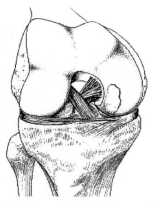

Partial discontinuity, stable on probing

ICRS OCD III

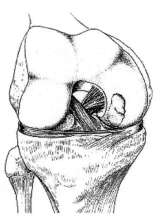

Complete discontinuity, "dead in situ", not dislocated.

ICRS OCD IV

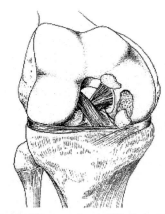

Dislocated fragment, loose within the bed or empty defect.> 10mm in depth is B-subgroup

C

FIGURE 29-1

(Continued)

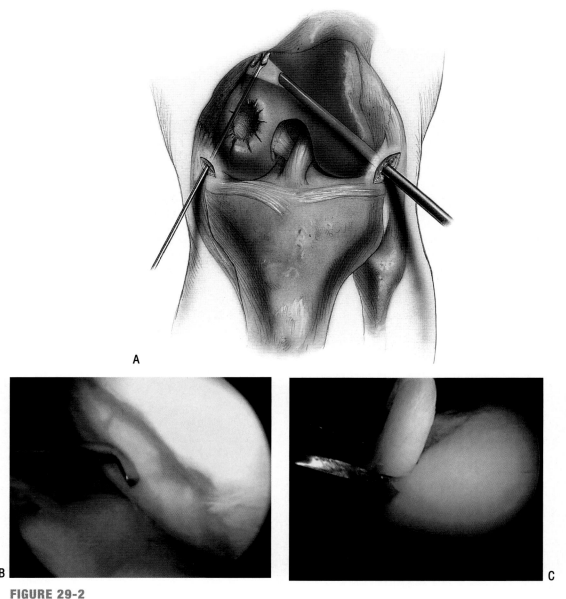

FIGURE 29-2

Schematic drawing of the cartilage harvest **(A)**. Arthroscopic pictures of a full-thickness cartilage lesion **(B)** and cartilage harvesting with a ring curette **(C)**.

- It is better to leave a 3 to 4 mm rim of cartilage of questionable quality than have a lesion bordering bone or synovium.
- Remove the damaged cartilage using a ring curette or a periosteal elevator.
- Be careful not to violate the subchondral bone and cause bleeding and possible fibrous ingrowth in the defect.
- The debrided defect should be as circular or oval as possible (Fig. 29-4).
- Measure the defect and use sterile aluminum foil or paper to make a template of the defect (Fig. 29-5).
- Check for any bleeding of the subchondral bone; at this time the tourniquet can be let down for easier detection.
- If there is a bleeding, place an epinephrine-wet sponge in the defect to stop it.
- Keep the explored cartilage moist throughout the procedure.

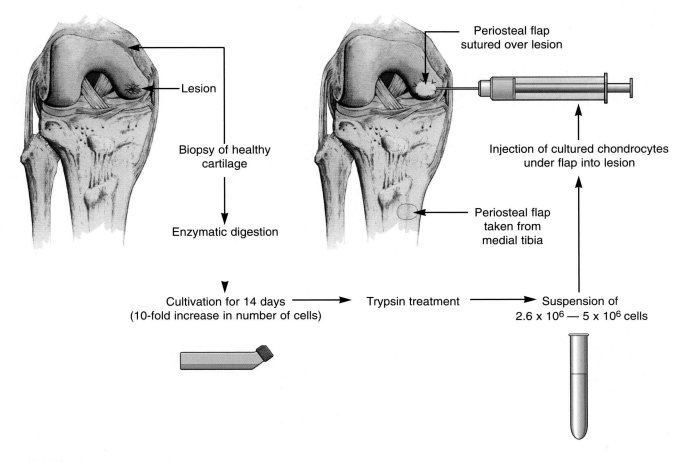

Lesion

Biopsy of healthy
cartilage

Enzymatic digestion

Periosteal flap
sutured over lesion

Injection of cultured chondrocytes
under flap into lesion

Periosteal flap
taken from
medial tibia

Cultivation for 14 days ——→ Trypsin treatment ——→ Suspension of
(10-fold increase in number of cells) $2.6 \times 10^6 — 5 \times 10^6$ cells

FIGURE 29-3

From the harvested cartilage slices the chondrocytes are isolated and cultured for 2 weeks, before the implantation can take place.

Periosteal Flap Harvest   It is then time for the harvesting of a periosteal flap to cover the cartilage defect. The periosteum is easily accessed at the proximal medial tibia, distal to pes anserinus and the medial collateral ligament insertion. The medial or lateral femoral condyles proximal to the articular cartilage can also be used as harvest sites but the periosteum is thicker, less elastic, and covered by numerous vessels, which may cause postoperative bleeding and arthrofibrosis if not taken care of. More adequate periosteum is found on the distal shaft of the femur proximal to the condyles. The steps for periosteal flap harvest are as follows:

- Incise to get good exposure.
- Dissect gently and remove the overlying fibrous tissue, fat, and crossing vessels covering the periosteal flap.
- Use the template to measure how a large flap you need (Fig. 29-6).
- Oversize the periosteal flap with 1 to 2 mm at the periphery of the template.
- Incise the periosteal flap using a knife with a No. 15 blade.
- Carefully dissect it with a periosteal elevator with small movements and lift with a nontoothed forceps.
- Go close down to the bone so the cambium layer of the periosteum is preserved and take care not to penetrate the flap. A healthy cambium layer interacts with the chondrocytes and is thus important.

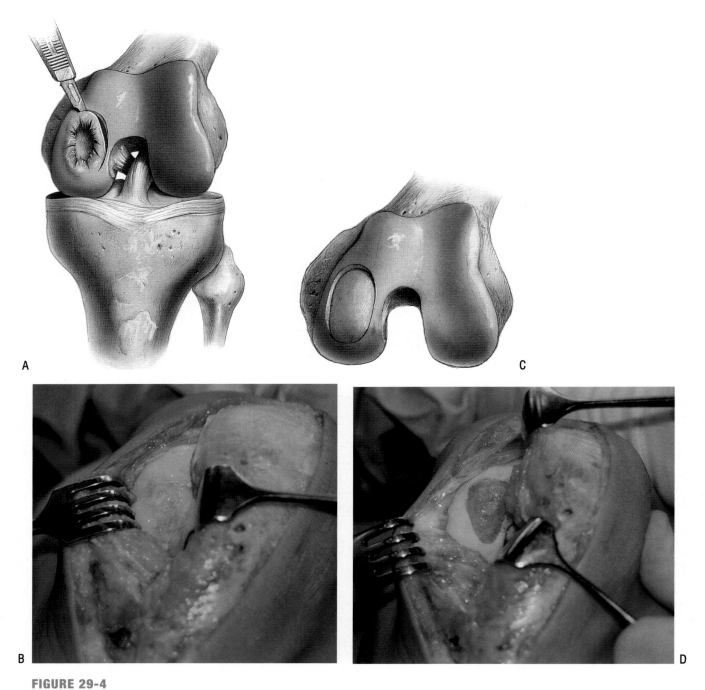

FIGURE 29-4

Drawings and photographs showing a femoral condyle defect before **(A,B)** and after **(C,D)** radical excision and debridement of all damaged and undermined cartilage.

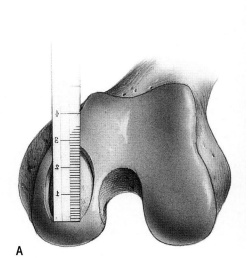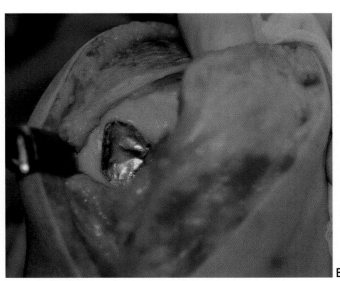

FIGURE 29-5

The debrided defect is measured **(A)** and a template of aluminum foil is made **(B)**.

- Mark the outside of the periosteal flap with a sterile pen for orientation at fixation.
- Be sure to keep the flap moist at all times.

Periosteal Flap Suturing
- Return to the debrided defect and inspect once again for bleeding.
- Cover the defect with the periosteal flap with the cambium layer facing the defect bed.
- Anchor the periosteal flap with one suture in each corner using a cutting needle with 6.0 resorbable sutures, soaked in glycerin or mineral oil (Fig. 29-7A,B).
- Place the knots over the periosteal flap.
- Tension the flap like a skin over a drum with interrupted sutures in a Z pattern.
- The distance between the sutures should be 3 to 5 mm (Fig. 29-7C,D).
- Leave an opening in the most superior portion for the injection of the chondrocytes.
- Use fibrin glue to seal the distances between the sutures.

A good periosteal fit and fixation is crucial for the surgical outcome. If the lesion is not contained by cartilage the periosteal flap has to be sutured to the synovium. If there is no synovial lining or osteophytes interfere, suture to small holes drilled through the bone or use resorbable minitacks.

Testing Watertightness   With a saline-filled tuberculin syringe and a plastic 18-gauge 2-inch angiocath, test the watertightness of the periosteum-covered defect.

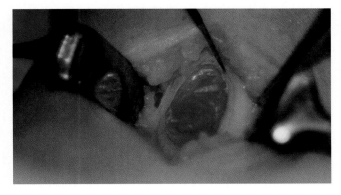

FIGURE 29-6

The template is used to excise a periosteal flap of the right size and form from the proximal medial tibia.

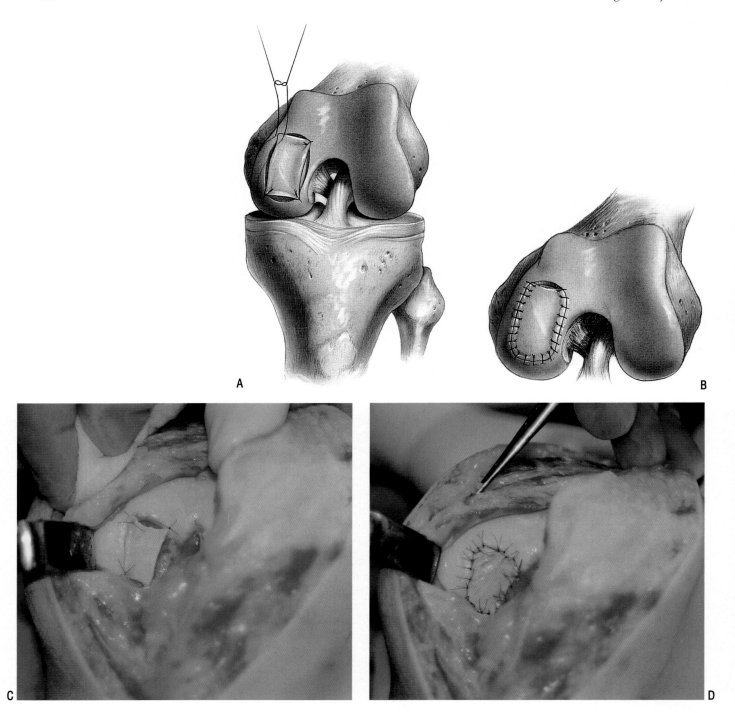

FIGURE 29-7
The flap is first anchored with one suture in one corner **(A,B)**. The flap is then sutured to the cartilage rim with interrupted sutures **(C,D)**.

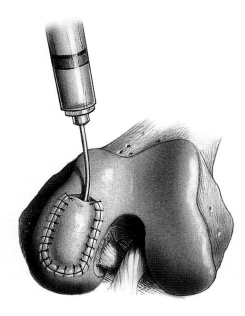

FIGURE 29-8

Test the watertight integrity by injecting saline under the periosteal flap.

- Gently insert the angiocath through the superior opening and slowly inject the saline (Fig. 29-8). Any leakage may easily be detected at the periosteum-cartilage border around the defect.
- If needed, add another suture and fibrin glue so watertight integrity is obtained.
- Check for leakage again.
- If satisfied, aspirate the saline but make sure that the periosteal flap does not stick to the defect bed.

Implantation of Cells   The defect is now ready for the chondrocyte implantation.
- Aspirate the chondrocytes in a tuberculum syringe using an 18-gauge or larger needle.
- Replace the needle with a plastic 18-gauge 2-inch angiocath.
- Start filling the inferior portion of the defect by placing the angiocath deep into the defect and gently inject the chondrocytes.
- Withdraw the angiocath as you inject the chondrocytes; the cells should be evenly distributed throughout the defect (Fig. 29-9).
- Close the superior opening with sutures and fibrin glue.

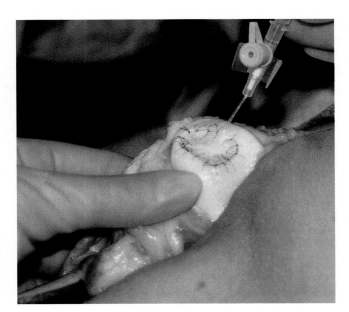

FIGURE 29-9

Patella defect showing the syringe placed deep into the defect and under withdrawal the chondrocytes are injected.

- If the defect is very large you may have to use an upper and a lower opening for proper filling of the defect. Inject through the lower opening, then close it before you start filling through the upper opening.

When the opening is sealed, the defect is contained and watertight, but the periosteal flap still allows diffusion of fluid and nutrition to the transplanted chondrocytes. Intra-articular drains should not be used as they could harm the periosteum and suck out the transplanted chondrocytes. If a drain must be used make sure it is without suction. Close the wound in layers and bandage the leg from the foot and up over the knee.

Postoperative Management   The patient usually stays in the hospital for 1 to 3 days depending on the severity of the case. Prophylactic antibiotics are used for 48 hours postoperatively. Continuous passive motion (CPM) is started 6 to 8 hours after the surgery. The chondrocytes can then be expected to have attached to the defect bed and the rim of healthy cartilage. Continuous passive motion is continued intermittently until the patient is released from the hospital. The day after surgery range of motion (ROM) and isometric quadriceps training are started. The patient is mobilized with crutches. Depending on the size and location of the defect, weight bearing to 20 kg or to the limit of pain is allowed for the first 6 weeks. Over the next 6 weeks, a gradual increase in weight bearing is allowed until full weight bearing is reached. After release from the hospital, the patient returns after 3 and 6 weeks and after 3 months for check-ups. Follow-ups are then as needed.

Concomitant Surgery

It is important to create an optimal environment for the repair tissue. This means correcting any background factors such as instability or malalignment, and if necessary, unloading the repair tissue. These procedures may be done separately, for example an anterior cruciate ligament (ACL) reconstruction or a tibial osteotomy, or at the same time as the biopsy is taken. Often it is done at the same time as the implantation. Pathologic mechanics in the joint reduce the chances of a successful repair. Patellar lesions are often related to an unstable patella, and the patella must thus be stabilized for a good healing. Stabilizing procedures may include anteromedialization of the tibial tuberosity, lateral release, proximal medial soft tissue shortening, and trochlear groove plasty (if it is dysplastic). In trochlear and patellar lesions, unloading with ventralization of the tibial tuberosity should be considered. A torn ACL is reconstructed after the cartilage lesion is debrided and covered with periosteum, but before the chondrocytes are injected. To unload the transplanted area when a varus or valgus malalignment is present, a high tibial or femoral osteotomy is performed. When these corrective surgeries are performed, a brace limiting the range of motion to 0 to 60 degrees is used postoperatively for 3 weeks and for the following 3 weeks with a ROM of 0 to 90 degrees.

Osteochondral Lesions (Osteochondritis Dissecans)

When treating osteochondritis dissecans with ACT, attention must be paid to the depth of the defect. If the bony defect is shallower than 6 to 8 mm, the lesion is treated the same way as a chondral lesion. Gently debride the sclerotic bottom of the defect, but be careful not to cause bleeding; and the cartilage is debrided to vertical edges to healthy cartilage. Cover the defect with a periosteal flap, seal, and check for leakage. Then implant the chondrocytes and close the last opening.

If the bony defect is deeper than 6 to 8 mm only ACT is not enough, concomitant autologous bone grafting is needed (Fig. 29-10A,B).

- Abrade away the sclerotic bottom of the defect to spongious bone and undercut the subchondral bone.
- Drill holes in the spongious bone with a 2-mm burr.
- Debride the cartilage to healthy cartilage with vertical edges (Fig. 29-10C,D).
- If the bony defect is small, use cancellous bone from the tibial or femoral condyle; but if the defect is larger, bone has to be harvested from the iliac crest.
- Start packing the defect from the bottom and contour the cancellous bone over the defect just below the subchondral bone level (Fig. 29-10E,F).
- Harvest a periosteal flap and cover the contoured bone grafted defect at the level of the subchondral bone with the cambium layer facing the joint.
- Anchor it with horizontal or mattress sutures into the cartilage or subchondral bone and use fibrin glue under the flap for fixation to the grafted bone.

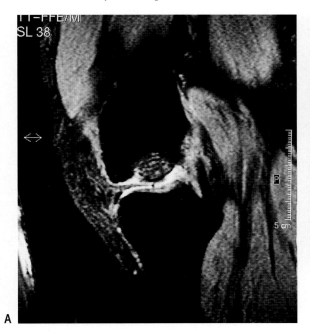

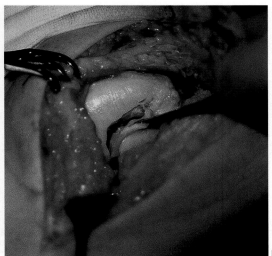

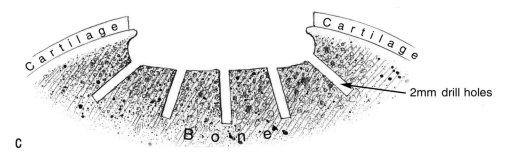

2mm drill holes

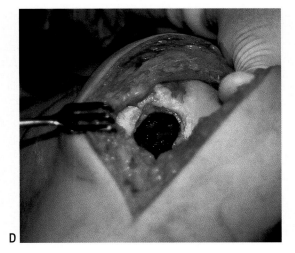

FIGURE 29-10

MRI **(A)** and photo **(B)** of an osteochondritis dissecans with a deep bony defect on the medial femoral condyle. The defect is abraded and multiple holes are drilled. The subchondral bone is undercut **(C,D)**.

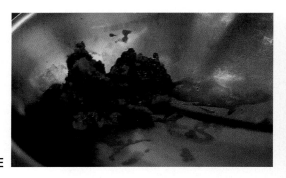

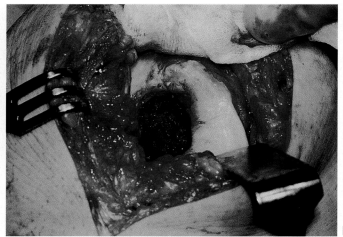

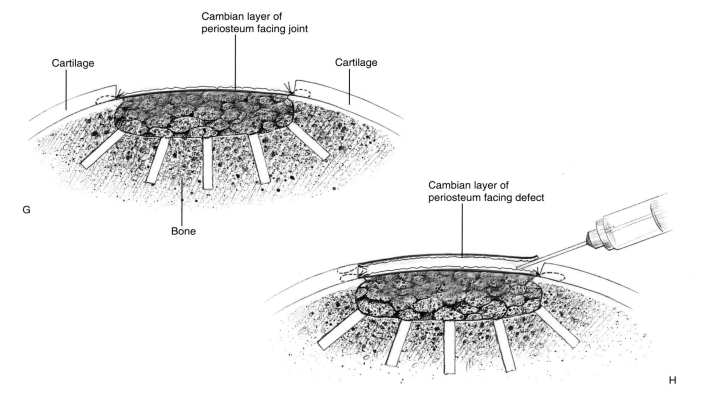

Cambian layer of
periosteum facing joint

Cartilage

Cartilage

Bone

Cambian layer of
periosteum facing defect

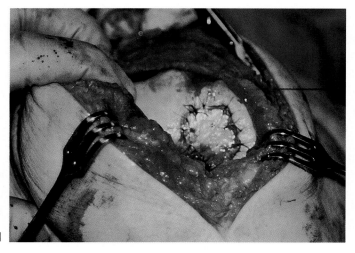

FIGURE 29-10

(Continued) Cancellous bone (**E**) is used to fill the bony
defect and should contour the subchondral bone (**F**). A
periosteal flap with the cambium layer facing the joint is
glued on top of the bone graft and sutured to the
surrounding cartilage (**G**). Another periosteal flap is
sutured to the cartilage rim with the cambium layer
facing the defect and the chondrocytes are injected
underneath (**H,I**).

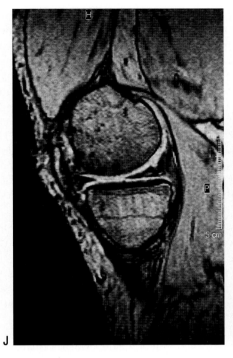

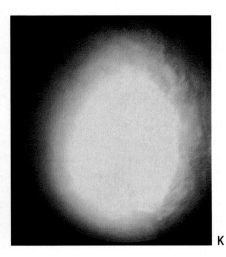

FIGURE 29-10

(Continued) MRI **(J)** 18 months after concomitant bone and chondrocyte transplantation, and arthroscopic picture of the transplanted area 2 years after the transplantation **(K)**.

- After depositing the glue richly between the bone graft and periosteal flap, compress the area with a dry sponge for 2 to 3 minutes to seal off the bone marrow cavity. This will avoid bleeding into the cartilage defect (Fig. 29-10G).
- Suture another periosteal flap to the cartilage edges, with the cambium layer facing the defect (Fig. 29-10H).
- Use fibrin glue to seal off the intervals between the sutures.
- Test the watertightness with a gentle saline injection.
- If there is no leakage, aspirate the saline and inject the chondrocytes (Fig. 29-10I).
- Close the opening and seal with fibrin glue.

Pearls and Pitfalls

Pearls   For a good result, only defects that fit the indications should be transplanted. Kissing lesions should not be transplanted other than as a salvage procedure. It is important that the surgeon performs the initial arthroscopy himself or herself, to be able to adequately decide if the patient is a candidate for ACT or not. At the time of implantation, excise the cartilage defect radically. All undermined, fissured, and damaged cartilage should gently be debrided to get a good fit of the periosteal flap. Accurate sizing, harvesting, and suturing of the flap are crucial for a good and durable outcome. There is definitely a learning curve for this procedure. Begin with at least ten simple cases to become comfortable with the technique before treating multiple lesions or cases combined with corrective surgery, such as ACL reconstruction.

Pitfalls

PERIOSTEUM   It is important that the flap used to cover the defect is of healthy periosteum. Atrophic periosteum may be found in inactive, obese, and older patients; it is also more common in females and smokers. A very thin and fragile periosteum must not be used; try to find periosteum of good quality at the femoral condyles. Incise the flap and carefully dissect thicker vessels, fat, and fibrous tissue off the flap. A clean and thin flap leaves more room for cell expansion and matrix filling of hyaline cartilage and causes less periosteal complications. Compress the fat away with a wet sponge but be careful not to harm the periosteum. After the flap is removed, use electrocoagulation to seal the vessels and thus avoid unwanted bleeding at the harvest site. Bleeding after harvest from the femoral condyles may cause problems with pain and arthrofibrosis with difficulties in regaining range of motion. If you find rifts or vessels penetrating the flap, close these with 6.0 resorbable sutures and fibrin glue after the flap has been sutured to the defect. In large defects you may have to use two flaps. Suture the two flaps separately. Then adapt the two flap borders with a few interrupted sutures and secure it with a running suture across.

DEBRIDEMENT When debriding the defect, be careful and meticulous so all pathologic cartilage is removed without causing bleeding. If bleeding occurs, place an epinephrine sponge in the defect during periosteal harvesting. If this is not enough, stop the bleeding by dripping a drop of fibrin glue and then press your fingertip over for 30 seconds, or carefully use punctual electrocoagulation (risk for bone necrosis).

If the cartilage defect has been previously treated with drilling, microfracture, abrasion, arthroplasty, or other procedures harming the subchondral bone, internal osteophytes can be present. If they interfere with the periosteal anchoring, they must be handled. Gently tap them down to the level of the surrounding subchondral bone (Fig. 29-11). You may gently debride a large and high osteophyte with a curette. Any resultant bleeding must be treated accordingly. Treatment penetrating the subchondral bone may also result in fibrous plugs; debride them down to the level of the surrounding subchondral bone.

What I Have Learned from Experience Radical excision is important. Incise in normal cartilage in the periphery, including pathologic cartilage. In the beginning I was not radical enough in the excision especially in patellar lesions. It is sometimes difficult to separate macroscopically normal from abnormal cartilage. Add a margin of 1 to 2 mm to include apoptotic chondrocytes in the border.

Suture with interrupted sutures, not running sutures, and grasp 4 to 6 mm into the cartilage to avoid cutting through with the sutures. If you loose one interrupted suture, it is not so bad but if you loose a

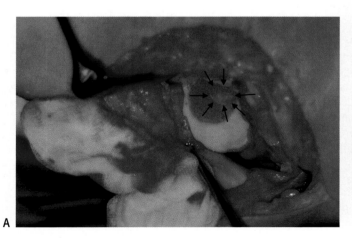
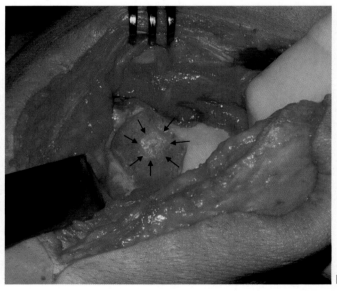

FIGURE 29-11

An intralesional osteophyte (**A**) that has been tapped down to the level of the subchondral bone (**B**).

running suture, it may cause delamination. Tie the suture with four knots, placed on the vertical edge of the cartilage over the periosteal flap. Three knots only may have a tendency to untie the suture.

Pay great attention to background factors such as ligament instability, varus-valgus deformities, patellar instability, and maltracking. The results are improved by correction of these factors. On large patellar or trochlear lesions, elevate the tibial tuberosity.

The meniscus has an important role and should be preserved and sutured when possible. Resection should be optimal but kept as conservative as possible. Total meniscectomy in the injured compartment may need meniscus replacement. Initial results when combining ACT with meniscus transplantation are promising.

An overly aggressive rehabilitation program with dynamic strength training in open kinetic chains, and too early weight bearing may cause pain, swelling, and periosteal complications. However, in contained isolated lesions, the increased weight bearing can start earlier—at about 3 weeks if no pain is experienced. If the patient experiences a clicking, snapping sensation, sometimes catching or locking, usually between 3 to 4 or 8 to 9 months, analyze the activity that elicits the symptoms and change the program accordingly. In half the cases the symptoms will disappear. If symptoms persist, arthroscopically examine and debride either hypertrophic periosteal tissue or intra-articular adhesions. Slow progress with ROM may occur postoperatively. Supervise the training and intensify the ROM exercises; frequent check-ups of progress are important. Usually the motion will increase, but slowly. Do not interfere during the first 4 months; any manipulation could jeopardize the repair or cause graft delamination. If it is necessary, use arthroscopy to visualize and remove adhesions and then gently mobilize the knee. Leave a drainage and start continuous passive motion (CPM) immediately.

POSTOPERATIVE MANAGEMENT

The rehabilitation following autologous chondrocyte transplantation is a slow process with gradual progression that extends over a long period of time. The new cartilage matures over time and must have the right amount of stimulation to form a durable tissue, able to withstand the forces in the knee. There is a large degree of individual variation in the rehabilitation process, and the program should be formed according to the patient's status and needs. Factors such as the size and location of the defect and possible concomitant corrective surgery are important to have in mind when forming the rehabilitation program. It is important that there is regular contact between the patient and physical therapist. An aggressive rehabilitation with too early or heavy dynamic strength training could jeopardize the transplanted area. Keys to a successful rehabilitation are mobility exercises, isometric strength training, functional exercises, and patience.

COMPLICATIONS

More then 1,300 transplantations have been made in Sweden since 1987, and there have been no major general complications such as intra-articular infections. Local complications from the periosteal flap or the graft of transplanted chondrocytes are not uncommon, but most of them can be corrected with only minor surgery. The periosteal flap covering the defect can become fibrillated and cause crepitations and swelling (Fig. 29-12A,B). As a response to the friction of joint movement, it may also become hypertrophic and cover the normal cartilage surrounding the defect in the direction of motion or become thicker (Fig. 29-12C). When symptomatic, this causes crepitations and clicking, and is sometimes associated with pain and swelling. All these periosteal complications should be evaluated arthroscopically. Examine the graft incorporation to the surrounding cartilage and the subchondral bone. If a fibrillated or hypertrophic periosteal flap causes the symptoms, shave or excise the flap down to the level of the surrounding cartilage.

A delaminated periosteal flap could cause early problems with catching or locking. The delamination could be either marginal (less than 10 mm), partial (less than 50% of the flap is delaminated), or total (more than 50% of the flap is detached) (Fig. 29-12D–F). A marginal or partial periosteal flap delamination is treated with a gentle debridement of the loose part. If the delamination is total and the periosteal flap appears as a loose body, it should be extracted; but if it is still attached to the underlying repair tissue, remove the whole flap. The remaining repair tissue is capable of filling the

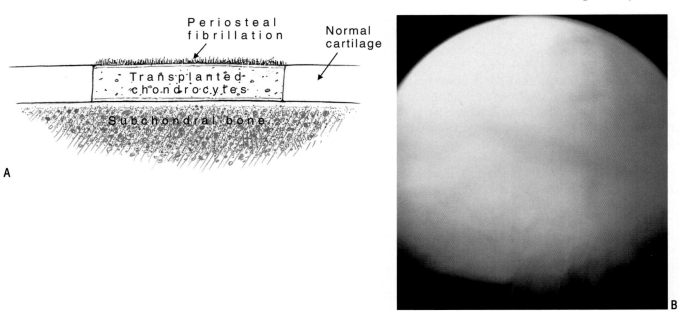

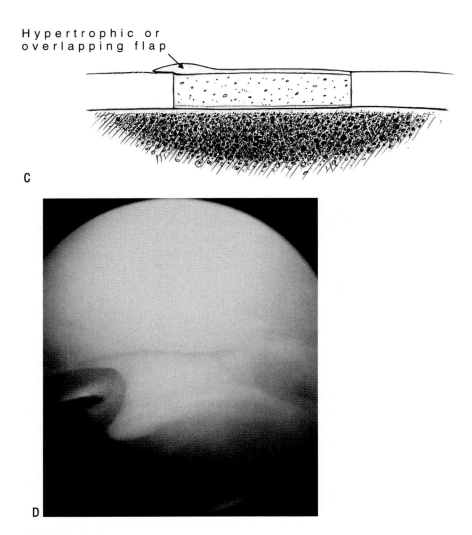

FIGURE 29-12

Periosteal complications: fibrillation **(A,B)**, periosteum overlaps surrounding cartilage **(C,D)**, marginal **(E)**, partial **(F)**, and total **(G)** periosteum delamination.

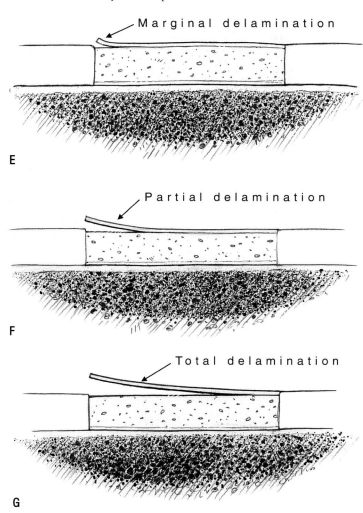

E

F

G

FIGURE 29-12
(Continued)

defect, but be careful with excessive loading of the repair tissue and encourage bicycling the first 6 to 8 weeks.

The graft of transplanted chondrocytes can also show incomplete incorporation to the surrounding cartilage and the underlying subchondral bone. A marginal delamination with less than 10 mm of the graft loosened (Fig. 29-13A) is excised and the subchondral bone of the failed area is microfractured. A partial delamination means that less than 50% of the graft is delaminated (Fig. 29-13B). This is treated with a gentle debridement, and cartilage for a retransplantation is harvested.

A total graft failure in which the whole graft is loose or only a rim is still attached is seldom seen (Fig. 29-13C). It could be caused by a distorsion of the knee or too aggressive rehabilitation and early return to sports. In this case, the patient experiences pain, swelling, and locking. Remove the graft and harvest chondrocytes for a new ACT.

RESULTS

You can expect hyaline-like repair tissue in 80% of cases. If you have a good/excellent result at 2-year follow-up, it will stay good/excellent at 5 to 11 years (mean 7.4). In femoral condyle lesions and OCD, you can expect 85% to 90% good/excellent results. In patellar lesions, there are about

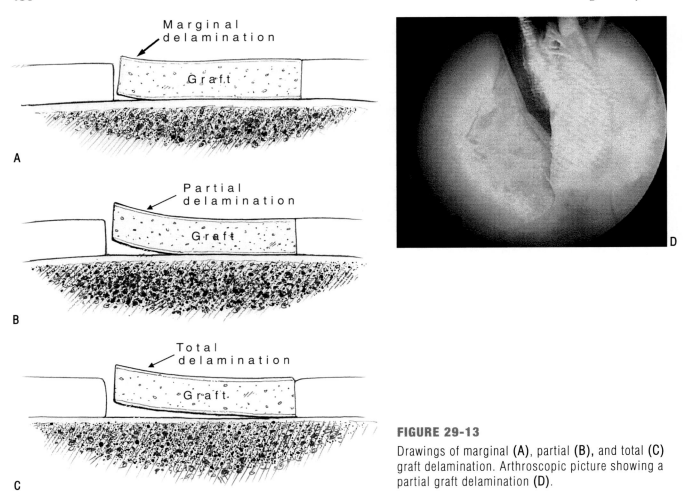

FIGURE 29-13

Drawings of marginal (**A**), partial (**B**,) and total (**C**) graft delamination. Arthroscopic picture showing a partial graft delamination (**D**).

70% good/excellent results. In salvage procedures in kissing lesions in the patellotrochlear or tibiofemoral joints, 3 out of 4 patients may improve (Fig. 29-14).

What to Tell Patients to Expect

Patients are told that this is a repair process starting with cultured chondrocytes in suspension injected into the defect. The cells undergo some mitosis to confluence, adhere to the subchondral bone and cartilage edges, and start to produce matrix. It is important that the collagen is anchored in the subchondral bone. At 3 months, the defect is filled with soft and compressive repair tissue. From 3 to 9 to 12 months, there is an ongoing maturation with improved organization of the cells and filling with matrix, and increased weight bearing stimulates this process. The maturation process continues slower after 12 months but is active at 2 to 3 years. The ultimate goal is that the turnover of repair cartilage is equal to the normal surrounding cartilage. There is a 5% to 10% rate of complications leading to reoperation; however, most complications are benign and can be handled with arthroscopic procedures (e.g., periosteal complications, adhesions, and arthrofibrosis).

Crutches are used and only partial weight bearing is allowed for 10 to 12 weeks. Walk increasing distances when full weight bearing is achieved. Bicycling is used with low resistance for stimulation and adaptation of the repair tissue. Expect a year before returning to impact sports activities. The patient should be followed by the surgeon throughout the whole rehabilitation period.

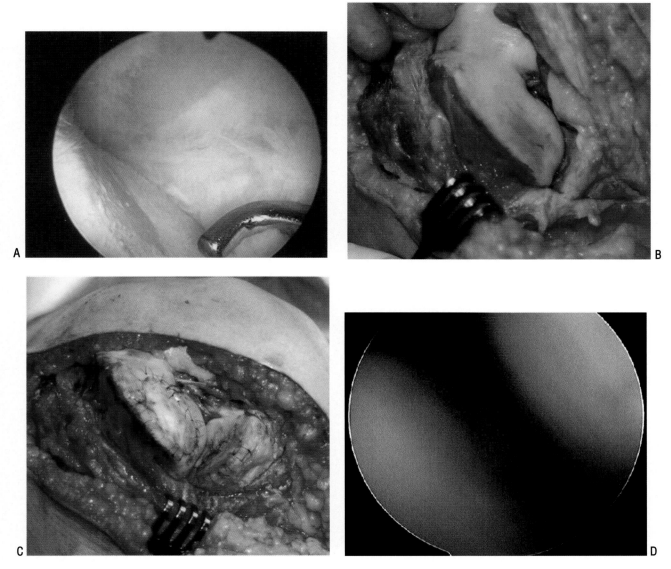

FIGURE 29-14
A 39-year-old female soccer player had total meniscectomy at age 16. Arthroscopy showing bipolar
lesions to medial femoral condyle and medial tibial condyle **(A)**, that were treated with ACT **(B,C)**
concomitant with high tibial osteotomy as a salvage procedure. Follow-up arthroscopy at 4 years
shows healing with good integration to the surrounding cartilage **(D)**.

RECOMMENDED READING

Brittberg M, Lindahl A, Nilsson A, et al. Treatment of deep cartilage defects in the knee with autologous chondrocyte trans-
    plantation. *New Engl J Med.* 1994;331:889–895.
Minas T, Peterson L. Advanced techniques in autologous chondrocyte transplantation. *Clin Sports Med.* 1999;18(1):13–
    44.
Peterson L. Cartilage cell transplantation. In: Malek MM, ed: *Knee surgery.* New York: Springer; 2001:440–449.
Peterson L. International experience with autologous chondrocyte transplantation. In: Insall JN, Scott WN, eds. *Surgery of
    the knee.* 3rd ed. New York: Churchill Livingstone; 2001:341–356.
Peterson L, Brittberg M, Kiviranta I, et al. Autologous chondrocyte transplantation: biomechanics and long-term durability.
    Am J Sports Med. 2002;30(1):2–12.
Peterson L, Minas T, Brittberg M, et al. Treatment of osteochondritis dissecans of the knee with autologous chondrocyte
    transplantation: results at two to ten years. *J Bone Joint Surg Am.* 2003;85-A(suppl 2):17–25.
Peterson L, Minas T, Brittberg M, et al. Two- to 9-year outcome after autologous chondrocyte transplantation of the knee.
    Clin Orthop Relat Res. 2000;374:212–234.

30 Opening Wedge Osteotomy— Proximal Tibia and Distal Femur

Giancarlo Puddu, Vittorio Franco, Massimo Cipolla, Guglielmo Cerullo, and Enrico Gianni

INDICATIONS/CONTRAINDICATIONS

Osteoarthrosis of the knee has many causes. Degenerative changes of the articular cartilage can occur through tension, compression, or shear. These changes are very much related to the forces exerted on the bearing surfaces. Genetic factors are known to play a part. Specific trauma and trauma from the overload caused by obesity or occupational factors are etiologically important. In essence, the biophysical cause of osteoarthrosis is an overload or a concentration of forces beyond the ability of the cartilage and subchondral bone to cope.

In any discussion of osteoarthrosis of the knee and its treatment, the operation of knee replacement (arthroplasty) versus knee realignment (osteotomy) is always pertinent. Historically, osteotomy preceded replacement by about 10 years. As replacement became a reality in the 1970s, the indications for each operation became clearer. While the annual number of osteotomies has remained stable, the proportional rate of total arthroplasties has increased dramatically since the early 1960s.

It follows that alignment of the lower extremity plays an important role in osteoarthrosis of the knee. Malalignment into a varus position overloads the medial condyles of the femur and tibia; valgus malalignment, similarly, overloads the lateral condyles. The rationale behind the osteotomy is to correct the angular deformity at the knee and therefore to decrease the excessive weight-bearing load across the affected compartment, which is the most involved by the degenerative process. Since alternative treatments for severe osteoarthrosis of the knee in the 1960s were limited, tibial osteotomy at the beginning was used for osteoarthrosis, rheumatoid arthritis, and secondary arthrosis, regardless of the etiopathogenesis and the magnitude of the angular deformity. After several years' experience, Coventry (1), Insall (3), and others narrowed the indications for tibial osteotomy. By the late 1970s, high tibial osteotomy was felt to be for the younger, more active patient in whom total knee replacement was thought to be unwise.

Now we think that the patients selected for proximal tibial/distal femur osteotomy should have mostly unicompartmental osteoarthrosis with axial malalignment. However, fracture and other trauma, congenital and acquired deformities, and idiopathic osteonecrosis are also reasons for osteotomy.

A patient is typically a candidate for high tibial osteotomy when the orthopaedic surgeon can clinically detect a varus standing alignment associated with a medial compartment arthritis in a stable knee; a medial compartment cartilage damage associated with anterior cruciate ligament (ACL), posterior cruciate ligament (PCL), posterolateral corner, or combined ligament deficiencies; a painful knee after a medial meniscectomy; articular cartilage defects requiring a repair technique; an osteochondritis dissecans lesion; or a patient who requires a meniscal allograft.

A typical candidate for distal femur osteotomy is young or middle-aged, athletic patient who has developed a disabling painful knee due to an early arthritis of the lateral compartment after lateral meniscectomy. Also candidate to the antivalgus procedure is the patient with chondral damages of the lateral femoral condyle associated with an ACL or PCL acute tear or chronic laxity; the patient with congenital valgus deformity often associated with overweight and lateral compartment arthritis; and the patient with a cyst of the lateral meniscus or with a discoid meniscus followed by a subtotal meniscectomy.

There is no definite patientage below which one should have an osteotomy, or above which one should have an arthroplasty. The age of 65 years is cited most often, but activity level, lifestyle, and general health must be considered. As long-term studies of arthroplasty demonstrate, age considerations may change. But the fact remains that osteotomy patients are generally younger than those who undergo knee arthroplasty.

Osteotomy is best done for unicompartmental osteoarthrosis in knees with generally well-maintained range of motion (ROM) (at least 90 degrees of flexion; less than 15 degrees of flexion contracture). Osteotomy should probably not be done in patients with rheumatoid arthritis, patients with very unstable knees, or those whose knees have greater than 20 degrees of varus deformity or 15 degrees of valgus deformity, according to Insall (2). These knees are complicated by an associated severe ligamentous laxity and subluxation; the latter is a relative contraindication. In fact, even if the correction of the mechanical axis in such a great deformity can result in a relaxed collateral ligamentous complex, often the knee finds a new functional stability so that many authors, including ourselves, do not routinely perform retightening of the ligamentous structures.

A patient who has varus deformity and ACL insufficiency may be treated with an ACL reconstruction in addition to the proximal tibial osteotomy. A technically demanding procedure, the osteotomy associated with the ligament reconstruction addresses the underlying disorder and corrects the problems. Because this is not a routine procedure, it will not be discussed here. However, the symptoms of pain and instability must be separated as clearly as possible, because when pain prevails, especially in sedentary patients, correction of alignment, with consequent relief of medial compartment pain, can be a satisfactory treatment.

The varus arthritic symptomatic knee very often shows articular cartilage lesions, Outerbridge (4) grades III and IV, that affect the involved medial compartment. Full-thickness chondral defects rarely heal without a direct intervention. Together with the modern proposals of treatment of the articular cartilage tears (autologous chondrocyte implantation and osteochondral autografts), the methods based on bone marrow stimulation are still in action. Historically, the first technique of marrow stimulation proposed was the Pridie drillings, introduced by the author in 1959. Presently, Steadman's (7) microfracture arthroplasty seems a more effective and safer option, as it is completely arthroscopic, and has the advantage, compared with the former, of not inducing local thermal necrosis. When performed together with the HTO, microfractures fully complement the surgical treatment, satisfying the necessity of a direct treatment of the intra-articular pathology, without increasing the risk of complications or lengthening time of surgery.

Overweight is a controversial topic. Obesity has a negative effect on the outcome of surgery in many orthopaedic operations. Most would agree that excess weight could make a patient a better candidate for osteotomy than for arthroplasty, but it is also true that obesity itself represents a negative factor in view of the possible general postoperative complications. When a patient is overweight, the weight should be brought to near normal before surgery, since osteotomy has a worse long-term outcome when the patient is obese.

Another contraindication to osteotomy is severe bone loss (more than a few millimeters) of the medial or lateral tibia or femur. When medial or lateral compartment bony support is insufficient, congruent weight bearing on both tibial plateaus following the osteotomy is impossible. In this situation tibiofemoral contact will teeter on the relatively prominent intercondylar tibial spines.

Severe varus or valgus deformity may be associated with lateral or medial subluxation of the tibia, respectively. Subluxation of more than 1 cm is an absolute contraindication to osteotomy, and some authors suggest that osteotomy should not be performed if any translation or subluxation is present.

Studies on the biomechanics of the dynamic gait accurately addressed the issue of varus or lateral thrust of the knee during ambulation. The term *adductor moment* was used to describe the amount of lateral or varus thrust of the knee observed during gait. Patients with high adductor moment have worse results following osteotomy than those with a low adductor moment. Furthermore, patients with a high adductor moment are more likely to have a recurrent varus deformity following valgus osteotomy. When osteotomy is chosen for those patients in spite of a high adductor moment, over-correction of the deformity may be helpful.

Osteotomy of the proximal tibia or distal femur is designed to relieve pain caused by medial or lateral tibiofemoral osteoarthrosis. Slight degenerative changes of the patellofemoral joint are not a contraindication to osteotomy. However, following proximal tibial osteotomy with a medial open-ing wedge, the anterior tibial tubercle is lowered to about one half of the angular correction; there-fore, the condition of "patella baja" is a contraindication to this kind of operation.

PREOPERATIVE PLANNING

The goal of knee osteotomy is to realign the mechanical axis of the limb, thereby shifting weight-bearing forces from a diseased compartment to a more normal compartment.

The alignment of the limb is best measured by full-length radiographs of the lower extremity.

The mechanical axis is determined by drawing a line from the center of the femoral head through the center of the knee to the center of the talus. The anatomic axis is depicted by drawing a line through the center of the shaft of the femur and through the center of the shaft of the tibia. In the nor-mal knee, the two lines cross each other in the center of the joint, making an angle of 5 degrees (phys-iologic valgus), and the mechanical axis passes through the center of the joint, or slightly varus (about 1 degree medially).

The deformity is measured by using these parameters as the reference points of "normality." With a varus knee we want to move the mechanical axis through the neutral alignment (approximately the center of the knee) up to a more lateral point at about two thirds (63%) of the tibial plateau to get 5 degrees of mechanical valgus alignment and thereby overcorrect the anatomic valgus from the "nor-mal" 5 degrees to 9 or 10 degrees (Fig. 30-1). Extensive experience has shown that overcorrection is absolutely essential if one wants to optimize a long-standing result from valgus osteotomy. It is inconvenient to correct to normal valgus that brings the extremity back to the position from which it originally became deformed, and that does not properly unload the medial compartment. In the normal knee, approximately 60% of the weight-bearing forces are transmitted through the medial compartment and approximately 40% are transmitted through the lateral compartment. Even in se-vere valgus deformity (up to 30 degrees valgus), the medial plateau load never falls below 30%.

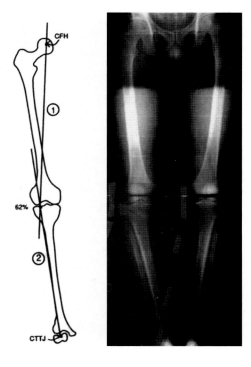

FIGURE 30-1

In the varus knee we want to correct the deformity, moving the mechanical axis up to a lateral point of the tibial plateau (62%, about two thirds of the articular surface) to get 10 degrees of anatomic valgus alignment (hypercorrection).

There is a controversy about full-length radiographs made with the patient supine compared with those made with the patient standing. Originally these radiographs were made with the patient supine. Then, some surgeons noted that, in this position, the amount of deformity was underestimated in certain patients who had osseous defects or ligamentous laxity, and this was presented as a cause of undercorrection by the osteotomy. For these reasons, most authors currently recommend that radiographs be made with the patient standing. However, two problems remain. First, because the patient can take the weight off the painful limb when standing and thus negate much of the benefit of this position, it could be better to take the radiographs with the patient standing on only the affected limb. Second, when there is severe ligamentous laxity, to plan the operation on radiographs made with the patient standing can lead to overcorrection, a potentially greater problem than undercorrection.

When we have a reasonable doubt from the physical examination, we calculate the joint line convergence angle (JLCA), which is formed by a line tangent to the distal femoral condyles and a line tangent to the tibial plateau. A single-leg weight-bearing full radiograph and a double-leg full radiograph, always in standing position, are obtained to measure the lower limb alignment. The difference in the JLCA between the two radiographs represents the component of malalignment associated with ligamentous laxity. To prevent overcorrection, the soft tissue laxity is subtracted from the overall valgus correction.

A young patient with a symptomatic congenital varus could be an early candidate for a valgus osteotomy, but the correction must not be an overcorrection, because in such patients it is sufficient to restore the physiologic alignment of the knee.

With the valgus knee, we want to reposition the mechanical axis to neutral alignment at approximately 0 degrees in the center of the joint. This means 5 degrees of anatomic and physiologic valgus (Fig. 30-2). The biomechanics of varus and valgus deformities of the knee differ. In fact, the intrinsic valgus angle between femur and tibia determines an asymmetric overload of the medial compartment, at about 60% of the whole, already in the normal knee. Thus, the overbalance of the knee toward a varus alignment will result in a functional disaster because of the additional overload of the medial compartment and the consequent, dramatic acceleration of the degenerative changes of the more normal side.

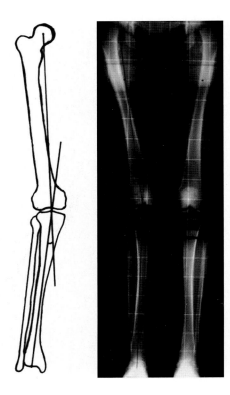

FIGURE 30-2

In the valgus knee we want to correct the deformity, moving the mechanical axis up to approximately the center of the tibial plateau to get 5 degrees of physiologic valgus alignment (normocorrection).

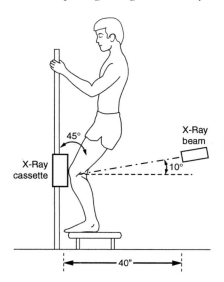

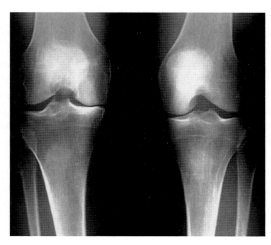

FIGURE 30-3

The Rosenberg view. Comparative posteroanterior weight-bearing knee radiograph at 45 degrees of flexion facilitates the diagnosis if the standard standing AP view is not sensitive enough.

The osteotomy we propose here is based on the opening wedge technique. Special plates with a spacer "tooth" were designed for this aim. We need to know the size of the base of the wedge, calculated in millimeters, to choose the plate and fix the osteotomy to the planned angle. Different widths of the tibia, at the level of the osteotomy cut, correspond to different wedge sizes, for the same degree of angular correction.

To complete evaluation of the knee, we look at the different radiographic views, including the standard lateral and the axial views of the patellofemoral joint.

The Rosenberg view, comparative posteroanterior weight-bearing radiograph at 45 degrees of knee flexion, facilitates the diagnosis in case the standard anteroposterior (AP) view is not sensitive enough (Fig. 30-3). The Rosenberg examination has a strong predictive value when the deformity is associated with a cruciate insufficiency, and therefore the chondral wear prevails in the posterior part of the tibial plateaus.

Most authors don't recommend computed tomography (CT) scans or magnetic resonance imaging (MRI) in studying a candidate for knee osteotomy; but we think that the stress reaction of the subchondral bone, detectable by MRI (Fig. 30-4), could be the only sign of a degenerative process at its earlier stage.

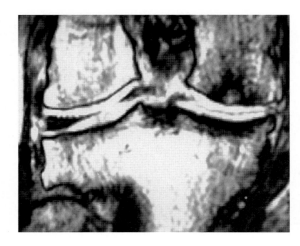

FIGURE 30-4

MRI can be positive for a stress reaction of the subchondral bone as the only diagnostic sign of an early degenerative process.

SURGERY

Dedicated Surgical Instrumentation

The object of valgus osteotomy is to obtain a new mechanical axis overcorrected up to 5 degrees of valgus. Our purpose with varus osteotomy is to reposition the lower limb to align to the physiologic 0 degrees of the neutral mechanical axis.

We present here our technique to perform the opening wedge osteotomy. To achieve more reproducible results with the fewest technical difficulties, the senior author (GP) developed a complete but simple and easy system of dedicated instruments and plates.

We get the valgus correction of the knee by means of proximal tibia osteotomy and the varus correction by means of distal femoral osteotomy. In varus deformity the tibiofemoral joint line is usually parallel to the floor. Proximal tibia osteotomy has been demonstrated to transfer load effectively from the medial to the lateral compartment. In valgus deformity, the joint line has a valgus tilt with a correspondent obliquity from superolateral to inferomedial direction. Although tibial varus osteotomy may realign a valgus limb, it cannot correct the joint-line tilt because the procedure is performed distally to the joint. The mechanical consequence of this, in patients with severe valgus deformities (more than 10 to 12 degrees according to various authors), is the effect of transferring the load transmission medially not more than the lateral portion of the tibial spine. The resultant increased valgus tilt of the joint line leads to greater shear forces and lateral subluxation during gait. However, distal femoral varus osteotomy may realign a valgus limb and correct valgus tilt of the joint line when used to treat lateral tibiofemoral osteoarthrosis with valgus deformity.

The plates specially designed for this osteotomy are butterfly shaped, with four holes for the tibia, and T shaped, with seven holes for the femur (Fig. 30-5) (Arthrex, Naples, FL). Their peculiarity is a spacer, a tooth as it were, available in many different sizes from 5 to 17.5 mm thick (up to 20 mm for the femur), with the tooth increasing one size for each additional millimiter. Tibial plates with trapezoidal spacers are also available to permit the correction of the coronal and, eventually, the sagittal deformity, the so-called tibial posterior slope, in one operation. The tooth enters the osteotomic line, holding the position and preventing a later collapse of the bone with the recurrence of the deformity. The thickness of the spacer must coincide with the desired angle of correction, calculated in the preoperative planning. The two upper holes of the tibial plate and the three of the horizontal lower arms of the femoral T plate allow the introduction of the AO 6.5-mm cancellous screws, and the lower holes of the tibial plate and the holes in the vertical arm of the femoral plate are cut for the AO 4.5-mm cortical screws.

The new plates are now made in a titanium alloy (see Figs. 30-14 and 30-22). The most important improvement from the former ones is the new special holes of the plate. Through them the screws can be freely oriented in every preferred direction and then even locked in the plate, like an internal mini fixator (thanks to a special device of the hole itself, created by the manufacturer). Dedicated cortical and cancellous screws for the new plates, also of titanium alloy, are now available.

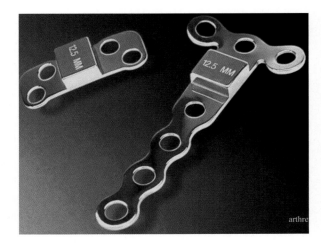

FIGURE 30-5

The plates are specially designed for opening wedge osteotomies in different shapes and sizes.

The crucial point of the operation is the opening of the metaphysis, where the osteotomy has cut the bone, at the desired angle of correction and holding the position to allow the introduction of the plate tooth. Recently we introduced a new innovative tool, the "opener jack" (Fig. 30-6), which greatly facilitates this step. Introduced into the osteotomic line, the jack gently retracts the bone to create the space for the plate and the grafts. It consists of two osteotomes coupling with a screw long enough to move away the blades and open the osteotomy. Then, a very simple "opener wedge" enters into the already prepared osteotomic site. It looks like a fork with two wedge-shaped tines, graduated to hold the opening at the correct rate, and a removable handle to allow the positioning of the plate.

The other two dedicated tools are the special Homan retractor for the vastus lateralis (Fig. 30-7), to be used in the femoral osteotomy, and a long rod guide with an ankle support to check intraoperatively the mechanical femorotibial alignment (Fig. 30-8).

Surgical Technique of Tibial Osteotomy

Step 1: Patient Position   We prefer a normal operating table with the patient in a supine position and the C-arm of an image intensifier set up opposite the surgeon. The patient is draped as usual in knee surgery; we also prepare the iliac wing and cover the foot using a very fine stockinette and a transparent adhesive drape to minimize the bulging at the ankle so that it will be possible to better realize the femorotibial alignment after the correction. The tourniquet may be inflated.

Step 2: Arthroscopy   Arthroscopy of the knee is carried out before the osteotomy to assess the relative integrity of the controlateral tibiofemoral compartment and that of the patellofemoral joint and to treat any intra-articular pathology.

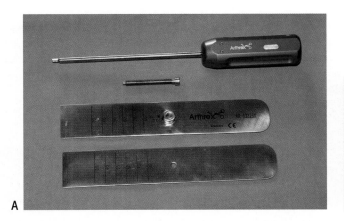

A

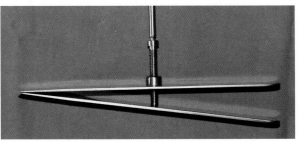

B

C

FIGURE 30-6

The "osteotomy jack" consists of two osteotomes coupling with a screw long enough to move away the blades and open the osteotomy.

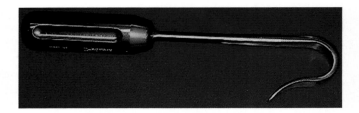

FIGURE 30-7

The special Homan is designed for the lateral femoral approach to retract the vastus lateralis.

After the careful arthroscopic examination has been completed, we perform all the other opportune procedures before microfracture arthroplasty. This caution is to prevent loss of visualization that could happen when droplets and blood enter the knee from the microfracture holes, after the penetration of the subchondral bone.

We dedicate particular attention to the treatment of meniscal tears and synovial pathology and, of course, removal of any eventual, loose body.

Then we examine the full thickness defects of the cartilage, candidate to the microfracture, to assess that the exposed bone is intact. It is critical to remove all loose or marginally attached flaps of cartilage in and surrounding the affected area to leave a lesion with a stable rim. Also very important is to remove the calcified cartilage layer that is often present but preserve an intact subchondral plate without violating it with a courette or motorized burr. The aim of this accurate preparation is the creation of a firm "cratere" with stable perpendicular edge of healthy cartilage that will trap in the clot formed by the bone marrow coming from the microfractures. The special surgical instrument to use is the dedicated awl, suggested by Steadman, with an angled tip, typically 30 or 45 degrees, that allows it to be perpendicular to the bone as it is advanced in the tibial, or femoral, tear. Chondral lesions up to 3 or 4 cm^2 are treated in this manner, and the holes must be approximately 3 to 4 mm apart, or about 4 or 5 holes per cm^2. The major advantage of this technique, compared to the older drilling procedure, is that the awl produces no thermal necrosis of the bone at all.

When the holes in a sufficient number have been made, marrow fat droplets and blood are released from the microfracture and form a pluripotential clot which fills in the chondral defect. The defect on the joint surface had been carefully prepared in advance to get the cratere with the firm perpendicular edge of healthy cartilage that becomes the ideal site for the clot and provides an optimal environment for the pluripotential marrow cells to differentiate into stable repairing tissue and cover the whole lesion. Moreover the awl produces, because of the microfractures, a roughened surface of the subchondral bone to which the clot can adhere more easily.

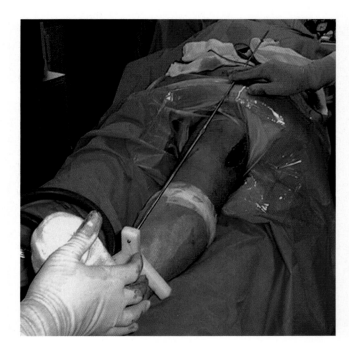

FIGURE 30-8

The long rod guide with an ankle support is dedicated to intraoperatively check the tibiofemoral alignment after the osteotomic correction.

When the cartilage that surrounds the critical area of the lesion is too thin, it may be impossible to create a stable rim with a well-defined perpendicular edge and, consequently, the technique is contraindicated.

Chronic degenerative chondral lesions commonly have extensive sclerotic bone with thickening of the subchondral plate. In these cases, it is very important to remove the sclerotic bone, using a motorized burr or an aggressive courette, until a punctuate bleeding of the surface appears; but the integrity of the subchondral plate should be always respected to preserve the joint surface's original shape and congruence.

The marrow clot, which Steadman named "superclot," promotes the healing process of the joint surface toward a neoformed tissue very close in substance and function to the normal articular cartilage.

Step 3: Incision and Exposure   We expose the anteromedial aspect of the tibia through a vertical skin incision centered between the medial border of the anterior tibial tubercle and the anterior edge of the medial collateral ligament and extending 6 to 8 cm distally to the joint line. Sharp dissection is carried to the sartorius fascia, and pes anserinus tendons are identified and detached from the bone. The pes anserinus is now retracted and the anterior half of the underlying superficial collateral ligament is cut horizontally (Fig. 30-9). There is no risk of instability because the deepest, and much more stabilizing, tibiomeniscal bundle of the ligament remains intact. A blunt retractor is placed dorsally, deep to the collateral ligament, to protect the posterior vessels and to clearly expose the posteromedial corner of the tibia. Anteriorly, a second retractor is placed under the patellar tendon. The procedure is facilitated by flexion of the knee.

Step 4: Osteotomy   The authors' preferred method is a "free" technique. With the knee in extension and under fluoroscopic control, a guide pin (Steinmann) is drilled, by the "free hand," through the proximal tibia from medial to lateral. This is oriented obliquely, starting approximately 4 cm distally to the joint line and directed across the superior edge of the tibial tubercle to a point 1 cm below the joint line (Fig. 30-10).

The original instruments system also provides an osteotomy guide assembly to help the surgeon in the proper placement of the guide pin and an osteotomy cutting guide to facilitate the use of the oscillating saw. The guide may be oriented to accommodate variations in size and anatomy. Different choices in tilting the osteotomy cut in both the coronal and sagittal planes are also possible.

The osteotomy is then performed, keeping the oscillating saw blade below and parallel to the guide pin, to prevent an intra-articular fracture. The saw is used to cut the medial cortex only. Then a sharp osteotome (Fig. 30-11) is used to finish the osteotomy, making certain that the all the cancellous metaphysis and especially the anterior and the posterior cortices are completely interrupted but preserving a lateral hinge of about 0.5 cm of intact bone. Fibular osteotomy is not necessary.

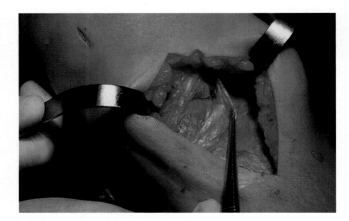

FIGURE 30-9
The pes anserinus tendons are retracted to expose the superficial collateral ligament.

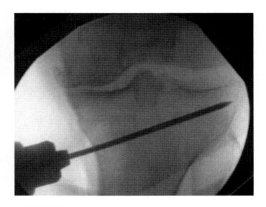

FIGURE 30-10
A guide Steinmann pin is drilled through the proximal tibia from medial to lateral, obliquely oriented and directed across the superior edge of the tibial tubercle to a point 1 cm below the joint line.

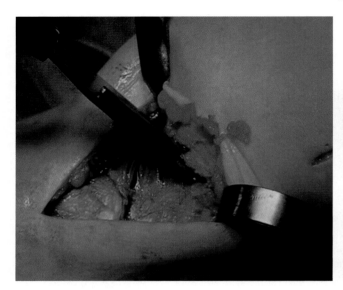

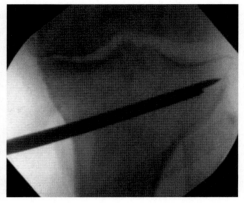

FIGURE 30-11

The osteotomy is performed, keeping the osteotome below and parallel to the guide pin to prevent an intra-articular fracture.

Step 5: Wedge Opening   The osteotomic line is easily opened by the help of the jack, which gently moves the tibial axis and realigns the knee. Then the opener wedge is introduced and slowly advanced into the metaphysis (Fig. 30-12). The surgeon measures the dimension of bone gap directly on the graduated tines of the wedge and chooses the plate.

Step 6: Plate Fixation   By removing the handle and, if necessary, one of the wedges, with the other one still into the osteotomy, the plate can be positioned easily on the medial cortex of the tibia

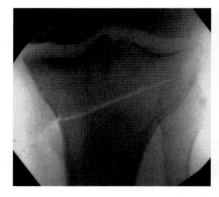

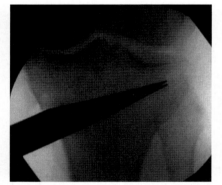

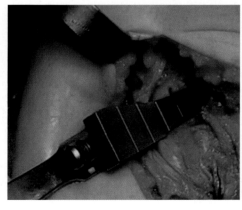

FIGURE 30-12

The opener wedge is introduced and slowly advanced until the osteotomy has been opened to obtain the planned realignment of the knee.

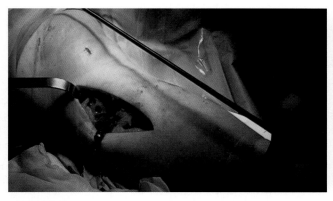
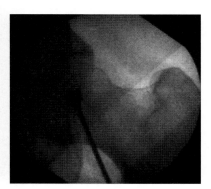

FIGURE 30-13

Before fixing the plate, we check under fluoroscopy the mechanical axis by means of the special guide rod, which is long enough to extend from the center of the femoral head through the knee to the center of the ankle.

with the spacer tooth introduced into the osteotomic line (Fig. 30-13). Before fixing the plate, we check the mechanical axis under fluoroscopy by means of the special guide rod, which is long enough to extend from the center of the femoral head through the knee to the center of the ankle (Fig. 30-14). When the rod crosses the knee at a lateral point about two-thirds (63%) of the tibial plateau, we know the angular correction corresponds to the 10 degrees of anatomic valgus we had planned in advance. But if the correction is under- or oversized, we can still change the plate, with one having a thicker or thinner tooth as needed. Next, the plate is fixed proximally with two 6.5-mm cancellous screws and distally with two 4.5-mm cortical screws. In the valgus knee, the medial side is the convex side so that the plate can act as a tension band device, obeying an important biomechanical principle for the effectiveness of the internal fixation.

Step 7: Bone Grafting   With a skin incision extended from the anterosuperior iliac spine 8 to 10 cm above the iliac crest, we take two or three corticocancellous bone grafts with the same wedge shape of the osteotomy. The larger one measures the full correction; the others are proportionately smaller. The grafts are press-fit and introduced to fill the defect. It is also possible to use different grafts, such as bone from the bank ; or bovine, freeze-dried bone; or, according to some other authors, no grafts at all. The correct position of the plate and grafts is confirmed with AP and lateral

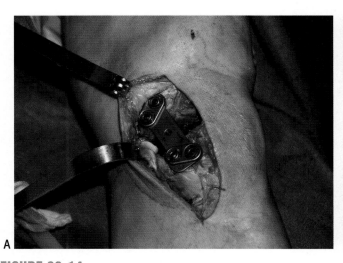
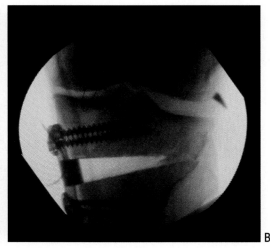

A   B

FIGURE 30-14

A new titanium plate positioned on the tibia medial cortex with the spacer tooth into the osteotomy and fixed to the bone with two proximal 6.5-mm cancellous screws and two distal 4.5-mm cortical screws.

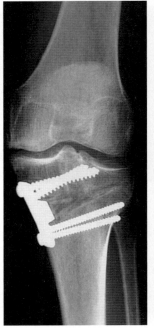
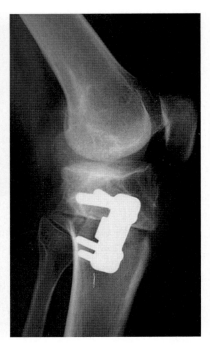

FIGURE 30-15
The correct position of the plate and grafts is confirmed by the postoperative AP and lateral radiographs.

radiographs (Fig. 30-15). One or two drains (the second, intra-articular, if needed) are prepared and the wound is closed in a routine fashion.

Surgical Technique of Femoral Osteotomy

Steps 1 and 2: Patient Position—Arthroscopy   There are no differences in positioning and preparing the patient for femoral osteotomy compared with the tibial procedure. The arthroscopy for the femoral osteotomy has the same justification and is performed with the same intentions as in the tibial procedure.

Step 3: Incision and Exposure   We expose the lateral aspect of the femur with a standard straight incision through the skin and the fascia, starting two finger-breadths distally to the epicondyle and extending the incision about 12 cm proximally (Fig. 30-16A). The dissection is carried

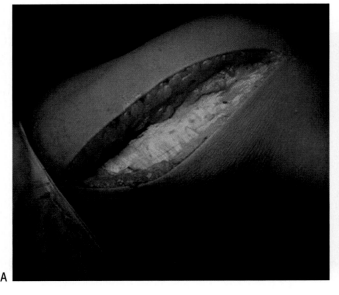
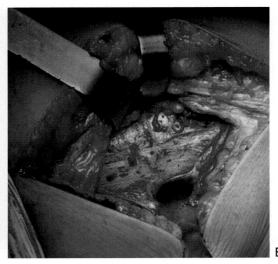

A   B

FIGURE 30-16
A: The lateral aspect of the femur is exposed with a standard straight skin incision. **B:** The dissection is carried down through the fascia to the lateral cortex, retracting the vastus lateralis with the special Homan.

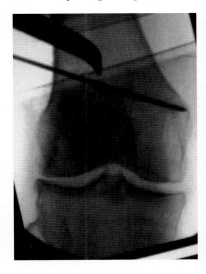 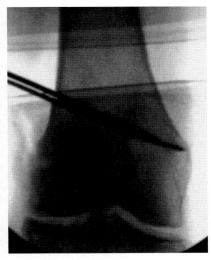

FIGURE 30-17

The Steinmann guide pin is drilled in a slightly oblique direction from lateral to medial, safely off from the troclear groove.

down to the vastus lateralis, which is retracted from the posterolateral intermuscular septum by the special dedicated Homan retractor placed ventrally (Fig. 30-16B). Perforating vessels are to be expected and should be controlled with ligature or electrocautery. We leave the joint capsule intact. The lateral cortex is now exposed. The procedure is facilitated by flexion of the knee.

Step 4: Osteotomy   Again the authors' preferred method consists of drilling the guide pin into the femur with the "free hand." The osteotomy guide assembly and the cutting guide may be helpful in properly positioning the guide pin when the oscillating saw must be used.

The Steinmann guide pin should be positioned in a slightly oblique direction (about 20 degrees) from a proximal point on the lateral cortex, three finger-breadths above the epicondyle, safely off from the trochlear groove, to a distal point on the medial cortex (Fig. 30-17). A second Homan is placed dorsally to avoid soft-tissue damage, and the osteotomy is started with the power saw just to cut the cortical bone. It is very important to do the osteotomy with the blade, the saw, and then the osteotome parallel and proximal to the guide pin to help prevent intra-articular fracture (Fig. 30-18).

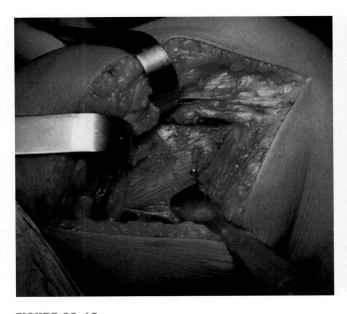 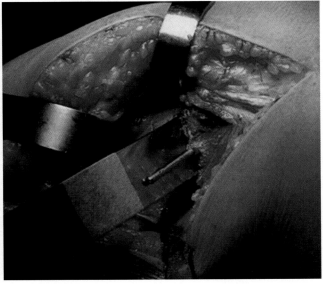

FIGURE 30-18

The osteotome must be kept parallel and proximal to the guide pin to help prevent intra-articular fracture.

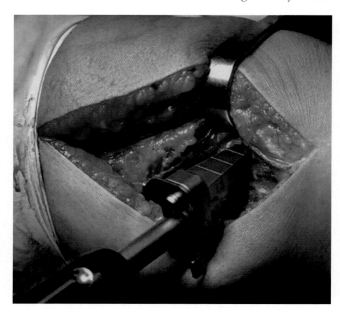

FIGURE 30-19

The wedge opener is inserted into the osteotomy and advanced until the opening corresponds to the planned correction.

After the first few centimeters with the saw, a sharp, flexible, thin osteotome is introduced and driven in all directions into the femur. This will preserve a hinge of intact bone by separating the cancellous bone and the anterior and posterior cortices, ending the osteotomy 0.5 cm before the medial cortex.

Step 5: Wedge Opening   After the distraction by the jack, the opener is introduced and slowly advanced until the osteotomy has been opened to obtain the planned realignment of the knee (Fig. 30-19); the handle is removed. The surgeon measures the dimension of bone gap directly on the graduated wedges of the opener and chooses the plate.

Step 6: Plate Fixation   By removing the handle of the opener, the plate can be easily positioned on the lateral cortex of the femur with the spacer tooth introduced into the osteotomic line (Fig. 30-20). If the plate does not fit the femur cortex properly, we must precontour it by modeling with the bending pliers. Before fixing the plate, we make an intraoperative control of the mechanical axis by means of the special guide rod, long enough to extend from the center of the femoral head to the center of the ankle, which we check under fluoroscopy at the passage on the knee joint, approximately the center of the tibial spine for neutral mechanical axis (Fig. 30-21). When the correc-

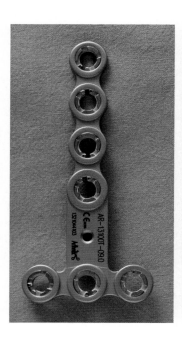
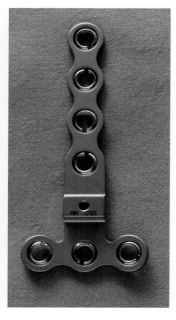

FIGURE 30-20

The new femoral titanium plate with the locking holes.

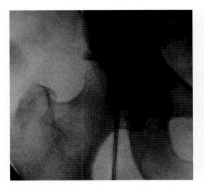 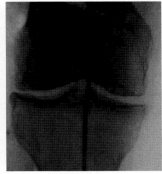 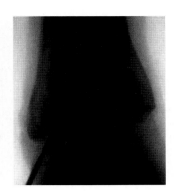

FIGURE 30-21

In distal femur varus osteotomy we check under fluoroscopy the mechanical alignment and move the axis to the center of the tibial plateau in a neutral position.

tion is under- or oversized, we choose a different plate with a thicker or thinner tooth as needed. We then fix the plate with four cortical screws proximal to the osteotomy and two (rarely three) cancellous screws distally (Fig. 30-22). We recommend a lateral plate instead of a medial one for an important biomechanical reason. When a normal knee with a valgus femorotibial angle is loaded in single-leg stance, the lateral femur is the tension side secondary to the extrinsic varus component of the body weight. In severe genu valgum, the mechanical axis moves laterally and therefore the convex medial side is subjected to tensile forces. After osteotomy, the mechanical axis is again moved medially, which returns the tension side of the knee to the lateral side. To act as a tension band, the plate must be applied to the lateral femur. Application of the plate to the medial femur after the osteotomy, as in the closing wedge osteotomy with the AO 90-degree angled blade plate, violates this principle and will probably lead to a high rate of failure.

Step 7: Bone Grafting   We always fill the osteotomic defect with autologous bone harvested from the omolateral iliac wing or grafts from the bank. According to other authors, bone grafting is recommended in all opening wedge osteotomies greater than 7.5 mm to prevent delayed union or nonunion and/or fixation failure. In osteotomies 7.5 mm or smaller, the decision to bone-graft should be individualized. The correct position of the plate and grafts is confirmed with AP and lateral radiographs (Fig. 30-23). One or two drains (one intra-articular) are prepared and the wound is closed in a routine fashion.

TECHNICAL PITFALLS AND COMPLICATIONS

The risk of intra-articular fracture always exists. This is more often due to a mistake in positioning the guide pin too close to the joint, leaving a very poor metaphysary bone stock between the osteotomy and the articular surface; or it may be due to imperfect finishing of the osteotomy without

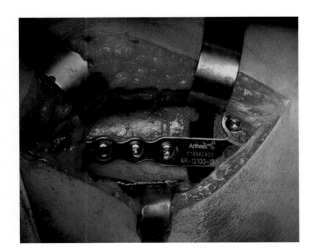

FIGURE 30-22

The plate is secured to the femur cortex with two (rarely three) distal cancellous screws and all four cortical screws.

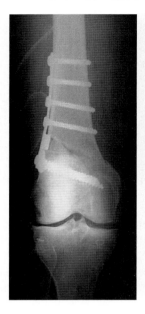
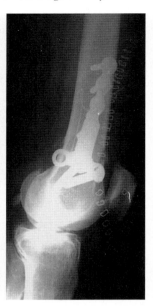

FIGURE 30-23

The correct position of the plate and grafts is confirmed by the postoperative

complete interruption of the anterior cortex. More often, however, an intact posterior cortex produces an articular fracture to stress the knee, in valgus or varus, and open the osteotomy. Most often it is possible, although not easy, to fix the fracture with the proximal screws in tibia, or the distal ones in femur, introduced as usual through the plate.

When the surgeon does not respect the hinge of intact bone, the osteotomy will dislocate. Checking the fixation and the alignment of the bone under fluoroscopy, the osteotomy angle looks subluxated with the tibia, or the femur, diaphysis, slipped laterally or medially, respectively. The way to prevent this technical problem begins with the proper choice of the site of the osteotomy cut that should be proximal enough, in the tibia, or distal in the femur, to avoid the maximum step-off of the bone profile and address a more stable fixation. Mainly, however, an intact bone hinge is essential for stability; when the hinge is correctly preserved, it prevents any dislocation. But if the undesired subluxation has occurred, then a possible solution is a staple fixation by a contralateral incision.

Failure of the hardware, especially the plates, should be a rare event. However, it can happen that a screw breaks when the patient returns to weight bearing too early postoperatively against the rehabilitation protocol. But sometimes, a screw breaks due to a technical pitfall. An imperfect congruence of the tooth plate into the osteotomic space overloads the screws with a lever arm that the screws cannot resist. An intact hinge maintains a sort of intrinsic elasticity and, as a spring, closes the osteotomy on the tooth making the system plate-bone congruent and tight; conversely, a fissured hinge misses to exert this elastic compression on the opposite side of the bone. The plate could be loose into the bone and the spacer tooth not in contact with both cortices. The screws have to support part of the effort to prevent the osteotomy collapse until the bone heals, but they break because of a fatigue fracture of the metal before the complete recovery.

The lateral positioning of the "T" plate is critical. The osteotomy has to be perfectly oriented in the sagittal plane, perpendicular to the longitudinal axis of the femur to have the long arm of the plate completely lying on the bone, just in the center of the diaphysis. In fact the spacer tooth forms a right angle with the plate that prevents the correct positioning of the long arm on the bone when the osteotomy is oblique with the femur. If the vertical arm is not parallel to the diaphysis, the last upper holes of the plate fall out from the bone, anteriorly or posteriorly to the cortex, making it very difficult to fix the all screws properly (Fig. 30-24).

Injuries to the vessels are infrequent. Accidental tears to the anterior tibial artery are reported in the literature, but only when an extensive lateral approach to the tibia is taken, or to the posterior vessels, which could be safely protected by correct use of a posterior Homan retractor and keeping the knee flexed during surgery.

Thrombophlebitis and infections are generic complications in common with all the other surgical procedures involving the inferior limb.

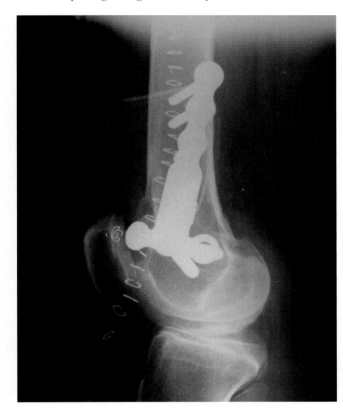

FIGURE 30-24
Badly oriented osteotomy, oblique to the longitudinal axis, leads to a malposition of the plate.

Delayed union may occur, but most osteotomies will go on to union with time and partially assisted early weight bearing. Nonunion is also a possibility. In our series (55 tibial and 21 femoral osteotomies with a minimum follow-up of 4 years) we had no nonunions. This probably is the result of the systematic use of bone grafts to fill the osteotomy.

Peroneal palsy was always a potential complication of tibial valgus closing wedge osteotomy. We have never seen this complication in opening wedge technique. However, in severe valgus deformities, when distal varus osteotomy is performed, a transitory peroneal apraxia can occur from overstretching the nerve.

It may be incorrect to include loss of the desired correction as a true complication. In opening wedge, the bone collapse of the grafts might determine a decrease of the angular correction, but the new plates have been demonstrated to be effective in preventing it. Of course continuing degenerative changes and high adduction moment contribute to a gradual loss of correction as time goes by.

POSTOPERATIVE MANAGEMENT

After the operation the knee is immobilized with a range-of-motion brace in full extension or at slight flexion of about 10 degrees that allows a full ROM when unlocked. Passive flexion and extension in a continuous passive motion device are started the day after surgery. The drains are removed 48 hours later. Patients are allowed to walk with no weight bearing on the operated limb from the second postoperative day, and they are dismissed from the hospital in 4 to 5 days. When postoperative knee pain and effusion have been minimized, restoring normal lower limb ROM and musculotendinous extensibility (with consideration for bi-articular muscles) is foundational to implementing an exercise program that integrates the trunk, hip, and ankle muscles into dynamic knee stabilization challenges while addressing isolated quadriceps femoris deficiencies. Physical therapy intervention with the knee osteotomy patient requires continual attention to the balance of protection and function. Although progressive weight bearing and ROM exercises are vital to recovery, early excessive joint loading and terminal knee flexion-extension with external loads can compromise the integrity of the surgical realignment. Usually within the first 4 weeks, the patients are able to completely flex the knee. After 4 weeks (6 weeks in femoral osteotomy), functional weight bearing is allowed. Full weight bearing is normally possible after 6 to 7 weeks (8 or 9 weeks in femoral osteotomy) when the radiographs show satisfactory healing of the bone. Then greater emphasis needs to be placed on restoring proprioceptive-kinesthetic normalcy at the involved lower limb. While the rehabilitation program progress to address both anaerobic and aerobic physiologic energy systems, increasing fatigue resistance as evidenced by prolonged maintenance of appropriate body control during functional exercises without apparent discomfort or movement-avoidance patterns assures the therapist that neuromuscular control for dynamic knee stabilization is improving. All progressions may need to be delayed for older patients, particularly if they have not recently participated in a physical exercises program, and rehabilitation should emphasize active ROM to facilitate articular cartilage nourishment and preservation.

RECOMMENDED READING

Puddu G. Osteotomies about the athletic knee. In: Drez D Jr, DeLee JC, eds. *Operative techniques in sports medicine*. Vol. 8, No. 1. Orlando: WB Saunders; 2000.

Puddu G, Fowler PJ, Amendola A. Opening wedge osteotomy system by Arthrex. Surgical technique. Naples, FL: Arthrex Inc.; 1998.

REFERENCES

1. Coventry MB. Osteotomy about the knee for degenerative and rheumatoid arthritis. *J Bone Joint Surg*. 1973;55:23–48.
2. Insall JN, Joseph DM, Msika C. High tibial osteotomy for varus gonarthrosis. *J Bone Joint Surg*. 1984;66:1040–1048.
3. Insall JN, Shoji H, Mayer V. High tibial osteotomy: a five-year evaluation. *J Bone Joint Surg*. 1974;56:1397–1405.
4. Outerbridge RE. The etiology of chondromalacia patellae. *J Bone Joint Surg* (Br). 1961;43:752–757.
5. Steadman JR, Rodkey WG, Singleton SB, et al. Microfracture techniquefor full-thickness chondral defects: technique and clinical results. *Op Tech Sports Med*. 1997;7:300–304.

31 Computer-Assisted Opening Wedge High Tibial Osteotomy

Douglas W. Jackson and Blaine Warkentine

After using computer assistance in various knee surgery applications, we found this technology particularly helpful in obtaining the desired alignment in an opening-wedge proximal tibial osteotomy. Prior to its use, intraoperative fluoroscopy, radiographs, and/or visual assessments were the tools to assist in trying to obtain the desired intraoperative alignment. Computer assistance offers real time alignment information related to rotation of the limb as well as the exact sagittal and coronal planes for the osteotomy. This information is obtained with less radiation exposure (to patient, staff, and surgeon) and has enabled us to use smaller incisions as well as decrease our overall operative time. This application of computer-assisted surgery is based on and draws heavily from the contributions and techniques described by Dr. Guancarlo Puddu (see Chapter 30).

INDICATIONS/CONTRAINDICATIONS

Indications

Our current indications for computer-assisted opening wedge proximal osteotomy reflect our practice's patient profile. This procedure is considered in our physically active patients and in combination with certain other knee procedures:

- The patient has pain and limitations primarily related to the knee's medial compartment.
- The patient is "physiologically" younger and wants to continue high-demand activities after surgery.
- The varus alignment is less then 12 degrees. In our experience caring for an active patient population, those requiring greater than 12 degrees of correction usually have more than unicompartment disease. In addition, those with larger corrections require significant bone grafting at the opening osteotomy site and run a higher risk of nonunion. In our experience, patients with high degrees of malalignment represent more individualized approaches; and while they may benefit from computer-assisted surgery applications, those techniques used are beyond the scope of this chapter.
- The opening wedge osteotomy is in combination with other surgical procedures in the knee where there is the desire to unload the diseased medial compartment of the knee. It is used in attempt to provide a more favorable environment for a desired biologic response or protected healing for another procedure. These include:
  - Microfracture
  - Chondrocyte transplantation, osteochondral autografts and allografts

- Meniscal allograft transplant
- Helping to reduce loads associated with varus and posterolateral ligament insufficiency and/or reconstructions
- Anterior cruciate ligament (ACL) reconstruction associated with symptomatic arthritic medial compartment

Contraindications

- Inflammatory arthritis
- Tricompartmental disease
- A flexion arc of less the 110 degrees (this and those contraindications below are in our patients whose objective is to remain physically active)
- Greater than a 5-degree flexion contracture
- Greater than 12 degrees of varus
- Tibiofemoral subluxation on standing radiograph
- Previous meniscectomy in the contralateral compartment

PREOPERATIVE PLANNING

The history and physical examination establish that the physiologically younger, active patient being evaluated has symptoms primarily related to the knee's medial compartment. The knee range of motion (ROM) is documented; weight-bearing radiographs allow joint space determinations. If an osteotomy is being considered in those patients with varus alignment that is felt to contribute to their current complaints or is over weighting their medial compartment, we obtain an overall leg alignment on long-standing weight-bearing radiograph. In the group of patients who are also being evaluated for other surgical procedure(s) of the knee, it is part of the initial evaluation. These include any biologic restoration of their cartilage surfaces or a meniscus replacement in the overloaded compartment. It is unlikely that a biologic replacement will survive any better than the native tissues if the abnormal forces continue to be present. In addition, we consider it in varus alignment associated with posterolateral and varus instability (see Chapter 24).

SURGERY

Patient Positioning

The patient is positioned on the operating room table in the supine position with a tourniquet (which we may or may not use for portions or all of the procedure) applied. The entire lower extremity is prepared and draped separately from the groin distally in the usual orthopaedic manner. We use an adhesive wrap on the leg to decrease the bulky surgical stocking, allowing better visualization of the leg alignment.

Technique

An arthroscopic examination is performed and the treatable intra-articular cartilage and meniscal pathology addressed before the osteotomy. It varies among patients, but it is common to remove, debride, and contour a portion of a degenerative medial meniscus and loose or fragmented articular cartilage in the medial compartment. In addition, loose bodies and intra-articular debris and localized chondroplasties may be performed (see Chapter 26). Exposed bone that meets the indications in Chapter 27 may be addressed with microfracture or chondrocyte transplantation (see Chapter 29). Autograft (see Chapter 28) and allograft (see Chapter 33) osteochondral transplantation, meniscal allograft (see Chapters 10 and 11) or ACL reconstruction (see Chapter 12) may be performed in conjunction with the tibial osteotomy (see Chapter 24).

There are several companies that offer computer chosen software to assist in proximal tibial osteotomy, and use different methods for acquiring the position and alignment of the limb. Ideally, newer versions will allow less invasive data acquisition methodology. We currently use a system that requires femur and tibia reference arrays. The distal femur array is placed along the lateral intermuscular septum. For the tibia they are placed percutaneously along the lateral aspect of proximal one-third of the tibia (Fig. 31-1). In addition, the system we currently use has a navigated drill guide (Fig. 31-2), a round tip surface pointer, and a sharp percutaneous pointer.

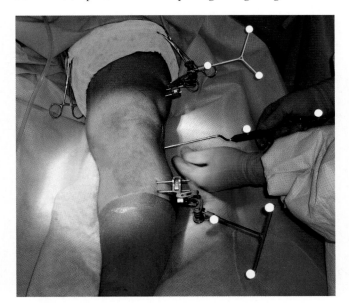

FIGURE 31-1

The femoral and tibial reference arrays are in place. A percutaneous pointer is being used to select the level of the osteotomy on the lateral side of the tibia.

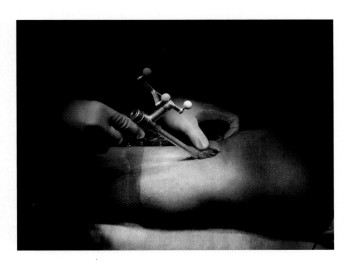

FIGURE 31-2

Using computer-assisted navigation, the reference guide is used to select the desired slope of the osteotomy and the exact level on the tibia. Once the position is chosen and confirmed, guides pins are inserted and used with the guide in making the osteotomy cut.

The operating room is arranged to facilitate the workflow and enhance the visibility of the reference rays by the camera. We place the computer and the associated infrared camera at the foot of the bed approximately 2 to 3 meters from the extremity (Fig. 31-3).

We prefer using a fluoroscopic mini C-arm because of the reduced radiation; it can be used without a radiology technician and we do not wear lead aprons during the procedure.

Registering Anatomic Landmarks   Eight anatomic landmarks are registered. The sequence of the registration points is shown in Figure 31-4.

The kinematic hip center is defined by the software as the femur is moved in a circular motion (Fig. 31-4A). This allows an accurate assessment of the center of femoral head, which is very helpful in obtaining the desired correction and confirming it.

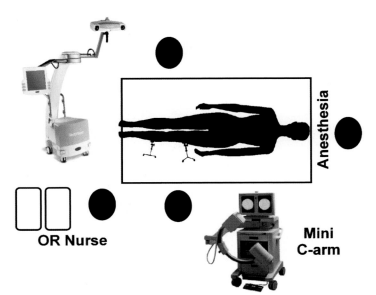

FIGURE 31-3

When performing the osteotomy on a left lower extremity, we place and drape the mini-image intensifier so that it can be moved into position for confirmation and site-selection registration. The infrared camera should have an unobstructed line of sight of the reference arrays.

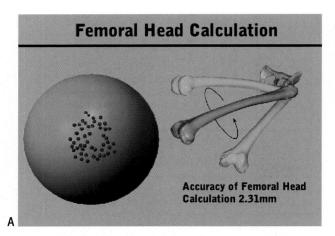

Femoral Head Calculation

Accuracy of Femoral Head
Calculation 2.31mm

A

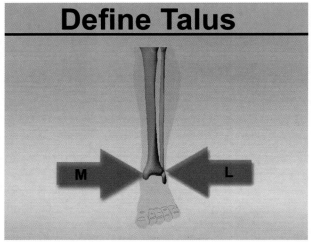

Define Talus

M   L

B

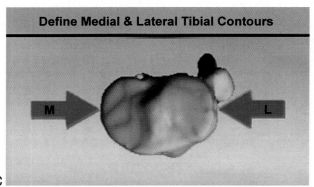

Define Medial & Lateral Tibial Contours

M   L

C

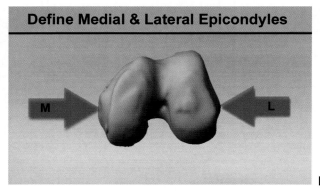

Define Medial & Lateral Epicondyles

M   L

D

FIGURE 31-4

The sequence of registering the eight anatomic
landmarks. **A:** The computer calculates three sets of
center points within the femoral head. These points are
compared, and the worst center point is discarded.
Distance between the remaining two center points is
calculated and read as the error of registration. In this
example the accuracy of the center of the femoral head is
2.31 mm. We prefer the accuracy for the femoral points to
be 3 mm or less. If it is not, we perform the pivoting
registration again until we have registered 3 mm or less.
This corresponds with a deviation of less then 0.7
degrees varus/valgus on a 33-cm femur. **B:** The medial
and lateral malleoli points are registered using the blunt
pointer. **C:** The tibial joint line is located at the
midcoronal point of both the medial and lateral tibial
plateau and registered using the blunt pointer. **D:** The
medial and lateral femoral epicondyles are located and
registered. **E:** The pointer's tip is placed at the tibial
tubercle and rotated to represent the rotation of the lower
limb. This establishes the axis that is important in
calculating the osteotomy correction.

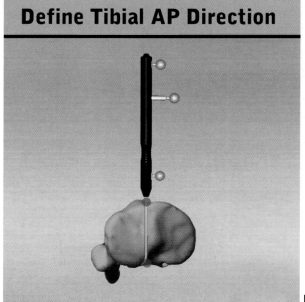

Define Tibial AP Direction

E

During the registration of the data to calculate the kinetic hip center, it is important that the pelvis is not moving. If we feel this is a problem in our accuracy, we use an assistant to stabilize the pelvis and re-enter the data. We start with small circles at approximately 90 degrees of hip flexion and gradually continue to do the circular motion until we reach full extension at the hip

Both medial and lateral malleoli points are registered using the blunt pointer. The software bisects these two points, which defines the distal point of the mechanical axis of the affected limb (Fig. 31-4B)

The tibial joint line is located with two points, at the midcoronal point of both the medial and lateral tibial plateau (Fig. 31-4C). The computer then bisects the medial and lateral registered points to give the center of the tibial mechanical axis.

The medial and lateral femoral epicondyles are located and registered (Fig. 31-4D). The software bisects these points to develop the distal mechanical axis of the femur.

The rotation for the tibia is registered. The pointer tip is placed at the tibial tubercle and rotated to represent the rotation of the lower limb. We use the second metatarsal as the landmark and the apex to the spine of the anterior tibia as an additional check (Fig. 31-4E).

This rotation must be known for the computer to calculate the midsagittal axis on which the osteotomy is calculated. The osteotomy is made in an oblique fashion, and this axis is the pivoting axis on which the software calculates the correction.

Initial Angle Definition   The leg is placed in the fully extended position, and the computer stores the preoperative leg alignment. Figure 31-5A demonstrates the several choices the surgeon

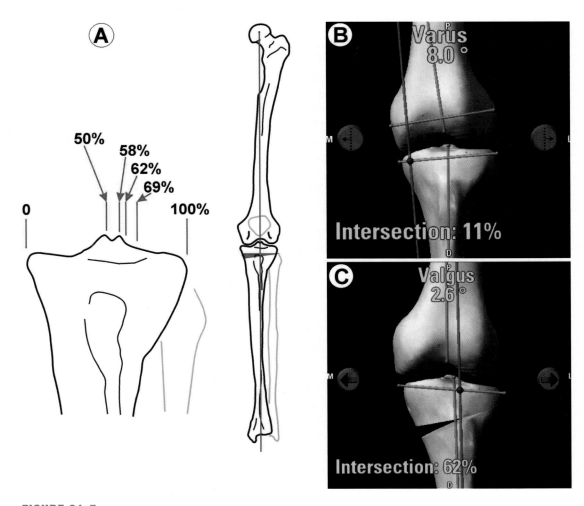

FIGURE 31-5

A: The software allows you to select your precise preference for the amount of correction desired. The surgeon can decide where the mechanical axis (Misculicz line) bisects the tibial plateau as it crosses the chosen point in the medial-lateral width of the tibia. **B:** Demonstrates where the mechanical axis bisects the tibial plateau in a patient with 8 degrees of genu varum. **C:** Demonstrates the degree of correction (2.6 degrees of valgus) if the surgeon chooses the mechanical axis to bisect the tibia at 62% of it width.

has in placing the point at which the mechanical axis will bisect the tibia. Noyes has recommended surgical corrections with the mechanical axis bisecting the tibia at 62% of the width, and Fujisawa has recommended a point at 69% of the width. Figure 31-5B shows a preoperative example of a patient with 8.0 degrees of genu varus and a mechanical axis (Misculicz line) that bisects the tibial plateau at 11 % of its total medial-lateral width. For example, achieving a correction to 2.6 degrees of genu valgus in this patient would occur by placing the mechanical axis bisecting the plateau at 62% of its width (Fig. 31-5C). We prefer using corrections between 58% and 62% when combining the osteotomy with other surgical procedures. Based on end points collected with the pointers, the software calculates the length of the osteotomy that will leave a 5-mm lateral cortical hinge (Fig. 31-6). After defining the exact point on the medial tibial cortex for the desired beginning point for the osteotomy, it is used as the mid point of our surgical incision and exposure to the medial tibia.

The software sets the cut plane of the osteotomy perpendicular to the mechanical axis according to the sagittal plane. If desired by the surgeon, additional slope can be fine-tuned into the planned osteotomy.

The computer will give the necessary data to correct the coronal plane so that the mechanical axis bisects the tibia at 62% of tibial width (which was defined by the two landmarks acquired at the joint line). This roughly represents between 2 to 4 degrees of valgus, depending on the length of the extremity, and can be fine-tuned to any position desired.

Tibia cutting plane navigation is defined from the start point and end point of the osteotomy. The software allows the use of a pre-calibrated K-wire drill guide to navigate two K-wires according to the trajectory given by these previously defined points (Fig. 31-7A,B).

Through the small surgical incision we use the navigated drill guide and two K-wires. We penetrate the far cortex with these wires to maintain stability of the K-wires and to stress relax the far cortex allowing plastic deformation of the far cortex instead of fracture. The unslotted low profile cutting block is slipped over the K-wires, and the osteotomy is cut to the desired length. The software has calculated this from the distance between start and end points minus the desired far cortical hinge. Our preference is to intermittently check the progression of the saw blade with the mini C-arm to confirm and assure ourselves of the exact location of the saw blade.

We then apply a valgus force slowly to the extremity until the desired correction is achieved. (Fig. 31-8).

We pack bone graft into the wedge and select an appropriately sized medial distraction plate. The real time alignment can be checked at anytime, and once it is chosen, the appropriate plate is selected. The final alignment is confirmed on the computer screen, and the correction is depicted prior to closure.

Using the mini C-arm we confirm the placement of the fixation and the length of the screws (Fig. 31-9). The ligament status, final ROM, and coronal and sagittal alignment are documented. The surgical wound is closed; a long leg support hose and a knee immobilizer are applied.

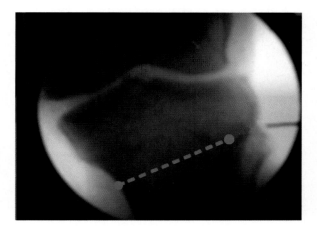

FIGURE 31-6

Using fluoroscopy (mini C-arm), the sharp percutaneous pointer defines and registers where we want the osteotomy (the oblique bone cut) to start (*point a*) and end (*point b*) in relation to the near and far cortex.

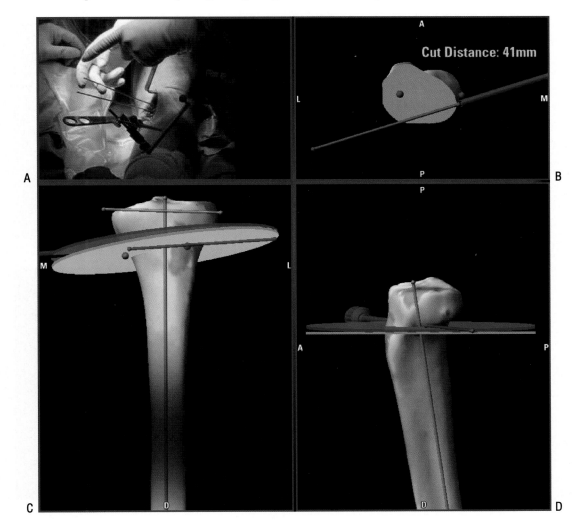

FIGURE 31-7

A–D: The precalibrated K-wire drill guide is used to navigate two K-wires according to the trajectory given by previously defined points. These pins are placed to achieve the wedge size and placement in both the coronal and sagittal plane. This aids the surgeon to prevent adversely affecting the slope of the tibia during the osteotomy. Through the small surgical incision we use the navigated drill guide and the two K-wires. The unslotted low-profile cutting block is slipped over the K-wires, and the osteotomy is cut to the desired length.

Pearls and Pitfalls

- The reference arrays fixed to the femur and tibia need to be rigid. The fixation pins need to be checked for any extraneous movement and may need to be advanced for better fixation. Care must be taken with the exact position of the tips of the fixation pins to prevent possible nerve and vascular injury.
- Errors in navigation may occur from poor fixation and if the reference arrays position are altered during the case.
- The camera should be positioned for easy and accurate visualization of the arrays. This point will eliminate a significant amount of frustration during the case if visualization is difficult or if the camera needs constant positioning adjustments.
- The registration of the required landmarks for high tibial osteotomy takes a few minutes but is critical. Each entry point has a purposeful use within the software's calculations for both the precise osteotomy bone cuts, the degree of correction, and the AP rotation of the tibia. When these are registered incorrectly, the information will be significantly altered.

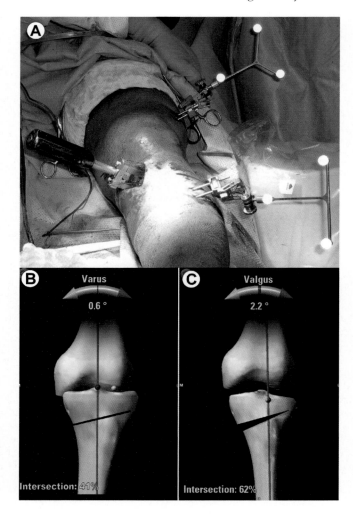

FIGURE 31-8

A: A wedge can be placed and used to open the osteotomy and check the correction. The computer screen will give the degree of progressive correction, and the point the mechanical axis is bisecting the tibia **(B,C)**.

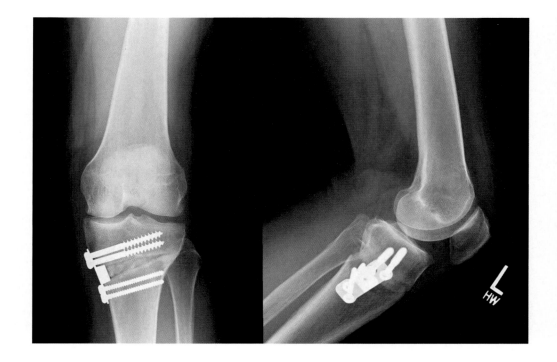

FIGURE 31-9

The fluoroscopic images are obtained to confirm the plate and screw placement. If these are as desired, the arrays are removed and the wounds closed.

- There are other options in the software for distal femoral osteotomy as well as closing wedge tibial osteotomy. This chapter has focused on the application of computer-assisted orthopedic surgery with the opening wedge proximal tibial osteotomy.
- Additionally, you can transfer the femoral array to the proximal wedge after the osteotomy has been accomplished. In this way you will now be tracking the true opening of the wedge as opposed to some instability within the knee. Our opinion is that if we axial load the knee in extension, this issue is negligible. If you decide to do this, then you must try your best to be as close to full extension as possible when assessing alignment.

POSTOPERATIVE MANAGEMENT

We currently prefer the patients be discharged the day following their osteotomy with touch weight bearing. It is possible some of these procedures can be done on an outpatient basis. We delay active ROM for 1 to 2 weeks until the patient returns to the office for their first postoperative evaluation. We take radiographs at their first postoperative office visit (Fig. 31-9), and again at 6 weeks postoperatively. Radiographs are then taken at 3 and 6 months to confirm bony union if necessary.

COMPLICATIONS AND PATIENT INFORMATION

- The patient should understand there is a period of limited weight bearing which depends on the degree of correction and the rate of time for the individual osteotomy to heal.
- There may be incomplete resolution of the patient's knee arthritic symptoms.
- There is a likely chance that the patient will undergo a later conversion to total knee arthroplasty (hopefully not needing that option for at least a 7- to 10-year period).
- Potential complications that may occur include delayed unions, nonunions, loss of correction, return of symptoms, peroneal nerve palsy, vascular injury, compartment syndrome, intra-articular fracture, patella baja, infection, and thromboembolism.

RESULTS

We have been using this technique since 2002 and have a limited number of patients. Our desired alignment corrections have been the best we have obtained to date. If one looks at the existing literature following proximal tibial osteotomies, it appears the results are better when the authors adhered to specific indications and obtain the desired surgical correction. Several long-term studies (primarily closing-wedge proximal tibial osteotomies) indicate that accurate correction has been the leading predictor for success. The reported initial high success rates of 70% to 90% seem to deteriorate with time. Some studies suggest that more than half of high tibial osteotomies have remained effective at 7 to 10 years. Undercorrection tends to cause failure from continued symptoms. Overcorrection produces a poor cosmetic result and can make later total knee replacement more difficult to perform.

There is very little literature on active patients undergoing osteotomy with concomitant surgeries. The many variables make it difficult to specifically address and randomize for comparisons. As our techniques improve and particularly for those active physiologically younger patients wishing to defer replacement, we find the opening wedge proximal tibial osteotomy with tibial varus is a strong consideration.

- The surgical incisions we use are 4.0 to 6.0 cm in length.
- Our operative time (including the limited intra-articular arthroscopic procedures and for the osteotomy) averages 68 minutes.
- Total fluoroscopy time averages 12 seconds using a mini C-arm.
- Follow-up radiographic assessment in the office setting confirms corrections within 2.0 degrees of the planned correction.

RECOMMENDED READING

Coventry MB, Ilstrup DM, Wallrichs SL. Proximal tibial osteotomy: a critical long-term study of eighty-seven cases. *J Bone Joint Surg Am.* 1993;75:196–201.

Insall JN, Joseph DM, Msika C. High tibial osteotomy for varus gonarthrosis: a long-term follow-up study. *J Bone Joint Surg Am.* 1984; 66:1040–1048.

Kessler OC, Jacob HA, Romero J. Avoidance of medial cortical fracture in high tibial osteotomy: improved technique. *Clin Orthop*. 2002;395:180–185.

Marti RK, Verhagen RA, Kerkhoffs GM, et al. Proximal tibial varus osteotomy: indications, technique, and five- to twenty-one-year results. *J Bone Joint Surg Am*. 2001;83:164–170.

Sprenger TR, Doerzbacher JF. Tibial osteotomy for the treatment of varus gonarthrosis: survival and failure analysis to twenty-two years. *J Bone Joint Surg Am*. 2003;85:469–47 Therapeutic study, level III-2 (retrospective cohort study).

32 Allograft Transplantation for Articular Defects of the Knee

Petros J. Boscainos, Catherine F. Kellett, and Allan E. Gross

INDICATIONS/CONTRAINDICATIONS

The use of fresh osteochondral allografts for osteochondral defects of the knee is based on a scientific rationale and on long-term clinical experience.

Fresh avascular osteochondral allografts, if harvested within 24 hours of death and preserved at 4° C, show 100% viability of cartilage at 4 days (7,12,33). Although freezing decreases the immunogenicity of the bone to some degree, it also results in decreased chondrocyte viability (13,38). Even cryopreservation and controlled rates of freezing and thawing will not achieve an acceptable degree of cartilage viability (13). The matrix that surrounds the chondrocytes isolates them from the host's immune cells and prevents host sensitization (23). The avascular bone remains structurally intact and mechanically strong until it is replaced by host bone by creeping substitution (30). Although the osteocytes will not survive unless the graft is vascularized, the use of immunosuppressive drugs to counter the increase in immunogenicity, that this would produce, cannot be justified in this setting. In a series of failed fresh osteoarticular allografts between 12 and 84 months after transplantation, none has demonstrated histologic evidence of transplant rejection (21). Long-term chondrocyte viability of fresh osteochondral allografts has been confirmed in a number of studies, even at 17 years after transplantation (9,11,26,30).

Based on that scientific rationale, cadaveric allografts with viable cartilage and avascular bone, which provides an intact structure until host bone replaces it by creeping substitution, provide a reconstructive solution for young, high-demand patients where implants or an arthrodesis is not desirable (Fig. 32-1) (17,36). Osteochondral allografts provide flexibility in terms of the size of defect that can be reconstructed. Both femoral and tibial defects can be addressed and where needed, the allograft meniscus can also be transplanted (17).

Appropriate patient selection is paramount to satisfactory outcome. A number of patient characteristics have been identified that are predictive of success.

Diagnosis

McDermott et al (25) reviewed the first 100 patients who received fresh, small-fragment osteochondral allografts for articular defects in and around the knee. Initially, these grafts were performed for uni-

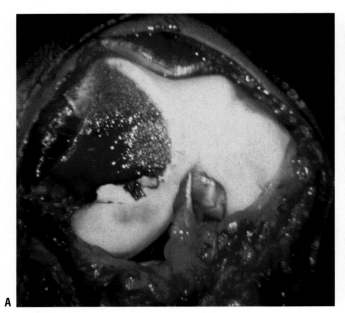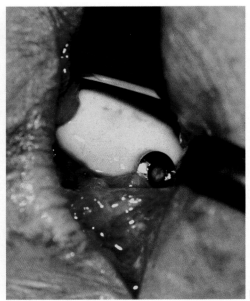

FIGURE 32-1

A: Intraoperative pictures of an osteochondral posttraumatic defect of a lateral femoral condyle of 5 cm diameter and 1.5 cm in depth. **B:** Intraoperative picture of the same knee 2 years after grafting. The graft appears healthy.

compartmental osteoarthritis, spontaneous osteonecrosis of the knee, steroid-induced avascular necrosis of the femoral condyles, osteochondritis dissecans, and most commonly, traumatic defects. Grafts performed for trauma had the best results (10). Those done for primary osteoarthritis had poor results. Meyers and coworkers also had poor results with fresh grafts placed into osteoarthritic knees (27). Garret (15) produced excellent midterm results in treating patients with osteochondritis dissecans.

It may be concluded that posttraumatic defects and osteochondritis dissecans of the knee are the best indications for fresh grafting (6,8,9,15,17,25,27,30,41).

It has been our experience that the best results with fresh osteochondral allografts are in patients with unipolar posttraumatic defects and osteochondritis dissecans of the knee. At our institution osteochondral allografts are no longer used for treating osteoarthritis, spontaneous osteonecrosis, or steroid induced osteonecrosis, or in patients with inflammatory arthropathy. If the posttraumatic defect has been present for long enough to cause severe degenerative changes in the opposing articular surface, the graft is contraindicated. Also the patient must be compliant and capable of rehabilitation.

Age

Beaver et al (3), using Kaplan-Meier survivorship analysis, demonstrated that patients younger than 60 years of age with posttraumatic defects had better results with osteochondral allografts than patients older than 60 years. Fortunately, the great majority of posttrauma patients are in their second and third decades.

Site

The use of allografts for bipolar lesions (femur and tibia) has not been reported to be as successful as unipolar transplants (3,8,17,25,30,40). Patients therefore should be referred for surgery before secondary changes occur on the nontraumatized side.

Size

Recent advances in other techniques for cartilage repair and resurfacing, such as microfracture technique, autologous chondrocyte transplantation, osteochondral autografts, and periosteal grafts (6,

24,28,29,31,37), have reduced the role of allograft transplantation to defects larger than 3 cm in diameter and 1 cm deep (20).

Deformity

Most osteoarticular defects have a concomitant malalignment of the limb. In order to unload the compartment that has received the transplant, this malalignment should be addressed with a realignment osteotomy of the tibia or femur, as appropriate (18,19). For this purpose, a lateral-closing wedge high tibial osteotomy is performed for valgus realignment and a medial-closing wedge, distal femoral osteotomy is used to realign the limb into varus (20) (Fig. 32-2). Lately, the senior author has been using a medial-opening wedge high tibial osteotomy for valgus realignment and fixation with a Puddu plate (32) (Fig. 32-3). If indicated, the osteotomy should be performed at the same time as the osteochondral graft transplantation. Delayed osteotomy could be reserved as a salvage procedure for a deteriorating graft when the mechanical axis passes through the grafted compartment in very young patients (20).

PREOPERATIVE PLANNING

The preoperative assessment includes a clinical and radiographic evaluation of the injured knee. The presence of previous scars or hardware that needs to be taken out might determine the configuration of the skin incision.

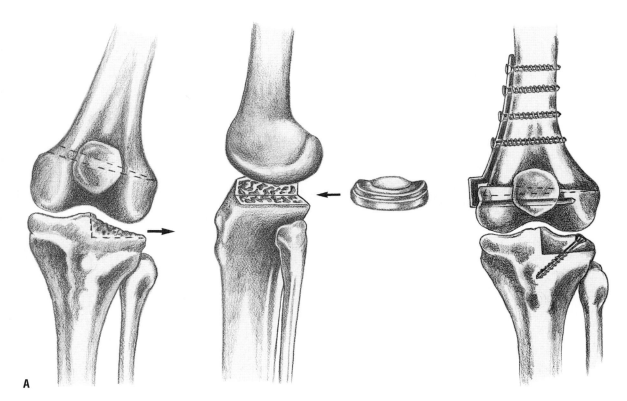

A   **B, C**

FIGURE 32-2

Lateral tibial plateau allograft and distal femoral varus osteotomy. **A:** Old fracture of lateral tibial plateau with secondary valgus deformity. **B:** The plateau is resected to healthy cancellous bone, and the lateral plateau osteochondral allograft is inserted. **C:** The lateral tibial plateau allograft is fixed with two 4.0-mm cancellous screws. A distal femoral varus osteotomy is performed to decompress the lateral compartment after the allograft is fixed.

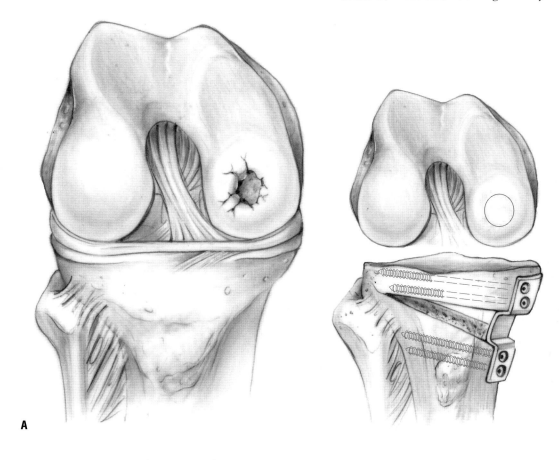

A

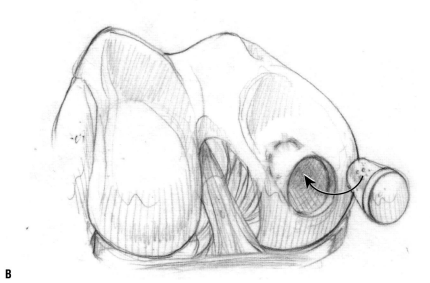

B

C

FIGURE 32-3

A: Osteochondral defect of the medial femoral condyle. **B:** Press-fit osteochondral allograft implantation in the defect. **C:** Medial-opening wedge high tibial osteotomy and fixation with a Puddu plate.

Routine views of the knee and a 3-foot standing radiograph will provide the data necessary to estimate the location, size, and structure of the defect and required graft. A careful assessment for the presence of degenerative changes and of the need to correct alignment must be done. The biomechanical axis is used to evaluate deformity and plan correction. Computed tomography (CT) scans and magnetic resonance imaging (MRI) are not required routinely but, if available, can help define the defect.

In some patients, previous arthroscopic data might help evaluate the size of the defect, secondary degenerative changes, and status of the opposing surface.

Graft Procurement and Handling

The local organ procurement agency (in our case The Trillium Gift of Life Network—Ontario's Organ and Tissue Donation Agency) identifies potential donors. The donor must meet the criteria outlined by the American Association of Tissue Banks (14). The donors must be less than 30 years old to provide healthy, viable cartilage and strong bone. Graft procurement is carried out within 24 hours of death, under strict aseptic conditions with the specimen consisting of the entire joint with the capsule intact. Before harvesting, standardized radiographs of the knee are obtained, and the recipient is matched to the donor with regard to size. Appropriate cultures (aerobic, anaerobic, fungal, and tuberculosis) and blood for serology are taken, but no tissue typing or HLA matching is performed. The graft is stored in a sealed container in sterile Ringer's lactate solution at 4°C with cefazolin (1 g) and bacitracin (50,000 U) per liter of solution.

The recipient patient is notified as soon as a donor has been located and is admitted to the hospital as prearranged. Implantation is performed within 48 hours of the harvest (graft procurement), but we are willing to extend it to 96 hours based on previous research (12,22,33,34).

SURGERY

Two surgical teams work simultaneously. One team performs the arthrotomy, while the other prepares the graft. The graft is prepared on a separate table with a separate set of instruments. At the time of soft-tissue removal, care must be taken to preserve the donor menisci and the articular cartilage. The osteochondral fragment is gradually shaped to fit the defect. It is kept in Ringer's lactate and antibiotics until implantation.

The patient is lying supine on a radiolucent table. One gram of cefazolin is given intravenously to the patient on induction of anaesthesia. The leg is prepared and draped to allow an extensile anterior approach, the old scars are marked, and the tourniquet is inflated. It is important after draping to have access to the anterior superior iliac spine by palpation and the ankle to evaluate alignment.

The Surgical Approach

A straight midline incision is performed if possible. This allows access to the defect site as well as permits a proximal tibia or distal femoral osteotomy, if one is indicated. Furthermore, the same midline incision can be used for possible future procedures, thus preserving the skin flap blood supply. If the knee has incisions other than midline, an alternative approach may be needed to avoid potential skin necrosis. The incision is approximately 25 to 35 cm long and is centered over the patella; proximally, it overlies the quadriceps tendon and distally, it overlies the tibial tubercle. Minor skin flaps are raised to facilitate later closure. A medial or lateral parapatellar arthrotomy is made, depending on the site of the defect. Where varus deformity exists, we prefer to perform a medial opening-wedge tibial osteotomy, but in the rare case where a lateral closing wedge is necessary, the skin incision is carried further distal to allow reflection of the muscles of the anterior tibial compartment. There is usually no difficulty doing a standard high tibial osteotomy through this approach. In the case of a distal varus femoral osteotomy, the medial aspect of the distal femur is approached through a midline skin incision and a subvastus approach is carried out.

Preparation of the Recipient Bed and Grafting

Once exposure is obtained, the reconstruction is straight forward and quite conservative. The articular defect is "squared off" with the goal of removing as little bone as possible. The resection is down to bleeding cancellous bone. Precise measurements are done and the graft is machined to fit the recipient bed accurately. The graft is orthotopic and the graft's articular surface has to lie flush

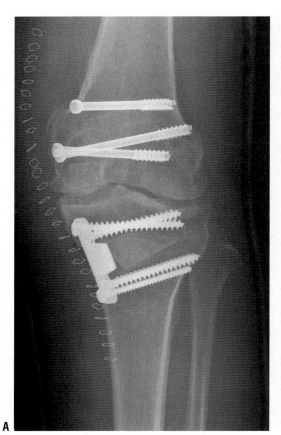
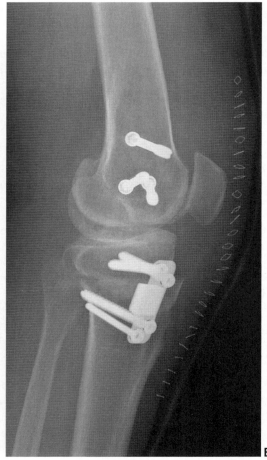

FIGURE 32-4

A: Anteroposterior knee radiograph of a medial femoral condyle allograft plug and an opening wedge high tibial osteotomy fixed with a Puddu plate. The distal femoral screws are from previous surgery. The opening wedge space has been filled with a mixture of cortical allograft and autologous bone. **B:** Lateral postoperative radiograph of the same knee.

with that of the host joint. Femoral allografts are usually inserted with a press-fit technique (Fig. 32-4), whereas tibial allograft stability has to be tested prior to fixation (Fig. 32-5). This is done by moving the knee slowly into full extension and flexion before internal fixation. If the graft fits well and is relatively stable in flexion and extension, it is fixed with two or three 4.0-mm partially threaded cancellous screws. Enough bone must be retained on the graft to accommodate screw fixation (at least 1 cm).

Realignment

According to the preoperative planning a realignment procedure should be carried out.

High Tibial Osteotomy (Medial-Opening Wedge)   If varus alignment exists, a lateral-closing wedge high tibial osteotomy is performed in concert with a medial femoral condyle graft for valgus realignment (19). Lately the senior author is using a medial-opening wedge high tibial osteotomy for valgus realignment and fixation with the Puddu plate (32) (see Fig. 32-4). The characteristic of this plate is that is has a spacer that fits into the osteotomy site. Calculating the degrees of correction will establish the width of the spacer to be used. It is important to aim for overcorrection from the physiologic valgus so that after the correction the mechanical axis of the lower limb passes 3 to 4 mm into the lateral tibiofemoral compartment.

A straight midline incision is performed from the upper pole of the patella to 4 to 6 cm distal to the tibial tubercle. Sharp dissection is done to the sartorius fascia, and the pes anserinus is retracted.

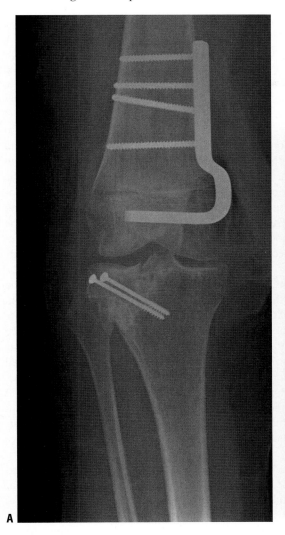
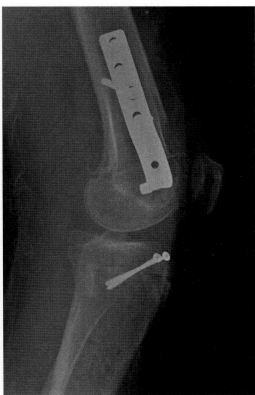

A   B

FIGURE 32-5

A: Anteroposterior knee radiograph of a lateral tibial plateau allograft and a distal femoral varus osteotomy showing screw fixation of the lateral tibial allograft. **B:** Lateral postoperative radiograph of the same knee.

A retractor is placed under the medial collateral ligament to expose the posteromedial aspect of the proximal tibia. This is further facilitated by knee flexion. Another retractor is placed under the patellar tendon.

A 3.0-mm osteotomy guide pin is inserted into the tibia from medial to lateral within 1 cm of the lateral cortex. The use of fluoroscopy is advised at this point. The pin should be 1 to 2 cm from the joint line. An osteotomy guide assembly is mounted onto the guidewire. A parallel guide sleeve assembly is inserted into the osteotomy guide in such a way so that it reproduces the existing anteroposterior slope of the tibia. Two distal pins are passed through the parallel guide sleeves (above the tibial tubercle) within 1 cm of the lateral tibia cortex. The sleeves and the osteotomy guide assembly are removed, and the cutting guide is placed over the pins. An oscillating saw is used to perform the osteotomy within 1 cm of the lateral cortex. Osteotome blades are used to complete the lateral aspect of the osteotomy but we aim to keep the lateral cortex intact. The osteotomy is confirmed by fluoroscopy. The osteotomy wedge is inserted with a mallet to the predetermined correction. Autologous bone graft from the iliac crest is packed into the osteotomy space. The plate is inserted between the wedge tines. The plate usually sits just anterior to the medial collateral ligament. Two 6.5-mm screws cancellous screws are inserted proximally. The tines are removed and two 4.5-mm cortical screws are inserted distally. More bone graft is packed in the osteotomy space if necessary. Anteroposterior and lateral radiographs are taken to confirm staple position and adequate correction.

Distal Femoral Varus Osteotomy   The distal femoral varus osteotomy that is performed concurrently with a lateral tibial plateau graft is a closing wedge osteotomy (18) (see Fig. 32-5). The medial aspect of the distal femur is approached through a midline skin incision and a subvastus approach is carried out. The fascia over the vastus medialis is incised. The muscle is dissected from the medial intermuscular septum and reflected anteriorly and laterally, exposing the medial aspect of the distal femoral shaft and the medial femoral condyle. A medial arthrotomy is made to enable visual control of the guidewires during the procedures.

The knee is flexed to 90 degrees· and a guidewire is inserted across the joint space from medial to lateral through the medial arthrotomy resting on the most distal aspect of the condyles. A second guidewire is inserted into the medial femoral condyle, parallel to the first guidewire and about 1 cm proximal to the femoral articulating surface. A third guidewire may be inserted through the patellofemoral compartment to mark the anterior part of the femoral articular surface. An anteroposterior radiograph or a view with an image intensifier is then made to confirm that the second guidewire is parallel to the articular surface. This is very important as the second wire guides the blade plate into the femoral condyles. The amount of correction achieved after the osteotomy depends on the angle of the blade plate with the condition that the blade is parallel to the femoral articular surface.

If the guidewire is in the correct position, three 4.5-mm drill holes are made on the cortex of the medial femoral condyle, along the line where the chisel will be inserted, to prevent comminution. The chisel is then inserted in the anterior half of the medial femoral condyle (to ensure that the plate is going to sit on the femoral shaft) at a point 2.0 to 2.5 cm from the distal femoral articular surface and to a depth of 50 to 70 mm, depending on the size of the distal part of the femur. The chisel is kept parallel to the second guidewire, which is parallel to the articulating surfaces. It is also aimed 10 to 15 degrees posteriorly to avoid cutting out at the anterior aspect of the lateral femoral condyle. The plate holder is used to guide the chisel and, as a guide, to obtain correct apposition of the plate to the long axis of the femur. After insertion of the chisel, anteroposterior and lateral radiographs are made if there is any doubt as to the position of the chisel. Visualization through the medial (or lateral) arthrotomy can confirm that the chisel has not penetrated the intercondylar notch or the anterior part of the femoral articular surface.

The femoral osteotomy is done from the medial side, just proximal to the adductor tubercle and the anterior part of the femoral articular surface, which may be easily palpated through the medial (or the lateral) arthrotomy. Using methylene blue, a line is drawn on the medial part of the femoral cortex parallel to the long axis of the femur, to extend proximally and distally to the line of the osteotomy. This line is used to ensure the correct rotational alignment of the femur after completion of the osteotomy.

The cut in the medial part of the femoral cortex is made with an oscillating saw. The lateral part of the cortex is perforated at several points with a drill bit and, if needed, a small osteotome. This allows easier correction of the deformity while it prevents lateral translocation of the proximal fragment. A medially based wedge of bone is then removed from the proximal femoral fragment. The base of the wedge should be 5 to 10 mm wide, or just wide enough to allow a 90-degree angle between the chisel and the medial part of the femoral cortex after the wedge is removed. With our technique, only a small wedge of bone is removed initially; the proximal cortical fragment can be easily impacted into the cancellous bone of the distal fragment because the diameter of the bone proximal to the osteotomy differs from that distal to the osteotomy. This allows an increase in the angle of the osteotomy if desired; it also provides more stability and promotes more rapid healing of the osteotomy.

The 90-degree offset dynamic compression blade plate is then inserted. Three sizes of the offset (10, 15, and 20 mm) are available. Therefore, selection of the plate depends on the length of blade and the degree of offset that is required, both of which can be measured from the radiographs, using the available templates for these plates. If, after inserting the blade, the plate cannot be brought into contact with the medial part of the femoral cortex, more bone is removed from the base of the wedge until contact is made. The bone that is removed from the wedge is cut into small pieces and used for grafting along the medial part of the femoral cortex. The screws are inserted according to the principles of the dynamic compression plate. The medial part of the femoral cortex and the distal femoral articular surface are then at 90 degrees to each other. This results in a tibiofemoral angle of approximately 0 degrees, which is the desired position. The vastus medialis is fastened back to the medial septum with interrupted sutures (Figs. 32-6 and 32-7).

Before closure, the knee is checked again for full range of motion, stability, and alignment.

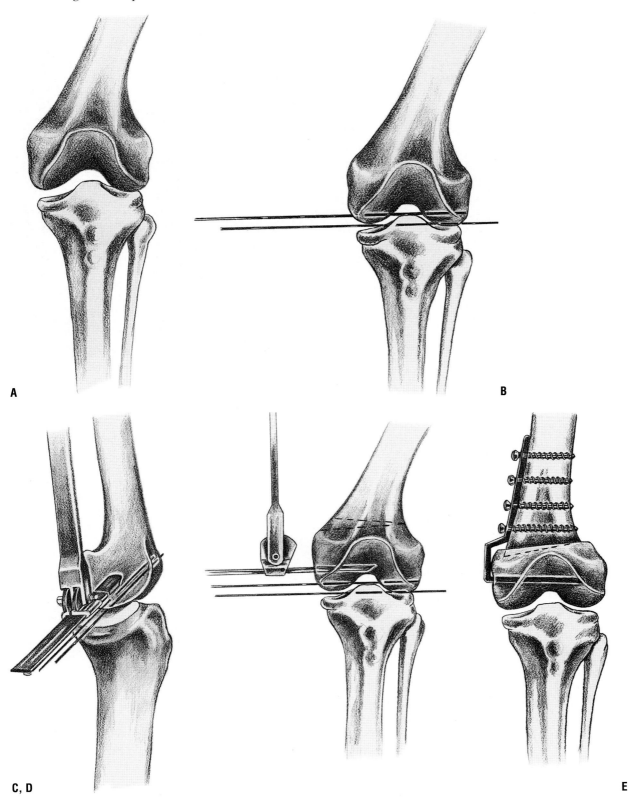

FIGURE 32-6

Technique of distal femoral varus osteotomy. **A:** Valgus knee. **B:** A guidewire is inserted parallel to the transcondylar axis of the distal femur 1 cm from the joint line and confirmed on a radiograph. **C:** Seating chisel for the blade plate is inserted 2.5 to 3 cm from the joint line, parallel to the guidewire. **D:** Osteotomy is performed parallel to the chisel at least 1.5 cm proximal and a 5-mm based wedge is removed. **E:** Osteotomy is held with a 90-degree offset blade plate.

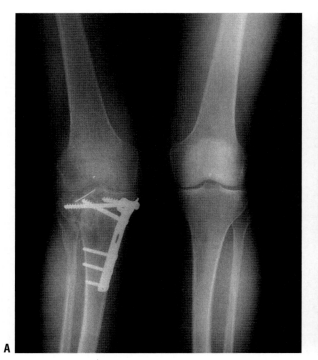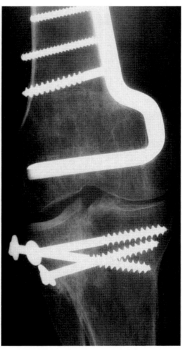

A

B

FIGURE 32-7

A: Anteroposterior radiographs of the right knee in a 31-year-old woman 2 years after open reduction and internal fixation of the lateral tibial plateau fracture. The lateral tibial plateau has collapsed, causing a secondary valgus deformity of the knee. **B:** Postoperative standing radiograph in the same patient at 8 years. A fresh lateral tibial plateau allograft has been fixed with three screws. A distal varus femoral osteotomy was done in conjunction with the allograft. The alignment of the knee is well corrected. The allograft is united and no evidence of resorption or fragmentation, and the joint space is maintained.

Closure

The tourniquet is deflated and careful hemostasis is done. The surgical site is well irrigated. The soft tissues are closed in layers with interrupted absorbable sutures over a vacuum drain. A Jones-type bandage is applied supplemented by an above knee full leg cast.

Pearls and Pitfalls

Tibial Graft Fixation When the graft is fixed to the recipient site with screws, we drill the first hole with a 2.5-mm drill bit and leave it in place while drilling the second hole. After inserting the screw into the second hole, the first drill bit is taken out and replaced by a screw. This sequence provides good stabilization of the small fragment while drilling the holes for the screws. Make sure that the screws do not interfere with other hardware, do not protrude into the soft tissues, and are not close to the articular surface.

Realignment Procedure The graft itself should not be used to correct alignment. This is achieved by an osteotomy either before or at the time of allograft implantation. This decision depends on whether the graft involves the same side of the joint as the osteotomy. When a realignment procedure is done at the same time of grafting, it should be carried out after graft fixation. If the realignment procedure involves the same side of the joint as the graft, is should be carried out several months before transplantation to allow sufficient time for revascularization of host bone.

POSTOPERATIVE MANAGEMENT

The drain is taken out after 24 hours, and the patient receives intravenous cefazolin for 5 days. The limb is placed in an above knee cylindrical fiberglass cast after 2 or 3 days. At 2 weeks the cast is removed, the patient is fitted with a hinged knee brace, and physiotherapy is begun. Physiotherapy consists of active and active-assisted range of motion exercises, isometric strengthening exercises, and non–weight-bearing ambulation with crutches for 3 months. No resisted exercises are performed until there is radiographic evidence that the osteotomy is healed.

RESULTS

The use of fresh osteochondral allograft for posttraumatic joint defects is based on long-term clinical and experimental evidence of maintenance of viability and function of chondrocytes as well as replacement of the grafted bone by host bone (17). Recent advances in other techniques for cartilage repair and resurfacing, such as microfracture technique, autologous chondrocyte transplantation, osteochondral autografts, and periosteal grafts (5,24,28,29,31,37), have reduced the indication of allograft tissue transplantation to defects larger than 3 cm in diameter and 1 cm in depth.

There are some disadvantages with the use of osteochondral allograft tissue. A well-organized transplant program is necessary. The surgery cannot be performed on an elective basis. Disease transmission in fresh allograft remains a concern. Risks are described to prospective recipients as equal to those for homologous blood transfusion (HIV 1:493,000 [39], HCV 1:103,000, HBV 1:63,000 [35]), although there are published estimates of lower risk (4). If the antigen test for viruses becomes precise enough to eliminate the window period for detection to less than 24 hours, then allograft tissue will become the tissue of choice for all the previously mentioned techniques because there is no sacrifice of host tissue and it is less expensive.

There are several advantages in using allograft tissue to repair osteochondral defects. There is no donor site morbidity. The exact size and shape of the osteochondral defect may also be duplicated using allograft tissue, and the use of multiple grafts is obviated.

Encouraging mid- to long-term results have been published related to the use of fresh osteochondral allograft for posttraumatic defect of the knee joint. In a recent report, survival of fresh femoral allografts has been reported to be 74% at 15 years with 61% of the patients achieving excellent or good functional outcomes. These results include development of degenerative joint disease as a cause of failure (20). Agnidis et al compared the Short Form-36 scores of 47 patients with transplants to large articular defects with normative data from an age-matched group. At an average of 12 years follow-up, the patients with transplants had favorable results in every category, and 93% considered their operation a success (1).

In an earlier study performed at the authors' institution (16), 126 knees of 123 patients with osteochondral defects secondary to trauma (111 cases) or osteochondritis dissecans (15 cases) were reviewed. The average age was 35 years (range, 15 to 64); there were 81 males and 42 females. The defects were located in the tibial plateau (55 lateral, six medial, and two combined medial and lateral), femoral condyle (27 medial and 23 lateral), bipolar tibial and femoral (seven lateral and one medial compartment) and patellofemoral (one in patellar groove of the femur and one in the patella). The grafts, which were between 8 and 40 mm thick, were fixed to good bleeding cancellous bone after resecting the defect. In 47 cases the meniscus was included in the transplant. Sixty-eight knees underwent osteotomy to correct alignment (37 distal femoral, 31 upper tibial). Patients were assessed clinically pre- and postoperatively, using a rating score based on subjective and objective criteria. Radiographic assessment included alignment, graft union, fracture and resorption, joint-space narrowing, and osteoarthritis.

The average follow-up was 7.5 years (range, 1 to 22). Failure was defined as a decrease in knee score or the need for further surgery. Kaplan-Meier survivorship analysis demonstrated 95% successful results at 5 years (95% confidence limits: 87 to 98), 71% at 10 years (95% confidence limits: 56 to 83), and 66% at 20 years (95% confidence limit: 50 to 81) (Fig. 32-8). Among 18 failures, one patient had an arthrodesis, eight had total knee replacement, one had removal of the graft, and eight experienced failure because of a decrease in score but still retain these grafts. The success rate was 85%.

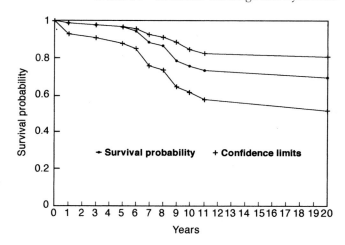

FIGURE 32-8

Kaplan Meier survivorship curve with 95% confidence limits (Greenwood's method).

COMPLICATIONS

In the previously described prospective cohort, five complications were noted and included three stiff knees, one wound hematoma, and one rupture of the patellar tendon. Long-range analysis reveals a statistically significant relationship of failure with bipolar grafts ($p < 0.05$) and patients receiving worker's compensation ($p = 0.0396$) but no significant relationship with other factors such as osteotomy, meniscus transplant, sex, and medial and lateral side of the knee.

In addition, analysis of variance in successful cases did not show any statistically significant effect of patient age or sex, postoperative complications, or preoperative scores. Radiographic assessment of 18 patients experiencing failure showed four collapsed grafts, seven patients with loss of joint space, and 10 with significant osteoarthritis.

Except for two instances of questionable union, all grafts solidly united to the host bone 6 to 12 months after surgery. Among clinically successful patients, we noted five instances of mild graft collapse (less than 3 mm), 11 of decreased joint space, and 18 of osteoarthritic changes.

Although most patients experiencing failure showed radiographic changes of collapse (four), joint-space narrowing (seven), and osteoarthritis (13), similar changes were found in some patients in whom the procedure was successful.

In a functional outcome study, the SF-36 scores of 47 patients with successful transplants were compared to normative data from an age-matched group (1). The greatest discrepancies in the SF-36 scores were in the categories of physical functioning and "role physical." Despite this, patients returned to a normal lifestyle, including leisure sports but not competitive sports.

A recent study was performed on 60 patients who were a minimum of 5 years (average, 10 years) from the time of transplantation of fresh osteochondral allografts of the femoral condyles (2). Excellent long-term survival has been demonstrated, with 85% (confidence limits, 41% to 100%) of cases surviving without further surgery at 10 years, and a projected survivorship of 74% at 15 years. Of the 12 patients with more than 15 years of follow-up, only four have failed. Of equal importance is the mean 10-year Hospital for Special Surgery (HSS) score of 83, with 84% of patients reporting good to excellent overall outcomes. The mean score for pain was 28 (mild pain requiring occasional analgesics), and most patients were able to walk more than 1 mile with few problems.

Overall, the high success rate in mid- to long-term follow-up of this procedure, which not only does not compromise salvage surgery but facilitates it by restoring bone stock, makes it an appropriate procedure for unipolar osteochondral defects of the knee secondary to trauma, or for osteochondritis dissecans in properly selected patients.

REFERENCES

1. Agnidis Z, Stimec J, Krajbich J, et al. Health-related quality-of-life following fresh osteochondral allograft of the knee: a minimum five-year follow-up. *J Bone Joint Surg.* 1999;81B(suppl 1):106.
2. Aubin PP, Cheah HK, Davis AM, et al. Long-term follow-up of fresh femoral osteochondral allografts for posttraumatic knee defects. *Clin Orthop Relat Res.* 2001;391(suppl):S318–S327.
3. Beaver RJ, Mahomed M, Backstein D, et al. Fresh osteochondral allografts for posttraumatic defects in the knee. A survivorship analysis. *J Bone Joint Surg.* 1992;74B:105–110.

4. Buck BE, Malinin TI, Brown MD. Bone transplantation and human immunodeficiency virus. An estimate of risk of acquired immunodeficiency syndrome (AIDS). *Clin Orthop Rel Res.* 1989;240:12–136.

5. Buckwalter JA, Mankin HJ. Articular cartilage repair and transplantation. *Arthritis Rheum.* 1998;41:1331–1342.

6. Bugbee WD, Converty FR. Osteochondral allograft transplantation. *Clin Sports Med.* 1999;18:67–75.

7. Campbell CJ, Ishida H, Takahashi H, Kelly F. The transplantation of articular cartilage. An experimental study in dogs. *J Bone Joint Surg.* 1963;45A:1579–1592.

8. Chu Cr, Convery FR, Akeson WH, et al. Articular cartilage transplantation. Clinical results in the knee. *Clin Orthop Rel Res.* 1999;360:159–168.

9. Convery FR, Akeson WH, Amiel D, et al. Long-term survival of chondrocytes in an osteochondral articular cartilage allograft. A case report. *J Bone Joint Surg.* 1996;78A:1082–1088.

10. Convery FR, Meyers MH, Akeson WH. Fresh osteochondral allografting of the femoral condyle. *Clin Orthop Relat Res.* 1991;273:139–145.

11. Czitrom AA, Keating S, Gross AE. The viability of articular cartilage in fresh osteochondral allografts after clinical transplantation. *J Bone Joint Surg.* 1990;72A:574–581.

12. DePalma AF, Tsaltas TT, Mauler GG. Viability of osteochondral grafts as determined by uptake of S^{35}. *J Bone Joint Surg.* 1963;45A:565–578.

13. Enneking WF, Mindell ER. Observations on massive retrieved human allografts. *J Bone Joint Surg.* 1991;73A:1123–1142.

14. Fawcett KJ, Barr HR, eds. Tissue banking. Arlington, VA: American Association of Blood Banks; 1987:97–107.

15. Garrett JC. Fresh osteochondral allografts for treatment of articular defects in osteochondritis dissecans of the lateral femoral condyle in adults. *Clin Orthop Relat Res.* 1994;303:33–37.

16. Ghazavi MT, Pritzker KP, Davis AM, et al. Fresh osteochondral allografts for post-traumatic osteochondral defects of the knee. *J Bone Joint Surg.* 1997;79B:1008–1013.

17. Gross AE. Use of fresh osteochondral allografts to replace traumatic joint defects. In: Czitrom AA, Gross AE, eds. *Allografts in orthopaedic practice.* Baltimore: Williams & Wilkins;1992: 67–82.

18. Gross AE, Hutchison CR. Realignment osteotomy of the knee. Part 1: Distal femoral varus osteotomy for osteoarthritis of the valgus knee. *Oper Tech Sports Med.* 2000;8:122–126.

19. Gross AE, Hutchison CR. Realignment osteotomy of the knee. Part 2: Proximal valgus tibial osteotomy for osteoarthritis of the varus knee. *Oper Tech Sports Med.* 2000;8:127–130.

20. Gross AE, Shasha N, Aubin P. Long-term follow-up of the use of fresh osteochondral allografts for posttraumatic knee defects. *Clin Orthop Relat Res.* 2005;435:79–87.

21. Kandel RA, Gross AE, Ganel A, et al. Histopathology of failed osteoarticular shell allografts. *Clin Orthop Relat Res.* 1985;197:103–110.

22. Kwan MK, Wayne JS, Woo SL, et al. Histological and biomechanical assessment of articular cartilage from stored osteochondral shell allografts *J Orthop Res.* 1989;7:637–644.

23. Langer F, Czitrom A, Pritzker KP, Gross AE. The immunogenicity of fresh and frozen allogeneic bone. *J Bone Joint Surg.* 1975;57A:216–20.

24. Mandelbaum BR, Browne JE, Fu F, et al. Articular cartilage lesions of the knee. *Am J Sports Med.* 1998;26:853–861.

25. McDermott AG, Langer F Pritzker KP, et al. Fresh small-fragment osteochondral allografts: Long-term follow-up study on first 100 cases. *Clin Orthop Rel Res.* 1985;197:96–102.

26. McGoveran BM, Pritzker KPH, Shasha N, et al. Long-term chondrocyte viability in a fresh osteochondral allograft. *J Knee Surg.* 2002;15:97–100.

27. Meyers MH, Akeson W, Convery FR. Resurfacing of the knee with fresh osteochondral allograft. *J Bone Joint Surg.* 1989;71A:704–713.

28. Moran ME, Kim HK, Salter RB. Biological resurfacing of full-thickness defects in patellar articular cartilage of the rabbit. Investigation of autogenous periosteal grafts subjected to continuous passive motion. *J Bone Joint Surg.* 1992;74B:659–667.

29. Newman AP. Articular cartilage repair. *Am J Sports Med.* 1998;26:309–324.

30. Oakeshott RD, Farine I. Pritzker KP, et al. A clinical and histologic analysis of failed fresh osteochondral allografts. *Clin Orthop Rel Res.* 1988;233:283–294.

31. O'Driscoll SW. The healing and regeneration of articular cartilage. *J Bone Joint Surg.* 1998;80A:1795–1812.

32. Puddu G, Franco V, Cipolla M, et al. Opening wedge osteotomy. Proximal tibia and distal femur. In Jackson DW, ed. *Master techniques in orthopaedic surgery: reconstructive knee surgery.* 2nd ed. Philadelphia: Lippincott Williams & Wilkins; 2000:375–390.

33. Rodrigo JJ, Thompson E, Travis C. Deep-freezing versus 4 degrees preservation of avascular osteocartilaginous shell allografts in rats. *Clin Orthop Relat Res.* 1987;218:268–275.

34. Schachar N, McAllister D, Stevenson M, et al. Metabolic and biochemical status of articular cartilage following cryopreservation and transplantation: a rabbit model. *J Orthop Res.* 1992;10:603–609.

35. Schreiber GB, Busch MP, Kleinman SH, et al. The risk of transfusion-transmitted viral infections. The Retrovirus Epidemiology Donor Study. *N Engl J Med.* 1996;334:1685–1690.

36. Shasha N, Aubin PP, Cheah HK, et al. Long-term clinical experience with fresh osteochondral allografts for articular knee defects in high-demand patients. *Cell Tissue Bank.* 2002;3:175–182.

37. Steadman JR, Rodkey WG, Briggs KK. Microfracture to treat full-thickness chondral defects: surgical technique, rehabilitation, and outcomes. *J Knee Surg.* 2002;15:170–176.

38. Stevenson S, Dannucci GA, Sharkey NA, et al. The fate of articular cartilage after transplantation of fresh and cryopreserved tissue-antigen-matched and mismatched osteochondral allografts in dogs. *J Bone Joint Surg.* 1989;71A:1297–1307.

39. Tomford WW. Transmission of disease through transplantation of musculoskeletal allografts. *J Bone Joint Surg.* 1995;77A:1742–1754.

40. Zukor DJ, Oakeshott RD, Gross AE. Osteochondral allograft reconstrucion of musculoskeletal allografts. Part 2: Experience with successful and failed osteochondral allografts. *Am J Knee Surg.* 1980;2:182–191.

41. Zukor DJ, Paitich B, Oakeshott RD, et al. Reconstruction of posttraumatic articular surface defects using fresh small-fragment osteochondral allografts. In: Aebi M, Regazzoni P, eds. *Bone transplantation.* New York: Springer-Verlag, 1989.

33 Allograft Osteochondral Plugs

William Bugbee

Fresh osteochondral allografts are becoming increasingly popular in articular cartilage reconstruction in the knee. The ability to restore diseased or damaged cartilage with mature hyaline cartilage tissue is attractive, and the surgical technique for implanting plugs or dowel-type grafts in simple femoral condyle lesions is fairly straightforward. A large body of basic science and clinical outcome data support the use of fresh osteochondral allografts in clinical practice (3).

INDICATIONS/CONTRAINDICATIONS

Fresh osteochondral allografts possess the ability to restore a wide spectrum of articular and osteoarticular pathology, as a result, the clinical indications cover a broad range of pathology. As is true for other restorative procedures, in addition to evaluating the particular articular lesion, the careful assessment of the entire joint, as well as the individual, is important. Many proposed treatment algorithms suggest the use of allografts for large lesions (>2 or 3 cm) or for salvage in difficult reconstructive situations where bone loss is also present. In our experience, allografts can be considered as a primary treatment option for osteochondral lesions greater than 2 cm (approximately) in diameter, as is typically seen in osteochondritis dissecans (OCD) and osteonecrosis. Fresh allografts are also useful as a salvage procedure when other cartilage-restorative procedures, such as microfracture, osteoarticular transfer system (OATS), and autologous chondrocyte implantation, have been unsuccessful.

Additionally, allografts often are used for salvage reconstruction of post traumatic defects of the tibial plateau or the femoral condyle. Other indications for allografting in the knee include treatment of patellofemoral chondrosis or arthrosis and in very select cases of unicompartmental tibiofemoral arthrosis (Table 33-1).

Relative contraindications to the allografting procedure include uncorrected joint instability or uncorrected malalignment of the limb. An allograft may be considered in combination or as part of a staged procedure in these settings. Allografting should not be considered an alternative to prosthetic arthroplasty in an individual with symptoms and acceptable age and activity level for prosthetic replacement. In the younger individual, bipolar and multicompartmental allografting have been modestly successful. The presence of inflammatory disease or crystal-induced arthropathy is considered a relative contraindication, as well as is any unexplained synovitis. The use of fresh osteochondral allografts in individuals with altered bone metabolism, such as is seen in chronic steroid use, smoking, or even nonsteroidal anti-inflammatory agents, has not been studied extensively. Unlike other cartilage procedures, relative size of the lesion (large or small) is not considered a contraindication to allografting.

PREOPERATIVE PLANNING

Common to all fresh allografting procedures is matching the donor with recipient. This is done on the basis of size. In the knee, an anteroposterior radiograph with a magnification marker is used, and a mea-

TABLE 33-1.   Major Indications for Fresh Osteochondral Allografting of the Femoral Condyle

1. Chondral lesions: traumatic or degenerative
2. Osteochondritis dissecans
3. Post fracture reconstruction
4. Osteonecrosis
5. Salvage of previous cartilage procedure (microfracture, OATS, autologous chondrocyte implantation)

surement of the medial-lateral dimension of the tibia, just below the joint surface, is made (Fig. 33-1). This corrected measurement is used, and the tissue bank makes a direct measurement on the donor tibial plateau. Alternatively, a measurement of the affected condyle can be performed. A match is considered acceptable at ± 2 mm; however, it should be noted that there is a significant variability in anatomy that is not reflected in size measurements. In particular, in treating OCD, the pathologic condyle typically is larger, wider, and flatter; therefore, a larger donor generally should be used. When using allograft plugs or dowels, one is generally safe with a larger donor. Small donor condyles lead to problems with matching radius of curvature, particularly for grafts over 20 mm in diameter. Most femoral condyle lesions can be treated using dowel-type grafts. Commercially available instruments (Arthrex, Naples, FL) simplify the preparation, harvesting, and insertion of these grafts, which may be up to 35 mm in size (Fig. 33-2). Perhaps the most important step in preoperative planning is understanding that one is using human tissue and performing a transplantation. Respect for the donation process, understanding the recovery, processing, and safety issues are minimum requirements necessary for the surgeon wishing to use fresh allograft tissue.

SURGERY

For most femoral condyle lesions, allografting can be performed through a miniarthrotomy. In most situations, a diagnostic arthroscopy has been performed recently and is not a necessary component of the allografting procedure. However, if there are any unanswered questions regarding meniscal status, or the status of the other compartments, a diagnostic arthroscopy can be performed prior to the allografting procedure. Examination under anesthesia is done in the standard fashion, as is the diagnostic arthroscopy when the surgeon feels this is indicated. Only rarely do we perform arthroscopy, as adequate data have typically been collected prior to beginning the process of graft acquisition.

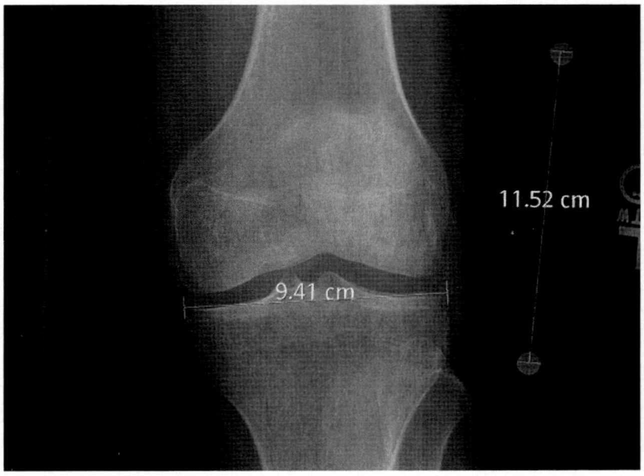

FIGURE 33-1

Radiographic technique for graft sizing. In this example the corrected tibial width is 81 mm (9.41 × 10/11.52).

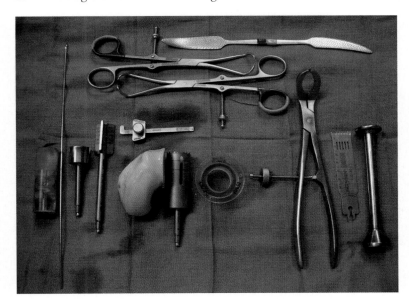

FIGURE 33-2
Commonly used instruments for allograft plug
technique.

Patient Positioning

The patient is positioned supine, with a tourniquet on the thigh. A leg holder is valuable in this procedure to position the leg in between 70 and 100 degrees of flexion, and to access the lesion (Fig. 33-3). At least one surgical assistant is necessary to provide adequate retraction and leg position for working through the mobile window of the small arthrotomy.

Technique

The fresh graft is inspected to confirm the adequacy of the size match and quality of the tissue prior to opening the knee joint. It is important to keep the graft moist during the procedure; generally, it is left in the packaging media when not being instrumented.

A midline incision is made with the knee in flexion from the center of the patella to the tip of the tibial tubercle. This incision is preferred in anticipation of further surgery in the patient's lifetime. This incision is elevated subcutaneously, either medially or laterally to the patellar tendon, depending on the location of the lesion (either medial or lateral). A retinacular incision is then made from the superior aspect of the patella inferiorly. Great care is taken to enter the joint and to incise the fat pad without disrupting the anterior horn of the meniscus. In some cases in which the lesion is posterior or very large, the meniscus must be detached and reflected; generally, this can be done safely, leaving a small cuff of tissue adjacent to the anterior attachment of the meniscus for later repair. This is most common for large OCD lesions of the lateral femoral condyle.

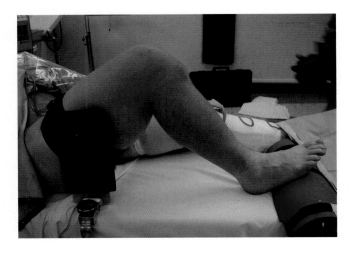

FIGURE 33-3

Position of the leg for access to a
typical medial femoral condyle
lesion.

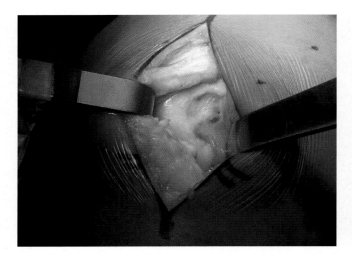

FIGURE 33-4

Miniarthrotomy with Z retractor and bent Hohman in notch, exposing the OCD lesion of the medial femoral condyle.

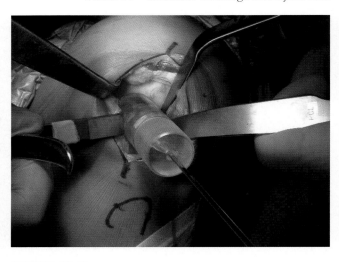

FIGURE 33-5

Guidewire in place and sizing dowel measuring lesion diameter.

Once the joint capsule and synovium have been incised and the joint has been entered, retractors are placed medially and laterally. Care is taken in the positioning of the retractor within the notch to protect the cruciate ligaments and the articular cartilage. This notch retractor is essential to adequate mobilization of the patella. The knee is then flexed and/or extended until the proper degree of flexion is noted that presents the lesion into the arthrotomy site (Fig. 33-4). Excessive degrees of flexion limit the ability to mobilize the patella. If access is difficult, extending the arthrotomy proximal is warranted. The lesion then is inspected and palpated with a probe to determine the extent, margins, and maximum size. After a size determination is made, a guidewire is driven into the center of the lesion, perpendicular to the curvature of the articular surface. It is critical to place the guidewire perpendicular to the joint surface. The size of the proposed graft is determined using sizing dowels (Fig. 33-5), the remaining articular cartilage is scored, and a coring drill is used to remove the remaining articular cartilage and 3 to 4 mm of subchondral bone (Figs. 33-6 and 33-7). In deeper lesions, the pathologic bone is removed until there is healthy, bleeding bone. In cases of very deep lesions, the depth of this coring should not exceed 10 mm, and bone grafting should be performed to fill any deeper or more extensive osseous defects. Our experience suggests that the minimal amount of allograft bone should be transplanted, and our grafts are rarely more than 5 to 8 mm in thickness.

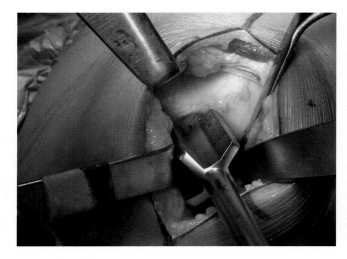

FIGURE 33-6

The cutting reamer placed over the guidewire with soft tissues well protected.

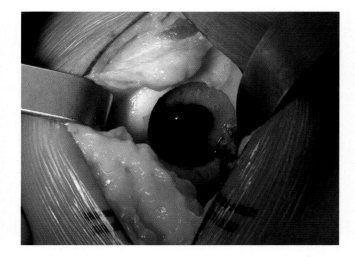

FIGURE 33-7

Recipient socket after preparation. Note the minimal depth.

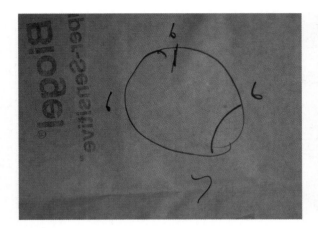

FIGURE 33-8

Depth map of recipient site. The position of the free edge is marked.

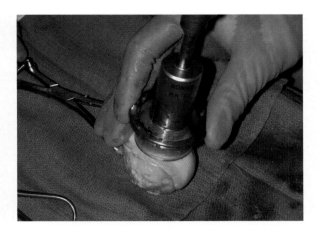

FIGURE 33-9

Harvesting of the plug from the allograft condyle. The graft and guide are held as one unit.

The guide pin then is removed, depth measurements are made in the four quadrants of the prepared recipient site, and a simple map is created (Fig. 33-8).The corresponding anatomic location of the recipient site then is identified on the graft. The graft is placed into a graft holder (or alternately, held with bone-holding forceps). A saw guide then is placed in the appropriate position, again perpendicular to the articular surface; and an appropriate sized tube saw is used to core out the graft (Figs. 33-9 and 33-10). Prior to removing the graft from the condyle, an identifying mark is made to ensure proper orientation. Once the graft is removed, depth measurements, which were taken from the recipient, are transferred to the graft; this graft then is cut with an oscillating saw, and then trimmed with a rasp to the appropriate thickness in all four quadrants (Figs. 33-11 and 33-12). Often, this must be done multiple times to ensure precise thickness and to match the prepared defect in the patient.

The graft now is irrigated copiously with a high-pressure lavage to remove all marrow elements, and the recipient site is dilated to ease the insertion of the graft and to prevent excessive impact loading of the articular surface when the graft is inserted. At this point, any remaining osseous defects are grafted.

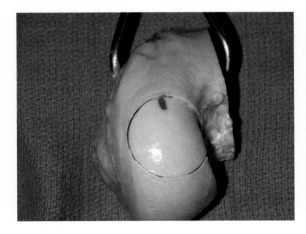

FIGURE 33-10

Allograft plug is marked and ready for removal from condyle.

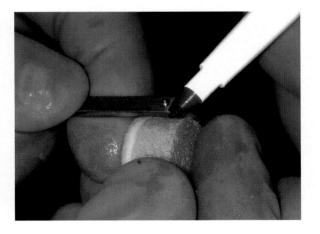

FIGURE 33-11

Depth measurements from the recipient socket are transferred to the plug.

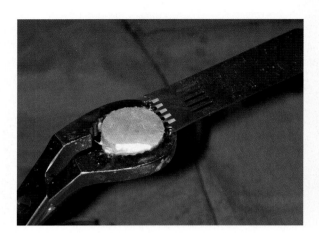

FIGURE 33-12
Allograft plug is trimmed carefully to the appropriate thickness.

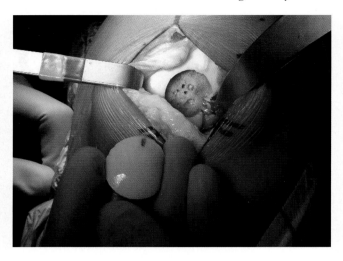

FIGURE 33-13
After lavage the graft is ready for implantation. Correct rotation is determined.

The graft is then inserted by hand in the appropriate rotation and is gently tamped in place until it is flush (Figs. 33-13 and 33-14). Recent studies have shown that impact loading during insertion of osteochondral grafts causes chondrocyte death (1). Thus, gentle manual pressure followed by joint range of motion may be a more reasonable method of graft insertion. If the graft does not fit, re-fashioning of either the recipient site (deepening or dilating) or the graft itself (tapering or thinning) is performed carefully. An excessively tight fit is not necessary. We accept mismatches of no more than 1 mm from flush with the surrounding joint surfaces and avoid countersinking of the graft.

Once the graft is seated, a determination is made whether additional fixation is required. If the graft is captured and not rocking with direct pressure, then no further fixation is generally required. Absorbable polydioxanone pins or chondral darts can be used, particularly if the graft is large or has an exposed edge within the notch (Fig. 33-15). We have used small diameter absorbable pins through the graft surface for years without any deleterious effect. Occasionally, the graft needs to be trimmed in the notch region to prevent impingement. The knee is then brought through a complete range of motion to confirm that the graft is stable and there is no catching or soft-tissue obstruction

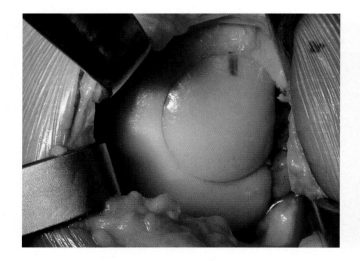

FIGURE 33-14
The graft is seated and rotation, step-off, and stability are checked. At this time the joint is carried through a range of motion to completely seat the graft.

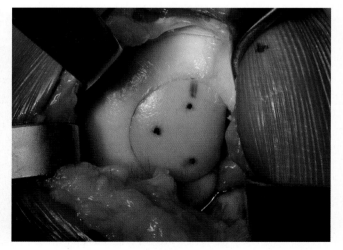

FIGURE 33-15
Three PDS pins have been placed through the graft for additional fixation.

noted. At this point, the wound is irrigated copiously, and routine closure is performed. We always use a small drain for 24 hours to prevent painful hemarthrosis from developing.

Lesions of the trochlea are approached in a similar manner; however, these are much more technically challenging, as the anatomy of the trochlea is much more complex, leading to technical issues in creating symmetric matching recipient sites and donor grafts. In this setting, extensive care must be taken to match the anatomic location and the angle of approach, as most larger grafts will end up being elliptical in shape due to the anatomy of the trochlear groove.

Pearls and Pitfalls

- Preoperative assessment of the biological and mechanical environment of the joint is critical. Be sure of the necessity of concomitant procedures, such as finding and removing loose bodies, meniscectomy or repair, anterior cruciate ligament reconstruction, and osteotomy.
- Adequate confirmation of appropriateness of the lesion for fresh osteochondral allografting is necessary. Don't be surprised by new or enlarging lesions.
- A careful, informed consent process, including risks of infection and disease transmission, should be in place.
- Confirm graft recipient match both in size and side. Do this before induction of anesthesia.
- Inspect the allograft before making an incision. If it is a small graft, don't try to make a big plug (30 mm) from it. The curvature will not match the recipient condyle.
- All cutting instruments should contact the condyle (recipient and graft) perpendicular to the articular surface.
- Use reamers rather than drills for all cutting and irrigate copiously.
- Save reamings for possible bone graft.
- For in-between sizes, always start preparing for the smaller graft. One can always enlarge the recipient site. Avoid removing too much normal cartilage.
- Two or more plug grafts can be placed overlapping for large lesions (snowman technique).
- Be prepared to use a freehand technique, if necessary, for large or posterior lesions.
- Minimize the osseous portion of the allograft at 3 to 6 mm. Use bone graft from the recipient site reaming (or the allograft) to fill any deeper defects.
- Always remove all soft tissue and perform pressurized lavage of graft prior to insertion.
- Avoid excessive impacting of the graft during insertion. Loose fitting grafts can be pinned.
- Use adjunctive fixation, including absorbable pins, chondral darts, or even screws.
- If the graft ends up too thin, remove it and add bone graft to the base of the recipient site. We prefer the graft flush, but 1 mm proud is better than 1 mm countersunk.
- Adequate and prolonged quadriceps rehabilitation is essential. Often these patients are multiply operated and have had a long period of disability prior to allografting.
- Nonunion of the graft is very rare. Late fragmentation is a more common event.

POSTOPERATIVE MANAGEMENT AND REHABILITATION

The rehabilitation of the knee allograft patient in the early postoperative period includes management of pain, swelling, restoration of limb control, and range of motion. Assuming rigid graft fixation, patients are allowed touch-down weight bearing for a minimum of 6 to 8 weeks postoperatively, or until bony union is determined by radiographs. For femoral condyle allografts, no bracing is needed; but if an osteotomy is performed, a hinged range-of-motion brace is used for protection until healing is apparent. Weight bearing is progressed slowly between the second and fourth month, with full weight bearing using a cane or crutch. Continuous passive motion is considered optional. The main objective is restoration of range of motion and strengthening of the quadriceps/hamstrings using isometric exercises and avoidance of open-chain exercises. We use the stationary bicycle at 4 to 6 weeks in addition to pool therapy if available.

Clinical follow-up includes radiographs at 4 to 6 weeks, 3 months, 6 months, and yearly thereafter. Careful radiographic assessment of the graft-host interface is important. Any concern of delayed healing should lead to a more cautious approach to weight-bearing and other high-stress activities.

Patients will typically experience continued improvement over the first postoperative year and often continue to demonstrate functional improvement between years 1 and 2. This often depends on patient motivation, desired activity level, and adherence to a rehabilitation program. Return to sports and recreational activities is individualized in the period between 4 months and 1 year (Table 33-2).

TABLE 33-2.   Postoperative Management of Femoral Condyle Allografts

1. Non–weight-bearing, 6 to 12 weeks
2. Range-of-motion exercises
3. Quadriceps sets
4. Stationary bicycle at 4 weeks
5. Progressive weight bearing beginning 8 to 12 weeks
6. Sports/recreation at 6 months

COMPLICATIONS

Early complications unique to the allografting procedure are few. There does not appear to be any increased risk of surgical site infection with the use of allografts as compared with other procedures. The most unique issue regarding possible postoperative complications with fresh allografts relates to transmission of disease from the graft itself. In our series of over 500 allografts, we have yet to record a graft-associated bacterial or viral infection.

The use of a miniarthrotomy in the knee decreases the risk of postoperative stiffness. Occasionally, one sees a persistent effusion, which is typically a sign of over use, but which may indicate an immune-mediated synovitis. Delayed union or nonunion of the fresh allograft is the most common early finding. This is evidenced by persistent discomfort and/or visible graft-host interface on serial radiographic evaluation. Delayed or nonunion is more common in larger grafts, or in the setting of compromised bone, such as in the treatment of osteonecrosis. In this setting, patience is essential, as complete healing or recovery may take an extended period. Decreasing activities, the institution of weight-bearing precautions, and possible use of external bone stimulators may be helpful in the early management of a delayed healing. In this setting, careful evaluation of serial radiographs can provide insight into the healing process. Magnetic resonance imaging scans are rarely helpful, particularly before 6 months postoperatively, as they typically show extensive signal abnormality that is difficult to interpret. It should be noted that with adequate attention to postoperative weight-bearing restrictions and adequate graft fixation, delayed or nonunion requiring repeat surgical intervention within the first year is extremely uncommon. The natural history of the graft that fails to osseointegrate is unpredictable. Clinical symptoms may be minimal, or there may be progressive clinical deterioration and radiographic evidence of fragmentation, fracture, or collapse. Typical symptoms of this type of graft failure include increase of pain or sudden onset, often associated with minor trauma. Effusion, crepitus, or focal, localized pain are commonly seen. Careful evaluation of serial radiographs typically will demonstrate collapse, subsidence, fracture, or fragmentation. Fresh osteochondral allografts rarely fail due to the cartilage portion of the graft; most failures originate within the osseous portion. It is important to note that the allografted joint may suffer from the same pathology that is present in any other joint, such as meniscus or ligamentous injury. It should also be noted that radiographic and magnetic resonance abnormalities are commonly noted, even in well-functioning allografts, and great care must be taken in interpreting and correlating the imaging studies with clinical findings.

Treatment options for failed allografts include observation, if the patient is minimally symptomatic and the joint is thought to be at low risk for further progression of disease. Arthroscopic evaluation and debridement also may be used. In many cases, revision allografting is performed and generally has led to a success rate equivalent to primary allografting. This appears to be one of the particular advantages to fresh osteochondral allografting, in that fresh allografting does not preclude a revision allograft as a salvage procedure for failure of the initial allograft.

RESULTS

We have reported the results of 69 knees in 66 patients with OCD of the femoral condyle, treated with fresh osteochondral allografts (Table 33-3). All allografts were implanted within 5 days of their recovery. Patients were prospectively evaluated using an 18-point modified D'Aubigne and Postel scale, which measures function, range of motion, and absence of pain, allotting 1 to 6 points each for a maximum of 18 points. Subjective assessment was performed with a patient questionnaire. There were 49 males and 17 females, with a mean age of 28 years (range, 15 to 54). Forty lesions

TABLE 33-3. Selected Outcomes—Osteochondral Allografting in the Knee					
Author	**Site of Lesion**	**Diagnosis/ Indication**	**Number of Patients**	**Mean Follow-up (Years)**	**Successful Outcome**
Meyers	Knee	Multiple	31	3.5	77%
Chu	Knee	Multiple	55	6.2	84% G/E
Ghazavi	Knee	Trauma	126	7.5	85% SVS
Aubin	Femur	Trauma	60	10.0	85% SVS
Görtz	Femur	Trauma	43	4.5	88% G/E
Garrett	Femur	OCD	17	2.9	94% G/E
Bugbee	Femur	OCD	69	5.2	80% G/E
Bugbee	Knee	Osteonecrosis	21	5.3	88% G/E
Park	Knee	Osteoarthrosis	37	5.3	76% G/E
Jamali	Patellofemoral	Multiple	29	4.5	52% G/E

G/E, good/excellent; OCD, osteochondritis dissecans; SVS, survivorship.
From Gortz S, Bugbee WD. Allografts in articular cartilage repair. *J Bone Joint Surg.* 2006;88:1374–1384. With permission.

involved the medial femoral condyle and 29 the lateral femoral condyle. An average of 1.6 surgeries had been performed on the knee prior to the allograft procedure. Allograft size was highly variable, with a range from 1 to 13 cm^2. The average allograft size was 7.4 cm^2. Six knees were lost to follow-up. Mean follow-up in the remaining 63 knees was 4.3 years (range 1 to 14). Overall, 50/69 (79%) knees were rated good or excellent, scoring 15 or above on the 18-point scale; 11/69 (17%) were rated fair; and 2/69 (3%) were rated poor. The average clinical score improved from 12.9 preoperatively to 16.1 postoperatively ($p < 0.01$). Six patients had reoperations on the allograft, one was converted to total knee arthroplasty, and five underwent revision allografting at 1, 2, 5, 7, and 8 years after the initial allograft. Thirty-six of 66 patients completed questionnaires: 95% reported satisfaction with their treatment; 86% felt they were significantly improved. Subjective knee function improved from a mean of 3.2 to 7.8 on a 10-point scale.

Between 1997 and 2004, 43 patients with isolated cartilage lesions of the femoral condyle were treated with fresh osteochondral allografting at our institution. The study population included 23 males and 20 females and had a mean age of 35 years. Twenty-nine lesions involved the medial femoral condyle, 13 the lateral femoral condyle, and one was bilateral. All patients had undergone prior surgery. Mean allograft area was 5.9 cm^2. Thirty-eight of 43 (88%) were considered successful (score 15 or greater on the 18-point modified D'Aubigne and Postel scale) at mean 4.5 years of follow-up.

SUMMARY

Fresh osteochondral allograft plugs are useful for a wide variety of chondral and osteochondral lesions of the femoral condyle of the knee. The surgical technique is straightforward but does require special instruments and careful attention to detail. Postoperative management is not complex and complications are uncommon.

RECOMMENDED READING

Gortz S, Bugbee WD. Allografts in articular cartilage repair. *J Bone Joint Surg.* 2006;88:1374–1384.
Görtz S, Ho A, Bugbee WD. Fresh osteochondral allograft transplantation for cartilage lesions in the knee. American Academy of Orthopaedic Surgeons 73rd Annual Meeting, Paper A151, 2006.

REFERENCES

1. Borazjani BH, Chen AC, et al. Effect of impact on chondrocyte viability during insertion of human osteochondral grafts. *J Bone Joint Surg Am.* 2006;88:1934–1943.
2. Emmerson BC, Jamali A, Bugbee WD. Fresh osteochondral allografting in the treatment of osteochondritis dissecans of the femoral condyle. *Am J Sports Med.* 2007;35:907–914.
3. Gortz S, Bugbee WD. Fresh osteochondral allografting: graft processing and clinical applications. J Knee Surg. 2006;19:231–240.

34 Osteochondritis Dissecans of the Knee

Frederick M. Azar and S. Terry Canale

Osteochondritis dissecans (OCD) of the knee is a common entity in both adults and children. Its incidence has historically been estimated to be between 0.02% and 0.03% based on knee radiographs, and 1.2% based on knee arthroscopy (5,11,27). More recent investigators have reported much higher frequencies (1,21). Osteochondritis dissecans occurs twice as often in males as in females. Osteochondritis dissecans is most common in the medial femoral condyle, followed by the lateral femoral condyle; its occurrence in the patella is rare. It primarily affects young athletic individuals and can significantly impair knee function and activity and lead to long-term disability (10).

The etiology of OCD is controversial and remains unclear. Theories include ischemia, repetitive microtrauma, familial predisposition, endocrine imbalance, epiphyseal abnormalities, accessory centers of ossification, growth disorders, osteochondral fracture, repetitive microtrauma with subsequent interruption of interosseous blood supply to the subchondral area of the epiphysis, anatomic variations in the knee, and congenitally abnormal subchondral bone.

It is important to distinguish OCD from acute osteochondral fracture (Fig. 34-1). In addition, an OCD lesion that has separated from a vascular bony bed should be distinguished from one that has separated from an avascular bony bed (osteonecrosis). Osteochondritis dissecans is more common in adolescents and young adults than is osteonecrosis.

Several classification schemes for OCD have been proposed. Bradley and Dandy (5) developed a classification for the knee and limited the term OCD to expanding concentric lesions of the medial femoral condyle that appear during the second decade of life and progress to concave, steep-sided defects. Cahill and Berg (6) proposed a classification scheme based on the appearance of the lesion on scintigraphy. Dipaola et al (12) classified lesions according to their appearance on magnetic resonance imaging (MRI) and associated specific findings with the potential for fragment detachment. Guhl (19) developed an intraoperative classification based on cartilage integrity and fragment stability noted at the time of arthroscopy.

Although the natural history of these lesions has not been conclusively defined, current evidence suggests that they persist and can lead to further cartilage degradation (32). Primary prognostic factors, in addition to the age of the patient, include progression, size, stability, amount of subchondral bone present, and location of the lesion, especially as it relates to weight bearing. Lateral femoral condylar lesions tend to be more posterior, larger, less stable, and more fragmented than medial lesions.

Although nonoperative treatment has a limited role in patients with symptomatic osteochondral lesions, multiple forms of nonoperative treatment have been described, including periods of immobilization, activity modification, and non-weight bearing. Prolonged immobilization should be avoided because joint motion affects articular cartilage attrition. Cahill et al (7) noted a 50% failure rate with conservative treatment in a juvenile population with OCD.

A number of operative procedures have been devised for treatment of OCD, ranging from simple debridement to autograft/allograft or chondrocyte implantation (Table 34-1). Arthroscopy is preferable to arthrotomy; however, it may be necessary to convert an arthroscopic procedure to an arthroscopic-assisted mini arthrotomy to obtain adequate fixation of an unstable lesion.

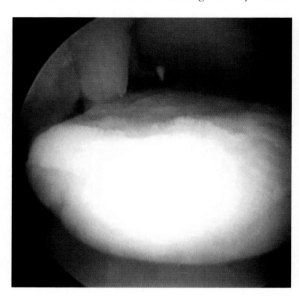

FIGURE 34-1
Unstable lesion that requires fixation.

INDICATIONS/CONTRAINDICATIONS

See Table 34-1 for surgical treatment options and their indications.

There are few contraindications to surgical treatment of OCD. Contraindications to specific surgical techniques may include the size of the lesion, with some procedures suited for only small (<2 cm^2) lesions; the activity demands of the patient (high vs. low demand), and the age of the patient (osteochondral allo- and autografts, autologous chondrocyte implantation usually not indicated in patients with open physes). The location of the lesion also may be a contraindication to a particular technique. Patient willingness to comply with postoperative weight-bearing restrictions also must be considered.

PREOPERATIVE PLANNING

History and Physical Examination

The most common complaint of patients with OCD is pain, which usually is difficult to localize and typically is present for several months. Patients also may report swelling or mechanical symptoms such as catching and popping if the lesion is partially or completely separated. Approximately 80% of juvenile patients have symptoms for an average of 14 months before initial presentation. A history of trauma to the knee is given by 40% to 60% of patients (8). Examination also may reveal effusion, joint line tenderness or tenderness over the lesion, limitation of motion, a positive McMurray's sign, and quadriceps atrophy. The patient may walk with an externally rotated gait to avoid contact of the medial femoral condyle with the medial tibial spine. A thorough history and physical examination are necessary to rule out other causes of knee pathology.

Imaging

Imaging techniques are important not only for diagnosis but for treatment decision-making. The size, location, and stability of the lesion are critical to choosing the appropriate technique.

Radiographs   Most OCD lesions can be easily identified on plain radiographs. Anteroposterior, lateral, notch or tunnel, and patellofemoral views are recommended. Most lesions occur in the lateral portion of the medial femoral condyle, and they are more clearly seen on the notch and lateral views. Lesions of the lateral femoral condyle tend to be more posterior than those in the medial

TABLE 34-1.	Surgical Treatment Options for Osteochondritis Dissecans of the Femoral Condyle		
Procedure	**Technique**	**Indications**	**Comments**
Arthroscopic debridement	Shaving of loose chondral flaps	Small defects (<2 cm^2) in areas of limited weight bearing	May provide short-term relief.
Internal fixation with K-wires, screws, biodegradable rods, or pins (arthroscopy or mini arthrotomy)	Removal of fibrous tissue from crater, antegrade or retrograde internal fixation. Cancellous graft from proximal tibia or femoral condyle can be added.	Unstable lesion, hinged or loose in crater.	Risk of hardware breakage or loosening, protruding hardware causing articular wear; second procedure may be needed for hardware removal.
Perichondral/periosteal graft	Graft harvested from distant (perichondrium) or adjacent (periosteum) site, implanted over defect to serve as joint buffer, source of mesenchymal stem cells	Small defect in non–weight-bearing area in young patient.	Long-term (5 to 10 year) results have been disappointing.
Abrasion chondroplasty/ microfracture	Arthroscopic drilling, microfracture with sharp awl, abrasion with a burr. Combined with removal of loose bodies and debridement of loose cartilage. Creation of bleeding surface to access pluripotential stem cells from marrow.	Younger patient Normal alignment Mechanical symptoms (catching, locking, swelling) Lesion <2 cm^2 with stable borders Good initial treatment	Results in mainly fibrocartilage matrix formation, which has more type I collagen, cannot withstand compressive and shear loads as well; may degenerate over time.
Osteochondral autograft (OATS, COR, mosaicplasty)	Transplantation of single or multiple plugs from areas with less weight-bearing to fill defects in areas with more weight-bearing function.	Defect ≤2 cm^2	Inability to treat large defects due to limited availability of donor cartilage. Potential problems from donor site.
Osteochondral allograft	Transplantation of single or multiple plugs from fresh allograft femoral condyles	Defect >2 to 3.5 cm^2 Isolated lesion Limited donor site Young patient	No morbidity from donor site, improved ability to shape and tailor graft. Risk of disease transmission.
Autologous chondrocyte implantation (ACI)	Cells obtained from arthroscopic cartilage biopsy, released from matrix and culture expanded, then placed in defect under periosteal patch.	Younger (15 to 55 years) patient Active patient Single or multiple defects 2 to 10 cm^2	Ligamentous or meniscal lesions, joint malalignment, patellofemoral instability must be corrected; complete meniscal deficit may be contraindication.

COR, chondral osseous replacement; OATS, osteochondral autograft transfer systems.

condyle (Fig. 34-2). The size of the lesion usually can be accurately determined on plain radiographs. Most small lesions are stable; lesions with a sclerotic margin of 3 mm or more and lesions larger than 0.8 cm^2 have an increased risk of being loose. Comparison radiographs should be obtained in juvenile and adolescent patients because an OCD lesion may be confused with ossification centers, which may cause transient symptoms but usually resolve spontaneously within 6 to 12 months. In addition, OCD is bilateral in approximately 30% of patients (Fig. 34-3).

Magnetic Resonance Imaging   Magnetic resonance imaging is recommended to determine the extent of the lesion. Common MRI characteristics include a high-signal-intensity line or cystic area beneath the lesion, a high-signal-intensity line through the articular cartilage, and a focal articular cartilage defect on T2-weighted spin echo and short tau inversion recovery (STIR) images

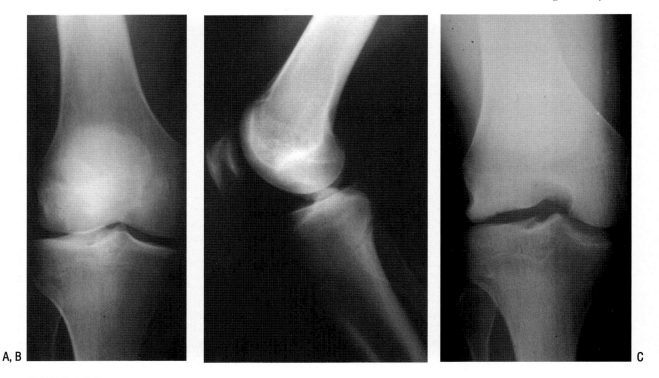

A, B   C

FIGURE 34-2

Recommended radiographic views for evaluation of OCD of the knee. **A:** Anteroposterior. **B:** Lateral. **C:** Tunnel.

(Fig. 34-4). Currently, a spoiled gradient (SPGR) echo sequence using fat suppression and three-dimensional acquisition is considered the optimal technique for evaluating articular cartilage lesions. The presence of fluid around the fragment or focal cystic areas beneath the fragment is the best indicator of instability; the absence of a zone of high-signal intensity at the interface of the fragment and the bone is a reliable sign of lesion stability (28). Magnetic resonance imaging also is useful for identification of associated ligamentous and meniscal injuries.

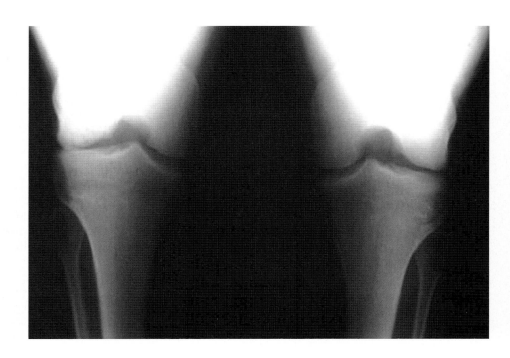

FIGURE 34-3

Bilateral OCD lesions of lateral femoral condyles.

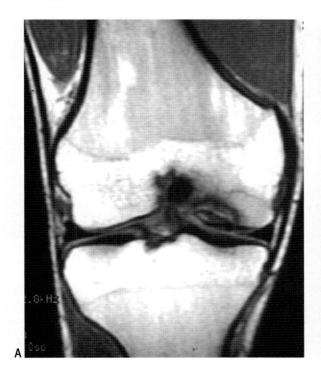
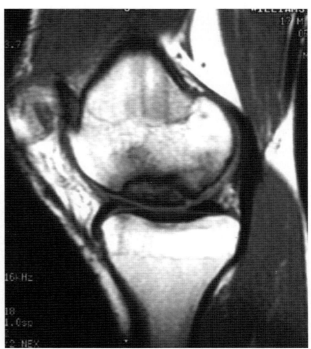

FIGURE 34-4
MRI evaluation of OCD. **A:** AP-coronal plane view. **B:** Lateral sagittal plane view.

Computed Tomography Scanning   Computed tomography (CT) scanning can delineate the bony contours and allow determination of the amount of cortical bone present in the osteochondral fragment (8). Healing potential is determined by the quantity of bone attached to the major fragment, and healing can be followed with tomograms until union.

Bone Scanning   Bone scanning (technetium bone scintigraphy) may be helpful to determine the extent of activity within the lesion and to monitor progress of healing (6,37). This has been shown to be more reliable in patients with open physes than in skeletally mature patients.

SURGERY

Patient Positioning

The patient is placed supine with the prepared and draped limb angled off the lateral aspect of the table; a leg holder or lateral post can be used.

Technique

- Typically, a 30-degree arthroscope is used, although a 70-degree arthroscope can sometimes be helpful when the lesion is posterior.
- A complete and systematic examination of the joint with the 30-degree arthroscope in the antero-lateral portal is the first step in any arthroscopic procedure about the knee. The articular surfaces of the femoral condyles should be inspected carefully. Moving the knee from 20 to 90 degrees of flexion during viewing will help with inspection of the posterior extent of the lesion.
- The articular surfaces should appear smooth except for a slightly raised irregularity at the borders of the lesion. A probe inserted through the anteromedial portal is used to carefully probe this irregular line to be sure there is no break in the continuity of the articular surface overlying the subchondral bone (Fig. 34-5).

Arthroscopic Drilling of the Intact Lesion

- If the lesion is intact, a 0.062-inch Kirschner wire is used to perforate it with multiple holes.
- The wire is positioned perpendicular to the articular surface, with the soft tissues protected by a sleeve or cannula over the wire.

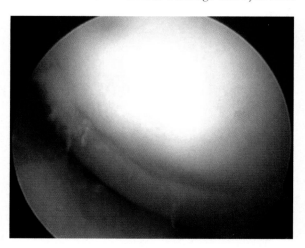

FIGURE 34-5
Arthroscopic view of OCD of knee.

- Drilling of inferior lateral lesions of the medial femoral condyle usually is done through the anterolateral portal; lateral central lesions may be better accessed with the wire through the anterolateral portal and the arthroscope in the anteromedial portal. Large lesions may require drilling through both portals.
- The wire should penetrate the articular surface, the subchondral lesions, and the underlying bone to a depth of 1 to 1.5 cm to ensure vascular access. In patients with open physes, imaging is recommended when drilling to avoid entering the physis (Fig. 34-6).

Arthroscopic Removal and Curettage/Microfracture   If the lesion does not have a salvageable fragment, it can be treated with curettage or abrasion arthroplasty, with or without microfracture for small lesions in non–weight-bearing areas where fibrocartilage growth may be satisfactory (Fig. 34-7).

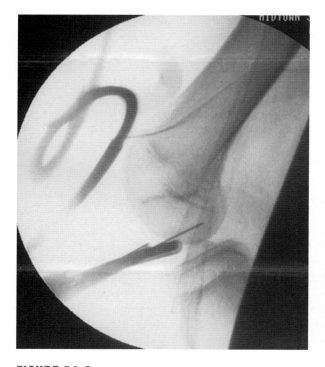

FIGURE 34-6
Intraoperative fluoroscopy helps avoid the physis in skeletally immature patients.

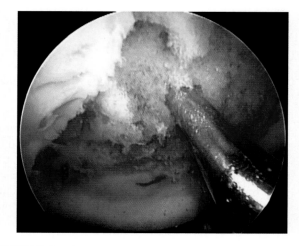

FIGURE 34-7
Microfracture of OCD lesion of knee.

Internal Fixation

- Two or three 0.062-inch threaded pins can be used for antegrade or retrograde fixation. The pins should be left long within the adjacent medial femoral condylar soft tissues so that they can be easily removed once healing has occurred.
- Headless metal screws with variable pitch also can be used but should be countersunk to the level of subchondral bone. Most authors recommend removal of screws once healing has occurred (Fig. 34-8). Bioabsorbable screws also can be used to avoid a second procedure for hardware removal (Fig. 34-9).
- For smaller, relatively stable lesions, we generally prefer to use an absorbable fixation device. Implant removal is not necessary, and loading stress on the fracture site is gradually increased as the implants degrade. The general technique for insertion is the same regardless of the exact device used (Fig. 34-10).

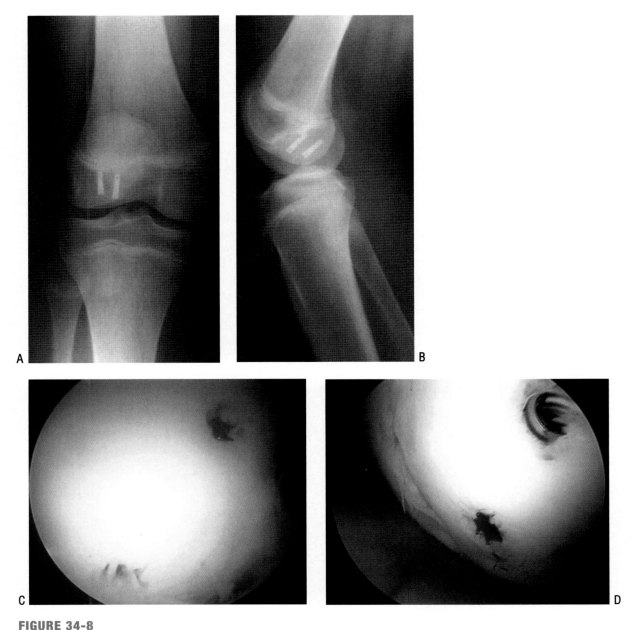

FIGURE 34-8

Arthroscopic internal fixation with cannulated headless screws. **A,B:** Radiographic appearance. **C,D:** Arthroscopic views. Screw head should be buried down to subchondral bone.

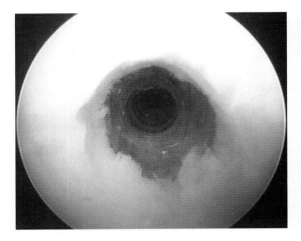

FIGURE 34-9

Bioabsorbable screw can be used for fixation.

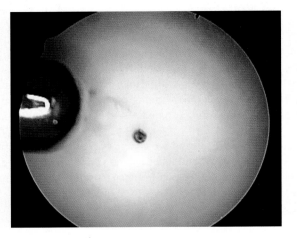

FIGURE 34-10

Insertion of bioabsorbable pin.

- Before reduction and fixation of partially or completely detached lesions, the bed and fragment must have all fibrous tissue debrided with a curet or shaver (Fig. 34-11). If bone grafting is indicated, cancellous bone grafts can be packed into the base of the crater to obliterate step-off. Cancellous graft can be obtained from the proximal tibia or a femoral condyle with a trephine coring needle or similar device.
- The graft is placed arthroscopically or through a mini arthrotomy behind the OCD lesion and packed to make a smooth surface before fixation. This also can be accomplished retrograde.

Osteochondral Autograft Transplantation

- The osteochondral defect is inspected arthroscopically, and the size of the lesion is measured.
- A set of sizer/tamps with varying head sizes is used to determine the exact diameter of the defect.
- A donor harvester is driven with a mallet into subchondral bone to a depth of approximately 15 mm, and a bone core is removed by axially loading the harvester and rotating the driver 90 degrees clockwise and then 90 degrees counterclockwise.
- The recipient harvester and protector caps are inserted into the driver and placed over the defect at a 90-degree angle to the articular surface to create the recipient socket.
- With the knee in a constant flexion angle, a mallet is used to drive the recipient tube harvester into subchondral bone to a depth of about 13 mm (2 mm less than the length of the donor core), and the recipient bone core is extracted in the same manner as the donor core; the depth of the core is measured and recorded.
- A calibrated alignment stick of the appropriate diameter is used to measure the recipient socket depth.

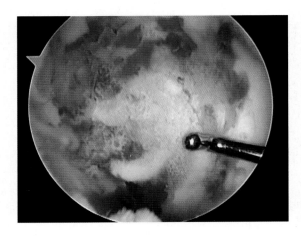

FIGURE 34-11

Debridement of OCD lesion on lateral femoral condyle.

- With the harvester stabilized, a mallet is used to lightly tap the end of the collared pin and drive the bone core into the recipient socket. A stable knee flexion angle and the position of the harvester must be maintained during this step.
- Multiple smaller autografts (4 to 8 mm) can be implanted (mosiacplasty) in the same manner for lesions less than 2 cm in diameter.

Osteochondral Allografting   Osteochondral allografts can be used for larger lesions (approx. 2 to 3.5 cm); however, they have some disadvantages: risk of transmission of disease and problems with storage and stabilization (Fig. 34-12). More recently, fresh articular allografts have been used, but time-dependent loss of chondrocyte viability is a concern. Malinin et al (31) reported a gradual, significant decrease in the number of chondrocytes after 9 days; cell outgrowth occurred from specimens stored for up to 15 days but not in samples stored for longer than 34 days. Using knee condyles from sheep, Williams et al (43) found 98% chondrocyte viability at 8 days, but only 80% at 15 days. In a canine model, Glenn et al (17) showed that fresh osteochondral autografts and allografts were not statistically different with respect to bony incorporation, articular cartilage composition, or

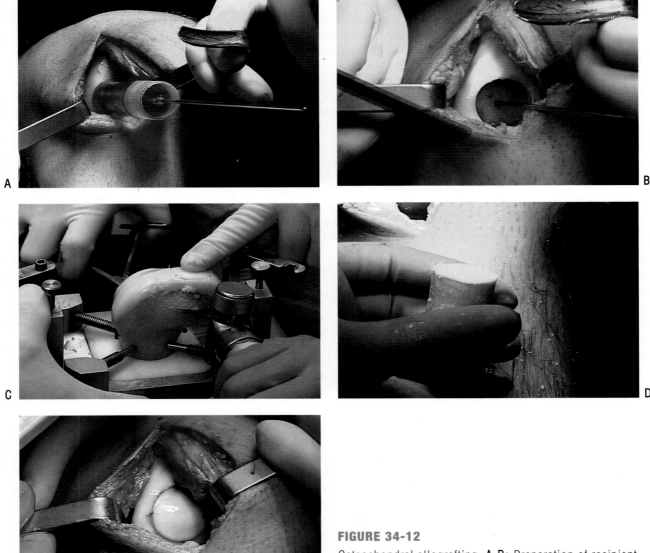

FIGURE 34-12

Osteochondral allografting. **A,B:** Preparation of recipient bed. **C:** Removal of graft from donor bone. **D:** Harvested allograft. **E:** Graft in place.

biomechanical properties up to 6 months after implantation. Shasha et al (41) reported 95% survival of fresh osteochondral allografts at 5 years, 71% at 10 years, and 66% at 20 years after implantation.

Autologous Chondrocyte Implantation Cartilage is harvested arthroscopically from the margin of the knee joint, cultured for 4 weeks, and then transplanted into the damaged area. The cells are held in position by a membrane of periosteum that is taken from the upper tibia and sutured into position over the cartilage defect before the cells are injected (Fig. 34-13). For deep osteochondral defects, staged open or arthroscopic bone grafting has been done, followed 4 to 9 months later by autologous chondrocyte implantation (ACI) (16,39). To avoid multiple operative procedures, Peterson (38) advocated an ACI "sandwich" technique in which cancellous bone graft is used to fill the bone defect, periosteum is sutured above the bone graft at the level of the subchondral bone with the cambium layer facing the joint, more periosteal membrane is sutured to the rim of the chondral defect with the cambium layer facing the defect, fibrin glue is used to secure a water-tight seal, and chondrocytes are injected between the membranes. Bartlett et al (2) described a variation of this sandwich technique using a porcine type I/III membrane rather than periosteum. The same authors described a matrix-induced autologous chondrocyte implantation (MACI) technique that uses a porcine collagen bilayer seeded with chondrocytes and secured directly to the base of a prepared chondral defect by fibrin glue.

Pearls and Pitfalls

- Flexing the knee as much as possible during arthroscopy can help expose lesions that may not be clearly visible with the knee flexed at 90 degrees.
- When drilling an intact lesion, care should be taken not to destabilize the lesion by drilling too many holes; the holes should be approximately 3 to 4 mm apart.
- When drilling an intact lesion in an adolescent with open physes, image guidance is recommended to avoid entering the physis.
- It is important to remove all fibrous tissue from the crater and the fragment to optimize healing potential.
- If fixation is done arthroscopically, the proper cannula must be used; a mini arthrotomy should be used if adequate fixation cannot be obtained arthroscopically.
- Screw heads should be buried down to subchondral bone to avoid abrasion.
- During autograft or allograft transplantation, when creating the recipient socket, a 90-angle to the articular surface is maintained to obtain and flush transfer, and the harvester must be rotated so that the depth markings can be seen.
- If an osteochondral autograft technique is used, the harvest tunnels should be 1 to 2 mm apart.

POSTOPERATIVE MANAGEMENT

A restricted motion brace is used, with the arc of motion controlled to prevent contact of the tibial articular surface with the lesion. Use of crutches with non–weight bearing is encouraged until early healing is seen on radiographs, usually 6 to 8 weeks. An unlocked functional brace is then recommended for an additional 2 to 4 months. Sports-specific exercises and return to unrestricted activity is allowed between 6 and 12 months after surgery, depending on the individual patient and his or her outcome. Postoperative management and rehabilitation may vary according to the exact procedure done and the individual patient (20).

OSTEOCHONDRITIS DISSECANS OF THE PATELLA

Osteochondritis dissecans of the patella is less frequent than involvement of the femoral condyles and typically has a worse prognosis. It usually occurs in the second and third decades and is most often located in the lower half of the patella. Involvement is bilateral in up to one third of patients and should be distinguished from dorsal defects of the patella. Fixation can be technically demanding. At present, arthroscopic excision, curettage, drilling, and debridement (Fig. 34-14) are recommended. Surgery is indicated for loose bodies and for lesions with sclerotic margins. Prognosis is believed to be related to the size of the lesion, with those in the 5- to 10-mm range reported to have good to excellent results. However, about half of patients have significant patellofemoral pain at

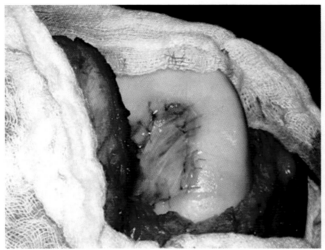

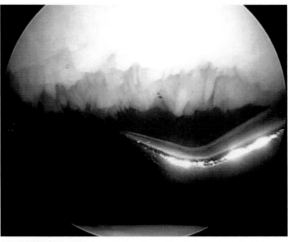

FIGURE 34-13
Autologous chondrocyte implantation. Cells held in position by periosteum sutured over defect.

FIGURE 34-14
Arthroscopic view of OCD of the patella.

long-term follow-up. Overall, the relationship between prognosis and skeletal maturity for patellar lesions is less clear than that for femoral lesions.

COMPLICATIONS

Complications, in addition to typical postoperative knee complications such as infection and hemarthrosis, include iatrogenic cartilage damage, hardware loosening, and abrasion of the articular cartilage by hardware. Aggressive drilling of an intact lesion can cause fragmentation of the lesion. Metallic screws that are prominent or become prominent as surrounding articular cartilage wears down can damage adjacent articular cartilage. Absorbable fixation devices have been reported to occasionally cause foreign-body reactions. Damage to adjacent articular cartilage has been attributed to loosening and failure of bioabsorbable screws that backed out, and unabsorbed screw heads have been found as intra-aticular loose bodies (13,40). LaPrade and Botker (25) reported two patients who had fibrocartilage hypertrophy at osteochondral autograft donor sites that caused knee pain and occasional locking; arthroscopic trimming of the fibrocartilge was required in both. Delayed union or nonunion of an internally fixed lesion may require an additional procedure if symptomatic.

RESULTS

Reported results of operative treatment of osteochondral lesions of the knee vary considerably among techniques and among authors. Levy et al (26) reported good and excellent results at 1-year follow-up in all 15 patients treated with debridement, while Mithoefer et al (37–39) reported 67% good and excellent results in 48 patients 24 months after microfracture. Makino et al (32) found stable fragments and intact smooth surfaces in 14 of 15 knees at second-look arthroscopy an average of 50 months after fixation with a Herbert screw.

Several series (9,23,24,29) have reported good and excellent results in 83% to 89% of patients after osteochondral autograft procedures. Karataglis et al (24) reported improvement in preoperative symptoms in 32 (86.5%) of 37 knees at 3-year follow-up, Ma et al (31) reported 89% good results in 18 patients at 42-month follow-up, and Chow et al (9) reported 83% good or excellent results in 33 patients at 45-month follow-up. The sizes of the lesions treated with autografts ranged from 1 to 4.1 cm.

In the largest series of mosiacplasty procedures (831 patients), Szerb et al (42) reported good to excellent results in 92% of femoral condylar lesions. Gudas et al (18), in a prospective randomized study, compared mosaic osteochondral autografting with microfracture in 57 young athletic individuals. Functional results were much better in those with autografts (96% good or excellent) than in those with microfracture (52% good or excellent); MRI showed more good results after auto-grafting (94%) than after microfracture (49%); and more patients returned to sports activities after autografting (93%) than after microfracture (52%). Bently et al (4), however, compared mosaic-plasty with ACI in 100 patients with an average defect size of 4.66 cm^2 and found 88% good and excellent clinical results after ACI and 69% after mosiacplasty; arthroscopic examination found 82% good and excellent results after ACI, compared to only 34% after mosiacplasty. In another prospective comparative trial, Horas et al (22) found that results were equally good after ACI and osteochondral cylinder transplantation, although recovery was slower after ACI.

Allografting procedures, generally reserved for larger lesions, were reported by Ghazavi et al (15) to be successful in 85% of 126 knees at 7.5 years after fresh allografts were implanted. Gross et al (16) reported failure of 12 of 60 allografts at 10-year follow-up. Mega-OATS procedures have been developed for very large lesions, but few reports of their results are available and follow-up is relatively short. Karataglis and Learmonth (24) reported functional improvements at 2.5 years after distal femoral allografts in 5 patients with large defects (average of 30 × 30 mm).

Autologous chondrocyte implantation procedures have been reported to be successful in 66% to 96% of patients. Peterson et al (38) reported successful clinical results in more than 90% of 48 patients at follow-up ranging from 2 to 10 years. Bentley et al (4), in a prospective randomized comparison, found excellent or good results in 82% of 58 ACI procedures and only 34% of 42 mosaic-plasty procedures at an average follow-up of 19 months. Fu et al (14) compared ACI (58 patients) to debridement (58 patients) for treatment of full-thickness chondral defects and found that those who had ACI obtained higher levels of knee function and had greater relief of pain and swelling at 3-year follow-up. Micheli et al (33) reported marked clinical improvements after ACI in 14 patients younger than 18 years who had OCD lesions of the knee. Bartlett et al (3) reported improvements in the clinical scores of 91 patients who had either ACI or MACI grafting procedures; the authors concluded that the clinical, arthroscopic, and histologic outcomes of the two procedures are comparable, but that longer follow-up is needed before MACI is widely adopted.

RECOMMENDED READING

Gross AE, Shasha N, Aubin P. Long-term followup of the use of fresh osteochondral allografts for posttraumatic knee defects. *Clin Orthop Rel Res.* 2005;435:79–87.

Kocher MS, Tucker R, Ganley TJ, Flynn JM. Management of osteochondritis dissecans of the knee: current concepts review. *Am J Sports Med.* 2006;34:1181–1191.

Marcacci M, Konn E, Zaffagnini S, et al. Multiple osteochondral arthroscopic grafting (mosiacplasty) for cartilage defects of the knee: prospective study results at 2-year follow-up. *Arthroscopy.* 2005;21:462–470.

REFERENCES

1. Aroen A, Loken S, Heir S, et al. Articular cartilage lesions in 993 consecutive knee arthroscopies. *Am J Sports Med.* 2004;32:211–215.
2. Bartlett W, Gooding CR, Carrington RWJ, et al. Autologous chondrocyte implantation at the knee using a bilayer collagen membrane with bone graft: a preliminary report. *J Bone Joint Surg Br.* 2005;87B:330–332.
3. Bartlett W, Skinner JA, Gooding CR, et al. Autologous chondrocyte implantation versus matrix-induced autologous chondrocyte implantation for osteochondral defects of the knee: a prospective, randomised study. *J Bone Joint Surg Br.* 2005;87B:40–45.
4. Bentley G, Biant LC, Carrington RW, et al. A prospective, randomized comparison of autologous chondrocyte implantation versus mosaicplasty for osteochondral defects in the knee. *J Bone Joint Surg Br.* 2003;85B:223–230.
5. Bradley J, Dandy DJ. Osteochondritis dissecans and other lesions of the femoral condyles. *J Bone Joint Surg Br.* 1989;71B:518–522.
6. Cahill BR, Berg BC. 99m-technetium phosphate compound joint scintigraphy in the management of juvenile osteochondritis of the femoral condyles. *Am J Sports Med.* 1983;11:329–335.
7. Cahill BR, Phillips MR, Navarro R: The results of conservative management of juvenile osteochondritis dissecans using joint scintigraphy. A prospective study. *Am J Sports Med.* 1989;17:601–605.
8. Cain EL, Clancy WG. Treatment algorithm for osteochondral injuries of the knee. *Clin Sports Med.* 2001;20:321–342.
9. Chow JC, Hantes ME, Houle JB, Zalavras CG. Arthroscopic autogenous osteochondral transplantation for treating knee cartilage defects: a 2- to 5-year follow-up study. *Arthroscopy.* 2004;20:681–690.
10. Crawford DC, Safran MR. Osteochondritis dissecans of the knee. *J Am Acad Orthop Surg.* 2006;14:90–100.
11. Curl WW, Krome J, Gordon ES, et al. Cartilage injuries: a review of 31,516 knee arthroscopies. *Arthroscopy.* 1997;13:456–460.
12. Dipaola JD, Nelson DW, Colville MR. Characterizing osteochondral lesions by magnetic resonance imaging. *Arthroscopy.* 1991;7:101–104.
13. Friederichs MG, Greis PE, Burks RT. Pitfalls associated with fixation of osteochondritis dissecans fragments using bioabsorbable screws. *Arthroscopy.* 2001;17:542–545.

14. Fu FJ, Zurakowski D, Browne JE, et al. Autologous chondrocyte implantation versus debridement for treatment of full-thickness chondral defects of the knee: an observational cohort study with 3-year follow-up. *Am J Sports Med.* 2005;33:1658–1666.
15. Ghazavi MT, Prtizker KP, Davis AM, Gross AE. Fresh osteochondral allografts for post-traumatic osteochondral defects of the knee. *J Bone Joint Surg Br.* 1997;79B:1008–1013.
16. Gillogly SD, Myers TH. Treatment of full-thickness chondral defects with autologous chondrocyte implantation. *Orthop Clin North Am.* 2005;36:433–446.
17. Glenn RE Jr, McCarty EC, Potter HG, et al. Comparison of fresh ostoechondral autografts and allografts: a canine model. *Am J Sports Med.* 2006;34:1084–1093.
18. Gudas R, Kalesinskas RJ, Kimtys V, et al. A prospective randomized clinical study of mosaic osteochondral autologous transplantation versus microfracture for the treatment of osteochondral defects in the knee joint in young athletes. *Arthroscopy.* 2005;21:1066–1075.
19. Guhl JF. Arthroscopic treatment of osteochondritis dissecans. *Clin Orthop Rel Res.* 1982;167:65–74.
20. Hambly K, Bobic V, Wondrasch B, Van Assche D, Marlovits S. Autologous chondrocyte implantation postoperative care and rehabilitation: science and practice. *Am J Sports Med.* 2006;34:1020–1038.
21. Hjelle K, Solheim E, Strand T, Muri R, Brittberg M. Articular cartilage defects in 1,000 knee arthroscopies. *Arthroscopy.* 2002;18:730–734.
22. Horas U, Pelinkovic D, Herr G, Aigner T, Schnettler R. Autologous chondrocyte implantation and osteochondral cylinder transplantation in cartilage repair of the knee joint. A prospective, comparative trial. *J Bone Joint Surg Am.* 2003;85A:185–192.
23. Karataglis D, Green MA, Learmonth DJ. Autologous osteochondral transplantation for the treatment of chondral defects of the knee. *Knee.* 2006;13:32–35.
24. Karataglis D, Learmonth DJ. Management of big osteochondral defects of the knee using osteochondral allografts with the MEGA-OATS technique. *Knee.* 2005;12:389–393.
25. LaPrade RJ, Botker JC. Donor-site morbidity after osteochondral autograft transfer procedures. *Arthroscopy.* 2004;20:69–73.
26. Levy AS, Lohnes J, Sculley S, LeCroy M, Garret W. Chondral delamination of the knee in soccer players. *Am J Sports Med.* 1996;24:634–639.
27. Linden B. Osteochondritis dissecans of the femoral condyles: a long-term follow-up study. *J Bone Joint Surg Am.* 1977;59A:769–776.
28. Loredo R, Sanders TG. Imaging of osteochondral injuries. *Clin Sports Med.* 2001;20:249–2778.
29. Ma HL, Hung SC, Wang ST, Chang MC, Chen TH. Osteochondral autografts transfer for post-traumatic osteochondral defect of the knee—2 to 5 years follow-up. *Injury.* 2004;35:1286–1292.
30. Makino A, Muscolo DL, Puigdevall M, Costa-Paz M, Averza M. Arthroscopic fixation of osteochondritis dissecans of the knee: clinical, magnetic resonance imaging, and arthroscopic follow-up. *Am J Sports Med.* 2005;33:1499–1504.
31. Malinin T, Temple HT, Buck BE. Transplantation of osteochondral allografts after cold storage. *J Bone Joint Surg Am.* 2006;88A:762–770.
32. Messner K, Maletius W. The long-term prognosis for severe damage to weight-bearing cartilage in the knee: a 14-year clinical and radiographic follow-up in 28 young athletes. *Acta Orthop Scand.* 1996;67:165–168.
33. Micheli LJ, Moseley JB, Anderson AF, et al. Articular cartilage defects of the distal femur in children and adolescents: treatment with autologous chondrocyte implantation. *J Pediatr Orthop.* 2006;26:455–460.
34. Mithoefer K, Minas T, Peterson L, Yeon H, Micheli LJ. Functional outcome of knee articular cartilage repair in adolescent athletes. *Am J Sports Med.* 2005;33:1147–1153.
35. Mithoefer K, Williams RJ III, Warren RF, et al. The microfracture technique for the treatment of articular cartilage lesions in the knee. A prospective cohort study. *J Bone Joint Surg Am.* 2005;87A:1911–1920.
36. Mithoefer K, Williams RJ III, Warren RF, Wickiewicz TL, Marx RG. High-impact athletics after knee articular cartilage repair: a prospective evaluation of the microfracture technique. *Am J Sports Med.* 2006;34:1413–1418.
37. Paletta GA, Bednarz PA, Stanitski CL, et al. The prognostic value of quantitative bone scan in knee osteochondritis dissecans: a preliminary experience. *Am J Sports Med.* 1998;26:7–14.
38. Peterson L. Chondrocyte transplantation. In: Jackson DW, ed.: *Master techniques in orthopaedic surgery: reconstructive knee surgery.* Philadelphia: Lippincott Williams & Wilkins, 2003;353–373.
39. Peterson L, Minas T, Brittberg M, Lindahl A. Treatment of osteochondritis dissecans of the knee with autologous chondrocyte transplantation:results at two to ten years. *J Bone Joint Surg Am.* 2003;85A(suppl 2):17–24.
40. Scioscia TN, Giffin JR, Allen CR, Harner CD. Potential complication of bioabsorbable screw fixation for osteochondritis dissecans of the knee. *Arthroscopy.* 2001;17:E7.
41. Shasha N, Aubin PP, Cheah HK, et al. Long-term clinical experience with fresh osteochondral allografts for articular knee defects in high demand patients. *Cell Tissue Bank.* 2002;3:175–182.
42. Szerb I, Hangody L, Duska Z, Kaposi NP. Mosaicplasty: long-term follow-up. *Bull Hosp Joint Dis.* 2005;63:54–62.
43. Williams RJ III, Dreese JC, Chen CT. Chondrocyte survival and material properties of hypothermically stored cartilage: an evaluation of tissue used for osteochondral allograft transplantation. *Am J Sports Med.* 2004;32:132–139.

35 Synovectomy for Pigmented Villonodular Synovitis

Edward Y. Cheng and Vineet Sharma

Pigmented villonodular synovitis (PVNS) is a unique condition affecting synovial tissues in joints, tendon sheaths, and bursa. The disease is classified into three categories: (a) extra-articular PVNS (also known as giant cell tumor of the tendon sheath), (b) localized intra-articular PVNS, and (c) diffuse intra-articular PVNS. It is unknown whether or not this disease is a true neoplasm or reactive in origin (24), but recent evidence of monoclonality suggests a neoplastic etiology (3,18). The disease may occur in either young adults or the elderly and commonly presents with symptoms related to the intra-articular nature of the mass. The knee is the most common joint involved but any synovial joint including the hip (Fig. 35-1) (33), ankle (Fig. 35-2) (13), shoulder (Fig. 35-3) (22), or elbow (30) may be affected. Polyarticular disease in children has also been reported (12,34). Pain and intermittent effusions, either traumatic or nontraumatic in origin, are caused by the inflammatory synovitis and recurrent hemarthroses that are typical. In the knee, locking may occur or the disease may be misdiagnosed as a popliteal cyst.

INDICATIONS/CONTRAINDICATIONS

The mainstay of treatment of PVNS is surgical excision by either open or arthroscopic means. No medical therapy is known to be effective at eradicating the disease. Untreated, some patients may develop stable disease but most patients will require treatment for symptomatic reasons or to prevent the eventual progression to periarticular erosive cyst formation and subsequent destruction of the cartilaginous joint surface. In about one third of cases, an aggressive course may ensue with multiple recurrences despite surgical resection (9). In these cases, radiation may be considered, administered by either external beam (26) or via intra-articular radiation synovectomy (11,16). Once joint destruction has occurred, total knee arthroplasty is the only means of addressing the disabling symptoms; however, a synovectomy must still be performed as recurrences after knee arthroplasty have been documented (1,14).

Indications

- Symptomatic PVNS
- Asymptomatic PVNS
- Locally recurrent PVNS

Contraindications (Relative)

- Multiply recurrent PVNS
- Medical comorbidities precluding surgery

499

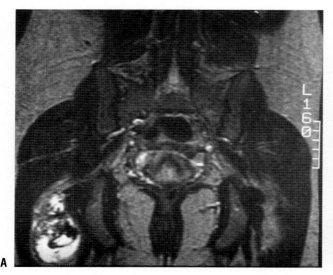

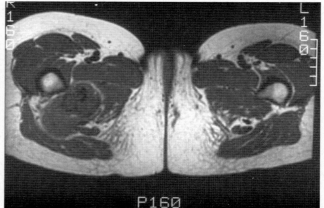

FIGURE 35-1

A: Coronal fat suppression MRI of PVNS of the hip. Note effusion and dark areas of hemosiderin deposition. **B:** Axial T1 MRI of PVNS of the hip. Note how the extent of disease is seen much more readily than on computed tomography scan **(C).**

PREOPERATIVE PLANNING

Examination and Evaluation

Patients with PVNS demonstrate evidence of an effusion or a hemarthrosis when minor trauma results in a hemorrhage. In the localized type, locking due to the presence of an intra-articular mass is common, and in both the diffuse and localized from, there may be limited joint arc of motion. A palpable mass is not usually appreciated unless there are extra-articular disease manifestations. Most commonly, the extra-articular disease occurs in the popliteal fossa or intercondylar notch (Fig. 35-4). In advanced cases, findings consistent with degenerative arthrosis are evident.

Imaging Studies

Plain radiographic findings in the early stage of disease are either normal or may show a displaced suprapatellar fat plane due to presence of an effusion. A capsular-based noncalcified soft tissue mass may be present (7). In later stages, periarticular cysts are present and cartilage thinning is seen (4). The findings on magnetic resonance imaging (MRI) are more dramatic and in many cases diagnostic. A soft tissue mass with alternating areas of bright signal and dark signal void on both T1 and T2 sequence represents the fluid (bright on T2) and fat (bright on T1) accumulation as well as hemosiderin deposits within the soft tissue (dark on both T1 and T2), respectively (Fig. 35-5). In the appropriate clinical setting, these findings are nearly diagnostic of PVNS, although rheumatoid arthritis may have a similar appearance (23,31). The nodular form may not always be localized to one location and instead may occur in multiple compartments within the joint. It is essential to pre-

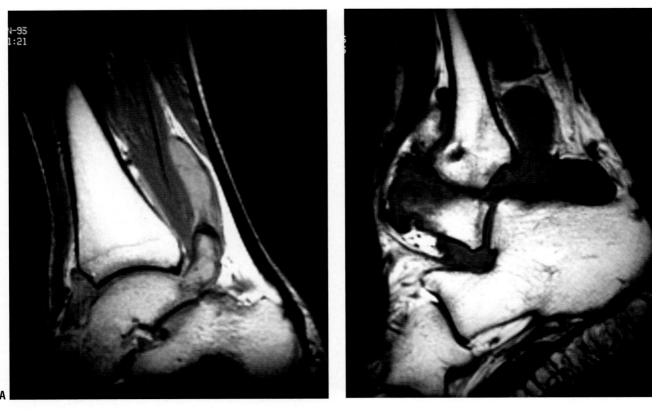

FIGURE 35-2

A: Sagittal T2 MRI image of PVNS of the tibio talar and subtalar joint. **B:** Sagittal T1 MRI image of PVNS of the tibio talar and subtalar joint.

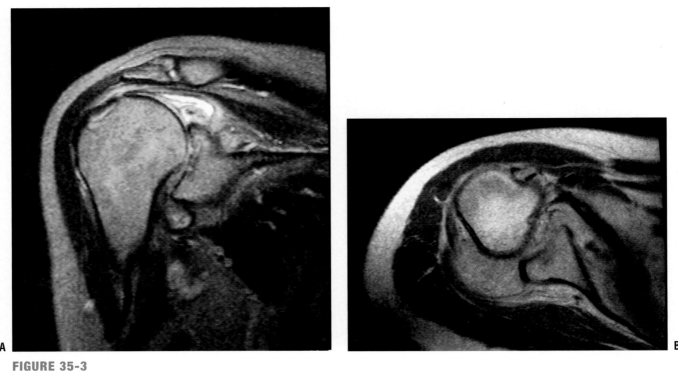

FIGURE 35-3

A: Coronal STIR (Short T1 inversion recovery) MRI image of PVNS of the glenohumeral joint. Note large effusion and synovial thickening. **B:** Axial T2 MRI image of PVNS of the glenohumeral joint. Note erosion into the glenoid fossa.

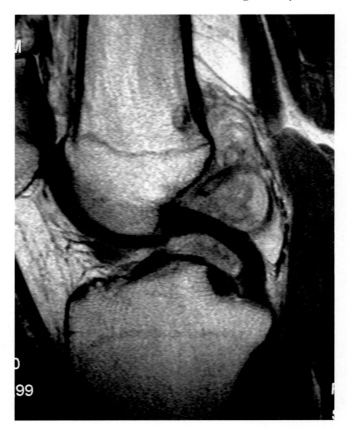

FIGURE 35-4

Sagittal T2 MRI image of PVNS in an extra-articular location extruding outward from the intercondylar notch.

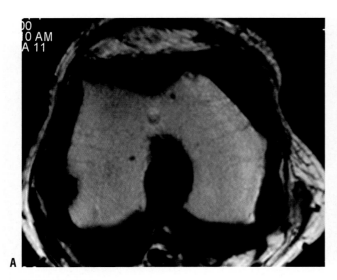

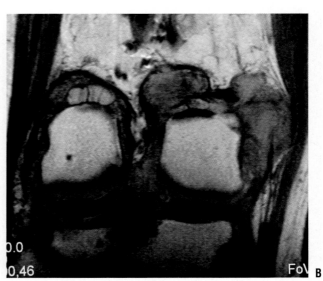

FIGURE 35-5

A: Axial T1 MRI. **B:** Coronal T2 MRI.

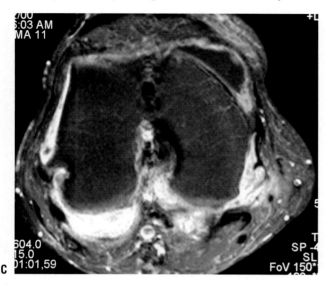

FIGURE 35-5

(Continued) **C**: Axial fat suppression MRI images of PVNS.

cisely determine the extent of the disease on MRI as this will directly affect the surgical approach to the disease. In doubtful cases, the diagnosis can be established with a biopsy.

Gross and Histologic Appearance

The intraoperative gross appearance of disease is characteristic. In the diffuse form, multiple fronds of reddish-brown pigment-stained synovial tissue represent villous projections floating in synovial fluid. In the nodular form, a thickened reddish-brown and yellow stained xanthomatous soft tissue mass with cavitary areas of fluid accumulation is seen and the mass may spread dramatically in the suprapatellar pouch (Fig. 35-6) or intercondylar notch.

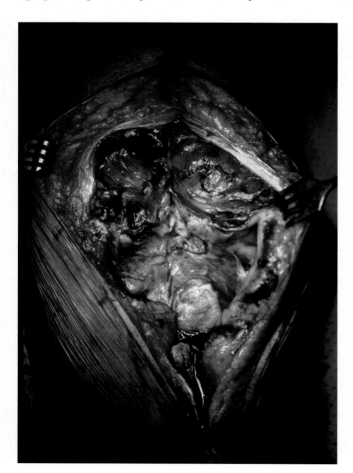

FIGURE 35-6

Clinical intraoperative photo of markedly thickened PVNS with reddish-brown pigmentation and xanthomatous appearance in the suprapatellar pouch.

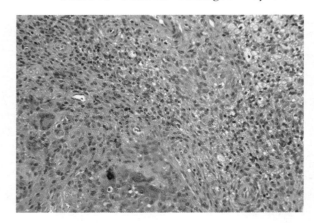

FIGURE 35-7

Histologic photomicrograph (20× power) of PVNS.

Histologically, PVNS is indistinguishable from a giant cell tumor of tendon sheath (nodular tenosynovitis). A proliferation of round synovial-like cells is present with occasional multinucleated osteoclast-type giant cells, xanthomatous cells, and inflammatory cells interspersed throughout the lesion (Fig. 35-7) (5,15).

Specific Approaches

The controversy regarding open versus arthroscopic synovectomy is difficult to resolve. With either technique, in the diffuse form, the recurrence rate ranges from 8% to 50% (10,25,32). The only factor which is conclusively known to prevent local recurrence is complete and aggressive resection of the affected tissues. The benefits of arthroscopic synovectomy are a quicker rehabilitation and avoidance of arthrotomy and postoperative knee stiffness. The disadvantages are related to performing an intralesional excision or debridement, potential for intra-articular spread of disease converting a localized form to diffuse disease, seeding of portal sites (Fig. 35-8), difficulty accessing posterior and extra-articular locations of disease, and difficulty in removal of markedly thickened

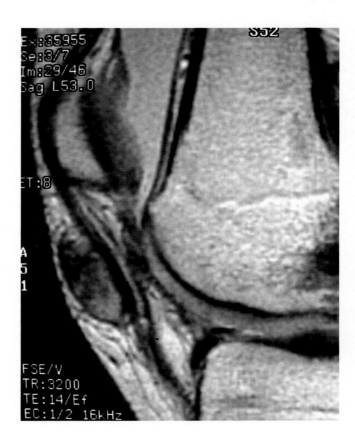

FIGURE 35-8

Axial T2 MRI image of local recurrence of PNVS in prior arthroscopic portal site adjacent to patellar tendon.

synovial tissue. Advantages of an open synovectomy over the arthroscopic technique are the ability to do a marginal or *en bloc* excision of the mass, complete a total synovectomy as opposed to a only a debridement, and the expeditious nature of an arthrotomy. Excellent results using cryosurgery in addition to open synovectomy have been reported (20). However, the open procedure can be technically challenging to perform adequately through a popliteal exposure and may result in postoperative adhesions if a normal arc of knee motion is not regained promptly after surgery. No prospective trials directly comparing these techniques have been performed, and they would be considerably difficult to power adequately due to the rarity of the disease.

Arthroscopic Approach
- Disease is limited to a single location
- Accessible arthroscopically
- Nodular form

Open Approach
- Extra-articular disease
- Posterior disease inaccessible arthroscopically
- Diffuse form (8,9,19,21).

SURGERY

Positioning, Draping, and Organizing the Operating Room

When open synovectomy is performed, the operative team must be prepared to undertake the surgical approach mandated by the anatomic location of disease. If both the anterior and posterior compartments of the knee are affected, an anterior and posterior synovectomy is required. In the supine position, a roll is placed beneath the buttock and a sandbag taped to the table at midcalf level to support the heel while the knee is flexed. In the prone position, blanket rolls or a spinal frame are adequate for positioning. It is helpful to have a second table to turn the patient onto after completion of the anterior portion of the surgery.

Details of Procedure and Avoiding Pitfalls

Anterior Exposure   The anterior arthrotomy is performed first through an exposure similar to total knee arthroplasty. Using a tourniquet facilitates visualization. Care must be taken to avoid injury to the menisci upon exposing the knee. Areas where an incomplete resection may occur include the medial and lateral gutters, beneath the menisci, and in between the anterior and posterior cruciate ligaments. A bone hook placed within the femoral notch to distract the femur assists exposing the ligaments. Flexing and rotation the tibia assist exposing the gutters. Once the anterior synovectomy is completed, the tourniquet is deflated, hemostasis secured, wound is closed, drapes removed, the patient is turned prone onto another table, and the knee is reprepped and draped (Fig. 35-9).

Posterior Exposure   The posterior exposure is usually more challenging for most surgeons as it is performed less frequently than the anterior exposure and one must dissect out the popliteal vessels, and tibial and peroneal nerves. With practice, however, one can become comfortable with this dissection and maneuver around the critical structures with ease. Under tourniquet control, a gentle "S" shaped curvilinear incision is made with care taken to avoid an abrupt turn in the corners resulting in a corner edge at risk for necrosis. Ideally, a turn no greater than 45 degrees is fashioned and the flaps are kept as thick as possible by keeping the plane of dissection deep to the popliteal fascia before raising the flap (Fig. 35-10). This greatly facilitates the wound closure as well. The incision can be based from either the lateral or medial border of the thigh depending on which side has the greatest extent of disease. The semitendinosis tendon is readily identified in the medial border of the incision (Fig. 25-10B and C). A few gentle spreading motions with the blunt-tipped scissors allow one to identify the popliteal vein and artery together. Similarly, the peroneal nerve is found coursing obliquely toward the biceps tendon. This can then be dissected proximally toward the tibial-peroneal bifurcation. Vessel loops are placed around the neurovascular structures to aid in retraction (Fig. 35-11A). Multiple small venous structures around the popliteal vein will need to be divided when skeletonizing the vein. It is necessary to dissect a sufficient distance to allow sufficient mobility for retraction without undue tension. Hemoclips aid in the speed of dissection but have the

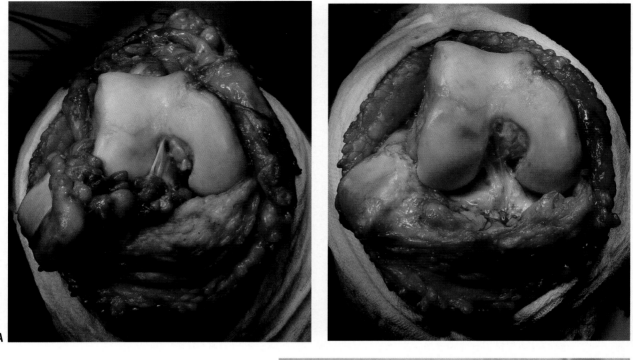

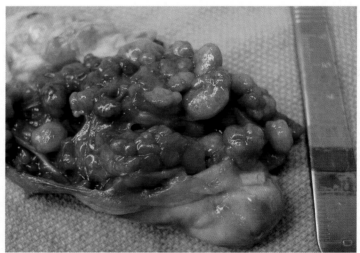

FIGURE 35-9

A: Intra-operative picture showing the anterior exposure with extent of synovitis. **B:** Same knee after complete anterior synovectomy. **C:** The synovial mass removed en masse.

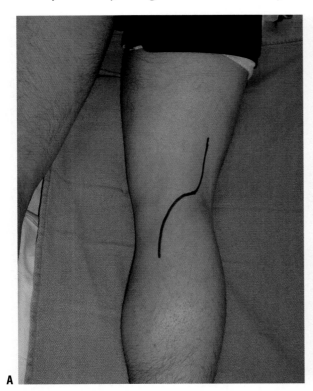

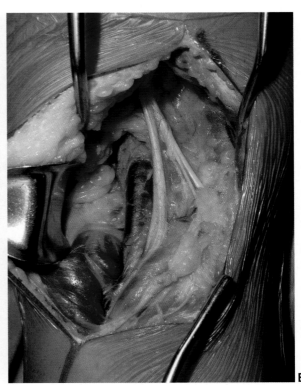

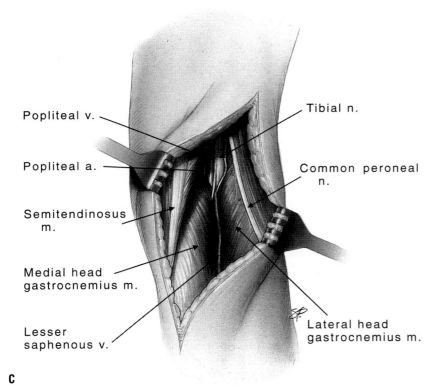

Poppliteal v.

Tibial n.

Popliteal a.

Common peroneal
n.

Semitendinosus
m.

Medial head
gastrocnemius m.

Lesser
saphenous v.

Lateral head
gastrocnemius m.

C

FIGURE 35-10

A: Intraoperative photo of incision. Note curvilinear incision avoids corner angles <135 degrees to prevent flap necrosis in corners. Intraoperative **(B)** and diagrammatic views **(C)** of superficial dissection keeping dissection deep to fascial layer, avoiding dissection through the subcutaneous tissue to keep the flap as thick as possible, thus avoiding necrosis.

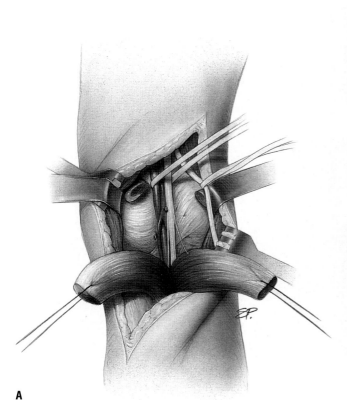

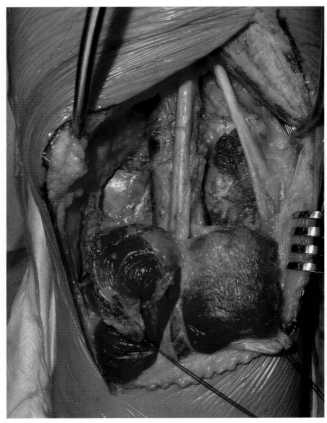

A   B

FIGURE 35-11

Line drawing **(A)** and intraoperative photo **(B)** of popliteal exposure with gastrocnemius muscle heads reflected from origin on posterior femur.

disadvantage of causing artifactual degradation of any subsequent MRI studies that will likely be necessary for postoperative surveillance. The distal extent of the vascular dissection is limited by the vessel branches to the gastrocnemius and the origin of the anterior tibial artery.

The key to exposing the posterior joint capsule adequately is taking down the gastrocnemius muscle origins (Fig. 35-11A,B). Depending on the lesion location on preoperative imaging, one or both gastrocnemius muscle heads will need to be divided. If there is any question, it is advisable to divide both as the MRI frequently underestimates the extent of disease in this locale. A right angle clamp is placed beneath the musculotendinous origin just proximal to the femoral condyle. Cautery is used to divide the tendon and separate the remaining muscle fibers from the posterior knee capsule. Extra-articular extensions of PVNS are frequently found in this location. Tagging sutures placed in the tendon are used to retract the muscle distally and away from the vessels. Homan retractors placed around the femoral condyle as well as slight knee flexion may aid in exposure. At this juncture, the posterior knee capsule should be fully exposed with the vessels coursing in the middle. Another extra-articular site frequently involved with PVNS is located in the intercondylar notch, posterior to the posterior cruciate ligament (Fig. 35-12). Retracting both gastrocnemius muscle origins to either side allows visualization of the ligament of Wrisburg and posterior cruciate ligament just beyond this structure. A small No. 15 scalpel blade is used to perform the capsulotomy along the periphery of the femoral condyle. This affords an intra-articular view of any disease that may be seen as fronds within the joint or attached to the synovial surface of the joint capsule (Fig. 35-13). The entire capsule and adjacent synovium can be resected leaving only the posterior cruciate ligament remaining behind the knee (Fig. 35-14). Again, the posterior menisci must be protected. The limits of the prior anterior dissection are now encountered in the gutters and intercondylar notch regions. These areas should be carefully inspected for any remaining tissue resembling PVNS.

After excising all abnormal tissue, the tourniquet is deflated to ensure satisfactory hemostasis. A drain is placed deep within the wound prior to reattaching the gastrocnemius muscles using a

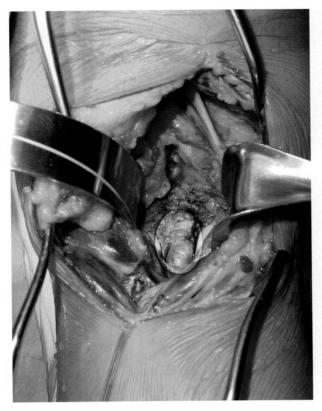

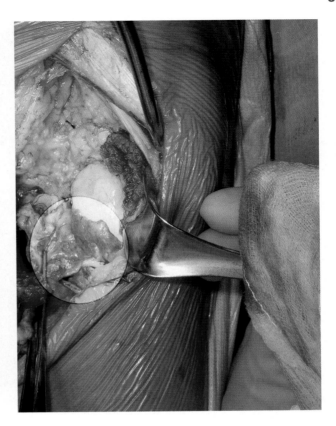

FIGURE 35-12

Intraoperative photo of PVNS tumor mass (*highlighted circle*) in the intercondylar notch adjacent to lateral femoral condyle.

FIGURE 35-13

Intraoperative photo of PVNS involving posterior joint capsule, reflected portion held in forceps (*highlighted circle*).

Kessler-type tendon suture and oversewing with No. 0 nonabsorbable sutures. The repair should be strong enough to withstand the tension applied when the knee is straight and the foot is placed in a neutral position. Approximating the popliteal fascia is facilitated by placing "far-near-near-far" type self-retention sutures to prevent tearing of the thin fascia. A sound fascial closure is important as this is the only layer of any significant tensile strength other than the skin, and the wound closure must be able to tolerate immediate motion postoperatively.

Arthroscopic Synovectomy Performing an adequate arthroscopic synovectomy is considerably more difficult than most arthroscopic procedures. The proliferative synovitis usually present makes visualization challenging. Using a tourniquet is essential, and a variable pressure pump for irrigating solution with epinephrine also is helpful. To afford sufficient visualization of the entire knee, additional portals other than the conventional 3-portal technique are required (Fig. 35-15). Both superior medial and lateral portals are needed to access the suprapatellar pouch, and switching among them with the arthroscope and operative instruments shaver allows complete excision of both sides of the pouch. While the standard anterior portals are used, using the midpatellar lateral or medial portal may assist in visualizing the lateral and medial gutters, respectively (28,29). The intercondylar notch can be accessed using conventional inferior medial and lateral portals. To see the posterior regions adequately, a 70-degree arthroscope is necessary, and a posterior medial or lateral portal allows the arthroscopist an additional port for operative instruments in addition to the arthroscope (Fig. 35-16). Illuminating the posterior portal sites and using a spinal needle may minimize an injury to the infrapatellar branch of the saphenous nerve or the peroneal nerve. A motorized full-radius shaver in oscillating mode is a necessity for performing the synovectomy. The larger 5.5-mm shaver is used as it is more aggressive, unless the anatomic confines of areas such as beneath the menisci or posterior recesses require using the smaller 4.5-mm shaver. Additional techniques helpful in the posterior recesses include flexing the knee and using the arthroscopic sheath for fluid inflow. If hemorrhage is considerable after tourniquet deflation, a drain should be considered.

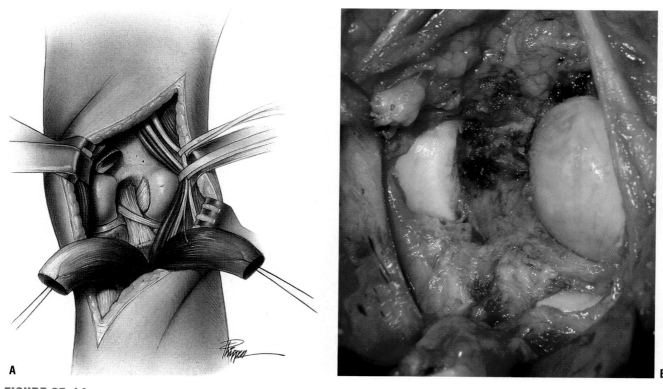

FIGURE 35-14

Line drawing **(A)** and intraoperative photo **(B)** of posterior knee joint after excision of the posterior joint capsule, synovium and PVNS.

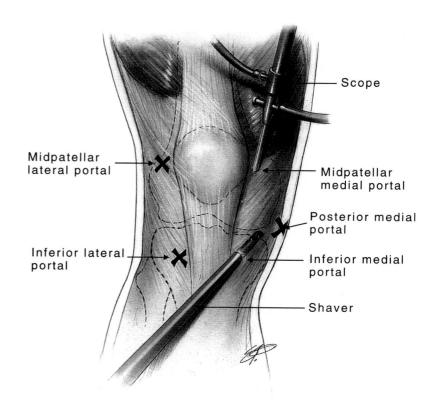

FIGURE 35-15

Arthroscopic portal sites for midpatellar lateral and midpatellar medial placement to facilitate visualization of lateral and medial gutters.

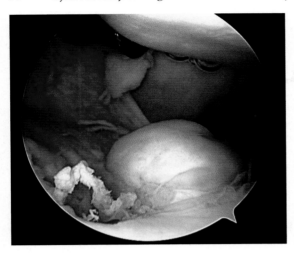

FIGURE 35-16
Arthroscopic view of PVNS.

POSTOPERATIVE MANAGEMENT

The postoperative management of the synovectomy patient depends on the type of procedure performed. For open synovectomy, the goals are as follows:

- Early and aggressive rehabilitation to gain range of motion
- Detection of any wound healing problems

The institution of early continuous passive motion devices the first day after surgery and an epidural catheter for some patients are quite beneficial. The drain is removed the first or second day after surgery. A supervised course of physiotherapy after hospital discharge is advisable until an arc from 0 to 90 degrees is attained and the patient is capable of a home therapy program. Protected weight bearing with crutches for 4 weeks is recommended until the gastrocnemius tendinous reattachment has healed sufficiently. Afterward, a strengthening program with progressive resistance exercises is commenced. Prophylaxis for deep venous thrombosis using anticoagulation is not routinely incorporated unless there are extenuating factors such as a hypercoagulable state or prolonged vascular retraction.

For the arthroscopic synovectomy patient, a compression dressing is left on for the first few days, followed by range of motion exercises. A long-acting anesthetic in instilled into the knee upon would closure. Immediate weight bearing is allowed as tolerated.

For either surgical procedure, careful assessment of the vascular and neurologic status of the limb after surgery is necessary. While more dissection takes place in the open procedure, the neurovascular structures are also at risk for injury during the arthroscopic procedure. An occult injury is more likely in a closed procedure and recognition may be especially problematic if the patient is discharged as an outpatient postoperatively.

Follow-up Surveillance

Pigmented villonodular synovitis has been reported to recur as late as 17 years after prior excision (27). A baseline MRI scan after the surgical changes in the knee have resolved, about 6 months postoperatively, is useful for comparison to any future studies that may be necessary if there is a question of recurrence. Recurrent pain or swelling of the knee most frequently will herald the onset of a relapse. Taking adequate time to educate the patient both pre- and postoperatively about the natural history of PVNS and its propensity for recurrence is the best means of monitoring for relapse and mitigating negative feelings on behalf of the patient.

If a local recurrence is diagnosed, management usually involves repeat excision. A careful assessment of the MRI is necessary to determine the extent of recurrence. If repeat excision is not a possibility, then radiation synovectomy or moderate dose external beam radiation are alternative means of treating this disease. Once joint destruction has already occurred, either arthrodesis or arthroplasty become considerations depending upon the age of the patient.

COMPLICATIONS

The main complications encountered with open synovectomy are:

- Wound healing issues with the posterior incision
- Arthrofibrosis and limitation of motion

If there is a localized area of flap necrosis despite taking the precautions described previously, conventional treatment with saline gauze dressing changes is usually satisfactory. If the patient has not regained a 0 to 90-degree arc of motion by the first month after surgery, a knee manipulation should be considered.

The main complications associated with the arthroscopic procedure are:

- Occult neurovascular injury
- Persistent pain and effusion

A vascular injury requires immediate attention and evaluation. Limiting activities and immobilizing the knee can manage any persistent pain and swelling that is bothersome.

RESULTS

- In the localized form of PVNS, recurrences are rare, regardless of type of excision (i.e., open vs. arthroscopic).
- In the diffuse form of PVNS, results vary according to extent of disease and completeness of excision.

The reported recurrence rate for diffuse PVNS in various studies is from 8% to 50% (6,10,25). This wide range in reported results is due to many reasons. Most studies are small retrospective series or case reports. Even among the larger reported series, there are numerous uncontrolled factors resulting in bias (such as nonuniform methods of treatment or usage of adjuvant radiation) and use of nonactuarial analysis to determine local recurrence rates. In addition, although most authors have distinguished between the localized and diffuse forms of disease, the criteria for these two types is poorly defined and at times, quite subjective. For the localized form of PVNS, the results of both open and arthroscopic treatment are good and the recurrence rate is low (6,17,21,25). Most of evidence supporting this conclusion is quite poor, consisting of mainly case reports and small retrospective studies.

For the diffuse form of PVNS, most centers have undertaken a more aggressive treatment approach. Flandry et al (10) reported a series of 23 patients with diffuse PVNS of the knee who underwent open total synovectomy. The recurrence rate was 8%; however, eight of the patients required a manipulation for loss of motion postoperatively. The outcome was good or excellent in 92% of the patients. Zvijac (35) reported on 14 patients with PVNS of knee treated with arthroscopic synovectomy. The average follow-up was 41.9 months. In the two patients with localized disease, there

TABLE 35-1.   Results of Surgical Treatment for Pigmented Villonodular Synovitis of the Knee at the University of Minnesota

Type of Disease	Treatment	Number of Patients	Mean Follow-Up (Months)	Recurrence (No. of patients/%)
Nodular	Arthroscopy.	2	24	None
	Open synovectomy	2	28	None
Diffuse	Open anterior and posterior	21	42.8	5 (23.8%)
	Arthroscopy and open posterior	6	40.3	2 (33.3%)
	Arthroscopy	3	30	3 (100%)
	Open anterior	3	16	None
	Open posterior	3	30	1 (33.3%)
	Observation	1	24	NA

was no recurrence; but in diffuse form, there was recurrence in 2 of 12 patients. De Ponti (6) has reported on 19 patients treated with arthroscopy with an average follow-up of 60 months. There were 15 patients with diffuse disease, seven treated with extended arthroscopic synovectomy and eight with partial synovectomy. The recurrence was 50% in patients treated with partial synovectomy, and 20% in patients with complete synovectomy at 2 years. Chin et al (2) reported on 40 cases treated with one of the three modalities, surgery alone (5 patients), surgery combined with intra-articular radiation synovectomy with use of dysprosium-165 (30 patients), and surgery with external beam radiation (5 patients). The overall recurrence rate was 18% (7 cases) at a mean follow-up of 5 years. Five recurrences were in patients who had surgery combined with intra-articular radiation synovectomy and two in the surgery and external beam radiation group.

We reviewed the results of surgery done at the University of Minnesota from 1990 to 2005 (unpublished data). A total of 41 patients were available for review. Postoperative MRI examinations were done to detect recurrence. Different methods of treatment were performed according to the disease extent and surgeon preferences. Recurrence rates are cited in Table 35-1.

REFERENCES

1. Ballard WT, Clark CR, Callaghan JJ. Recurrent spontaneous hemarthrosis nine years after a total knee arthroplasty. A presentation with pigmented villonodular synovitis. *J Bone Joint Surg Am.* 1993;75(5):764–767.
2. Chin KR, Barr SJ, Winalski C, et al. Treatment of advanced primary and recurrent diffuse pigmented villonodular synovitis of the knee. *J Bone Joint Surg Am.* 2002;84-A(12):2192–2202.
3. Choong PF, Willen H, Nilbert M, et al. Pigmented villonodular synovitis. Monoclonality and metastasis—A case for neoplastic origin? *Acta Orthop Scand.* 1995;66(1):64–68.
4. Cotten A, Flipo RM, Chastanet P. et al. Pigmented villonodular synovitis of the hip: review of radiographic features in 58 patients. *Skeletal Radiol.* 1995;24(1):1–6.
5. Darling JM, Goldring SR, Harada Y, et al. Multinucleated cells in pigmented villonodular synovitis and giant cell tumor of tendon sheath express features of osteoclasts. *Am J Pathol.* 1997;150(4):1383–1393.
6. De Ponti A, Sansone V, Malchere M. Result of arthroscopic treatment of pigmented villonodular synovitis of the knee. *Arthroscopy.* 2003;19(6):602–607.
7. Dorwart RH, Genant HK, Johnston WH, et al. Pigmented villonodular synovitis of synovial joints: clinical, pathologic, and radiologic features. *Am J Roentgen.* 1984;143(4):877–885.
8. Eisold S, Fritz T, Buhl K, et al. Pigmented villonodular synovitis. Case reports and review of the literature. *Chirurg.* 1988;69(3):284–290.
9. Flandry F, Hughston JC. Pigmented villonodular synovitis. *J Bone Joint Surg Am.* 1987;69(6):942–949.
10. Flandry FC, Hughston JC, Jacobson KE, et al. Surgical treatment of diffuse pigmented villonodular synovitis of the knee. *Clin Orthop Relat Res.* 1994;300:183–192.
11. Franssen MJ, Boerbooms AM, Karthaus RP, et al. Treatment of pigmented villonodular synovitis of the knee with yttrium-90 silicate: prospective evaluations by arthroscopy, histology, and 99mTc pertechnetate uptake measurements. *Ann Rheum Dis.* 1989;48(12):1007–1013.
12. Garcia Sanchez A, Utrilla Utrilla M, Casals Sanchez JL, et al. Pigmented villonodular synovitis with polyarticular presentation. *Anales de Medicina Interna.* 1996;13(7):341–343.
13. Ghert MA, Scully SP, Harrelson JM. Pigmented villonodular synovitis of the foot and ankle: a review of six cases. *Foot & Ankle International.* 1999;20(5):326–330.
14. Hamlin BR, Duffy GP, Trousdale RT, et al. Total knee arthroplasty in patients who have pigmented villonodular synovitis. *J Bone Joint Surg Am.* 1998;80(1):76–82.
15. Jaffe HL, Lichtenstein L, Sutro CJ. Pigmented villonodular synovitis, bursitis, and tenosynovitis: a discussion of the synovial and bursal equivalents of the tenosynovial lesions commonly denoted as xanthoma xanthogranuloma, giant cell tumor, or myeloplaxoma of the tendon sheath, with some consideration for the tendon sheath lesion itself. *Arch Pathol.* 1941;31:731.
16. Kat S, Kutz R, Elbracht T, et al. Radiosynovectomy in pigmented villonodular synovitis. *Nuklearmedizin.* 2000;39(7):209–213.
17. Kim SJ, Shin SJ, Choi NH, et al. Arthroscopic treatment for localized pigmented villonodular synovitis of the knee. *Clin Orthop Relat Res.* 2000;(379):224–230.
18. Kobayashi H, Kotoura Y, Hosono M, et al. Case report: uptake of pentavalent technetium-99m dimercaptosuccinic acid by pigmented villonodular synovitis: comparison with computed tomography, magnetic resonance imaging and gallium-67 scintigraphy. *Brit J Radiol.* 1994;67(802):1030–1032.
19. Le Tiec T, Hulet C, Locker B, et al. Villonodular synovitis of the knee. Analysis of a series of 17 cases and review of the literature. *Revue de Chirurgie Orthopedique et Reparatrice de l Appareil Moteur.* 1998;84(7):607–616.
20. Mohler DG, Kessler BD. Open synovectomy with cryosurgical adjuvant for treatment of diffuse pigmented villonodular synovitis of the knee. *Bulletin—Hospital for Joint Diseases.* 2000;59(2):99–105.
21. Moskovich R, Parisien JS. Localized pigmented villonodular synovitis of the knee. Arthroscopic treatment. *Clin Orthop Relat Res.* 1991;(271):218–224.
22. Mulier T, Victor J, Van Den Bergh J, et al. Diffuse pigmented villonodular synovitis of the shoulder. A case report & review of literature. *Acta Orthopaedica Belgica.* 1992;58(1):93–96.
23. Muscolo DL, Makino A, Costa-Paz M, et al. Magnetic resonance imaging evaluation and arthroscopic resection of localized pigmented villonodular synovitis of the knee. *Orthopedics (Thorofare, NJ).* 2000;23(4):367–369.
24. Neale SD, Kristelly R, Gundle R, et al. Giant cells in pigmented villo nodular synovitis express an osteoclast phenotype. *J Clin Pathol.* 1997;50(7):605–608.
25. Ogilvie-Harris DJ, McLean J, Zarnett ME. Pigmented villonodular synovitis of the knee. The results of total arthroscopic synovectomy, partial, arthroscopic synovectomy, and arthroscopic local excision. *J Bone Joint Surg Am.* 1992;74(1):119–123.

26. O'Sullivan B, Cummings B, Catton C, et al. Outcome following radiation treatment for high-risk pigmented villonodular synovitis. *International Journal of Radiation Oncology, Biology, Physics.* 1995;32(3):777–786.

27. Panagiotopoulos E, Tyllianakis M, Lambiris E, et al. Recurrence of pigmented villonodular synovitis of the knee 17 years after the initial treatment. A case report. *Clin Orthop Relat Res.* 1993;(295):179–182.

28. Patel D. Proximal approaches to arthroscopic surgery of the knee. *Am J Sports Med.* 1981;9(5):296–303.

29. Patel D. Superior lateral-medical approach to arthroscopic meniscectomy. *Orthop Clin North Am.* 1982;13(2):299–305.

30. Pimpalnerkar A, Barton E, Sibly TF. Pigmented villonodular synovitis of the elbow. *Journal of Shoulder & Elbow Surgery.* 1998;7(1):71–75.

31. Poletti SC, Gates HS III, Martinez SM, et al. The use of magnetic resonance imaging in the diagnosis of pigmented villonodular synovitis. *Orthopedics (Thorofare, NJ).* 1990;13(2):185–190.

32. Rader CP, Barthel T, Hendrich C, et al. Pigmented villonodular synovitis of the knee joint—long-term follow-up and therapeutic concept. *Zentralblatt fur Chirurgie.* 1995;120(7):564–570.

33. Sharafuddin MJ, Sundaram M, McDonald D. Progression from simple joint effusion to extensive pigmented villonodular synovitis of the hip within 2 years: demonstration with MR imaging [letter]. *Am J Roentgen.* 1995;165(3):742.

34. Vedantam R, Strecker WB, Schoenecker PL, et al. Polyarticular pigmented villonodular synovitis in a child. *Clinical Orthopaedics & Related Research.* 1998; (348):208–211.

35. Zvijac JE, Lau AC, Hechtman KS, et al. Arthroscopic treatment of pigmented villonodular synovitis of the knee. *Arthroscopy.* 1999;15(6):613–617.

Index

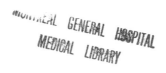